FIFTH EDITION

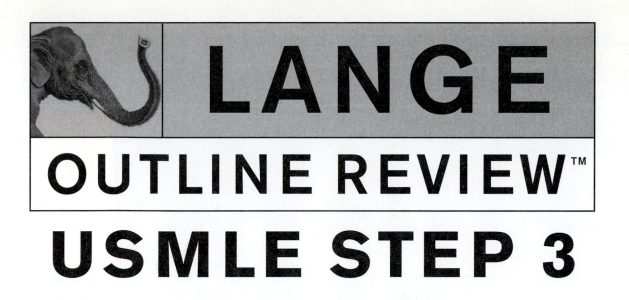

LANGE
OUTLINE REVIEW™
USMLE STEP 3

Joel S. Goldberg, DO
Assistant Professor of Medicine
Department of Medicine
Drexel University College of Medicine
Philadelphia, Pennsylvania

McGraw-Hill
Medical Publishing Division

New York   Chicago   San Francisco   Lisbon   London   Madrid   Mexico City   Milan
New Delhi   San Juan   Seoul   Singapore   Sydney   Toronto

Lange Outline Review: USMLE Step 3, Fifth Edition

Copyright © 2006 by The McGraw-Hill Companies, Inc. All rights reserved. Printed in the United States of America. Except as permitted under the United States Copyright Act of 1976, no part of this publication may be reproduced or distributed in any form or by any means, or stored in a data base or retrieval system, without the prior written permission of the publisher.

Previous editions copyright © 2004, 2001 by The McGraw-Hill Companies, Inc.; copyright © 1997, 1995 by Appleton & Lange.

1 2 3 4 5 6 7 8 9 0   QPD/QPD   0 9 8 7 6

ISBN 0-07-145193-5

This book was set in Palatino by Rainbow Graphics.
The editor was Marsha Loeb.
The production supervisor was Sherri Souffrance.
Project management was provided by Rainbow Graphics.
The cover designer was Aimee Nordin.
Quebecor World Dubuque was the printer and binder.

This book is printed on acid-free paper.

Library of Congress Cataloging-in-Publication Data

Lange outline review. USMLE step 3 / [edited by] Joel S. Goldberg.— 5th ed.
    p. ; cm
  Rev. ed. of: Appleton & Lange outline review for the USMLE step 3. 4th ed. 2004.
  Includes bibilographical references and index.
  ISBN 0-07-145193-5
  1. Medicine—Examinations, questions, etc. 2. Medicine—Outlines, syllabi, etc. I. Title:
USMLE step 3. II. Goldberg, Joel S. III. Appleton & Lange outline review for the USMLE
step 3.
  [DNLM: 1. Medicine—Examination Questions. 2. Medicine—Outlines. WB 18.2 L2739 2006]
R834.5.l55 2006
610.7'6—dc22
                             2005054046

For My Children, Dan and Kasey

Contents

Contributors

Amy C. Brodkey, MD
Clinical Associate Professor
Department of Psychiatry
University of Pennsylvania School of Medicine
Philadelphia, Pennsylvania
Chapter 15, "Psychiatry"

Christina M. Clay, MD
Attending Physician
Division of Hematology and Oncology
Crozer-Chester Medical Center
Upland, Pennsylvania
Chapter 5, "Hematology and Oncology"

Michael J. Costanza, MD
Assistant Professor of Surgery and Radiology
SUNY Upstate Medical University College of Medicine
Department of Veterans Affairs
VA Healthcare Network Upstate New York at Syracuse
Syracuse, New York
Chapter 18, "Surgical Principles"

Thomas Fekete, MD
Professor of Medicine
Section of Infectious Diseases
Departments of Internal Medicine and Microbiology
Temple University School of Medicine
Philadelphia, Pennsylvania
Chapter 8, "Infectious Disease"

Natali Franzblau, MD
Assistant Professor
Department of Obstetrics and Gynecology
UMDNJ–Robert Wood Johnson School of Medicine
Camden, New Jersey
Chapter 11, "Male and Female Reproduction"
Chapter 12, "Obstetrics"

Vivian Gahtan, MD
Professor of Surgery
Chief, Section of Vascular Surgery
SUNY Upstate Medical University College of Medicine
Department of Veterans Affairs
VA Healthcare Network Upstate New York at Syracuse
Syracuse, New York
Chapter 18, "Surgical Principles"

Jeffrey I. Greenstein, MD
Chairman
Department of Neurology
Graduate Hospital
Philadelphia, Pennsylvania
Chapter 10, "Neurology"

Victor A. Heresniak, DO
Chairman
Department of Emergency Medicine
Crozer–Chester Medical Center
Upland, Pennsylvania
Chapter 7, "Injuries, Wounds, Toxicology, and Burns"

Morris D. Kerstein, MD, FACS
Professor of Surgery
Jefferson Medical College of Thomas Jefferson
    University
Philadelphia, Pennsylvania
Chief of Staff
The VA Hospital
Wilmington, Delaware
Chapter 18, "Surgical Principles"

Thomas Klein, MD
Chief
Division of Allergy and Immunology
Delaware County Memorial Hospital
Drexel Hill, Pennsylvania
Chapter 6, "Immunology and Allergy"

S. Bruce Malkowicz, MD
Associate Professor
Co-director, Urology–Oncology Program
Division of Urology
University of Pennsylvania School of Medicine
Philadelphia, Pennsylvania
Chapter 17, "Diseases of the Renal and Urologic Systems"

Joseph R. McClellan, MD, FACC, FACP
President, Caritas Clinic
Caritas Christi Health Care System
Boston, Massachusetts
Chapter 1, "Cardiovascular Medicine"

Pekka A. Mooar, MD
Associate Professor
Department of Orthopedic Surgery
Temple University School of Medicine
Philadelphia, Pennsylvania
Chapter 9, "Musculoskeletal and Connective Tissue Disease"

Robin Perry, MD
Co-Division Head, Maternal-Fetal Medicine
Cooper University Hospital
UMDNJ—Robert Wood Johnson Medical School
Camden, New Jersey
Chapter 12, "Obstetrics"

Charles A. Pohl, MD, FAAP
Clinical Associate Professor of Pediatrics
Associate Dean of Student Affairs
Jefferson Medical College of Thomas Jefferson
    University
Philadelphia, Pennsylvania
Chapter 14, "Pediatrics"

Daniel L. Ridout III, MD
Clinical Assistant Professor
Division of Gastroenterology
Department of Medicine
Temple University School of Medicine
Philadelphia, Pennsylvania
Chapter 4, "Diseases and Disorders of the Digestive System"

Edward S. Schulman, MD
Professor of Medicine
Director, Division of Pulmonary and Critical Care
    Medicine
Drexel University College of Medicine
Philadelphia, Pennsylvania
Chapter 16, "Pulmonary Medicine"

Michael Sherman, MD
Associate Professor
Division of Pulmonary and Critical Care Medicine
Drexel University College of Medicine
Philadelphia, Pennsylvania
Chapter 16, "Pulmonary Medicine"

Richard L. Spielvogel, MD
Clinical Professor of Dermatology
Department of Dermatology
Drexel University College of Medicine
Philadelphia, Pennsylvania
Chapter 2, "Dermatology"

Dorota Wilson, MD
Resident Physician
Department of Dermatology
Drexel University School of Medicine
Philadelphia, Pennsylvania
Chapter 2, "Dermatology"

Preface

The typical review book is written in a question-and-answer-type format. It has long existed as the sole product for student examinations, until now. In 1992, I formulated my concept of a rapid-reading review manual, conceived out of the tremendous need for a succinct, yet complete review text. The key component was the extensive coverage of the USMLE "high-impact" disease list, with the inclusion and incorporation of all pertinent test material. In addition, it was necessary to present this material in a concise, easily assimilated format, to allow for a swift and highly effective review.

This text, *Lange Outline Review: USMLE Step 3,* Fifth Edition, exists as a result of the tremendous popularity and widespread use of the Step 2 text, called *The Instant Exam Review for USMLE Step 2.* After the Step 2 text received extraordinary acceptance and acclaim by students and educators across the United States and abroad, I was asked to create a new study book for the Step 3 exam. Thus, *Lange Outline Review: USMLE Step 3!*

In this review manual, my original concept and ideals remain unchanged. Once again, the material in this book encompasses the key test facts, diseases, and disorders listed by the National Board of Medical Examiners for the new Step 3 examination. Our categories in this revised edition have changed to reflect the new examination content, with each chapter encompassing the Board's new list of diseases and disorders.

Finally, I have enlisted as contributors an exceptional group of physicians, widely renowned for their clinical and educational proficiency. These authors have completely revised this book.

Please note that this book was not designed to teach general medicine, nor was it to be a substitute for accepted methods of medical education. Like its predecessor, it was designed as a unique study tool to assist you, the student, in passing the Step 3 examination.

Joel S. Goldberg, DO
Philadelphia, Pennsylvania

Acknowledgments

I would like to extend my sincere appreciation to Ms. Catherine Johnson, Ms. Marsha Loeb, and the all the staff at McGraw-Hill for their assistance with this project. They were always available for counsel and support during the task of manuscript preparation, copyediting, review of page proofs, and production of bound books. I would also like to thank David Hommel at Rainbow Graphics for his fine work in preparation of the final product.

I wish to thank my coauthors for their willingness to participate in this complex endeavor and for investing extensive time and effort in the construction of their chapters, despite their busy professional and personal schedules. They are a group of physicians dedicated to medicine, and their commitment to education is clear.

Finally, I would like to express my gratitude to the staff and faculty of Drexel University College of Medicine for their assistance and unselfish dedication to both the clinical practice of medicine and the education of young physicians in training.

How to Use This Book

This book is an innovative and practical study guide designed to be used in both the initial phase of USMLE Step 3 examination preparation as a comprehensive study outline and in the final few days and hours before the exam as a quick review manual.

USING THE BOOK AS A STUDY OUTLINE

When you begin to study, turn to the Contents to obtain an overview of this text. Review the material supplied by your school and the National Board of Medical Examiners, including the "Step 3 General Instructions, Content Description, and Sample Items." It is important to have a full understanding of the design of the exam and the type of questions that will be asked. Sample test questions and topics may also be found at www.usmle.org.

Once you begin to study, *do not* omit any chapters in this text; instead, start at the beginning and read the book in its entirety. Notice that the outline format is streamlined to allow the rapid assimilation of facts in a minimal amount of reading time. Because extraneous and time-consuming information and phrasing have been omitted, working with *Lange Outline Review: USMLE Step 3* for 1 hour will provide a database equivalent to that procured from several hours' study of any other review text. Because the text is concise, it is vital that you be well rested and in a proper frame of mind for study and concentration. A quiet, comfortable, bright study area without glare is vital (with plenty of snacks nearby, of course!).

USING THE BOOK AS A QUICK REVIEW

In the final several weeks and days prior to your examination, *Lange Outline Review: USMLE Step 3* will serve as a rapid review tool. As in the Step 2 text, this revolutionary new format, which completely covers the "high impact" fact list, will allow the handbook to be read quickly, with successful, easy assimilation of the core facts necessary for exam success.

Cardiovascular Medicine 1

I. ISCHEMIC HEART DISEASE

A. Acute

1. Unstable Angina

▶ **H&P Keys**

Anginal pain with accelerating pattern including new onset or rest symptoms. Midsternal squeezing or heaviness that may radiate to the left shoulder or arm, jaw, neck, etc. Symptoms may be similar to those present previously; however, usual alleviating factors (e.g., nitroglycerin [NTG], rest) may no longer be effective. Diaphoresis, nausea, dyspnea, are common.

With coexisting left ventricular (LV) dysfunction an S_3 or S_4 may be heard. In the presence of global ischemia or LV dysfunction, a dyskinetic cardiac impulse may be palpated, and papillary muscle dysfunction may cause the murmur of mitral regurgitation (MR). Ischemia-induced elevations in cardiac filling pressures often cause pulmonary congestion and rales.

▶ **Diagnosis**

Electrocardiogram (ECG): ST depression or elevation or T wave inversion. Exercise tolerance testing (ETT; not performed in patients with unstable angina) or pharmacologic stress testing is combined with an imaging agent, such as thallium, that permits the visualization of myocardial perfusion. Coronary angiography is indicated for patients with high-risk clinical features.

▶ **Disease Severity**

High-risk clinical features are advanced age, ST segment depression, heart failure, and elevation of biomarkers of cell damage (troponins). Response to therapy and duration of symptoms dictate evaluation. Patients not medically stabilized or whose symptoms reemerge on therapy and those with prominent ischemic ECG findings usually undergo coronary angiography. Location and severity of stenoses (e.g., left main, three-vessel) dictate management.

▶ **Concept and Application**

The vast majority of patients with unstable angina have underlying coronary atherosclerosis (CAD). Unstable symptoms are usually caused by plaque rupture with superimposed thrombosis. Platelet aggregation at site of plaque rupture with release of vasoconstricting mediators plays an important role.

▶ **Treatment Steps**

1. Continuous ECG monitoring.
2. Bed rest, mild sedation, and treatment of extracardiac precipitants of increased oxygen demand (e.g., hypoxia, sepsis, anemia, uncontrolled hypo- or hypertension, etc.).
3. Intravenous nitrates, heparin, thienopyridines, and aspirin (acetylsalicylic acid [ASA]) and IIB/IIIA inhibitors are of proven efficacy. Thienopyridines, especially clopidogrel, reduce adverse events including death, myocardial infarction (MI), and stroke. Agents that block the platelet glycoprotein IIB/IIIA receptor substantially reduces mortality and the occurrence of acute MI primarily in patients who undergo coronary intervention. Intravenous NTG often is successful when other routes fail. β-Blockers are useful and also reduce the incidence of acute MI (AMI).

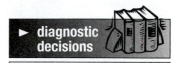

▶ **diagnostic decisions**

ISCHEMIC HEART DISEASE

Acute Myocardial Infarction
Sudden onset of typical squeezing or crushing substernal chest pain; ECG with ST segment elevation in two or more leads; increased CPK-MB isoenzymes and troponins.

Angina Pectoris
Chest pain lasting 1–15 minutes, precipitated by exertion, relieved by rest; associated ECG changes with ST segment depression. Abnormal exercise stress test or abnormal perfusion on nuclear scan.

Unstable Angina
Angina that increases in frequency or severity, is of new onset or occurs at rest. Coronary angiography defines the extent and severity of disease and need for intervention; exercise testing with perfusion imaging useful for risk stratification and treatment decisions.

4. Calcium channel blockers can provide symptomatic relief but do not decrease event rates.
5. Intra-aortic balloon counterpulsation (IABP) is often used as a bridge to percutaneous transluminal coronary angioplasty (PTCA) or coronary artery bypass graft (CABG) and is effective in stabilizing medically refractory patients.
6. Lipid-lowering therapy with hydroxymethylglutaryl coenzyme A (HMG CoA) reductase inhibitors should be started for patients with low-density lipoprotein (LDL) > 100 mg/dL.

2. Myocardial Infarction

► H&P Keys

Chest pain, often midsternal squeezing or crushing. The pain may radiate to the neck, jaw, shoulders, arms, etc. Diaphoresis is frequent. Approximately 20% of episodes occur in the absence of pain (silent). Displaced and even dyskinetic cardiac impulse can be palpated. Ischemia-induced papillary muscle dysfunction may cause a MR murmur. Associated right ventricular (RV) infarction, may cause jugular venous distention (JVD). Elevations in cardiac filling pressures often cause pulmonary congestion, allowing auscultation of pulmonary rales.

► Diagnosis

ECG: ST segment elevation MI (STEMI) and T wave inversions with subsequent evolution of Q waves. Non-STEMI: ST depression and T wave inversions are seen. Elevations in cardiac enzymes: creatine kinase (CK), specifically CK-MB isoforms, peaks at 24 hours; troponins I and T, and myoglobin detect cell injury early in the course of MI. L-lactate dehydrogenase (LDH) peaks at 3–5 days after MI. Two-dimensional (2-D) echocardiography and technetium nuclear scans can be valuable in detecting abnormalities in heart function and blood flow.

► Disease Severity

Mortality increases with the number of ECG leads showing ST segment elevation. Cardiac imaging with echocardiography (echo) or radionuclide ventriculography (RVG) can help assess the extent and prognosis of infarction by measuring LV systolic function and ejection fraction. Echo aids in diagnosis of MI complications, e.g., LV thrombus or aneurysm, pericardial effusion, free wall and septal rupture, and MR.

► Concept and Application

MI results from the abrupt cessation of myocardial blood flow. The vast majority of cases of MI are due to CAD. Plaque rupture, platelet aggregation, and release of vasoactive mediators leads to thrombosis, spasm, and coronary occlusion. Elevation of myocardial oxygen demand (e.g., tachycardia) can increase myocardial cell damage. Irreversible cell death occurs, usually within 6 hours, if therapy is not given to restore blood flow or if spontaneous improvement does not occur. Nonatherosclerotic causes of MI, such as embolism, trauma, vasculitis, or hypercoagulable states, are less common.

► Treatment Steps

1. Supplemental oxygen, and continuous monitoring to detect potentially lethal dysrhythmias are important first steps.
2. Analgesia as necessary.
3. Primary angioplasty of occluded artery optimum. Thrombolysis if PTCA unavailable.

► management decisions

ISCHEMIC HEART DISEASE

Acute Myocardial Infarction

Open the occluded artery to restore cardiac blood flow with thrombolytic therapy or angioplasty; monitor and treat serious dysrhythmias, aspirin to decrease clot formation, β-blockers to decrease myocardial oxygen needs, oxygen and pain relief.

Angina Pectoris

Drug therapy with nitrates, β-blockers, aspirin to prevent acute MI; calcium antagonists are second-line therapy. Intervention with bypass surgery or coronary intervention for patients with refractory symptoms or severe coronary disease.

Unstable Angina

Drug therapy for stabilization with intravenous nitroglycerin, aspirin, heparin, clopidogrel, glycoprotein IIB/IIIA inhibitors, and β-blockers. Coronary interventions and coronary bypass surgery for severe coronary disease.

4. Aspirin should be given on day 1 of AMI to all patients without a contraindication.
5. Heparin and ASA are useful in conjunction with thrombolysis.
6. Intravenous NTG is helpful in decreasing oxygen demand and increasing supply.
7. β-Blocker therapy should be administered to all patients without a contraindication within 12 hours of the onset of the MI.
8. Coronary angiography and revascularization wih PTCA or CABG if the patient is in shock, has a large infarct, or is unresponsive to medical therapy. Catheterization may also be required for the diagnosis and treatment of complications.

3. Spasm (Prinzmetal's or Variant Angina)

► H&P Keys

Anginal-type chest pain, typically occurring at rest. High percentage of patients with isolated coronary spasm are cigarette smokers or cocaine abusers. Patients tend to be younger than those with exertional angina. The cardiac exam is usually normal.

► Diagnosis

ECG typically shows ST elevation during symptomatic periods.

► Concept and Application

Most patients have CAD, and spasm occurs in close proximity to a diseased segment, although approximately one-third have angiographically normal coronaries. Diseased coronary vasculature loses the ability to manifest endothelial-dependent vasodilation and may react paradoxically to what are normally vasorelaxant stimuli.

► Treatment Steps

1. Avoid smoking and cocaine.
2. Nitrates and calcium channel blockers are usually effective; the effect of β-blockers is unpredictable; in some they can precipitate spasm.
3. α-Adrenergic β-blockers (e.g., prazosin) can be helpful.

B. Chronic

1. Stable Angina Pectoris

► H&P Keys

Episodic chest discomfort, often described as heaviness or squeezing lasting 1–15 minutes. Pain may radiate to the jaw, neck, shoulder, or the left arm. Symptoms typically are precipitated by exertion, cold weather, or emotional upset, and relieved by rest. Family history of premature CAD, diabetes, hyperlipidemia, hypertension, cigarette smoking. Exam may be normal, but if the patient is examined during an ischemic episode, an S_3 or S_4 may be heard.

► Diagnosis

ECG may be normal if patient is asymptomatic, but evidence of a prior MI or ischemic ST and T wave changes may be noted. ETT, pharmacologic stress testing, and exercise echo are useful.

► Disease Severity

Global ECG changes suggest multivessel CAD. Quantitation of ischemic burden can be accomplished with perfusion imaging. Coronary arteriography documents presence, extent, and severity of CAD and suitability for revascularization.

► Concept and Application

Angina results from myocardial oxygen supply–demand imbalance. Obstructive coronary lesions limit the blood flood to myocardial segments. Dilatation of myocardial arteriolar resistance vessels mitigates ischemia, but this mechanism eventually is inadequate as stenosis severity increases. Angina can be precipitated in the absence of CAD in patients with augmented myocardial oxygen demand, e.g., thyrotoxicosis, hypertrophy, or aortic stenosis.

► Treatment Steps

1. Reduction of ischemic precipitants and treatment of coexisting illnesses (e.g., hyperthyroidism) that increase oxygen demand.
2. Sublingual NTG is valuable for prompt relief.
3. Aspirin reduces the risk of future adverse events by 33%.
4. Lipid-lowering therapy with HMG CoA reductase inhibitors also substantially reduce the risk of future fatal and nonfatal MI.
5. β-Blockers stimultaneously improve angina and ischemia while also preventing MI and death.
6. Calcium channel blocking drugs also relieve ischemic symptoms.
7. PTCA and CABG relieve symptoms and improve outcomes in appropriate patients.

2. Silent Ischemia

► H&P Keys

Patients are asymptomatic, and the physical exam is usually normal.

► Diagnosis

Holter monitoring and ETT can uncover ST segment changes indicative of ischemia.

► Disease Severity

Degree of ST segment depression and number of leads involved can suggest disease extent; nocturnal ST segment depression often means multivessel CAD.

► Concept and Application

Most patients with symptomatic angina have episodes of silent ischemia. Silent ischemia is more common in diabetics, who often have an abnormality in pain perception.

► Treatment Steps

1. Medical therapy, as outlined for angina pectoris, is often used; however, specific therapy depends on extent of disease, patient's age, occupation, etc.
2. Most patients develop symptomatic angina before additional adverse events occur.

II. HEART FAILURE (HF)

A. Left-Sided

1. Low Output

► H&P Keys

History may elicit cause, e.g., CAD, prior MI, hypertension, or valvular disease. Symptoms: fatigue, weakness, reduced exercise tolerance, exertional or rest dyspnea, paroxysmal nocturnal dyspnea (PND), orthopnea, nocturia. Physical findings: displaced cardiac impulse; S_3 murmurs, especially MR; rales; rarely Cheyne–Stokes respiration.

►Diagnosis

Most often made by history and exam. Cardiac enlargement or dysfunction detected by chest x-ray (CXR), echo, or radionuclear angiogram (RNA).

►Disease Severity

Determined by degree of symptomatic incapacity and LV impairment.

►Concept and Application

In systolic dysfunction, the heart delivers inadequate oxygen to meet metabolic needs; in diastolic dysfunction, ventricular filling is abnormal. Systolic and diastolic dysfunction commonly coexist. In predominantly systolic dysfunction, activation of sympathetic nervous system, renin–angiotensin–aldosterone axis, and hormonal (antidiuretic hormone [ADH]) elaboration occurs.

►Treatment Steps

1. Search for precipitating causes of decompensation (infection, MI, uncontrolled hypertension, dietary indiscretion, etc.). Correct underlying diseases, e.g., valvular disease, ischemia, arrhythmia.
2. Pharmacologic therapy is tailored to the stage of the disease (A, high risk to develop congestive heart failure [CHF]; B, structural disease without symptoms; C, prior or current symptoms; D, refractory symptoms requiring special intervention).
3. Most symptomatic patients should be managed with a combination of four drugs: diuretics, angiotensin-converting enzyme (ACE) inhibitors, β-blockers, and digitalis.
4. Diuretics decrease symptoms related to volume overload.
5. ACE inhibitors reduce afterload, increase cardiac output, and decrease mortality (Stages B–D).
6. Digoxin augments contractility and reduces symptoms but does not improve prognosis (Stages C and D).
7. β-Blockers help modulate neurohumoral activation, blunt excess sympathetic tone, and are used in all stable, symptomatic patients (Stages C and D).
8. With severe decompensation, sympathomimetic amines (dobutamine) or phosphodiesterase inhibitors (milrinone) are used.
9. β-Natriuretic hormone therapy is also valuable to rapidly relieve symptoms and improve hemodynamics.
10. Stage D patients may require cardiac transplantation or an LV assist device.

2. **High Output**

►H&P Keys

Signs of hyperdynamic circulation, e.g., brisk pulses. Dyspnea, orthopnea often present. Angina in patients with CAD.

►Disease Severity

Assessed primarily on degree of disability.

►Concept and Application

Patients often have an underlying syndrome causing elevation in metabolic demands and/or cardiac output, e.g., arteriovenous fistulas, Paget's disease, hyperthyroidism, anemia.

►Treatment Steps

Treatment of underlying cause.

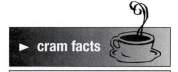

►**cram facts**

TREATMENT DECISIONS

Heart Failure

Left-Sided Heart Failure
Find and treat or correct any precipitating or underlying cause, e.g., valvular heart disease. Medical treatment with angiotensin-converting enzyme inhibitors, diuretics, digoxin, and β-blockers. Anticoagulation with severe dysfunction. Severe decompensation may require sympathomimetic agents, a left ventricular assist device or cardiac transplantation.

High-Output Heart Failure
Find and treat the underlying cause, e.g., thyrotoxicosis and/or arteriovenous fistula; diuretics.

Right-Sided Heart Failure
Correct underlying problems that resulted in pulmonary obstruction or hypertension; diuretics and treatment similar to left-sided failure.

B. Right-Sided

▶ H&P Keys

Seen with history of LV failure, RV infarction, lung disease, pulmonic stenosis, pulmonary emboli, myocarditis, etc. Clinical findings: fatigue, RV heave and gallops, JVD, hepatomegaly, ascites, edema, atrial arrhythmias.

▶ Diagnosis

Signs and symptoms of RV or biventricular failure in setting of predisposing condition. ECG may show RV or right atrial (RA) hypertrophy. Echo may show RV dilatation and hypokinesis.

▶ Disease Severity

Often suggested by degree of edema and JVD on exam. Ascites suggests more severe decompensation. Echo and RVG can quantitate the degree of functional impairment and dilatation

▶ Concept and Application

RV outflow obstruction (e.g., pulmonic stenosis), pulmonary hypertension resulting from chronic LV failure, obstructive lung disease, chronic pulmonary emboli (cor pulmonale), etc., lead to chronic overload of the RV. LV cardiac output is also reduced. Elevated pressures in systemic vasculature lead to accumulation of fluid in the extravascular space. See Figure 1–1.

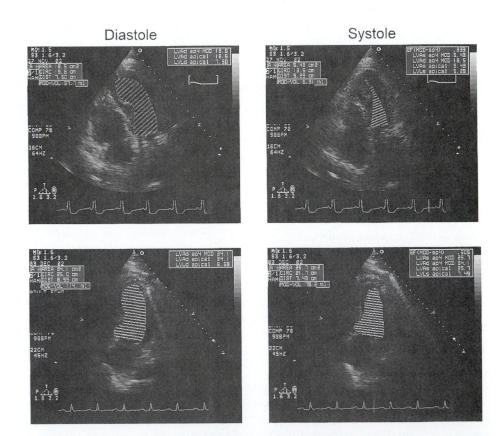

Diastole · Systole

Figure 1–1. Echocardiograms recorded in end-diastolic and end-systolic in a normal ventricle (upper panel) with uniform systolic contraction and a normal ejection fraction and an abnormal ventricle with reduced contraction during systole. The cross-hatched areas outline the left ventricular cavities.

▶ **Treatment Steps**
1. Treatment of underlying condition.
2. Diuretics lead to symptomatic improvement.
3. Oxygen supplementation.
4. ACE inhibitors.
5. Antiarrhythmics, anti-ischemics, anticoagulation as needed.

III. HYPOTENSION AND ACUTE CIRCULATORY COLLAPSE (SHOCK)

Occurs in a wide array of conditions that ultimately lead to inadequate oxygen delivery to the organs, tissues, and cells. Impairment in oxygen transport results from increases in demand or inability to maintain normal oxygen supply. Shock is classified by the primary hemodynamic derangement as cardiogenic, hypovolemic, obstructive, and distributive. In all forms, physical examination reveals hypotension defined as mean pressure < 60 mm Hg with evidence of peripheral hypoperfusion, including vasoconstriction, with cool and mottled extremities and poor organ perfusion, including abnormal mentation and decreased urine output.

A. Cardiogenic Shock

Inadequate cardiac output as a result of an abnormality in intrinsic cardiac function or an anatomic derangement in cardiac structure, e.g., acute valvular heart disease.

▶ **H&P Keys**
During an MI, patients will have typical features. Other entities, e.g., acute valvular endocarditis, will produce a characteristic clinical picture and new cardiac murmurs.

▶ **Diagnosis**
ECG to confirm MI, echo to evaluate global LV function, regional abnormalities, and structural abnormalities, e.g., ventricular septal defect or acute MR. Hemodynamic monitoring with Swan–Ganz catheter.

▶ **Disease Severity**
Level of blood pressure, organ perfusion including urine output, mentation, and metabolic acidosis.

▶ **Concept and Application**
With fatal cardiogenic shock, 40% of the functioning myocardium is lost. Reduction in coronary perfusion pressure leads to a downward spiral, with progressive loss of contractility. Mechanical derangements, including rupture of the ventricular septum or mitral valve apparatus at any level, e.g., papillary muscle or chordae, result in elevation of venous pressure, pulmonary congestion, reduced cardiac output, and organ hypoperfusion.

▶ **Treatment Steps**
1. The most effective therapy for MI is acute restoration of blood flow with coronary angioplasty.
2. Hemodynamic management is guided by placement of a balloon flotation catheter with determinations of pulmonary capillary wedge pressure and cardiac output.
3. If wedge pressure is low, volume is administered.

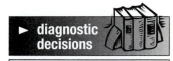

▶ **diagnostic decisions**

HYPOTENSION AND ACUTE CIRCULATORY COLLAPSE

Cardiogenic Shock
Diagnosis of acute MI or severe acute valvular heart disease with ECG and echocardiogram also useful to define severity of cardiac dysfunction and extent of valvular disease. Hemodynamic monitoring with balloon flotation catheter to define therapy, immediate surgery may be necessary.

Hypovolemic Shock
Hypotension or postural hypotension with tachycardia; blood loss evidenced by a low hemoglobin; illness resulting in fluid loss, e.g., severe diarrhea.

Obstructive Shock
Echocardiogram to diagnose pericardial effusion and cardiac tamponade; ventilation–perfusion lung scan or pulmonary angiogram for suspected pulmonary embolus.

Distributive Shock
Source of acute infection, blood cultures, WBC, or source of anaphylaxis. Hemodynamic monitoring to characterize cardiac output.

4. If wedge pressure is high and cardiac output is low, treatment is needed to augment cardiac output and improve organ perfusion at reduced filling pressures.
5. Intra-aortic balloon pump augments coronary perfusion and produces systolic unloading of the ventricle.
6. Dopamine or dobutamine may be helpful to produce augmentation of cardiac output and maintenance of peripheral perfusion. Oxygenation must be maintained. Mortality remains high, in spite of modern management techniques, unless effective myocardial blood flow can be restored or a mechanical complication is repaired.

B. Hypovolemic Shock

Inadequate circulatory volume caused by hemorrhage or dehydration. Common with trauma, surgery, vomiting, diarrhea, and some skin disorders.

▶ H&P Keys

Weakness, postural light-headedness in setting of blood loss or fluid loss, e.g., history of hemorrhage, melena. Postural hypotension and tachycardia, low jugular venous pressure.

▶ Diagnosis

Measurement of postural blood pressure and heart rate changes, nasogastric aspiration, hemoglobin, blood urea nitrogen (BUN):creatinine ratio.

▶ Disease Severity

Level of blood pressure, severity of impaired organ perfusion, mentation, hourly urine output.

▶ Concept and Application

Cardiac output is dependent on preload or venous return. An initial reduction in volume is compensated by an increase in heart rate and arterial and venous vasoconstriction. As volume reduction progresses, compensatory mechanisms fail and the blood pressure falls.

▶ Treatment Steps

1. Acute, rapid volume restoration with blood, crystalloid, or colloid solutions.
2. Temporary maintenance of peripheral perfusion pressure with vasoconstrictors.
3. Identification and treatment of the cause or source of blood loss or fluid loss.

C. Obstructive Shock

Impairment of venous return to the right ventricle or left ventricle occurs secondary to obstruction in the venous system, pulmonary artery, or pericardium. Observed with acute pulmonary embolus or tamponade with a pericardial effusion. Effusion is caused by trauma, infections, malignancy, connective tissue disease, and renal failure.

▶ H&P Keys

Dyspnea, orthopnea, elevated venous pressure, chest pain, hemoptysis, pulsus paradoxus, faint and distant heart sounds, or pulmonary hypertension.

► Diagnosis

Echo for effusion or tamponade, ECG with electrical alternans, analysis of pericardial fluid for etiology. Analysis for source of embolus, venous Doppler probe, ventilation–perfusion lung scan.

► Concept and Application

During pericardial tamponade, elevation of the intrapericardial pressure raises pressure in the cardiac chambers, leading to a reduction in venous return to the right and left heart and reduced cardiac output. Venous obstruction or pulmonary artery embolus also prevents adequate flow and venous return to the left heart.

► Disease Severity

Level of blood pressure, mentation, peripheral perfusion.

► Treatment Steps

1. Acute volume administration.
2. Administration of β-agonist to increase heart rate and stroke volume.
3. Definitive therapy requires drainage by pericardiocentesis, guided by hemodynamic monitoring or 2-D echo, or subxiphoid or anterior pericardiectomy. Pulmonary embolus with shock has a high mortality. Thrombolytic therapy with streptokinase infusion over 24 hours is favored over acute embolectomy.

D. Distributive Shock

Characteristic of sepsis, also anaphylaxis and neurogenic, toxic, or endocrinologic shock.

► H&P Keys

Fever, chills, rigor, respiratory alkalosis, bee sting or toxic ingestion, hypotension, peripheral vasodilation with warm extremities.

► Disease Severity

Level of blood pressure, evidence of poor organ perfusion.

► Diagnosis

Blood cultures, white blood count (WBC), ABG, pH, lactate, toxin screen, hemodynamic monitoring.

► Concept and Application

Diffuse arterial and venous dilatation in response to endotoxins, exotoxins, and cytokines. Other mediators include kinins, histamine, and prostaglandins. Cardiac output is increased and peripheral oxygen demand also markedly increased. Inadequate tissue oxygen delivery and failure of microcirculation, with inappropriate vasodilatation and vasoconstriction. Later, sepsis leads to depression in myocardial function.

► Treatment Steps

1. Antibiotic coverage, including two bactericidal agents for likely organisms.
2. Initial rapid volume infusion with crystalloid and colloid solutions and blood to maintain hemoglobin- and oxygen-carrying capacity.
3. Vasoactive drugs including dopamine to maintain perfusion pressure of 60 mm Hg.
4. Initial characterization of the site of infection and appropriate treatment, e.g., drainage of an abscess.

IV. MYOCARDIAL DISEASES

A. Dilated Cardiomyopathy

▶ **H&P Keys**

Symptoms suggest low cardiac output and congestion of systemic and pulmonary vasculature: dyspnea, fatigue, orthopnea, PND, edema. Exam often reveals hypotension; tachycardia; cool extremities; pulmonary rales; displaced cardiac impulse, often of diminished intensity; and S_3, mitral, or tricuspid murmur. Signs of RV failure (edema, ascites, elevated JVD) often present.

▶ **Diagnosis**

CXR often shows cardiomegaly, often with signs of congestion, possibly with pleural effusions. ECG often shows signs of ventricular or atrial enlargement, atrial fibrillation; premature ventricular complexes (PVCs) are often seen. Echo and RNA often show ventricular or four-chamber enlargement with diffuse hypocontractility and reduced cardiac output.

▶ **Disease Severity**

Symptoms may correlate poorly with degree of ventricular impairment. Echo and RNA document degree of ventricular dilatation and dysfunction. Echo documents associated valvular abnormalities. Cardiac catheterization documents degree of hemodynamic abnormality and presence of CAD. In absence of CAD, catheterization rarely alters therapy.

▶ **Concept and Application**

Various etiologies, most common being idiopathic. Other etiologies include ischemic (postinfarction), viral (e.g., coxsackie), peripartum, toxic (e.g., alcohol, doxorubicin). Myocyte injury occurs, causing reduction in contractility, leading to ventricular dilation, with compensation by activation of sympathetic nervous system and renin–angiotensin–aldosterone axis.

▶ **Treatment Steps**

1. Removal of inciting cause (e.g., discontinue alcohol) if one can be found.
2. Remainder of treatment plan as detailed in section II.

B. Hypertrophic Cardiomyopathy (HCM)

▶ **H&P Keys**

Often, patients are younger; history of sudden death of a relative during exertion may be obtained. Symptoms: exertional dyspnea, chest pain, syncope, light-headedness, sudden death, especially during exertion. Exam may reveal S_4, double or triple apical impulse, a crescendo–decrescendo systolic murmur that is increased by the Valsalva maneuver and by rising from recumbency, decreased by squatting.

▶ **Diagnosis**

ECG may show left ventricular hypertrophy (LVH) and possibly large Q waves in inferior and lateral leads; giant negative T waves are occasionally seen in the midprecordium. Characteristic echo findings are: (1) asymmetric septal thickening or hypertrophy (ASH), (2) systolic anterior motion of the anterior mitral leaflet, and (3) MR. Holter monitoring may document atrial fibrillation, which is poorly tolerated, or ventricular arrhythmias, which may precede sudden death.

▶ Disease Severity

Echocardiography can quantitate the degree of hypertrophy, especially with ASH, the most common form. The presence and magnitude of a pressure gradient can also be documented in the cardiac catheterization lab.

▶ Concept and Application

A massively hypertrophied LV wall results in a noncompliant, stiffened chamber with impaired filling. Increased myocardial mass leads to increased myocardial oxygen demand and frequently angina. Patients with ASH often have dynamic LV obstruction and frequently MR.

▶ Treatment Steps

1. β- and calcium channel blockers are effective in decreasing the intraventricular gradient, myocardial oxygen demand, and ventricular stiffness.
2. Competitive sports are generally prohibited because of the risk of sudden death.
3. Dual-chamber pacing has been shown to be effective in decreasing the amount of outflow obstruction in these patients.
4. Surgery (septal myectomy) is effective in patients with obstructive HCM.
5. Implanting a cardiac defibrillator may help to prevent sudden cardiac death.

C. Restrictive Cardiomyopathy

▶ H&P Keys

Patient may have an underlying disease (e.g., hemachromatosis, sarcoidosis, amyloidosis, or cancer). Symptoms: fatigue, weakness, dyspnea. Physical findings as described for diastolic dysfunction. ECG often shows low voltage.

▶ Disease Severity

Echo shows LV thickening and systolic impairment (if any). Doppler and cardiac catheterization can show augmented early diastolic filling. Catheterization demonstrates lowered cardiac output and abnormal RV filling. RV biopsy can identify a specific cause.

▶ Concept and Application

Restrictive cardiomyopathy is the least common of the cardiomyopathies. Systemic disorders (e.g., hemachromatosis, sarcoidosis, amyloidosis, metastatic cancer), patients with thoracic radiation or with other disorders (e.g., endomyocardial fibrosis) caused by myocardial infiltration, fibrosis, etc. have elevated filling pressures, which lead to signs and symptoms of right and left heart congestion. Reduced cavity size causes decreased cardiac output.

▶ Treatment Steps

1. Identify and treat the underlying illness if possible (e.g., steroids in sarcoidosis or chelation therapy in hemachromatosis).
2. Symptomatic treatment includes diuretics and salt restriction. Digitalis is often not helpful and may be harmful in these disorders.
3. The prognosis depends on the severity of the underlying condition.

V. CARDIAC ARRHYTHMIAS

A. Supraventricular Arrhythmias

Rhythm disturbances involving sinus node, atria, and atrioventricular (AV) node.

1. Bradyarrhythmias

a. Sinus Node Dysfunction (Sick Sinus Syndrome)—Heart rates < 60 beats per minute (bpm) or inappropriate rise in rate for level of activity (chronotropic incompetence). Includes sinus arrest, sinus exit block, bradycardia–tachycardia syndrome (rapid atrial fibrillation or flutter with long pauses).

► **H&P Keys**

Fatigue, dizziness, weakness, syncope, low rhythm and pulse.

► **Diagnosis**

ECG, cardiac rhythm monitoring, electrophysiologic studies.

► **Disease Severity**

Depressed mental status, fatigue, limitation of activity, shortness of breath.

► **Concept and Application**

Disruption of normal structures and conduction pathways resulting from collagen deposition, hypertension, ischemia, atrial stretch, idiopathic causes, autonomic nervous system.

► **Treatment Steps**

1. Acute symptomatic: Temporary intravenous pacemaker or external pacing device.
2. Chronic symptomatic: Permanent pacemaker, withdrawal of offending drugs.

b. AV Node

First-Degree AV Block—PR interval > 0.20 seconds. May or may not be associated with bradyarrhythmia.

Second-Degree AV Block—Intermittent failure of atrial activity to reach ventricles:

- Mobitz Type I (Wenckebach). Usually at level of AV node, progressive PR prolongation prior to blocked QRS. Does not include blocked premature atrial contraction.
- Mobitz Type II Block. Usually distal to AV node (bundle of His). High risk for complete AV block. Often associated with wide QRS.

Complete (Third-Degree) AV Block—May be at level of AV node, bundle of His, or bundle branches. Atrial and ventricular activity are independent. QRS usually wide. Often associated with symptoms.

► **H&P Keys**

Fatigue, shortness of breath, CHF, dizziness, syncope. Slow or irregular pulse.

► **Diagnosis**

ECG, cardiac rhythm monitoring, electrophysiologic studies.

► **cram facts**

TREATMENT DECISIONS

Cardiac Arrhythmias

Bradyarrhythmias
Withdrawal of medications that produce bradycardia; temporary intravenous or external pacemaker for acute management; permanent pacemaker for definitive treatment.

Atrial Fibrillation
β-Blockers, calcium channel blockers for rate control; anticoagulation with Coumadin if underlying structural heart disease; DC cardioversion or antiarrhythmic drugs such as amiodarone or sotalol to restore sinus rhythm. Catheter-based radiofrequency ablation techniques are also useful in restoring and maintaining sinus rhythm.

Ventricular Tachycardia
Immediate DC cardioversion if patient is hemodynamically unstable; drugs including lidocaine, procainamide, amiodarone, or pronestyl. Implantable defibrillator to treat high-risk patients.

Ventricular Fibrillation
Immediate DC cardioversion.

► Disease Severity

Heart rate, blood pressure, mentation, level of activity.

► Concept and Application

Influence of autonomic nervous system, medications, hypertension, associated valve diseases (calcific), ischemic heart disease, Lev's and Lenegre's degenerative diseases of the conduction system, electrolyte disturbances (potassium).

► Treatment Steps

1. Temporary pacemaker in unstable patients.
2. Withdrawal of offending medications.
3. Permanent pacemakers for patients with symptomatic bradycardia or asymptomatic Mobitz II or third-degree heart block.

2. Tachyarrhythmias

a. Premature Atrial Complex (PAC)—Found in over 60% of normal adults. Usually benign and asymptomatic. May be associated with the initiation of atrial fibrillation, flutter, or atrial tachycardias.

b. Premature Junctional Complex (PJC)—Early beat originating in AV node. Narrow QRS.

c. Sinus Tachycardia—Rate > 100 bpm. Normal or abnormal response to metabolic demand.

d. Atrial Fibrillation—Relatively common disorder characterized by irregularly irregular rhythm and absence of identifiable P waves. Sometimes seen in normal patients, often associated with various cardiac abnormalities and thyroid disease.

e. Atrial Flutter—Usually associated with atrial fibrillation. Organized atrial activity with rates 250–300 bpm. Sawtooth atrial activity on ECG. Variable conduction to ventricles (2:1, 3:1, 4:1).

f. Atrial Tachycardia—Rates > 100 bpm inappropriate for activity level. Originate from within left or right atrium.

g. AV Reentry (AVRT; Wolff–Parkinson–White Syndrome) and AV Nodal Reentrant Tachycardias (AVNRT)—Reentrant arrhythmias dependent on the AV node. Classic models for reentry.

► H&P Keys

Palpitations: Rapid heart rate is irregularly irregular for atrial fibrillation and often regular for other forms of sustained supraventricular tachycardia. Fatigue, shortness of breath, dizziness, syncope.

► Diagnosis

Long-term ECG recording, electrophysiologic studies.

► Disease Severity

Frequency of symptoms, including fatigue, lethargy, dizziness, chest pain, shortness of breath, syncope. Stroke is associated with atrial fibrillation.

► Concept and Application

Automatic mechanism for PACs, PJCs, and some atrial tachycardia. Reentry is a predominant mechanism for most supraventricular tachycardia. May be congenital (Wolff–Parkinson–White) or associated with other forms of structural heart disease, e.g., hypertension, ischemic heart disease, congenital heart disease (atrial septal defect). May be seen in normal patients.

▶ Treatment Steps
1. Direct-current (DC) cardioversion if unstable, radiofrequency ablation to maintain or convert to sinus rhythm.
2. Digoxin, calcium channel blockers, and β-blockers for rate control.
3. Antiarrhythmic drugs, e.g., amiodarone and sotalol.
4. Maintenance of sinus rhythm or control of ventricular rate.

B. Ventricular Arrhythmias
Disorders of rhythm isolated to ventricles.

1. Bradyarrhythmias
Conduction disturbances within the His–Purkinje system and bundle branches. Often symptomatic. Usually caused by second- and third-degree heart block.

▶ H&P Keys
Light-headedness, fatigue, syncope, intermittent cannon A waves in jugular venous pulse exam (third-degree heart block), slow pulse (intermittent or chronic).

▶ Diagnosis
ECG, auscultation (dissociation of atrial [S_4] and ventricular [S_1 and S_2] activity), electrophysiologic studies.

▶ Disease Severity
Frequency of symptoms including dizziness, light-headedness, fatigue, shortness of breath, chest pain, syncope. Trifascicular block may be asymptomatic but predictive of complete heart block.

▶ Concept and Application
Lenegre's disease (sclerodegenerative disease of the conduction system), MI, cardiomyopathies, drugs, infections (myocardial abscess).

▶ Treatment Steps
1. Temporary pacemaker for stabilization of symptomatic patients.
2. Withdrawal of offending medications.
3. Permanent pacemaker for patients at high risk of developing third-degree heart block, patients with trifascicular block, or symptomatic bradycardia.

2. Tachyarrhythmias
PVCs may be seen in normal patients. Often associated with ischemic heart disease, CHF, electrolyte abnormalities, and cardioactive drugs.

a. Ventricular Tachycardia (VT)—May be nonsustained, e.g., 3 beats ≤ 30 seconds, or sustained, e.g., > 30 seconds. May be uniform (regular); or polymorphic (irregular). Rate > 100 bpm and usually < 250 bpm.

b. Ventricular Fibrillation (VF)—Chaotic VT with rate > 250 bpm. Most common cause of cardiac arrest.

▶ H&P Keys
Palpitations, sudden-onset weakness, dizziness, syncope, and cardiac arrest. Often associated with ischemia, CHF, cardiomyopathy. Cardiac arrest victim is pulseless and without respirations.

► Diagnosis

ECG, signal-averaged ECG, invasive electrophysiologic studies.

► Disease Severity

Cardiac arrest has a high recurrence rate if untreated. Prognosis related to LV function, CAD. 2-D echo, cardiac catheterization to assess severity of LV dysfunction.

► Concept and Application

Most ventricular arrhythmias are due to reentry and are associated with acute or chronic ischemic heart disease or CHF. Rarely seen in structurally normal heart. Other forms (automatic, triggered activity) are associated with medications or electrolyte abnormalities (torsade de pointes) or are idiopathic.

► Treatment Steps

Sustained Ventricular Tachycardia

1. Low-energy cardioversion (50–200 J).
2. Antiarrhythmic drugs, including lidocaine, amiodarone, bretylium, and procainamide.

Ventricular Fibrillation

1. Rapid defibrillation with 200–360 J.

Chronic Management

1. Stabilization of underlying disease.
2. Correction of electrolyte imbalances.
3. Antiarrhythmic drugs, especially amiodarone.
4. Implantable cardioverter defibrillator in patients at risk for sudden death.

VI. PERICARDIAL DISEASES

A. Acute Pericarditis

Most common pericardial disorder, consisting of acute inflammation of the pericardium from a wide variety of causes.

► H&P Keys

Retrosternal and left precordial sharp chest pain, often radiating to the back and left trapezius, with strong pleuritic component. Dyspnea is common. Symptoms often are worse in supine position, alleviated by sitting forward. Friction rub (three-component) best heard in left precordium with patient sitting forward during held exhalation.

► Diagnosis

ECG can show evolutionary changes consisting of widespread ST elevations with upward concavity and depressed PR interval, reduction of T wave amplitude or T wave inversion; with large associated pericardial effusions, reduction and respiratory variation in R wave amplitude (electrical alternans). Tests for etiology, e.g., antinuclear antibody (ANA), purified protein derivative (PPD).

► Disease Severity

The underlying disease is an important determination of outcome. Echo used to assess for presence and degree of associated pericardial effusion.

► Concept and Application

Pericardial inflammation caused by a variety of factors. Most common cause is idiopathic, although serologic studies have suggested these cases may be due to viral infection. Tuberculous pericarditis now reemerging, especially in acquired immune deficiency syndrome (AIDS) patients. Purulent (bacterial) pericarditis is a fulminant disease with a poor prognosis. Other causes are post-MI injury (Dressler's syndrome), malignant neoplasia, radiation, uremia, and collagen vascular diseases.

► Treatment Steps

1. In idiopathic or viral cases, anti-inflammatory agents are used.
2. Rarely, steroids are used in recalcitrant cases.
3. Large effusions producing hemodynamic compromise require drainage.
4. Purulent pericarditis requires complete drainage and antibiotics.
5. Other treatment depends on the specific etiology.

B. Pericardial Effusion

Fluid accumulation in the pericardial space. The amount of fluid and the rapidity of accumulation of the effusion determines the observed signs and symptoms.

► H&P Keys

Symptoms of pericarditis, or patient may be asymptomatic. Previously present friction rub may diminish in intensity. In large effusion, heart sounds may be muffled.

► Diagnosis

CXR shows cardiomegaly with "water bottle" shape. ECG, especially in large effusions, shows reduced QRS amplitude; electrical alternans may be seen. Echo for direct visualization of size and presence of effusion.

► Disease Severity

Determined by rapidity of accumulation and size of effusion. Echo documents size of effusion and extent of the hemodynamic impairment; hemodynamic effects can be also documented by cardiac catheterization.

► Concept and Application

Any cause of pericarditis can lead to the formation of a pericardial effusion. Pericardial effusion can also occur with a variety of systemic disorders such as hypothyroidism.

► Treatment Steps

1. Pericardiocentesis for diagnosis and treatment.
2. Treatment of underlying cause.
3. Removal of the pericardium may be required to prevent recurrent tamponade.

C. Cardiac Tamponade

An accumulation of pericardial fluid under high pressure, which limits the ability of the heart to fill.

► H&P Keys

May have antecedent history of pericarditis or chest trauma. Symptoms: dyspnea, fatigue. Physical findings: JVD, hypotension, shock, distant heart sounds, tachycardia, pulsus paradoxus.

► Diagnosis

Echo documents effusion, often with diastolic collapse of right atrium and right ventricle. Cardiac catheterization documents elevated pericardial pressure and equivalence of this pressure to the diastolic pressures in all four chambers.

► Disease Severity

Can be assessed by degree of symptomatic or hemodynamic impairment.

► Concept and Application

Pericardial fluid under high pressure compresses the heart, impairing its ability to fill. This leads to signs and symptoms of pulmonary and systemic venous congestion and ultimately obstructive shock.

► Treatment Steps

1. Immediate pericardiocentesis or surgical drainage with removal of the fluid, usually during echocardiographic and hemodynamic monitoring.
2. In recurrent cases, pericardiectomy may be necessary.

D. Constrictive Pericarditis

Obliteration of pericardial space or scarring of pericardial tissue, causing cardiac enclosure, resulting in compromised cardiac filling.

► H&P Keys

Symptoms: fatigue, hypotension, weakness. Physical signs: ascites, edema, JVD, often with Kussmaul's sign (elevation of venous pressure during inspiration), pericardial knock in diastole, reduced amplitude of apical impulse.

► Diagnosis

ECG may show a low-voltage QRS complex with diffuse T wave changes. CXR may show pericardial calcification, present in approximately 50% of patients. Echo and Doppler demonstrate normal cavity size with enhanced early diastolic filling. Pericardial thickening can be suggested by echo; however, computed tomography (CT) and magnetic resonance imaging (MRI) are more accurate in diagnosis.

► Disease Severity

Hemodynamic features seen during catheterization include elevation and equalization of all diastolic pressures; LV and RV pressure tracings are equal in diastole and have a dip and plateau configuration (square root sign); RA pressure tracing shows an M configuration with prominence of the Y descent.

► Concept and Application

Historically, tuberculosis was the most common cause; current common causes are idiopathic and radiation. The scarred encasing pericardium restricts cardiac filling, leading to signs of reduced cardiac output and systemic venous congestion.

► Treatment Steps

1. Pericardial resection is the definitive therapy.
2. Diuretics can afford symptomatic improvement. Risks of the operation and prognosis postoperatively depend on the degree of involvement of the epicardium in the scarring, calcific process.

VII. VALVULAR DISEASES

A. Acute

1. Rheumatic Fever

Delayed sequela to pharyngeal infections with group A streptococci. Pathology involves the heart, joints, central nervous system (CNS), skin, and subcutaneous tissues.

2. Endocarditis

Native valve endocarditis usually with prior valve pathology; endocarditis in prior drug users; and prosthetic valve endocarditis are the most common forms. May be acute or subacute. Acute endocarditis is often caused by *Staphylococcus aureus* and is rapidly destructive, and often fatal (if untreated) in < 6 weeks. Subacute endocarditis has a longer, smoldering course and is frequently caused by viridans streptococci. Without effective treatment, death usually occurs in 2–6 months.

3. Ischemic

Acute valvular decompensation resulting from ischemic heart disease, e.g., acute ischemia or myocardial infarction: may lead to cardiac decompensation and death. Usually acute MR caused by posterior papillary muscle ischemia or infarct.

► H&P Keys

Acute Rheumatic Fever—Arthritis, heart murmurs, CHF, fever, arrhythmias, CNS disorders, subcutaneous nodules, and skin rash.

Endocarditis—Fever, malaise, weakness, CHF, cardiac murmurs, splinter hemorrhages under fingernails, skin manifestations (Osler's nodes, Janeway lesions), embolic episodes, and petechiae.

Ischemic-Related Acute Valvular Decompensation—Acute-onset CHF, hypotension, and shock; new cardiac murmur may not be heard.

► Diagnosis

Blood cultures, elevated WBC, erythrocyte sedimentation rate (ESR), liver and muscle enzyme levels. Streptococcal antibody titer for rheumatic fever. Echocardiography, cardiac catheterization.

► Disease Severity

Depends on the chronicity, extent, and severity of valvular damage. Frequently involves multiple valves. Organism causing the endocarditis often key to severity. Degree of involvement of subvalvular apparatus (papillary muscle) determines severity of CHF in patients with ischemia-related MR.

► Concept and Application

Destruction of valvular and subvalvular apparatus, and the production of inflammatory myocarditis. Systemic embolization, as well as involvement of other organ systems, with both the infecting agent and inflammatory response responsible for other disease manifestations. Acute volume overload results from acute mitral or aortic valve rupture.

► Treatment Steps

1. Penicillin to prevent recurrent rheumatic fever.
2. Prolonged course of appropriate antibiotics for endocarditis.
3. Hemodynamic stabilization in the acutely ill patient.

4. Surgical valve replacement in patients with progressive valvular heart disease.

B. Chronic

Degeneration of cardiac valvular structures over a prolonged time. Progressive dilation of the LV or RV. Chronic degenerative disorders including mitral valve prolapse (myxomatous degeneration) and calcific valvular disease in the elderly. Mitral and aortic valves are most commonly involved in endocarditis and degenerative valvular disorders including MR, aortic regurgitation (AR), aortic stenosis (AS). Acquired mitral stenosis (MS) occurs almost exclusively from rheumatic fever. Pulmonary and tricuspid valves less often involved. Bicuspid aortic valve is a common congenital abnormality predominantly in men, and is associated with AS later in life.

► H&P Keys

CHF, shortness of breath, fatigue, pedal edema, cardiac murmurs consistent with severe stenotic or regurgitant lesions, elevated JVP, pulse alterations, e.g., delayed upstroke with aortic stenosis, bounding pulse with aortic insufficiency.

► Diagnosis

CXR, echo, cardiac catheterization.

► Disease Severity

Heart rate, respiratory rate, auscultatory findings, peripheral edema, pulmonary rales, blood pressure, oxygen saturation, level of consciousness.

► Concept and Application

AS—Obstruction of LV ejection producing pressure overload, LV hypertrophy, and ultimately reduced cardiac output.

MS—Obstruction of blood flow resulting in elevated left atrial (LA) and pulmonary pressures, plumonary edema, and impaired cardiac output.

AR—Dilated aorta, hypertension; large volume of blood in reverse direction from aorta to left ventricle resulting in LV dilation and reduced forward flow.

MR—Mitral valve prolapse; large volume of blood in reverse direction from left ventricle to left atrium and pulmonary veins resulting in pulmonary congestion, pulmonary edema, and reduced cardiac output.

► Treatment Steps

Acute MR and AR
1. Diuretics.
2. Afterload reduction.
3. IABP for MR but contraindicated in AR.
4. Valve replacement surgery.

Chronic MR and AR—In less severe cases,
1. Diuretics.
2. Afterload reduction.

Symptomatic AS and MS
1. Treated surgically with valve replacement.
2. MS can also be treated with catheter-based balloon dilation of the stenotic valve.

VIII. CARDIAC TRANSPLANTATION

Reserved for patients who are severely compromised by CHF despite maximal medical therapy. Major contraindications to cardiac transplantation include factors that increase short- and intermediate-term morbidity or mortality, e.g., associated diseases such as diabetes with end-organ complications or lung disease with pulmonary hypertension.

Immunosuppression is critical in preventing rejection in the post-transplant period, and cyclosporine has been a major advancement since its introduction in 1980. Sequential endomyocardial biopsies are performed to assess transplant rejection; based on biopsy results, doses of cyclosporine, prednisone, and azathioprine are adjusted. Severe rejection is often treated with short courses of T-cell suppression. One- and 5-year survival rates continue to improve and are now over 90% and 70%, respectively.

Complications associated with cardiac transplantation include rejection, infection, accelerated atherosclerosis, and hypertension.

IX. CONGENITAL HEART DISEASE

Result of aberrant embryonic development of a normal structure or failure of such structure to develop beyond early stage of embryonic or fetal development. Malformations are complex and multifactorial and include genetic (chromosomal), environmental (e.g., maternal rubella infection), and toxic (e.g., anticoagulants) factors.

A. Ventricular Septal Defect (VSD)

One or more openings in the membranous or muscular septum. Most common congenital heart disease in adults.

▶ H&P Keys

Harsh systolic murmur at left sternal border radiating to right precordium, palpable thrill over precordium. Large left-to-right shunt associated with CHF. Pulmonary hypertension causes reversal of flow (right-to-left shunt), resulting in the Eisenmenger syndrome characterized by cyanosis, pedal edema, syncope, and CHF.

▶ Diagnosis

Physical exam, CXR, oxygen saturation of blood in the ventricles, 2-D echo, cardiac catheterization, and angiography.

▶ Disease Severity

Mentation, heart rate, cyanosis, growth retardation. In children, 30–50% spontaneous closure. May be asymptomatic if shunt is small.

▶ Concept and Application

The size of the defect and the amount of blood shunted between the chambers determines the physiologic consequences.

Left-to-Right Shunt—Large volume of blood from left ventricle to right ventricle causes volume overload of pulmonary circulation and decreased LV output.

Right-to-Left Shunt—Large volume of unsaturated blood from right ventricle to left ventricle and systemic circulation, causing cyanosis, fatigue, right heart failure, embolic phenomenon.

► Treatment Steps
1. Small shunts do not require treatment.
2. Large shunts should undergo surgical repair.
3. Endocarditis prophylaxis is warranted.

B. Atrial Septal Defect (ASD)

Persistent opening in the septum in the region of fossa ovalis (secundum), in the lower septum (primum), or in or near the sinus node (sinus venosum).

► H&P Keys

Often asymptomatic. Murmur heard at upper left sternal border. Associated with fixed and widely split S_2. May be associated with trisomy 21. Dyspnea, fatigue, atrial arrhythmias, right heart failure. May be associated with severe pulmonary hypertension and Eisenmenger's syndrome. Primum ASD may be associated with mitral and tricuspid valve disorders.

► Diagnosis

Physical exam, CXR, ECG (RV hypertrophy), 2-D echo, cardiac catheterization.

► Disease Severity

CHF, pedal edema, elevated jugular venous pulse, fatigue, palpitations, dizziness, paradoxic emboli.

► Concept and Application

Shunting of blood at level of atria. Again, the size of the defect and amount of blood shunted between the chambers determines the consequences. Usually, a left-to-right shunt develops, but reversal of flow may develop if pulmonary artery and RV pressure increases. Disease severity correlates with size of shunt and symptoms.

► Treatment Steps
1. Observation of small shunts in asymptomatic patients but systemic emboli are a risk.
2. Closure for larger or symptomatic shunts.
3. Current catheter-based techniques allow less traumatic closure for many defects.

C. Tetralogy of Fallot

Most common congenital heart lesion over the age of 1 year characterized by the following four signs:

1. VSD
2. RV outflow narrowing
3. Overriding aorta
4. RV hypertrophy

► H&P Keys

Growth retardation, cardiac murmurs, cardiac arrhythmias, polycythemia and cyanosis, exercise limitation with squatting maneuver to restore normal breathing, clubbing, thrill at left sternal border.

► Diagnosis

Physical exam, CXR, ECG (RV hypertrophy), 2-D echo, cardiac catheterization.

► Disease Severity

Activity level, growth, ABG, mentation, heart rate, cyanosis and pedal edema, heart size, CHF, syncope.

► Concept and Application

Caused by the combination and severity of characteristic abnormalities; the degree of obstruction at the right ventricular outflow tract (RVOT), shunting at the level of the VSD, amount of blood from right ventricle and left ventricle to the aorta.

► Treatment Steps

1. Total surgical correction.
2. Bacterial endocarditis prophylaxis.

D. Coarctation of the Aorta

Narrowing of aortic lumen, usually at level just below left subclavian artery (ligamentum arteriosum).

► H&P Keys

More common in males. Differential development of upper and lower body, differential pulses in upper and lower extremities, a cause of secondary hypertension.

► Diagnosis

Brachial and femoral artery pulses, blood pressure in upper versus lower extremities, CXR (rib notching), 2-D echo in children, aortography, CT scan.

► Disease Severity

Depends on extent of luminal narrowing. Severe hypertension may result, producing headache, CHF, CNS hemorrhage. Lower extremity claudication, aortic rupture possible. May be associated with bicuspid aortic valve (AS or AR).

► Concept and Application

Congenital. Narrowing of aorta at the level of the ligamentum arteriosum.

► Treatment Steps

1. Surgical correction optimally at age 4–8.
2. Bacterial endocarditis prophylaxis.

X. CARDIAC LIFE SUPPORT

Cardiopulmonary arrest is the cessation of effective cardiac function resulting in hemodynamic collapse. In children, a pulmonary etiology is most common, whereas in adults a cardiac etiology (e.g., VT or ventricular fibrillation [VF]) is the most common.

► H&P Keys

Dizziness, dyspnea, palpitations, chest pain may precede cardiac arrest and loss of consciousness that is not spontaneously terminated. Examination: cyanotic, pulseless, unconscious, or unarousable patient with absent or agonal respirations. Children often are cyanotic.

► Diagnosis

Most cardiopulmonary arrests occur outside the hospital and are fatal. Only 25% of cardiopulmonary arrest victims survive to hospital admission. Cardiopulmonary arrest victims are identified as unresponsive and pulseless patients. ECG, electrolytes, myocardial enzymes, and cyanosis.

► Disease Severity

Duration of cardiopulmonary arrest time.

► Concept and Application

Children—Sudden infant death syndrome (SIDS) may be multifactorial; pulmonary failure may be secondary to obstruction of airways.

Adult—VT or VF secondary to acute and chronic CAD. Often associated with depressed LV function resulting from acute or prior MI.

► Management

Basic Life Support (BLS)—ABC
1. Airway: Check for patency and obstruction.
2. Breathing: Ventilate.
3. Circulation: Reestablish with external compression.
4. Repetitive cycles of ventilation and external compression, punctuated by assessing for spontaneous ventilation and pulse, continued until Advanced Cardiac Life Support team available.

Advanced Cardiac Life Support (ACLS)
1. Arrhythmia recognition ("quick look" with defibrillator paddles or ECG) and appropriate treatment with electrical cardioversion (VT: 50–200 J) or defibrillation (VF: 200–360 J).
2. Continued BLS.
3. Use of adjunctive equipment including performing endotracheal intubation for improved ventilation and placement of intravenous lines.
4. Initiation of pharmacologic therapy, including IV fluids (normal saline), epinephrine (1:10,000), lidocaine, procainamide, amiodarone, dopamine, norepinephrine.

XI. HYPERTENSION

Hypertension is defined as a diastolic pressure > 90 and a systolic pressure > 140. Severe hypertension includes a diastolic blood pressure > 115. Hypertension is an important public health problem and a major cause of CHF. Uncontrolled hypertension is associated with a marked reduction in life expectancy.

A. Essential Hypertension

The etiology is unknown in 95% of patients with essential hypertension. There is a strong family occurrence.

► H&P Keys

The vast majority of patients are asymptomatic. Symptoms of occipital headache are seen with severe hypertension. Other associated symptoms reflect end-organ damage, e.g., hematuria, blurring of vision, CHF. Exam is tailored to detect evidence of end-organ damage, e.g., retinal hemorrhages, S_4, S_3.

► Diagnosis

All patients with hypertension should have urinalysis for protein, blood, potassium, creatinine, BUN, and an ECG for evidence of LV hypertrophy. Other testing is performed to exclude a suspected secondary cause.

▶ Disease Severity

Evidence of end-organ damage including CNS, renal, and cardiac dysfunction.

CNS—Lacunar infarcts and stroke.

Renal—Elevated creatinine, BUN.

Cardiac—LV hypertrophy, cardiomegaly. CHF, MI, aortic enlargement, and aortic dissection. Natural history depends on the level of blood pressure and the extent and severity of organ involvement.

▶ Concept and Application

The cause of essential hypertension remains unknown. Possible mechanisms include complex multifactorial genetic factors as well as abnormal responsiveness to sodium and calcium. Associated with diabetes and obesity.

▶ Treatment Steps

Both isolated systolic and diastolic hypertension should be treated.

1. In general, weight reduction in the obese patient and some restriction in salt are often very valuable in control. Step therapy has been evaluated over a 25-year period, with evidence of improved life expectancy.
2. Diuretics and β-blockers improve outcomes and are recommended as the initial drug choices.
3. Other agents including ACE inhibitors and calcium antagonists are useful as secondary agents.
4. As severity increases, antiadrenergic drugs such as clonidine and vasodilators (e.g., minoxidil) may be valuable.

B. Secondary Hypertension

A host of disease entities produce hypertension, including endocrine abnormalities, such as adrenal cortical hyperfunction (Cushing's disease), primary hyperaldosteronism, and pheochromocytoma; neurogenic, renovascular, and parenchymal diseases; and entities associated with increasing stroke volume, e.g., hyperthyroidism and aortic insufficiency.

▶ H&P Keys

Wide-ranging disease process may be detected such as cushingoid features, episodic marked elevation in blood pressure in pheochromocytoma, polyuria, polydipsia, and muscle weakness secondary to hypokalemia.

▶ Diagnosis

BUN, creatinine level, thyroid-stimulating hormone (TSH) level, renal artery Doppler flow studies or angiography, urine and plasma catecholamine levels, plasma renin activity, serum and urine catecholamine levels.

▶ Disease Severity

Depends on specific etiology and its natural history as well as response of the blood pressure to therapy.

▶ Concept and Application

Elevations of catecholamine levels, activation of the renin–angiotensin system with vasoconstriction, excessive sodium retention in primary and secondary aldosteronism, and excessive glucocorticoid production.

► **Treatment Steps**
1. Renal artery stenosis may respond to angioplasty or surgery, especially in patients with high renin from the affected kidney and suppression of renin production in the uninvolved kidney.
2. Other secondary forms, e.g., pheochromocytoma and Cushing's disease, can be cured with surgical removal of the tumor.
3. ACE inhibitors may worsen renal functions in patients with bilateral renal artery stenosis, and renal function must be followed in everyone who receives these agents.

C. Malignant Hypertension

Sudden and severe elevation of blood pressure with evidence of acute end-organ damage. Includes hypertensive encephalopathy, rapidly deteriorating renal function, and acute CHF.

► **H&P Keys**

Visual disturbances, severe headache, confusion, coma, seizures, edema, dyspnea, blood pressure > 200/115, papilledema, hemorrhage, spasm on ophthalmoscopic exam, S_3 gallop, oliguria.

► **Diagnosis**

BUN, creatinine levels, peripheral smear for microangiopathic hemolytic anemia, chest roentgenographic evidence of CHF.

► **Disease Severity**

Depends on the extent and severity of end-organ damage and may include stroke, refractory pulmonary edema, and progressive oliguric renal failure.

► **Concept and Application**

The trigger for malignant hypertension is unknown. There is widespread fibrinoid necrosis of the arterial walls. Cerebral autoregulation is impaired and cerebral blood flow is increased, which contributes to the encephalopathy.

► **Treatment Steps**
Acute
1. Nitroprusside infusion in doses of 0.5–8 mg/kg/min can produce rapid, graded control of blood pressure and is recommended initial therapy.
2. Also, continuous labetalol infusion in doses in the range of 2 mg/min have been effective.

Long-Term—Other agents for long-term control are needed.
1. Diuresis is useful to contract volume and decrease blood pressure and also to assist with CHF and encephalopathy.
2. β-Blockers, ACE inhibitors, and calcium antagonists are all effective. Renal function may deteriorate in the early phase of treatment, but persistent blood pressure control is needed to resolve the arterial lesions.

XII. LIPOPROTEINS AND ATHEROSCLEROSIS

A. Hyperlipoproteinemia

A wide array of disorders resulting from abnormalities in metabolism of the lipoproteins that transport exogenously and endogenously produced cholesterol and triglycerides. The major lipoproteins are chylomicrons and very-low-density lipoprotein (VLDL), which transport triglycerides (TG), and intermediate-, low-, and high-density lipoproteins (IDL, LDL, HDL), which primarily transport cholesterol. Hyperlipoproteinemias occur as a result of a genetic defect in synthesis or degradation or secondary to diabetes, hyperthyroidism, and excessive alcohol ingestion. Classification is based on the recognized abnormality in lipoproteins and the type of lipid that accumulates in the serum (see Table 1–1).

Most important are accumulations in LDL, which are associated with premature atherosclerosis (see Figure 1–2 for relative risk).

► H&P Keys
Cutaneous, tendinous, tuberous, and eruptive xanthomas; premature atherosclerosis; lipemia retinalis; and pancreatitis.

► Diagnosis
Examination of serum for creamy, chylomicron layer, measurement of serum lipids, e.g., cholesterol, TG, HDL, and LDL. High LDL is associated with an increased risk of atherosclerosis and MI. Occasionally, lipoprotein electrophoresis is required for definitive characterization.

► Disease Severity
The extent of atherosclerosis and its complications include MI, stroke, peripheral vascular disease. Patients with high level of TG frequently develop recurrent pancreatitis.

► Concept and Application
In familial hypercholesterolemia, premature, accelerated atherosclerosis and MI occurs in the third or fourth decade. The hyperlipoproteinemias are genetically transmitted as a result of single or multiple gene disorders.

► Treatment Steps

General
1. Dietary restriction of fats and weight reduction.
2. Control of secondary factors, e.g., cessation of alcohol, optimum control of diabetes.
3. Elimination of other risk factors for CAD.

Drug Therapy—Dependent on lipid abnormality, severity, other coronary risk factors, and associated disease. In patients with known atherosclerosis or significant, multiple risk factors, lipid therapy should be considered when LDL is > 100 mg/dL. HMG CoA reductase inhibitors are the most effective agents and have been demonstrated to substantially reduce atherosclerotic event rates and are widely used for both primary and secondary prevention. Available agents include:

1–1

LIPOPROTEIN ABNORMALITY TYPES		
Type	Lipoprotein Abnormality	Lipid Accumulation
I	Chylomicrons	TG
IIA	LDL	Cholesterol
IIB	LDL and VLDL	Cholesterol and TG
III	Chylomicrons and IDL	TG and cholesterol
IV	VLDL	TG
V	VLDL and chylomicrons	TG and cholesterol

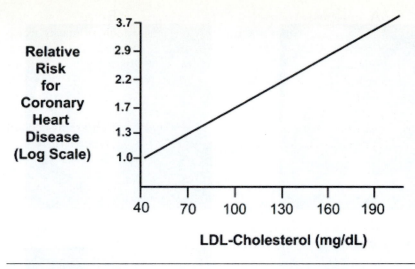

Figure 1–2. Relative risk for coronary heart disease.

1. HMG CoA reductase inhibitors—lower LDL by blocking endogenous cholesterol biosynthesis.
2. Ezetimibe—selective cholesterol absorption inhibition.
3. Nicotinic acid—reduces production of VLDL by liver and lowers LDL, HDL, and TG.

B. Atherosclerosis

Results as a response to injury of vascular endothelium with thrombus formation. Initially, isolated macrophages or foam cells infiltrate endothelium. Later, lipid-rich lesions with smooth muscle and fibrous collagen cap form mature atheromatous plaque. Acute coronary syndromes (unstable angina and MI) occur when there is acute plaque rupture and thrombus formation.

▶ H&P Keys
Anginal chest pain, stroke syndromes with neurologic deficits, including motor or sensory abnormalities, intermittent claudication, reduction in peripheral pulses and pressure.

▶ Diagnosis
ECG, stress testing, and myocardial perfusion imaging, noninvasive vascular assessment, including carotids, arterial Doppler, cardiac catheterization, and angiography (Fig. 1–3).

▶ Disease Severity
Extent of motor and sensory deficit after stroke, impairment in cardiac function after MI, exercise limitation, claudication.

▶ Concept and Application
The development of atherosclerosis is multifactorial and related to injury of the endothelium as well as the factors that enhance thrombosis. Endothelial cells produce a variety of substances that cause vasoconstriction and smooth-muscle proliferation. Acute plaque disruption occurs as a result of alterations of stress at the plaque surface. Exposure of damaged vessel wall leads to the adherence of platelets, development of thrombus, and, ultimately, occlusion of the vessel.

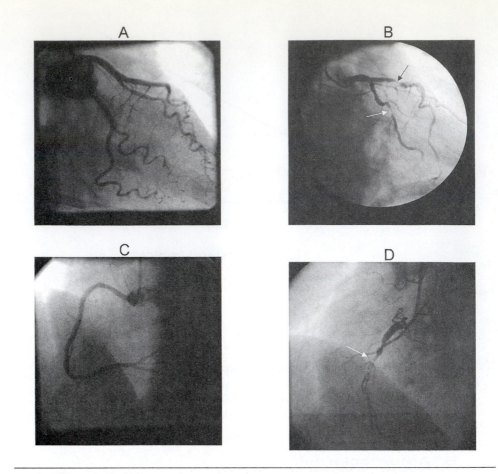

Figure 1–3. Normal coronary angiogram of left coronary (A) and right coronary (C). Figure B and D arrows point to atherosclerotic narrowing in abnormal left and right coronary arteries.

▶ **Treatment Steps**

1. Prevention of atherosclerosis and plaque rupture with thrombosis is complex and requires multiple interventions. Major risk factors include cigarette smoking, hypertension, diabetes, and elevated cholesterol. Management is directed at eliminating these risk factors. Thrombosis is enhanced by catecholamines (stress), cigarette smoking, and familial predisposition.

2. Aspirin therapy is effective in both primary and secondary prevention.

XIII. PERIPHERAL ARTERIAL VASCULAR DISEASE

A. Chronic Atherosclerotic Occlusion

Associated with generalized atherosclerosis and frequently coexists with CAD as well as cerebrovascular disease.

▶ **H&P Keys**

Intermittent claudication (exertional calf, thigh, and buttocks discomfort), rest pain with more severe reduction in blood flow, subclavian steal syndrome, reduction in blood pressure in affected limb (or limbs), decreased or absent pulses, vascular bruits over subclavian aorta or femoral arteries. Elevational pallor, dependent rubor, and prolonged venous filling time of the legs. Ulcers and gangrene.

► Diagnosis

Doppler pressure measurements before and after exercise and calculation of ankle-brachial index, pulse volume recordings (PVRs), peripheral angiography, CT, and magnetic resonance angiography.

► Disease Severity

Severe if ankle-brachial index is < 0.4. Resting ischemia, ulcerations, and gangrene. Recurrent neurologic symptoms with subclavian steal syndrome.

► Concept and Application

Progressive atherosclerotic lesions produce reduction in blood flow to the affected limbs. Associated with generalized atherosclerosis.

► Treatment Steps

Medical

1. Control of atherosclerotic risk factors.
2. Smoking cessation most important.
3. Exercise may stimulate collateral blood flow. Vasodilators are generally ineffective.
4. Pentoxifylline improves exercise ability in approximately one-third of patients.

Surgical

1. Revascularization with bypass procedure or angioplasty for limiting symptoms or for limb salvage.
2. Sympathectomy for pain relief.
3. Amputation for severely damaged ischemic limbs.

B. Acute Arterial Occlusion

Sudden cessation of blood flow as a result of an embolus, acute thrombosis, or vasospasm.

► H&P Keys

Appropriate setting with sudden onset of pain, then loss of sensation; paralysis; and cool, cyanotic, mottled limb.

► Diagnosis

Doppler studies, angiography, 2-D echo to evaluate thrombolytic source.

► Disease Severity

Occlusion of an artery to an extremity leads to paralysis, cyanosis, and loss of viability, with tissue necrosis, ulceration, and gangrene.

► Concept and Application

Majority of emboli are from cardiac sources. Intracardiac thrombosis occurs in MI and atrial fibrillation; also in valvular disease, especially MS and prosthetic valves. Acute and chronic bacterial endocarditis and vegetations may embolize. A "paradoxical" embolus may occur with an ASD. Large-vessel occlusion occurs with bulky vegetations, especially in fungal endocarditis. Acute thrombosis occurs in some infectious diseases, especially rickettsial, e.g., Rocky Mountain spotted fever, connective tissue disease, and hypercoagulable states.

► Treatment Steps

1. Heparin administration.
2. Prompt evaluation with arteriography and embolectomy.
3. After reperfusion, especially in the leg muscle compartments, fasciotomy may be necessary to relieve compressive symptoms.

4. Additional therapy may be required after the source of embolus is identified, e.g., valve replacement for MS or acute endocarditis.

C. Vasculitis Syndromes

Encompasses a wide variety of conditions, characterized by inflammation of the blood vessel wall. The syndromes include:

1. Necrotizing vasculitis: polyarteritis nodosa.
2. Hypersensitivity angiitis.
3. Giant cell arteritis: Takayasu's, temporal arteritis.
4. Other: thromboangiitis obliterans; mucocutaneous lymph node syndrome.

▶ H&P Keys

Wide-ranging because arterial thrombosis can affect any organ system. Systemic signs and symptoms include fever, weight loss, arthritis, organ dysfunction from occlusion of cerebral vessel limb or digital arteries, absent or decreased pulses, differential blood pressures, vascular bruits. Also, elevated sedimentation rate, leukocytosis.

▶ Diagnosis

Arterial biopsy, e.g., in temporal arteritis to confirm vessel inflammation. Arterial Doppler studies, PVR, and aortography.

▶ Disease Severity

Dependent on extent and severity of organ dysfunction or compromising blood flow to the limbs. Patients may develop stroke, gangrenous bowel, MI, ischemia to limbs and digits.

▶ Concept and Application

In general, vasculitis occurs because of immune injury. There is a deposition of immune complexes in the arterial wall, which initiates an acute inflammatory response that leads to thrombosis. There also may be cell-mediated vascular injury.

▶ Treatment Steps

1. Many of these entities respond partially to treatment with systemic glucocorticoids, e.g., temporal arteritis and Takayasu's disease.
2. Occasionally, responses are seen from other cytotoxic agents.
3. Cessation of smoking in thromboangiitis.
4. Sympathectomy is of value to relieve pain.

XIV. PERIPHERAL VENOUS VASCULAR DISEASES AND PULMONARY EMBOLISM

A. Venous Thrombosis

Occurs in a wide variety of settings. Predisposing factors include trauma or surgery, especially orthopedic, prolonged bed rest for any reason, pregnancy, and a variety of neoplasms. The disease commonly affects the lower extremities, although upper extremities can be involved.

▶ H&P Keys

Recognition of the appropriate setting and predisposing factors. Clinical signs (calf swelling, tenderness, and warmth) are nonspecific and frequently missed.

Superficial Venous Thrombosis—Hot, red, swollen visible vein.

Chronic—Leg swelling and superficial varicosities.

► Disease Severity

Acute—Pulmonary embolus is the primary risk; however, recurrent deep vein thrombosis (DVT) can lead to a chronic state.

Chronic—Refractory edema, stasis ulceration with superimposed chronic cellulitis.

► Diagnosis

Impedance plethysmography, Doppler ultrasonography, ventilation–perfusion lung scan, spiral CT, and pulmonary angiography.

► Concepts and Application

Virchow described the triad of venous thrombosis: (1) abnormality of the vascular wall; (2) stasis of blood flow; and (3) hypercoagulable state. Thrombosis may occur because of deficiency of antithrombin III or fibrinolytic proteins C and S, a circulating lupus anticoagulant, and homocystinuria.

► Treatment Steps

Acute

1. Heparin in continuous infusion for 7–10 days, adjusted so partial thromboplastin time (PTT) is approximately two times control value.

Chronic

1. Anticoagulation for 6–12 months with warfarin, longer (indefinite) if DVT recurs.
2. Elevation of legs when possible.
3. Full waist-length, graduated compression stockings.
4. Meticulous skin care.

Prophylaxis

1. With 5,000 U heparin every 8–12 hours in high-risk clinical situations needs to be initiated prior to surgical procedure.
2. Below-the-knee thrombosis can be followed if no proximal venous disease is detected; anticoagulation may not be required.

B. Pulmonary Embolism

A common event in hospitalized patients, frequently unrecognized, with high morbidity and mortality.

► H&P Keys

Sudden dyspnea, pleuritic chest pain, hemoptysis, syncope, unexplained tachycardia, supraventricular dysrhythmias, pulmonary hypertension with a right ventricular lift; wide, persistent splitting; and loud pulmonic component of the second heart sound.

► Diagnosis

ECG—Nonspecific ST-T wave changes, right axis deviation.

CXR—Dilatation of pulmonary artery, abrupt cutoff. Ventilation–perfusion lung scan, pulmonary angiogram, detection of DVT.

► Disease Severity

The size of the embolus and the resultant extent and severity of obstruction of the pulmonary arteries. Hemodynamic deterioration can occur with shock and peripheral hypoperfusion and is more severe with preexisting heart or lung disease. Impairment of gas exchange and arterial hypoxemia.

▶ Concept and Application

The majority of pulmonary embolisms occur in the setting of DVT. Embolization of clot from below the knee is unusual. The best approach to the disease is prophylaxis, prevention, early detection, and treatment of DVT.

▶ Treatment Steps

1. Heparin, with initial dose of 5,000 U and continuous infusion to maintain PTT approximately two times control.
2. Intermittent regimens can be employed.
3. With recurrent embolization or contraindication to anticoagulant therapy, venal caval filter or plication is effective in prevention of further emboli.
4. If severe hemodynamic compromise occurs, thrombolytic therapy with streptokinase (initial bolus of 250,000 U and 24-hour infusion) is favored over acute embolectomy.

XV. DISEASES OF THE AORTA

A. Aneurysms

Pathologic dilatation of a segment of a blood vessel. A true aneurysm involves all three layers of the vessel wall and is distinguished from a pseudoaneurysm, which involves only the intima and media. Classified by their location and gross appearance: thoracic versus abdominal, and fusiform versus saccular.

▶ H&P Keys

Most aneurysms are asymptomatic. Symptoms of pain may be produced by expanding aneurysms; often a harbinger of rupture and an acute medical emergency. Acute rupture may occur without warning and is always life threatening. Compression of contiguous blood vessels may result in other symptoms, including stroke from compression of carotid vessels in thoracic aortic aneurysms and impairment of lower-extremity blood flow in expanding abdominal aortic aneurysms.

Abdominal Aortic Aneurysms—Presence of palpable, pulsatile, and tender abdominal mass with abdominal bruit.

Thoracic Aortic Aneurysms—Tracheal deviation, hoarseness, and CHF because of aortic dilatation and resulting aortic regurgitation. Patients with abdominal aneurysms may also have distal arterial embolization and lower-extremity claudication. Most abdominal aneurysms occur distal to the renal arteries.

▶ Diagnosis

Radiography including CXR and abdominal films may demonstrate the enlarged aorta sometimes outlined by calcium. More definitive studies include thoracic and abdominal ultrasonography, CT, MRI, or invasive angiography.

▶ Disease Severity

Determined by location, size of aneurysm, and rate of dilatation. For abdominal aneurysms exceeding 6 cm in diameter, the 2-year mortality related to rupture is approximately 50%, and for those 4–6 cm in diameter, 25%.

► Concept and Application
Atherosclerosis is the most common cause of aortic aneurysm. Abdominal aortic aneurysms are almost always due to atherosclerosis, whereas those of the ascending thoracic aorta may be caused by cystic medial necrosis, atherosclerosis, syphilis, bacterial infections, or rheumatic aortitis. Aneurysms of the descending thoracic aorta that are contiguous with infradiaphragmatic aneurysms are usually due to atherosclerosis.

► Treatment Steps
1. Location and extent of the aneurysm using radiographic imaging techniques.
2. Followed by operative excision of the aneurysm and replacement with graft and reimplantation of branch vessels.

B. Aortic Dissection
Caused by a transverse or circumferential tear of the aortic intima in areas with high shear forces (left subclavian artery and right lateral ascending aortic wall).

- Type 1: Dissection in proximal aorta, may extend into the arch.
- Type 2: Dissection limited to aortic arch.
- Type 3: Dissection begins distal to left subclavian artery and extends for variable distance inferiorly.

► H&P Keys
Acute dissection is characterized by a sudden onset of severe and tearing pain associated with diaphoresis. Pain usually from front of chest to interscapular area. May be associated with syncope, dyspnea, or weakness. Blood pressure may be high or low. Other signs include differential pulses, pulmonary edema, neurologic symptoms (stroke or spinal cord compression), aortic regurgitation producing CHF. Abdominal aortic dissection may be accompanied by bowel ischemia and hematuria, whereas thoracic dissection may be accompanied by superior vena caval syndrome, hoarseness, airway compromise, dysphagia, inferior MI with hemopericardium and cardiac tamponade.

► Diagnosis
CXR, ECG, CT scan, MRI, and aortography.

► Disease Severity
Physical examination for involvement of brain, peripheral arteries, kidneys, spinal cord, heart. Continued pain or symptoms of compromise to major arterial branches indicate active propagation of dissection. Hypotension or shock, oliguria, mentation.

► Concept and Application
Disruption of aortic intima, possibly related to medial hemorrhage at areas with high shear forces. Pulsatile flow dissects along elastic laminar plates of aorta, creating false lumen. Underlying condition may be related to cystic medial necrosis of aortic wall or collagen dysfunction (Marfan syndrome).

► Treatment Steps
1. Emergency operation is indicated for patients with symptoms indicating propagating dissection. Emergency operation carries a

high mortality, but active propagation is often fatal if not stabilized.

2. Stabilization with medical therapy, including β-blockers and afterload-reducing agents (nitroprusside), is preferred for ≥ 14 days if possible before surgical correction.

3. For patients with stable and uncomplicated distal aortic dissection, medical therapy is preferred and includes long-term use of β-blockers and orally administered afterload-reducing agents.

C. Aortic Occlusion

Chronic occlusive disease that generally involves the distal abdominal aorta below the renal arteries.

► H&P Keys

Claudication, impotence in males (Leriche's syndrome). Symptoms vary depending on presence and adequacy of collateral blood flow. Physical findings include absent or depressed femoral and distal pulses and presence of bruits over abdominal aorta and femoral arteries. Lower-extremity skin loss, atrophic skin changes, cool extremities, peripheral skin ulcerations.

► Diagnosis

Physical examination, noninvasive Doppler evaluation of arterial blood flow, ankle-brachial index (ABI) (sphygmomanometry). Abdominal aortography to define anatomy prior to revascularization.

► on rounds

CARDIOLOGY AT A GLANCE

Myocardial Infarction
- Chest pain, diaphoresis, 20% without pain
- Transmural or Q wave has ST segment elevation and T wave inversions
- Nontransmural has ST segment elevation and T wave inversions.
- CK-MB peaks at 24 hours
- AST or SGOT peaks at 48–72 hours
- LHD peaks at 3–5 days

Prinzmetal's or Variant Angina
- Angina at rest
- Younger patients
- ECG positive for ST elevation during symptoms
- Gold standard diagnostic test: Spasm on angiography
- Treatment: Nitrates, calcium channel blockers, stop smoking, avoid cocaine

Signs of Heart Failure

Left Side, Low Output
- Fatigue, dyspnea, PND, orthopnea
- S_3 or S_4, displaced cardiac impulse, CXR, echo

Left Side, High Output
- Brisk pulse, dyspnea, orthopnea, hyperdynamic circulation

Right Side
- Fatigue, RV heave, JVD, hepatomegaly, atrial arrhythmias
- ECG may show RV or RA hypertrophy
- Echo may show RV dilation and hypokinesis

► **Disease Severity**

Dependent on collateral blood flow.

► **Concept and Application**

Atherosclerotic; nonatheromatous disease may be associated with smoking (Buerger's disease or thromboangiitis obliterans) or homocystinuria, especially in young adults.

► **Treatment Steps**

1. Preoperative assessment by aortography and surgical revascularization.
2. Cessation of smoking and modification of diet are important in stabilizing this progressive disease.

D. Aortitis

Syphilitic, rheumatic.

1. Syphilitic Aortitis

Usually affecting the proximal aorta, resulting in aortic root dilatation and aneurysm formation.

► **H&P Keys**

Often asymptomatic. As it progresses, may cause compression and erosion into adjacent structures; rupture may occur.

► **Diagnosis**

CXR, 2-D echo, cardiac catheterization, immunologic screening, rapid plasma reagin (RPR), Venereal Disease Research Laboratory (VDRL).

► **Disease Severity**

Long latency period: 15–30 years after initial infection. Symptoms may occur from aortic regurgitation or narrowing of coronary ostia or from compression to adjacent structures (esophagus), or rupture. Serologic tests confirm diagnosis. Evaluation includes CXR, ultrasonography, CT scan, MRI, and aortography.

► **Concept and Application**

Destruction of collagen elastic tissue, leading to dilatation of aorta with scar formation and calcification, is due to obliterative endarteritis of the vasa vasorum in the adventitia. This is an inflammatory response to invasion of the adventitia by spirochetes.

► **Treatment Steps**

1. Antibiotic treatment (penicillin).
2. Surgical excision and repair.

2. Rheumatic Aortitis

Includes rheumatoid arthritis, ankylosing spondylitis, psoriatic arthritis, Reiter's syndrome, Behçet's syndrome, relapsing polychondritis, and inflammatory bowel disorders.

BIBLIOGRAPHY

ACC/AHA Guidelines
1. Guidelines for the management of patients with ST-elevation myocardial infarction—executive summary. *Circulation* 2004;110:588–636.
2. Guideline update for the management of patients with unstable angina and non-ST segment elevation myocardial infarction. *J Am Coll Cardiol* 2002;40:1366.
3. Guidelines for the evaluation and management of chronic heart failure in the adult. *Circulation* 2001;104:2996.

4. Implications of recent clinical trials for the National Cholesterol Education Program Adult Treatment Panel III Guidelines. *Circulation* 2004;110:227–239.

Braunwald E. *Heart Disease: A Textbook of Cardiovascular Medicine,* 7th ed. Philadelphia: W.B. Saunders, 2005.

Fuster V, et al (eds.). *Hurst's The Heart,* 11th ed. New York: McGraw-Hill, 2004.

Loh E, McClellan JR. Congestive heart failure. In: Conn RB, et al (eds.). *Current Diagnosis.* Orlando, FL: W.B. Saunders, 1997.

McClellan JR. Clinical approach to the patient in shock. In Chizner M (ed.). *Classic Teachings in Clinical Cardiology.* Cedar Grove, NJ: Laennec Publishing, 1996.

Dermatology | 2

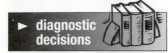
I. ACUTE EXANTHEMS

A. Varicella (Chickenpox)

► H&P Keys
Rash begins on face and scalp and rapidly spreads to trunk, with relative sparing of extremities. Typical lesions are vesicles with a pink base, but presence of lesions at all stages of development (macules, papules, vesicles, pustules, crusted lesions) is characteristic. Fever, chills, malaise, and headache may accompany. Mucous membranes may be affected.

► Diagnosis
History and physical exam. Confirm if necessary with Tzanck smear demonstrating multinucleated giant cells, viral culture, direct fluorescent antibody test.

► Disease Severity
Mildest cases in infants and most severe cases in adults. Fever correlates with disease severity. Prolonged fever may be associated with complications such as pneumonia. Scarring is more likely in adults.

► Concept and Application
Humoral and cellular immune response terminates viremia; immunity is complex, and antibody alone does not guarantee total immunity. A live attenuated vaccine is available.

► Treatment Steps
1. Symptomatic.
2. Antibiotics if secondary infection develops. Acyclovir or derivative for infections in adult or immunocompromised. Varicella-zoster immune globulin can be used in immunocompromised patients up to 3 days after exposure.

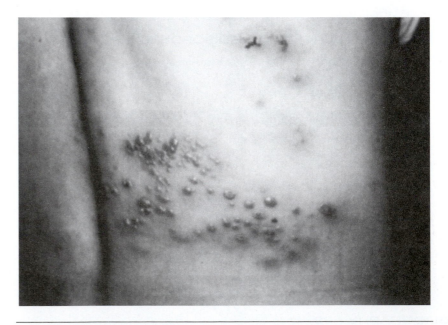

Figure 2–1. Varicella-zoster. Some lesions in this example are hemorrhagic.

B. Varicella Zoster (Shingles)

▶ **H&P Keys**

Prodrome of pain and paresthesia in involved dermatome; typical rash is localized, unilateral, does not cross midline, grouped vesicles on a pink base that evolve into pustules and crusts (Fig. 2–1).

▶ **Diagnosis**

Same as varicella.

▶ **Disease Severity**

Pain is more severe in elderly patients; disease is more severe in immunocompromised (skin necrosis and scarring, postherpetic neuralgia, dissemination).

▶ **Concept and Application**

Infection is a recrudescence of latent infection with varicella-zoster virus (VZV); increased incidence of infection in patients with human immunodeficiency virus (HIV) or defects in cellular immunity.

▶ **Treatment Steps**

1. Acyclovir or derivative for 7 days, analgesics.
2. Postherpetic neuralgia: capsaicin cream, tricyclic antidepressants, gabapentin. For severe pain, consider nerve blocks.

II. OTHER SKIN INFECTIONS

A. Mycoses

1. Dermatophytosis

▶ **H&P Keys**

Contact with infected person or animals, typical annular reddish scaly plaques with central clearing (tinea corporis), hair loss with scalp involvement (tinea capitis); fissures, scales, or blisters with foot involvement (tinea pedis).

▶ **Diagnosis**

Potassium hydroxide (KOH) preparation, fungal culture, Wood's light (some cases of tinea capitis).

▶ **Disease Severity**

Toenails involved (onychomycosis) usually with tinea pedis; hand infection usually accompanied by tinea pedis; extensive or chronic involvement in immunodeficiency states and endocrine disorders (Cushing's diabetes).

▶ **Concept and Application**

Infection dependent on climatic conditions (tinea pedis more common where occlusive footwear is used; tinea corporis more common in hot, humid climates under occlusive garments), host factors (men are more susceptible), virulence of organisms.

▶ **Treatment Steps**

1. Topical antifungals for most limited infections, oral agents (e.g., griseofulvin) for extensive disease and tinea capitis. Onycomycosis can be treated with itraconazole or terbinafine.
2. Recurrence or treatment failure: add or switch oral agent, check culture.

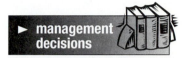

▶ **management decisions**

FUNGAL INFECTIONS

Tinea Capitis
Topicals ineffective. Treat with systemic agents for 4–8 weeks or until cultures are negative. Griseofulvin is the gold standard, but other oral agents, itraconazole, terbinafine, and fluconazole, are alternatives. Addition of shampoo such as selenium sulfide improves outcome.

Tinea Corporis, Tinea Pedis, Tinea Manuum
Mild, localized cases respond to treatment with topical imidazole or allylamine. More extensive disease requires systemic treatment.

Onychomycosis
Topical therapies not effective. Itraconazole pulse dosed (first week of the month for 3 months) or terbinafine daily for 6 weeks (fingernails) or 12 weeks (toenails).

Tinea Versicolor
Mild or localized cases often respond to topical treatment with ketoconazole and/or selenium sulfide, zinc pyrithione or sulfur shampoos. For more extensive disease, oral ketoconazole or itraconazole.

2. Candidiasis, Cutaneous

▶ **H&P Keys**

Acute—Inflammatory plaques with satellite pustules in moist, macerated folds of skin (e.g., axillae, submammary).

Chronic—Same as acute, but also can develop heavily crusted lesions on skin and thickened nail plate.

▶ **Diagnosis**

KOH preparation, culture, pathologic studies.

▶ **Disease Severity**

Acute—Increased predisposition in obesity, diabetes, and certain occupations (wet work: waitresses, dishwashers, housecleaners).

Chronic—Associated with endocrinopathies (hypoparathyroidism, hypoadrenalism, hypothyroidism), circulating autoantibodies, chronic active hepatitis, thymoma.

▶ **Concept and Application**

In chronic types, cell-mediated immune defect selective for *Candida.*

▶ **Treatment Steps**

1. Nystatin powder, topical imidazole (clotrimazole, econazole).
2. Fluconazole or itraconazole.

B. Bacterial Infections

1. Cellulitis, Abscess, or Other Local Infections

▶ **H&P Keys**

Cellulitis—Local area of redness, tenderness, warmth, and edema; may be accompanied by constitutional symptoms.

Abscess—Local pus collection with tenderness and fluctuation.

▶ **Diagnosis**

Culture, Gram stain.

▶ **Disease Severity**

Systemic toxicity suggests bacteremia.

▶ **Concept and Application**

Cellulitis—Breaks in skin allow entry of organism; β-hemolytic *Streptococcus* or *Staphylococcus* common in adults (erysipelas); *Haemophilus influenzae* seen in children under 2.

Abscess—Most often arises from an infected hair follicle (furuncle); *Staphylococcus* most common organism.

▶ **Treatment Steps**

1. β-Lactamase-resistant penicillin intravenously. Add gram-negative coverage in the case of underlying disease such as diabetes mellitus. Incision and drainage for abscess.
2. Adjust oral antibiotic according to culture results.

2. Impetigo

▶ **H&P Keys**

Golden-yellow, crusted lesions on face, nose, or around mouth (β-hemolytic *Strep, Staph*); bullous variant (*Staph*) (Fig. 2–2).

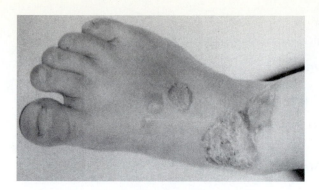

Figure 2–2. Bullous impetigo.

► Diagnosis
Bacterial culture, Gram stain.

► Disease Severity
Spread by close contacts. Secondary infection of preexisting skin lesions is common.

► Concept and Application
Highly communicable infection. Crowding, poor hygiene, neglected wounds, and minor trauma contribute to spread. Bullous variant caused by phage group II type 71 *Staphylococcus*.

► Treatment Steps
Topical antibiotic ointments, including mupirocin. β-Lactamase–resistant antibiotics for bullous type.

C. Viral Infections

1. Verrucae (Warts)

► H&P Keys
Common wart (verruca vulgaris), palmoplantar wart (verruca palmaris/plantaris), flat wart (verruca plana), genital wart (condyloma acuminatum); spread by trauma.

► Diagnosis
History and physical exam; biopsy confirmatory.

► Disease Severity
Disseminated lesions associated with immunodeficiency; certain viral types (16, 18, 31, 33) associated with squamous cell carcinoma.

► Concept and Application
Human papillomavirus (HPV) infection. Most treatment modalities involve destruction of involved tissue. Imiquimod induces a specific immune response locally.

► Treatment Steps
1. Topical acids (e.g., salicylic acid) daily. Imiquimod for genital warts.
2. Liquid nitrogen, paring, topical acids.
3. Excision, laser.

2. Molluscum Contagiosum

► H&P Keys
Discrete umbilicated pearly papules in children and adults; may be transmitted sexually.

► Diagnosis

History and physical exam, biopsy confirmatory.

► Disease Severity

Numerous, large, and disfiguring in acquired immune deficiency syndrome (AIDS) patients.

► Concept and Application

DNA poxvirus infection.

► Treatment Steps

Same as for warts.

3. Herpes Simplex

► H&P Keys

Grouped vesicles on base of erythema. Occurs anywhere on the skin, but mostly perioral or genital. Local discomfort and possible prodrome or systemic symptoms (Fig. 2–3).

► Diagnosis

History and physical exam. Vesicle for culture or direct fluorescent antibody assay, polymerase chain reaction (PCR). Tissue biopsy.

► Disease Severity

Herpetic keratoconjunctivitis can lead to blindness. Erythema multiforme minor usually related to outbreak of orolabial herpes. Dissemination to central nervous system (CNS) seen mostly in immunosuppressed.

► Concept and Application

Herpes simplex virus (HSV) is a DNA virus spread by physical contact. HSV-1 causes most orolabial disease and almost all adults are seropositive. HSV-2 associated with genital herpes with 20% seropositivity.

► Treatment Steps

1. Acyclovir or derivative PO at first sign of outbreak. Local care.
2. Suppressive therapy with daily acyclovir if more than six episodes per year.

Figure 2–3. Herpes simplex. (Reproduced, with permission, from Fitzpatrick TB, et al. *Dermatology in General Medicine,* 6th ed. New York: McGraw-Hill, 2003.)

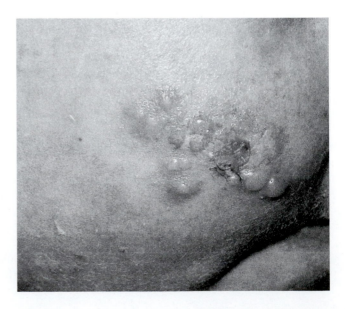

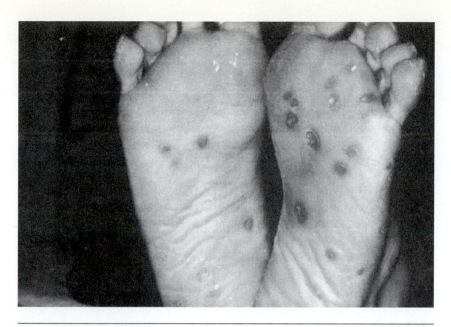

Figure 2–4. Secondary syphilis.

D. Secondary Syphilis

► H&P Keys

Lesions appear 6–12 weeks after onset of chancre (primary stage). Associated lymphadenopathy. Great imitator—many cutaneous expressions: macules, brownish-red papules, variable scale. Palms and soles often involved (Fig. 2–4).

► Diagnosis

History and physical exam, darkfield microscopy, serology, biopsy.

► Disease Severity

Associated findings: mucous patches, condylomalta, pharyngitis, iritis, periostitis, arthralgias, hepatosplenomegaly.

► Concept and Application

Sexually transmitted disease caused by the spirochete *Treponema pallidum*. Untreated, it may progress to tertiary phase (granulomas, gummas).

► Treatment Steps

1. Benzathine penicillin (tetracycline or doxycycline in penicillin allergic). Beware of Jarisch–Herxheimer reaction (acute exacerbation of disease with treatment).
2. Sexual partners should be screened.
3. HIV test recommended for all patients with syphilis.

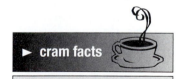

► cram facts

Secondary syphilis Rx: benzathine penicillin 2.4 million units IM × 3 doses administered q 7 days.

III. SKIN ERUPTIONS

A. Inflammatory Conditions of Skin

1. Psoriasis

► H&P Keys

Well-demarcated reddish plaques with adherent silvery scale (Fig. 2–5). Typically chronic, symmetric, and familial. Variable itching, shows Koebner's phenomenon (lesions occur after trauma). Sites: el-

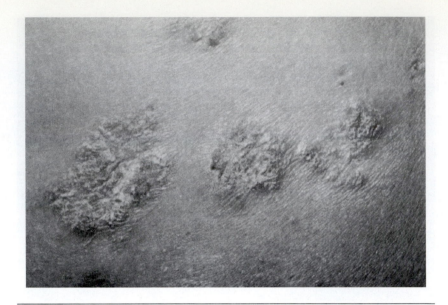

Figure 2–5. Plaques of psoriasis.

► **management decisions**

PSORIASIS

Topical halogenated corticosteroids are a principal mode of therapy; however, prolonged use is associated with skin atrophy. Topical retinoids, keratolytics, calcipotriene (vitamin D derivative), and tars are useful alone or in combination with a steroid. Resistant psoriasis usually responds to the addition of UVB or PUVA. If still no significant response, consider systemic treatment with acitretin, methotrexate, or cyclosporine. Etanercept indicated for psoriatic arthritis.

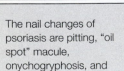

► **cram facts**

The nail changes of psoriasis are pitting, "oil spot" macule, onychogryphosis, and onycholysis.

bows, knees, scalp, buttocks, nails. Variants: pustular, erythrodermic, guttate, palmoplantar.

► **Diagnosis**
History and physical exam, biopsy to confirm.

► **Disease Severity**
Arthritis may be associated. Pustular and erythrodermic variants associated with systemic toxicity. Guttate psoriasis triggered by *Strep* pharyngitis. Some drugs (β-blockers, lithium, withdrawal of systemic steroids) cause flare.

► **Concept and Application**
Hyperproliferation of epidermis. Recent research indicates a strong role for cell-mediated immunity.

► **Treatment Steps**

Topical—Tars, corticosteroids, anthralin, calcipotriene ointment, topical retinoids, keratolytics, emollients.

Phototherapy—Ultraviolet B (UVB), psoralen plus ultraviolet A (PUVA).

Systemic—Acitretin, methotrexate, cyclosporine. Etanercept for psoriatic arthritis.

1. Start with topicals. If guttate, add course of antibiotic that covers *Strep*. If pustular, start acitretin.
2. Add phototherapy. If pustular disease unresponsive to acitretin, consider other systemic agent.
3. Start systemic agent.

2. **Seborrheic Dermatitis**

► **H&P Keys**
The mildest form is flaking of scalp (dandruff). Scale is yellowish and greasy. Variable erythema. Also affects external ear canal, eyebrows, nasal crease. Occasionally involves presternal area, axillae, umbilicus, and groin. In infant, referred to as cradle cap.

▶ Diagnosis

History and physical exam. Biopsy excludes other disorders.

▶ Disease Severity

May be severe and treatment resistant in HIV patients. More frequent and severe in neurologic disorders (e.g., Parkinson's disease).

▶ Concept and Application

Oily skin is a predisposing factor. Worse in fall and winter. The yeast *Pityrosporum ovale* is abundant in lesions and may be a trigger.

▶ Treatment Steps

1. Ketoconazole 2% cream and shampoo and/or shampoo containing selenium sulfide or zinc pyrithione. Low-potency steroid.
2. Tars, salicylic acid, sulfur compounds.

3. Contact Dermatitis

▶ H&P Keys

A type of eczematous dermatitis with linear, pruritic, erythematous plaques with or without blisters. Toxicodendron plants (poison ivy, oak, sumac) most common cause. Nickel (costume jewelry) (Fig. 2–6), neomycin (Neosporin), and fragrances (perfumes) are frequent causes. Twenty-four- to 48-hour delay from contact to development of rash.

▶ Diagnosis

History and physical exam, biopsy, patch tests.

▶ Disease Severity

May be generalized. Pruritus can be severe. Can become chronic if precipitating cause not eliminated. Frequent cause for work disability.

▶ Concept and Application

Type IV delayed hypersensitivity. Occasionally type I hypersensitivity (contact urticaria to foods, latex).

▶ Treatment Steps

1. Topical steroids for acute flare, systemic for severe cases; avoidance of precipitating antigen; antihistamines.
2. Consider patch testing.

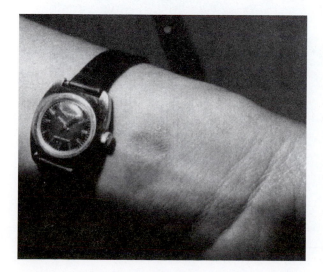

Figure 2–6. Allergic contact dermatitis from nickel.

4. Atopic Dermatitis

► H&P Keys

Personal or family history of atopy. Marked pruritus. May begin in infancy. Erythematous, vesicular or crusted plaques (see Fig. 2-7) in antecubital and popliteal fossae, posterior neck. Redundant eyelid fold, hyperlinear palmar creases, dry skin, and cataracts are associated findings.

► Diagnosis

History and physical exam, biopsy, blood eosinophilia, immunoglobulin E (IgE) levels.

► Disease Severity

May generalize (erythroderma). *Staphylococcus aureus* is a frequent colonizer and may trigger flares. Increased susceptibility to herpes infection (Kaposi's varicelliform eruption) and fungal infection.

► Concept and Application

A type of eczematous dermatitis with an unknown cause. In some patients, allergens (e.g., foods) may provoke itching, dermatitis, and bronchospasm.

► Treatment Steps

1. Moisturizers, topical corticosteroids, sedating antihistamines, avoidance of irritants. Antibiotics if secondary infection present or if staphylococcal-related flare suspected.
2. Tar preparations, higher-potency topical steroids. Topical tacrolimus and pimecrolimus.
3. UVB, PUVA, systemic steroids only rarely.

5. Urticaria (Hives)

► H&P Keys

Acute or chronic (> 6 weeks). Lesions are fleeting. Pruritic, pink, edematous papules (wheals).

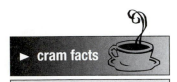

► cram facts

Nummular dermatitis is another eczematous dermatitis that often arises in patients with dry skin or a history of atopic dermatitis (see Fig. 2–8).

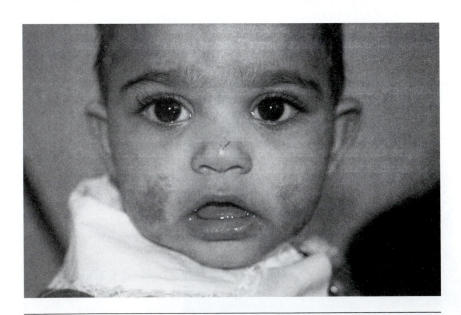

Figure 2–7. Atopic dermatitis.

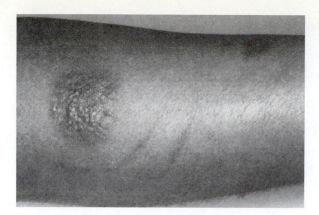

Figure 2–8. Nummular dermatitis.

► Diagnosis

History and physical. Biopsy in chronic cases to rule out vasculitis. Differentiate from dermographism (hives occurring after scratching).

► Disease Severity

May be associated with laryngeal spasm or bronchospasm. Angioedema (deep swelling in skin) may be associated (if prominent feature, rule out hereditary angioedema associated with C1 esterase inhibitor deficiency).

► Concept and Application

Numerous causes. Both type I and II hypersensitivity implicated. Mast cell degranulation leads to edema and vascular permeability.

► Treatment Steps

1. Elimination of cause if known (drugs, foods, insect bites most common), oral antihistamines, avoid systemic corticosteroids.
2. Switch antihistamine to H_1/H_2 blocker (doxepin) or add H_2-blocking antihistamine; consider patch testing.

6. Drug Reactions

► H&P Keys

Variable presentation. Disseminated pruritic pink macules and papules (morbilliform) are typical (e.g., mononucleosis patient given amoxicillin). Time course of rash usually corresponds to offending medication. Other presentations: urticaria, erythema multiforme (targetoid lesions), photosensitivity, vasculitis, fixed (lesions recur in same spot with rechallenge).

► Diagnosis

History and physical exam. Biopsy. Some drugs are more frequent offenders (trimethoprim–sulfamethoxazole, phenytoin, thiazides, penicillins).

► Disease Severity

May generalize (erythroderma). Itching may be severe. Erythema multiforme (Stevens–Johnson syndrome, toxic epidermal necrolysis) may be life threatening. Systemic vasculitis may be associated with cutaneous lesions (palpable purpura).

► Concept and Application

Immunologic (types I–IV) and nonimmunologic mechanisms.

► Treatment Steps

1. Cessation of offending medication.
2. Antihistamines, soothing topical emollient lotions, topical steroids. Systemic corticosteroids should be used with caution.

B. Blistering Diseases

1. Bullous Pemphigoid

► H&P Keys

Elderly patients; pruritus; large, tense blisters and urticarial plaques; negative Nikolsky's sign (cannot induce blister with blunt pressure).

► Diagnosis

Biopsy for routine studies and direct immunofluorescence, serum for indirect immunofluorescence (to detect circulating autoantibody).

► Disease Severity

Blisters can be large and leave large eroded areas; mucosal lesions are painful; pruritus can be severe.

► Concept and Application

Autoimmune mechanisms with immunoglobulin G (IgG) and complement infiltrating skin; immunosuppressives used for treatment. Rarely, may be caused by drugs (furosemide).

► Treatment Steps

1. Local skin care; superpotent topical corticosteroids for limited disease.
2. Systemic steroids, tetracyclines, or other immunosuppressives for generalized disease.
3. Taper as tolerated.

2. Herpes Gestationis

► H&P Keys

Clinical presentation identical to bullous pemphigoid except occurs in second or third trimester of pregnancy.

► Diagnosis

History and physical exam, skin biopsy and immunofluorescence (differentiate from pruritic urticarial papules and plaques of pregnancy [PUPPP], which begins on abdomen [usually striae] and occurs late in pregnancy).

► Disease Severity

May increase fetal mortality or premature delivery; fetus may be born with skin lesions.

► Concept and Application

Autoimmune mechanism. Oral contraceptives may exacerbate disease in patients with documented disease.

► Treatment Steps

Some cases of mild disease can be managed with antihistamines and topical steroids. Most patients require systemic steroids.

3. Pemphigus

► H&P Keys

Two types: superficial (foliaceus) and common (vulgaris). Vulgaris type shows fragile blisters and Nikolsky's sign. Oral lesions are common and often presenting feature. Lesions usually tender or painful, not pruritic. Increased frequency in people of Jewish or Mediterranean origin (Fig. 2–9).

► Diagnosis
History and physical exam, skin biopsy for histology and direct immunofluorescence, serum for indirect immunofluorescence.

► Disease Severity
Oral lesions may interfere with intake of solid foods; large eroded raw surfaces may develop; can be fatal if diagnosis and treatment are not established.

► Concept and Application
Autoimmune mechanism with antibodies to intercellular substrate of epithelium (skin and mucosae). Immunosuppressives mainstay of treatment. Pemphigus associated with malignant neoplasms (paraneoplastic pemphigus) can resemble erythema multiforme.

► Treatment Steps
1. High-dose systemic steroids, local skin care, antibiotics for secondary infection.
2. Add "steroid-sparing" agent such as azathioprine, dapsone.
3. Taper steroid as tolerated.

4. Dermatitis Herpetiformis

► H&P Keys
Markedly pruritic dermatosis characterized by symmetric grouped blisters (often excoriated) on extensor surfaces of skin (elbows, knees, scalp, back). Associated with gluten-sensitive enteropathy (usually subclinical).

► Diagnosis
History and physical exam; skin biopsy for histology and immunofluorescence.

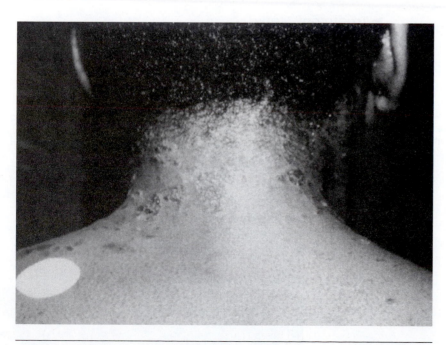

Figure 2–9. Fragile blisters and erosions in pemphigus vulgaris.

► **Disease Severity**

Itching usually severe. Associated steatorrhea, anemia.

► **Concept and Application**

Strong human leukocyte antigen (HLA) predisposition identical to that seen in celiac disease. Immunoglobulin A (IgA) in skin probably has gut origin.

► **Treatment Steps**

1. Dapsone. Gluten-free diet is beneficial and may reduce need for dapsone.
2. Taper dapsone as tolerated.

C. Other Diseases of the Skin and Subcutaneous Tissues

1. Erythema Multiforme

► **H&P Keys**

Target lesions (irislike) are typical. Lesions usually on palms and soles but can involve remainder of skin. May show central blister. Two forms: minor and major (Stevens–Johnson syndrome). Major form involves two or more mucosal surfaces and systemic symptoms (Fig. 2–10).

► **Diagnosis**

Physical examination, skin biopsy.

► **Disease Severity**

Major form causes significant morbidity. Toxic epidermal necrolysis (TEN) produces widespread denudation, and it is associated with mortality from fluid loss and infection.

► **Concept and Application**

Minor form usually associated with orolabial herpes simplex infection (immune complexes found in skin). Major form associated with drugs and *Mycoplasma* infection.

► **Treatment Steps**

1. Local skin care; antihistamines; chronic, suppressive dose of acyclovir or derivative if associated with herpes simplex infection.

Figure 2–10. Targetoid lesions of erythema multiforme.

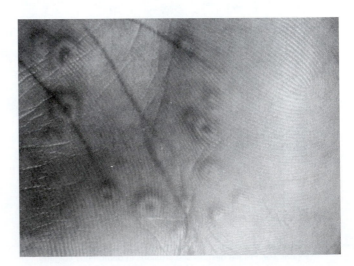

2. Admit patients with major form or TEN to burn center.

3. Use of systemic steroids controversial. Intravenous immune globulin (IVIG) preferred in major form/TEN.

2. Erythema Nodosum

▶ **H&P Keys**

Tender, red, warm nodules on legs; may show bruising; nonulcerating; heal without scarring.

▶ **Diagnosis**

Incisional biopsy for confirmation in atypical cases. To search for underlying cause: antistreptolysin-O (ASO) titer, throat culture (*Strep*), chest x-ray (sarcoidosis), purified protein derivative (PPD) (tuberculosis).

▶ **Disease Severity**

Extratibial sites occasionally involved. Associated fever, chills, malaise, arthralgias.

▶ **Concept and Application**

Immunologic.

▶ **Treatment Steps**

Bed rest, nonsteroidal anti-inflammatory drugs (NSAIDs), potassium iodide, systemic steroids if etiology not infectious.

D. Symptoms Involving the Skin

1. Pruritus (Itching), Generalized

▶ **H&P Keys**

Excoriations (no primary lesions) in accessible areas. No rash in nonreachable areas (e.g., midback "butterfly sign"). Examine for lymphadenopathy and signs for systemic cause.

▶ **Diagnosis**

When unaccompanied by rash, drugs or systemic causes are possible. If systemic cause considered, rule out uremia, hepatobiliary obstruction, polycythemia vera, hyperthyroidism, and Hodgkin's disease.

▶ **Disease Severity**

Severe pruritus interferes with quality of life and sleep. Secondary psychiatric disease (e.g., depression) may be present.

▶ **Concept and Application**

Cause undetermined in many cases.

▶ **Treatment Steps**

1. Treatment of underlying condition, if known. For unknown causes, antihistamines (hydroxyzine, doxepin), emollient lotions.

2. UV light is helpful in refractory cases.

3. Pruritus, Localized

▶ **H&P Keys**

Acute—Excoriations.

Chronic—Nodules (prurigo nodularis) or scaly plaques (lichen simplex chronicus).

▶ **Diagnosis**

History and physical exam, biopsy will confirm.

► **Disease Severity**

Disfiguring scars. In factitial dermatitis (self-inflicted), bizarre configuration of lesion is characteristic.

► **Concept and Application**

In some cases, an inciting event (insect bite, rash) leads to self-perpetuating itch–scratch cycle.

► **Treatment Steps**

1. Break the itch–scratch cycle, corticosteroids (triamcinolone acetonide) injected into nodules. Superpotent topical corticosteroids for lichen simplex chronicus.
2. Reinject as necessary. Psychological counseling in severe cases.

E. Ectoparasites

1. Scabies

► **H&P Keys**

Marked pruritus (especially in the evening); papules, vesicles, and burrows in typical sites (interdigital web spaces, volar wrists, axillae, areolae, umbilicus, genitals, knees, ankles) (Fig. 2–11).

► **Diagnosis**

Skin scraping with a drop of mineral oil on slide will demonstrate mites or their products.

► **Disease Severity**

Variant (Norwegian scabies) produces crusted, scaly lesions and is found in elderly, mentally retarded, or immunocompromised patients.

► **Concept and Application**

May be sexually transmitted.

► **Treatment Steps**

1. Permethrin 5% cream or Lindane 1% (associated with neurotoxicity in kids) lotion. Antihistamines and topical steroids for itching. Treat contacts. Consider HIV testing if sexually transmitted.
2. Repeat course if necessary or ivermectin PO.

2. Pediculosis

► **H&P Keys**

Pruritus, excoriation, and secondary infection of affected sites. Head lice (*Pediculosis capitis*), pubic lice (*Pediculosis pubis*) (Fig. 2–12), body lice (*Pediculosis corporis*). Nits on hair. Adult lice can be seen with hand lens.

► **Diagnosis**

Presence of nits or adult lice on physical examination.

► **Disease Severity**

Lice can transmit some rickettsial diseases.

► **Concept and Application**

Transmitted by casual or sexual contact. Often epidemic in schools (head lice).

► **Treatment Steps**

1. Elimite 5% or 1%, nit removal, 1% malathion powder to clothing for body lice, treat contacts.
2. Lindane 1% if above treatment ineffective.

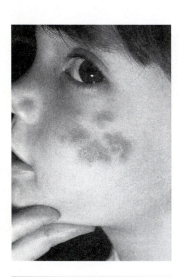

Figure 2–11. Burrow typical of scabies.

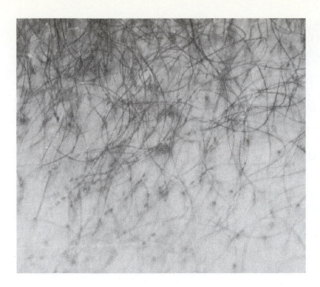

Figure 2–12. *Pediculosis pubis* with nits and lice.

IV. HAIR AND HAIR FOLLICLE DISORDERS

A. Chloracne

▶ **H&P Keys**

History of occupational/environmental exposure to halogenated aromatic hydrocarbons (e.g., dioxin).

▶ **Diagnosis**

History and physical exam. See multiple closed comedones and straw-colored cysts over malar crescents and retroauricular folds.

▶ **Disease Severity**

As toxicity increases, more skin is involved. Cosmetic disfigurement; scarring.

▶ **Concept and Application**

There is a delay of 2 weeks to 1 month before the appearance of lesions following exposure. Liver disease, peripheral neuropathy, hyperlipidemia, porphyria cutanea tarda have been reported depending on the level of chemical exposure. Possible increased risk of soft tissue sarcoma.

▶ **Treatment Steps**
1. Keratolytics (e.g., salicylic acid), topical retinoids, oral antibiotics, and topical benzoyl peroxide.
2. Oral isotretinoin if recalcitrant, acne surgery.

B. Rosacea

▶ **H&P Keys**

Adult onset, women predominate, associated with flushing; telangiectasia (dilated blood vessels), papules, pustules symmetrically distributed on face (Fig. 2–13); no comedones.

▶ **Diagnosis**

History and physical exam; may resemble malar erythema of lupus erythematosus.

▶ **Disease Severity**

Keratitis may be associated. Rhinophyma (hypertrophy of sebaceous glands) may result.

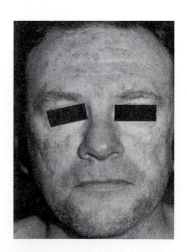

Figure 2–13. Rosacea.

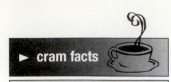

ACNE VULGARIS

Keratolytics (salicylic acid) and topical retinoids control comedones (beware photosensitivity while using retinoids—sunscreen important), mild soaps minimize irritation. If there is an inflammatory component, add antibiotic, topical (clindamycin, erythromycin, benzoyl peroxide) if mild, oral (tetracycline or derivative, erythromycin) if more severe. If acne is persistent, consider hormonal workup/ treatment. Severe cystic acne usually responds well to a course of oral isotretinoin. Need to monitor triglycerides and liver function tests (LFTs).

► Concept and Application

Flushing with increase in skin temperature provoked by hot liquids, spicy foods, and alcohol.

► Treatment Steps

1. Reduction or elimination of provoking factors. Topical metronidazole or sulfur lotions.
2. Add oral tetracycline, rarely, isotretinoin.

C. Alopecia Areata

► H&P Keys

Localized round or oval patches of hair loss without visible skin inflammation (see Fig. 2–14); children or adults; any hair-bearing area can be affected; can be stress provoked.

► Diagnosis

History and physical exam, biopsy.

► Disease Severity

Can involve entire scalp (alopecia totalis) or entire body (alopecia universalis); associated with other autoimmune disorders (Hashimoto's thyroiditis, vitiligo).

► Concept and Application

Autoimmune lymphocytes react against hair follicles, treatment difficult.

► Treatment Steps

1. Superpotent topical steroid.
2. If no response, intralesional triamcinolone, consider topical minoxidil, anthralin.

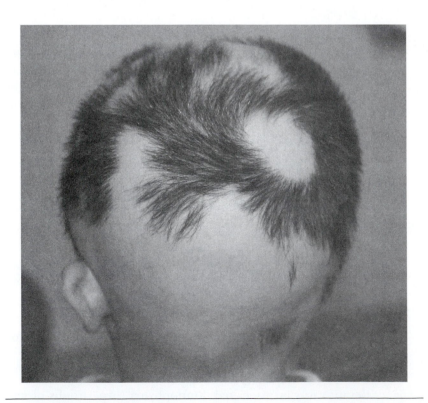

Figure 2–14. Alopecia areata.

V. TUMORS OF THE SKIN

A. Premalignant and Malignant Neoplasms of Skin

1. Actinic Keratosis (Solar Keratosis)

► **H&P Keys**

Sign of chronic sun damage; light-complected individuals (northern European); multiple discrete, rough, adherent, scaly, mildly erythematous patches and plaques on sun-exposed areas.

► **Diagnosis**

History and physical (other signs of sun damage: wrinkling, lentigines, etc.); biopsy.

► **Disease Severity**

May be associated with frank skin cancer (basal or squamous cell carcinoma).

► **Concept and Application**

Chronic sun exposure causes malignant keratinocyte transformation confined to lower layers of the epidermis. Sunscreens are protective.

► **Treatment Steps**

1. Destruction with liquid nitrogen.
2. Excision. Topical 5-fluorouracil or diclofenac for more extensive disease.
3. Surveillance for new lesions, recurrence.

2. Squamous Cell Carcinoma

► **H&P Keys**

Enlarging indurated papule or nodule with variable adherent scale on sun-exposed sites (skin and mucosa) in older people.

► **Diagnosis**

History and physical exam, biopsy.

► **Disease Severity**

May arise from preexisting actinic keratosis (low incidence of metastasis). When occurs de novo, higher rate of metastasis. Tumors on lower lip, particularly, have increased risk of metastasis (Fig. 2–15A). In-situ lesions called Bowen's disease or erythroplasia of Queyrat on the penis.

► **Concept and Application**

Numerous factors: sunlight, x-rays, arsenic ingestion, immunosuppression, chronic ulcers, burns, smoking.

► **Treatment Steps**

1. Excision.
2. Surveillance for recurrence, new lesions.

3. Basal Cell Carcinoma

► **H&P Keys**

Slowly growing pearly papule or nodule, often with telangiectasias, on sun-exposed skin (Fig. 2–15B); most common form of skin cancer; lesions often ulcerate (rodent ulcer) and have rolled borders.

► **Diagnosis**

History and physical exam, biopsy.

SKIN CANCERS

Actinic Keratosis
Rough, scaly, faintly erythematous thin plaques on sun-exposed/damaged skin, fair skinned individuals, can progress to invasive squamous cell carcinoma, related to chronic sun exposure, atypical keratinocytes, but not full-thickness.

Basal Cell Carcinoma (BCC)
Dome-shaped pearly papule or nodule with central ulceration and rolled edge, telangiectasias, sun-exposed/damaged skin, most common skin cancer, typically the face, ears, and trunk, several variants, e.g., pigmented (resembles malignant melanoma), slow growing, metastasis rare, often destructive locally.

Squamous Cell Carcinoma (SCC)
Enlarging scaly papule without sharp borders on sun-exposed/damaged skin, older lesions can ulcerate, locally invasive, may arise in actinic keratoses, chronic ulcers and scars, metastasis more common in de novo lesions and those on lower lip, Bowen's disease is SCC in situ, usually red to brown scaly plaque, anogenital and periungual SCC linked to HPV.

Malignant Melanoma (MM)
Enlarging asymmetric, variably colored (red, white, blue, black, and brown), large (> 6 mm) patch with irregular borders, may bleed and ulcerate, sometimes pruritic, related to intermittent intense sun exposure, aggressive neoplasm with frequent metastasis, prognosis based on tumor depth.

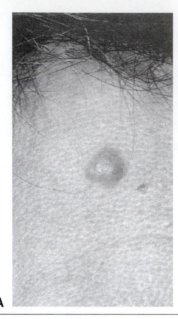

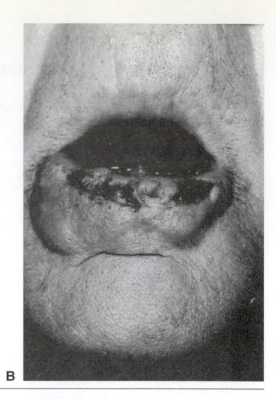

Figure 2–15. (A) Squamous cell carcinoma of lower lip. (B) Basal cell carcinoma.

► Disease Severity
Locally invasive. Metastasis rare.

► Concept and Application
Malignant tumor of skin related to chronic sun injury.

► Treatment Steps
1. Excision, destruction (electrical, freezing).
2. Mohs' surgery if cosmetically sensitive site.
3. Surveillance for recurrence, new lesions.

4. Malignant Melanoma

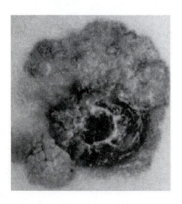

Figure 2–16. Melanoma.

► H&P Keys
Enlarging, asymmetric, irregularly bordered, variably colored, large (> 6 mm) pigmented patch. Black color is suspicious. Initially is flat (radial growth), then becomes nodular (vertical growth) (Fig. 2–16). May bleed and ulcerate. Family history and/or history of blistering sunburns.

► Diagnosis
Excisional biopsy.

► Disease Severity
Aggressive tumor with high propensity to metastasize widely. Prognosis related to depth of skin invasion (Clark's and Breslow's levels). Lesions < 1 mm have good prognosis, > 3 mm have poor prognosis.

► Concept and Application
Can develop from congenital nevi or chronic sun exposure (lentigo maligna). Superficial spreading is most common; nodular is worst prognostically; acrolentiginous (hands, feet, mucosae) is most common in blacks.

► Treatment Steps
1. Excision, with surgical margins determined by depth of tumor invasion. Lymph node dissection controversial. Interferon-α2b (INF-α2b) indicated for adjuvant therapy in patients with high risk for metastasis.
2. Examination and lab screening for metastasis. Treatment for metastatic disease unsatisfactory.
3. Close monitoring.

B. Benign Neoplasms

1. Lipoma

► H&P Keys
Single or multiple, rubbery or compressible subcutaneous masses, most often on trunk, posterior neck, or forearms. Angiolipomas are often multiple and painful.

► Diagnosis
Physical exam, excisional biopsy.

► Disease Severity
Rarely infiltrates into skeletal muscle. May occur in Gardner's syndrome. Midline back lesions can be associated with spinal dysraphism.

► Concept and Application
Benign tumor of adipose tissue.

► Treatment Steps
None if asymptomatic, excision.

2. Atypical (Dysplastic) Nevus

► H&P Keys
Familial or sporadic, large, irregularly bordered, pigmented macules and papules. Family history.

► Diagnosis
History and physical exam; biopsy.

► Disease Severity
Multiple familial atypical nevi associated with greatly increased risk of melanoma. Lesions themselves are not necessarily precursors.

► Concept and Application
Proliferation of melanocytes with varying cytologic atypia.

► Treatment Steps
Excision if melanoma is a diagnostic consideration; sun precaution and sunscreens; semiannual complete skin exams.

3. Hemangioma

► H&P Keys
Capillary or strawberry nevus (congenital), cavernous (bluish-purple subcutaneous), senile (red papules on trunk of elderly person).

► Diagnosis
History and physical exam.

► Disease Severity
Multiple cutaneous lesions may be associated with internal organ involvement (CNS, gastrointestinal [GI] tract, liver). Large cavernous

lesions may be associated with consumption of clotting factors. Kasabach–Merritt syndrome: hemangiomas and thrombocytopenia.

► Concept and Application

Localized proliferation and dilatation of capillaries.

► Treatment Steps

1. Capillary hemangiomas may self-involute.
2. Systemic steroids or surgical/laser treatment for cosmetically disfiguring or deep lesions or lesions that impede vision or eating.

4. Pyogenic Granuloma

► H&P Keys

Rapidly developing, bleeding, bright-red pedunculated papule or nodule (Fig. 2–17). Usually in young people, related to preceding trauma.

► Diagnosis

History and physical exam, biopsy.

► Disease Severity

None; differentiate from other tumors (melanoma, carcinoma).

► Concept and Application

Overproliferation of granulation tissue in response to injury. Drug-induced type (isotretinoin, indinavir).

► Treatment Steps

Excision, laser.

5. Seborrheic Keratosis

► H&P Keys

Most common benign skin lesion. Warty, light to dark brown stuck-on plaques. Usually multiple, in various stages of development (Fig. 2–18).

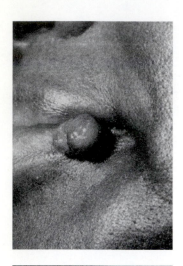

Figure 2–17. Pyogenic granuloma.

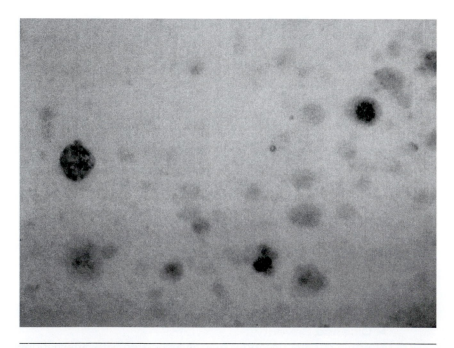

Figure 2–18. Numerous seborrheic keratoses.

▶ Diagnosis

History and physical exam, biopsy to confirm or rule out skin cancer.

▶ Disease Severity

Multiple pruritic, eruptive seborrheic keratoses may be sign of internal malignant neoplasm (sign of Leser–Trélat).

▶ Concept and Application

Proliferation of keratinocytes.

▶ Treatment Steps

None; excision if irritated.

VI. OTHER CONDITIONS

A. Acquired Keratoderma (Tylosis)

▶ H&P Keys

Localized or diffuse thickening of skin on palms and soles.

▶ Diagnosis

History and physical exam.

▶ Disease Severity

May be sign of internal malignant neoplasm (esophagus). May appear at menopause (keratoderma climacterium).

▶ Concept and Application

Unknown.

▶ Treatment Steps

1. Lubrication, elimination of aggravating factors.
2. Add keratolytic agents (salicylic acid, urea) if insufficient response.

B. Ulcer of Lower Limbs

1. Stasis Ulceration

▶ H&P Keys

Minimally painful, superficial, well-demarcated ulcer with red base and variable crust (Fig. 2–19). Typically on medial side of ankle. Associated stasis dermatitis, hyperpigmentation, and varicose veins.

▶ Diagnosis

Clinical exam; biopsy in atypical lesions.

▶ Disease Severity

Multiple or large ulcers may occur; secondary cellulitis.

▶ Concept and Application

Ischemia from venous back pressure, preventing capillary flow.

▶ Treatment Steps

1. Bed rest, leg elevation, hydrocolloid dressings, compression stockings, diuresis.
2. Compression bandage, surgical treatment for varicosities.

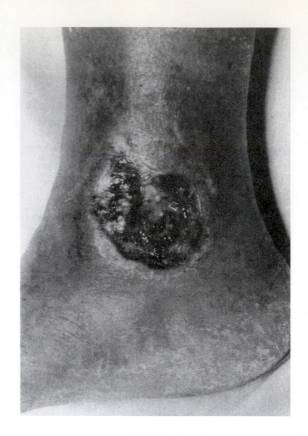

Figure 2-19. Stasis ulcer.

2. Arteriosclerotic Ulcer

▶ H&P Keys

Markedly painful, dry, shallow necrotic ulcer on foot or lateral leg. Foot is cold and hypoesthetic. Rest pain, claudication, or other signs and symptoms of atherosclerosis.

▶ Diagnosis

Palpation of peripheral pulses, Doppler studies, arteriography.

▶ Disease Severity

Significant associated large and small arterial disease.

▶ Concept and Application

Chronic obstruction of small and large vessels by atheromas.

▶ Treatment Steps

1. Address underlying disease, smoking cessation, antiplatelet agents, pentoxifylline.
2. Check ankle-brachial index.

3. Pyoderma Gangrenosum

▶ H&P Keys

Painful nodule or pustule that rapidly ulcerates, with a tender, undermined border. Associated with ulcerative colitis, Crohn's disease, arthritis, paraproteinemia, and leukemia.

▶ Diagnosis

History and phyiscal exam, biopsy, rule out associated underlying diseases.

▶ Disease Severity

Lesions may be large and involve sites other than legs. Ulcers usually indicate activity of bowel disease.

▶ Concept and Application

Disturbance in immunoregulation.

▶ Treatment Steps

Systemic steroids, dapsone, local care, treat underlying disease, if any.

C. Cutaneous Manifestations of Systemic Disease

1. Lupus Erythematosus

▶ H&P Keys

Three types: acute (systemic), subacute, chronic (discoid) (Fig. 2–20).

Acute—Malar erythema (butterfly rash), Raynaud's phenomenon, oral ulcers, alopecia, vasculitis.

Subacute—Annular or polycyclic (resembling tinea or psoriasis), photosensitivity.

Chronic—Scarring, red, scaling plaques, primarily on sun-exposed areas. Review-of-systems check.

▶ Diagnosis

History and physical exam; laboratory studies may include: complete blood count, antinuclear antibody (ANA), urinalysis, SMA, Ro (SS-A), La (SS-B); skin biopsy, immunofluorescence.

▶ Disease Severity

Acute may have serious renal or CNS manifestations. Subacute is associated with a low risk of CNS or renal disease. Chronic is usually limited to the skin.

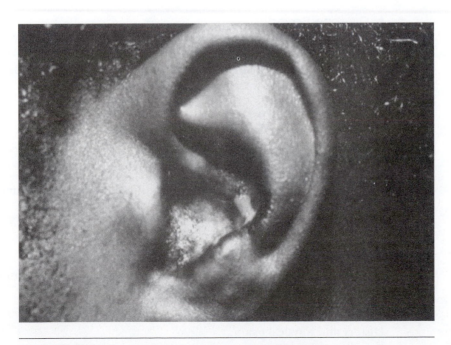

Figure 2–20. Discoid lupus erythematosus of the external auditory canal.

► **Concept and Application**
Autoimmune disease involving vasculature and connective tissue.

► **Treatment Steps**
1. Topical steroids for chronic, systemic and/or antimalarials for acute and subacute, broad-spectrum sunscreens.
2. Add intralesional steroids for persistent chronic cutaneous lesions.

2. Dermatomyositis

► **H&P Keys**
Proximal muscle weakness, heliotrope rash (eyelid erythema), Gottron's papules (purple papules on knees and knuckles).

► **Diagnosis**
History and physical exam, creatine phosphokinase (CPK), aldolase, skin and muscle biopsy, electromyogram (EMG).

► **Disease Severity**
In adults may herald internal malignant neoplasms.

► **Concept and Application**
Multisystem disorder with autoantibodies.

► **Treatment Steps**
Topical and systemic steroids, rest, cytotoxic agents.

3. Scleroderma

► **H&P Keys**
Localized: morphea. Diffuse: progressive systemic sclerosis. Latter also associated with Raynaud's phenomenon, dysphagia, masklike face. Skin is tight, woody, bound down.

► **Diagnosis**
History and physical exam, skin biopsy, ANA, anticentromere antibody, Scl-70 (anti-topoisomerase).

► **Disease Severity**
Progressive systemic sclerosis associated with multisystem involvement: renal, lung, esophagus. Variant: CREST = calcinosis, Raynaud's, esophageal dysfunction, sclerodactyly, telangiectasia. Better prognosis; associated with anticentromere antibody.

► **Concept and Application**
Unknown etiology. Excessive collagen deposition in skin and other organs.

► **Treatment Steps**
Symptomatic, physical therapy, immunosuppressives. Penicillamine (controversial).

4. Livedo Reticularis

► **H&P Keys**
Mottled, netlike vascular erythema; aggravated by cold exposure; most common in women < 40 years old.

► **Diagnosis**
History and physical exam.

► **Disease Severity**

Associated disease: arteriosclerosis, collagen vascular disease, endocrine disorders, antiphospholipid antibodies, drugs (amantadine).

► **Concept and Application**

Vasospasm of arterioles.

► **Treatment Steps**

Avoidance of cold exposure, treatment of associated medical conditions.

5. Amyloidosis, Systemic

► **H&P Keys**

Specific—Waxy papules or nodules on face, macroglossia.

Nonspecific—Purpura (most common), especially after proctoscopy, alopecia.

► **Diagnosis**

Exam, biopsy (amyloid stained with Congo red shows apple green birefringence when viewed with polarized light).

► **Disease Severity**

Systemic organ involvement, associated myeloma.

► **Concept and Application**

Immunoglobulin-related amyloid deposited in skin and other organs.

► **Treatment Steps**

Symptomatic, melphalan, or prednisone.

6. Behçet's Disease

► **H&P Keys**

Triad—Aphthous ulcers, genital ulcers, uveitis.

Skin Lesions—Erythema nodosum, ulcers.

► **Diagnosis**

Clinical exam.

► **Disease Severity**

Associated findings: arthritis, retinal vasculitis, cardiovascular and neurologic effects.

► **Concept and Application**

No known etiology; more frequent in men. Lesions develop at sites of trauma (pathergy).

► **Treatment Steps**

Systemic steroids, colchicine, azathioprine, chlorambucil, cyclophosphamide.

7. Tuberous Sclerosis

► **H&P Keys**

Autosomal dominant, seizures, retardation. Skin lesions: white spots (ash-leaf macule, earliest lesion), adenoma sebaceum (Fig. 2–21), connective tissue nevi (shagreen patch), periungual fibrous tumors.

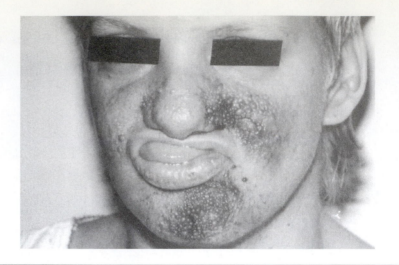

Figure 2–21. Adenoma sebaceum.

► Diagnosis

History and physical exam, biopsy of adenoma sebaceum.

► Disease Severity

Variable expression. Some patients may show cutaneous features only.

► Concept and Application

Genetic multisystem disease.

► Treatment Steps

Supportive management, magnetic resonance imaging (MRI) of the head to rule out CNS involvement.

8. Necrobiosis Lipoidica

► H&P Keys

Yellow-brown atrophic plaques on shins, may ulcerate.

► Diagnosis

History and physical exam, biopsy.

► Disease Severity

Most cases associated with diabetes.

► Concept and Application

Necrosis of the lower dermis, with granulomatous inflammation and vasculitis.

► Treatment Steps

Topical and intralesional corticosteroids, antiplatelet agents, check glucose.

9. Porphyria Cutanea Tarda

► H&P Keys

Photosensitivity, blisters on backs of hands, scars, increased hair growth (werewolf), hyperpigmentation.

► Diagnosis

Urine will fluoresce under Wood's light; blood, urine, stool studies for porphyrins; skin biopsy.

► Disease Severity

May be hereditary, but induced by hepatitis C infection, ethanol, estrogens, chloroquine, chlorinated phenols, iron. Diabetes in 25%.

► Concept and Application

Uroporphyrinogen decarboxylase deficiency.

► Treatment Steps

1. Discontinue provoking drugs or chemicals. Liberal use of broad-spectrum sunscreen, titanium dioxide/zinc oxide.
2. Phlebotomy and/or antimalarials.

D. Cutaneous Signs of Internal Malignant Neoplasms

1. See dermatomyositis, sign of Leser–Trélat (seborrheic keratoses), keratoderma (tylosis).
2. Acanthosis nigricans (Fig. 2–22): velvety brown patches on axillae and neck; associated with GI carcinomas (stomach), lung cancer, as well as obesity, endocrine disease.
3. Sweet's syndrome: tender, vesicular papules and plaques on face, extremities, and upper trunk; may be associated with leukemia.
4. Cowden's syndrome (multiple hamartoma syndrome): warty lesions on face (trichilemmomas), gums, hands, and feet; associated with breast cancer, thyroid tumors.
5. Gardner's syndrome (see lipomas): large epidermal cysts, fibromas, lipomas, osteomas; autosomal dominant; polyps and carcinoma of GI tract.
6. Peutz–Jeghers syndrome: freckle-like pigmented spots on lips, nose, fingertips; autosomal dominant; hamartomatous GI polyps; low frequency of malignancy.
7. Muir–Torre syndrome: benign and malignant sebaceous tumors of skin; high incidence of colon cancer; possibly autosomal dominant.

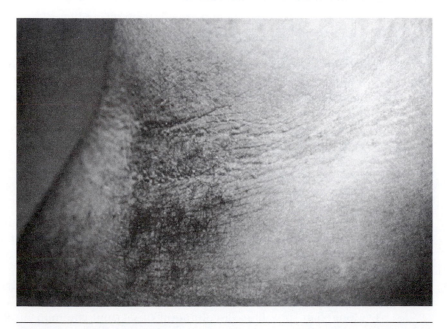

Figure 2–22. Acanthosis nigricans.

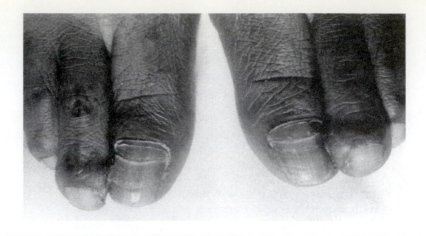

Figure 2–23. Beau's lines (patient had ruptured berry aneurysm 6 months previously).

8. Multiple mucosal neuroma syndrome: multiple neuromas (whitish nodules) on lips and anterior tip of tongue; medullary carcinoma of thyroid, pheochromocytoma, parathyroid adenomas (multiple endocrine neoplasia [MEN] type 2b); autosomal dominant.

9. Glucagonoma syndrome: necrolytic migratory erythema (erosive, annular, intense erythema) around orifices, abdomen, thighs, and distal extremities; α-cell tumor of pancreas.

E. Nail Signs and Disease

1. Onycholysis: nail plate lifts off nail bed; associated with trauma, psoriasis, hyperthyroidism.
2. Terry's nails: proximal two-thirds of nail is white; associated with low serum albumin, cirrhosis, congestive heart failure.
3. Splinter hemorrhages: streaks of blood under distal portion of nail plate; associated with trauma, subacute bacterial endocarditis (SBE).
4. Beau's lines: horizontal nail depressions (Fig. 2–23); associated with temporary arrest of nail growth from severe illness.
5. Clubbed nails: overcurvature of nail plate and loss of nail-digit angle; associated with cardiopulmonary disease, cancer.
6. Muehrcke's nails: two horizontal white stripes; associated with low albumin, nephrosis.
7. Yellow nails: yellow discoloration of nail plate, no cuticles, associated with lymphedema, pulmonary effusion.
8. Half-and-half nails: white proximal half, distal brown nail; associated with chronic renal failure.

F. Diseases and Disorders of Newborns

1. Erythema toxicum neonatorum: pinkish macules, papules, and pustules; self-limited.
2. Port-wine stain (nevus flammeus): most often on face or neck (stork bite), flat vascular patch; associated with Sturge–Weber syndrome, particularly if it involves the upper eyelid; treatment with laser.
3. Café au lait macules: presence of more than five is associated with neurofibromatosis.
4. Mongolian spot: blue discoloration of sacrum; common in black races; no clinical significance or treatment.

5. Miliaria: pruritic red papules from occlusion of sweat duct; aeration is critical; mild topical steroids.

6. Ataxia–telangiectasia: telangiectasia of bulbar conjunctiva and skin; ataxia, bronchiectasis, IgA deficiency; autosomal recessive.

BIBLIOGRAPHY

Fitzpatrick TB, et al. *Dermatology in General Medicine,* 6th ed. New York: McGraw-Hill, 2003.

Odom RB, James WD, Berger TG. *Andrews' Diseases of the Skin, Clinical Dermatology,* 9th ed. Philadelphia: W.B. Saunders, 2000.

Wolf K, et al. *Fitzpatrick's Color Atlas & Synopsis of Clinical Dermatology,* 5th ed. New York: McGraw-Hill, 2005.

Endocrinology | 3

I. THYROID GLAND DISORDERS

A. Hyperthyroidism

► **H&P Keys**

Most commonly autoimmune etiology (Graves' disease). Can also be toxic adenoma, toxic multinodular goiter, iodine induced or factitious.

Weight loss, palpitations, nervousness, muscle weakness, heat intolerance, dyspnea, increased bowel movements, change in menstrual function, eye symptoms (burning, tearing, diplopia). Family history of thyroid disease.

Thyroid enlargement common, thyroid bruit, proptosis, tremor, tachycardia, hyperactive reflexes, systolic hypertension, pretibial myxedema, onycholysis, proximal myopathy, ophthalmopathy (Fig. 3–1).

Hyperthyroidism in the elderly often presents with apathetic rather than hyperkinetic symptoms. Cardiac manifestations are common (atrial fibrillation, congestive failure).

► **Diagnosis**

Elevated levels of total or free thyroxine (T_4), triiodothyronine (T_3), and resin uptake (T_3RU). Suppressed levels of thyrotropin (TSH). Estrogen in pills or pregnancy increases T_4 binding globulin: in this situation the T_4 is increased and the T_3 uptake is decreased. Assay of thyroid antibodies may be performed to exclude Hashimoto's thyroiditis. An iodine (^{123}I) uptake and scan can be performed if the diagnosis is not secure or if radioactive iodine therapy is considered.

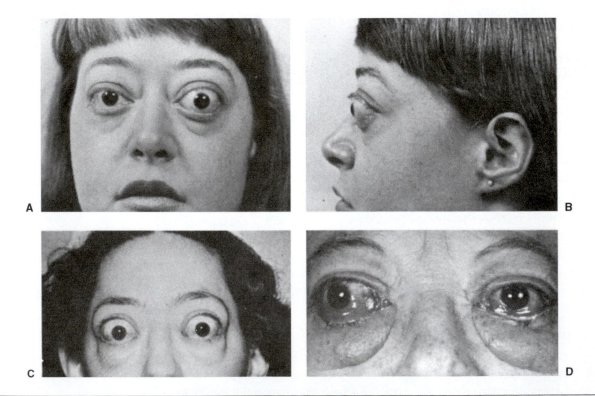

Figure 3–1. Photographs of three patients with ophthalmopathy due to Graves' disease. A, B. A young woman with moderate asymmetric proptosis, with marked left eyelid retraction. This patient has few manifestations of ocular inflammatory disease. **C.** A young woman with marked periorbital edema, bilateral lid retraction, and proptosis. **D.** A middle-aged woman with marked infraorbital edema, conjunctival injection and chemosis, and muscle restriction of the right eye, but little proptosis. (Reproduced, with permission, from Felig P. *Endocrinology and Metabolism,* 4th ed. New York: McGraw-Hill, 2001.)

► Disease Severity

Tachyarrhythmias, atrial fibrillation, severe weight loss, mental status change, and fever as in thyroid storm.

► Concept and Application

Hypermetabolism and hyperkinesis resulting from autonomous thyroid hormone secretion. Decreased thyroid hormone production with antithyroid drugs and decreased autonomic nervous system hyperactivity with β-blocking drugs.

► Treatment Steps

1. β-Blockade with propranolol, metoprolol, or atenolol to decrease sympathetic nervous system symptoms.
2. Antithyroid medications, methimazole, or propylthiouracil, especially in women of childbearing age and severe disease.
3. Radioactive iodine ablation if patient older, less severe thyroid disease, or intolerance to antithyroid medications.
4. Surgery if contraindications to medications or radioactive iodine.

B. Hypothyroidism

► H&P Keys

Usually secondary to chronic autoimmune (Hashimoto's) thyroiditis, radioactive iodine therapy, head or neck irradiation, or thyroid surgery. Family history of thyroid disease, fatigue, weakness, cold intolerance, sleepiness, dry skin, hoarseness, constipation, depression, slow mentation, menstrual irregularities, infertility, weight gain.

On physical examination, a firm goiter with multiple nodules (Hashimoto's disease) or a nonpalpable gland; bradycardia; slow, hoarse speech; cool, dry, thick skin; delayed relaxation of deeptendon reflexes; yellow skin (carotenemia); loss of scalp hair and eyebrows (see Fig. 3–2).

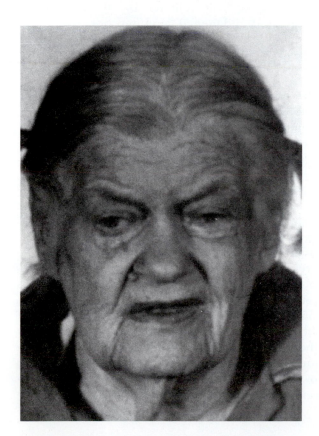

Figure 3–2. Photograph of a patient with hypothyroidism, showing facial puffiness and periorbital edema. (Reproduced, with permission, from Felig P. *Endocrinology and Metabolism,* 4th ed. New York: McGraw-Hill, 2001.)

► Diagnosis

Elevated level of TSH, low total or free T_4 level; T_3 levels and ^{123}I uptake and scans not helpful in diagnosis. Assays for thyroid peroxidase antibodies (previously antimicrosomal antibodies) or antithyroglobulin antibodies to confirm Hashimoto's thyroiditis. If positive, these patients and their families have an increased incidence of other autoimmune diseases such as Graves', pernicious anemia, vitiligo, rheumatoid arthritis, adrenal insufficiency, and premature menopause.

► Disease Severity

Mental status: confusion, dementia, stupor, or coma; decreased ventilation and abnormal blood gases; hypothermia, cardiomyopathy, ataxia.

► Concept and Application

Hypometabolic state caused by decrease or lack of thyroid hormone.

► Treatment Steps

Uncomplicated Hypothyroidism
1. Begin L-thyroxine replacement at 0.075–0.150 mg daily. Elderly patients should be started on 0.0125–0.025 mg daily.
2. Check TSH level in 6 weeks after any dose adjustment.
3. Avoid concomitant use of cholestyramine, antacids, and iron supplements that interfere with T_4 absorption in the gastrointestinal tract.

Myxedema Coma
1. Respiratory support.
2. Hydocortisone 100 mg IV every 8 hours; first dose must proceed T_4 replacement.
3. L-thyroxine IV 2 μg/kg load, followed by 100 μg every 24 hours until respiratory and mental status improve.

C. Neoplasms of the Thyroid Gland

► H&P Keys

Most thyroid nodules are benign. The most common cancer is papillary, followed by follicular, medullary, and the most aggressive, anaplastic (more common in the elderly).

Family history of thyroid cancer, head or neck irradiation as a child, radiation exposure. New-onset hoarseness: indirect laryngoscope needed to rule out recurrent laryngeal nerve involvement. May be a solitary thyroid nodule or a large nodule in a multinodular gland.

► Diagnosis

Fine-needle aspiration for histocytopathologic examination. If specimen inadequate, repeat the aspiration. Assay of T_4, TSH, and thyroid antibodies to determine if patient has Hashimoto's thyroiditis with a lumpy thyroid. Baseline thyroid ultrasonogram to check nodule size and rule out a cyst. ^{123}I thyroid uptake and scan will reveal if the nodule is "cold" (nonfunctioning), or "hot" (hyperfunctioning) and less likely to be malignant. A thyroglobulin level is occasionally helpful as a tumor marker. If elevated, it can be rechecked after surgery, and followed for recurrence of the tumor. Elevated calcitonin levels are seen in medullary thyroid carcinoma.

► Disease Severity

Nodule size, distant metastases, hoarseness. Past history of head or neck irradiation. Anaplastic classification.

► Concept and Application

None.

► Treatment Steps

1. Surgical removal of the thyroid and tumor, along with any obvious nodal involvement.
2. ^{131}I ablation of remaining thyroid tissue or metastatic disease.
3. Suppression of the TSH level (to < 0.3 μIU/mL) with exogenous L-thyroxine replacement.

II. PARATHYROID GLAND DISORDERS

A. Hypercalcemia

► H&P Keys

Family or personal history of hypercalcemia, renal stones, multiple endocrine neoplasia (MEN) type 1 or 2, or malignancy. Many are asymptomatic. Common symptoms: fatigue, lethargy, nocturia, weakness, constipation, depression, or renal colic from kidney stones. History of calcium, vitamin D or vitamin A intake, use of thiazides or lithium.

► Diagnosis

Elevation of calcium levels corrected for albumin. Primary hyperparathyroidism will have low levels of phosphorus and normal to elevated parathyroid hormone (PTH) assays (intact PTH assays most reliable). Sestamibi parathyroid scan to localize adenoma or hyperplasia. Suppression of PTH levels in face of hypercalcemia suggests nonparathyroid source. Chest x-ray (CXR), parathyroid-related protein assay in smoker with hypercalcemia. Serum protein electrophoresis to evaluate for multiple myeloma. 1,25-dihydroxyvitamin D levels elevated in lymphoma and granulomatous diseases (sarcoidosis, leprosy). T_4 and TSH to exclude hyperthyroidism.

► Disease Severity

Calcium levels > 12 mg/dL. Kidney stones, osteoporosis, pancreatitis, lethargy, confusion, stupor or coma.

► Concept and Application

Overproduction of parathyroid hormone in primary hyperparathyroidism (single adenoma or hyperplasia of all four glands), may be familial (autosomal dominant), part of MEN 1, which includes tumors of the pituitary and pancreas (insulinoma, gastrinoma), or MEN 2, which includes hyperparathyroidism, pheochromocytoma, and medullary thyroid carcinoma.

In malignancy-associated hypercalcemia, production of humoral bone resorbing factors (i.e., PTH-related protein, or direct bone destruction by tumor). Excess vitamin D intake or production.

► Treatment Steps

Severe Hypercalcemia

1. Intravenous hydration with 0.9% (normal) saline solution.
2. Intravenous furosemide to promote calciuresis.

HYPERCALCEMIA

Primary Hyperparathyroidism
Surgery indicated if osteoporosis or kidney stones are present; if Ca^{2+} > 12 mg/dL, or if patient < 50 years of age. Familial hypercalcemic hypocalciuria must be excluded prior to surgery.

Hypercalcemia of Malignancy
Intravenous hydration and furosemide, followed by salmon calcitonin and bisphosphonates. Treatment of the underlying malignancy if possible.

Vitamin D Intoxication
Removal of vitamin D source if possible, hydration, glucocorticoids.

3. Salmon calcitonin subcutaneously every 6–12 hours for rapid lowering of Ca^{2+} level.
4. Intravenous bisphosphonates (pamidronate or etidronate) for prolonged control.
5. Treatment of underlying source.

III. PITUITARY GLAND DISORDERS

A. Anterior Pituitary

1. Overproduction Syndromes

► H&P Keys

Galactorrhea, amenorrhea, infertility (prolactinomas); enlargement of hands, jaw, feet (acromegaly); moon facies, dorsocervical and supraclavicular fat pads, striae (Cushing's disease). May be a non-functioning adenoma presenting with visual changes, hypogonadism, fatigue, loss of axillary and pubic hair.

► Diagnosis

Assays of T_4, TSH (rule out primary hypothyroidism, which may elevate prolactin levels). Prolactin level (exclude use of medications that act on the central nervous system and elevate prolactin, e.g., phenothiazines).

Obtain a growth hormone and insulin-like growth factor-1 (IGF-1) level (somatomedin C) to evaluate for acromegaly. (See Fig. 3–3.) Corticotropin (ACTH)-producing tumors can be screened for with an overnight dexamethasone suppression test (AM cortisol level

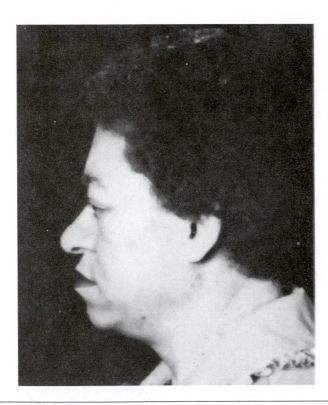
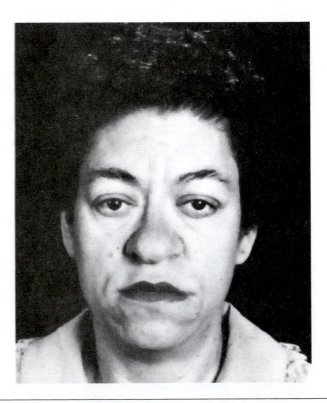

Figure 3–3. Facial appearance of a 43-year-old woman with acromegaly whose disease had been present for 15 years. Soft tissue overgrowth about the eyes, nose, and mouth has resulted in coarsening of the features. Lacrimal overgrowth is evident, as is thickening of the skin folds and the presence of fibroma molluscum (acrochordon). (Reproduced, with permission, from Felig P. *Endocrinology and Metabolism,* 4th ed. New York: McGraw-Hill, 2001.)

should be < 4). Perform a magnetic resonance imaging (MRI) scan with gadolinium of the pituitary and hypothalamus. Petrosal sinus sampling for Cushing's disease.

► Concept and Application

Tumors may be functioning, producing prolactin, growth hormone, corticotropin (ACTH), or TSH. Tumors of the pituitary stalk (craniopharyngiomas) may disinhibit prolactin and cause levels to increase. Large tumors can compress the optic chiasm and cause visual disturbance.

► Treatment Steps

1. Bromocriptine or cabergoline for prolactinomas and some growth hormone/prolactin producing tumors. Microprolactinomas (< 10 mm) need only medical management.
2. Transsphenoidal surgery for macroprolactinomas with visual changes, and all other tumors.
3. Postoperative radiation therapy for residual tumor.
4. Octreotide for partially treated/recurrent acromegaly.

2. Underproduction Syndromes

► H&P Keys

History of prior pituitary surgery or irradiation, history of sinus irradiation, postpartum hemorrhage. Severe headache (acute), inability to breast-feed, fatigue, amenorrhea, sexual dysfunction, testicular atrophy, signs of hypothyroidism, hypotension.

► Diagnosis

Measurement of serum T_4 and TSH levels. TSH will be low or normal in face of a low T_4 level. Measurement of estrogen or testosterone and FSH/LH. Low morning cortisol level, inappropriate adrenal hormone stimulation with insulin or metyrapone challenge. Insufficient stimulation of growth hormone with hypoglycemia. MRI of pituitary with gadolinium showing hemorrhage, necrosis, tumor, or granulomatous infiltration (sarcoidosis, tuberculosis).

► Concept and Application

Loss of one or more anterior pituitary hormones, leading to insufficiency of end-organ hormone production.

► Treatment Steps

1. Hydrocortisone replacement with split dosing morning and evening, or long-acting glucocorticoid (prednisone, dexamethasone) daily.
2. L-thyroxine replacement; cannot follow TSH levels to determine adequacy of dose, follow free T_4.
3. Estrogen replacement (oral or transdermal) or testosterone replacement (intramuscular or transdermal).
4. Growth hormone (GH) replacement in children; controversial in adults.

B. Posterior Pituitary

1. Diabetes Insipidus

► H&P Keys

Failure to concentrate urine, hypernatremia with thirst, polydipsia, polyuria.

► Diagnosis

Measure volume of fluid intake and urine output, serum electrolytes, urine and serum osmolality; water deprivation test.

► Concept and Application

Deficiency of vasopressin caused by brain trauma, neurosurgery, sarcoidosis, brain tumors (pinealoma, craniopharyngioma), histiocytosis. Nephrogenic diabetes insipidus (no response to vasopressin) should be ruled out.

► Treatment Steps

1. Hydration and normalization of electrolytes.
2. Aqueous vasopressin injections or nasal spray desmopressin (DDAVP). Chlorpropamide in mild cases.

2. Syndrome of Inappropriate Antidiuretic Hormone Secretion (SIADH), Hyponatremia

► H&P Keys

Mental confusion. History of cerebrovascular accident, tumor; use of chlorpropamide, phenothiazines; malignancies, pulmonary disease.

► Diagnosis

Urine hypertonic to plasma. Exclude adrenal insufficiency, diuretic therapy, nephrosis, cirrhosis, hypothyroidism, compulsive water drinking.

► Concept and Application

Inappropriate release of vasopressin causing an inability to dilute urine despite hyponatremia, extracellular fluid expanded without edema.

► Treatment Steps

Acute

1. 3% saline solution intravenously until Na^+ 125 mEq/L.
2. Intravenous furosemide.
3. Normal saline solution (NSS) if further hydration required.

Chronic

1. Fluid restriction 800–1,200 mL/day.
2. Demeclocycline.

IV. ADRENAL GLAND

A. Adrenal Insufficiency

► H&P Keys

Fatigue, weight loss, anorexia, nausea, vomiting, abdominal pain, hyperpigmentation, and volume depletion.

► Diagnosis

Electrolyte determination for hyponatremia, hyperkalemia, hypoglycemia. Low morning cortisol level. Cosyntropin (Cortrosyn) stimulation test.

► Disease Severity

Hypotension or circulatory collapse, hypoglycemia, hyperkalemia, fever.

► Concept and Application

Adrenal gland destruction of autoimmune, infiltrative, or infectious etiology. Underproduction of cortisol.

► Treatment Steps

Acute

1. Intravenous 5% dextrose/NSS.
2. Intravenous hydrocortisone 100 mg, followed by 100 mg every 8 hours.
3. If diagnosis not secure, IV dexamethasone pending cortisol testing.

Chronic

1. Hydrocortisone split dose morning and evening, or long-acting glucocorticoid (prednisone, dexamethasone) daily.
2. Florinef started at 0.1 mg daily, dose titrated to normalization of electrolytes and plasma renin activity.
3. Increased glucocorticoid dosing with febrile illness, surgery, or trauma.
4. Increase F and NaCl in hot weather.

B. Cushing's Syndrome

► H&P Keys

Central obesity, violaceous striae > 1 cm wide, general and proximal muscle weakness, easy bruising, dorsocervical and supraclavicular fatty deposition, moon facies, plethora, menstrual irregularities, hirsutism, sexual dysfunction, hyperpigmentation (Fig. 3–4).

► Diagnosis

Elevated late afternoon cortisol levels. Baseline 24-hour urinary free-cortisol elevation. Normal or elevated ACTH level. Dexamethasone suppression tests: overnight: 1 mg at 11 PM, serum cortisol at 8 AM;

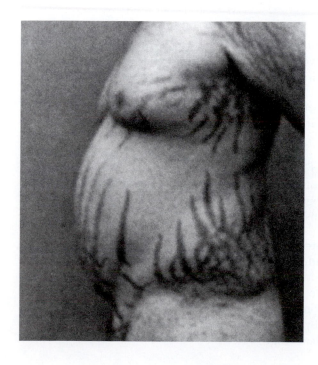

Figure 3–4. Marked striae in a patient with Cushing's syndrome. (Reproduced, with permission, from Felig P. *Endocrinology and Metabolism,* 4th ed. New York: McGraw-Hill, 2001.)

low-dose: 0.5 mg every 6 hours for 48 hours, with 24-hour urine collection for cortisol and 17-hydroxysteroids: high-dose: 2 mg every 6 hours for 48 hours, with 24-hour urine collection for cortisol and 17-hydroxysteroids. Computed tomographic (CT) scan or MRI of pituitary. CT of chest and abdomen. Petrosal sinus sampling.

► Disease Severity
Rapidity of symptom onset, hypokalemia, congestive heart failure, paper-thin skin, and osteoporosis.

► Concept and Application
Overproduction of cortisol: ACTH-producing pituitary or carcinoid tumor, cortisol-producing adrenal adenoma, and exogenous steroid use.

► Treatment Steps

Acute

1. Removal of source of excess hormone (transsphenoidal hypophysectomy, adrenal adenectomy, removal of carcinoid tumor).
2. Pituitary irradiation for residual or recurrent pituitary adenoma.
3. Replacement dose steroids until adrenal pituitary axis resumes function.

Chronic

Ketoconazole, aminoglutethimide, metyrapone, or mitotane for nonoperative cases.

C. Hirsutism

► H&P Keys
Age of onset, rate of progression, family history. Terminal hair growth in central location (upper lip, chin, neck, chest), clitoromegaly, male pattern baldness, menstrual irregularities, male body habitus.

► Diagnosis
Cosyntropin-stimulated 17-hydroxyprogesterone, and 17-hydroxypregnenolone levels, dehydroepiandrosterone sulfate (DHEAS), testosterone, cortisol levels. Thyroid function tests. CT of abdomen.

► Disease Severity
Rapid onset of hair growth, menstrual irregularities, virilization, prepubertal or older age of onset.

► Concept and Application
Overproduction of androgens of adrenal or gonadal origin (hyperplasia, tumor, exogenous); hypersensitivity of hair follicles to normal levels of androgens.

► Treatment Steps
1. Removal of androgen source if possible.
2. Oral contraceptives.
3. Spironolactone or cyperoterone acetate (contraindicated if chance of becoming pregnant).
4. Replacement hydocortisone if congenital adrenal hyperplasia.
5. Electrolysis, bleaching.

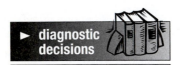

► diagnostic decisions

CUSHING'S SYNDROME

Cushing's Disease
Basophilic adenoma of pituitary, normal to slightly elevated ACTH, elevated serum/urine cortisol. Suppresses with high-dose but not low-dose dexamethasone. Unilateral ACTH elevation with petrosal sinus sampling.

Adrenal Adenoma
Elevated urine/serum cortisol, suppressed ACTH, adrenal nodule on MRI/CT. No suppression with high-dose dexamethasone.

Ectopic ACTH
Rapid onset symptoms, elevated cortisol levels and ACTH levels. No suppression with low-dose dexamethasone, rarely suppressed with high dose. ACTH levels equal bilaterally with petrosal sinus sampling.

D. Pheochromocytoma

► **H&P Keys**

Episodes of pallor, palpitations, and headaches; orthostatic hypotension, tachycardia, labile hypertension, panic attacks. Personal or family history of medullary carcinoma of the thyroid, hyperparathyroidism, or other endocrine tumors.

► **Diagnosis**

Supine and standing blood pressures, 24-hour urine collection for catecholamines, metanephrines, and vanillylmandelic acid (VMA); CT of adrenals or MRI of abdomen; methyliodobenzylguanidine imaging.

► **Disease Severity**

Persistent severe hypertension, frequent episodes, increased duration of episodes.

► **Concept and Application**

Tumor of enterochromaffin cells, which produce excessive amounts of catecholamines.

► **Treatment Steps**

Acute

1. Phentolamine or nitroprusside for hypertensive crisis.
2. α-Blockade: phenoxybenzamine (dose adjusted to cessation of paroxysms and hypertension) for 10–14 days.
3. β-Blockade added only after establishment of α-blockade.
4. Surgery to remove tumor.

Chronic

1. Phenoxybenzamine.
2. β-Blockers.
3. Metyrosine (catecholamine synthesis inhibitor).

E. Congenital Adrenal Hyperplasia

► **H&P Key**

Family history of congenital adrenal hyperplasia, dehydration, hypotension, and salt wasting (in infants), ambiguous genitalia, virilization, and hypertension.

► **Diagnosis**

Elevated levels of adrenal androgens, cortisol precursors, or mineralocorticoid precursors (depending on the specific enzyme abnormality).

► **Disease Severity**

Hypotension, salt wasting, failure to thrive in infants; severe genital ambiguity.

► **Concept and Application**

Complete or partial dysfunction of one of the enzymes used in the production of cortisol from cholesterol (21-hydroxylase, 11β-hydroxylase, 17α-hydroxylase, 3β-hydroxysteroid dehydrogenase, or cholesterol side-chain cleavage enzyme). May be due to an absolute or relative absence of the enzyme or abnormal enzyme structure of function. Backup of enzyme substrates causes the clinical sequelae associated with each specific enzyme abnormality.

► Treatment Steps

Acute
1. Aggressive intravenous fluid repletion.
2. Hydrocortisone 100 mg intravenously every 8 hours.

Chronic (Infants and Children)
1. Assignment of gender.
2. Replacement dose steroids (lowest possible dose to ensure adequate hormone concentrations and minimize growth-retarding potential of steroid therapy).
3. Surgical reconstruction of genitalia toward assigned gender.

Chronic (Adult: Partial Enzyme Blocks)
1. Glucocorticoids to decrease adrenal androgen production if menstrual irregularities interfere with fertility.
2. Spironolactone for hirsutism (cannot use if pregnancy planned).

V. CLINICAL LIPOPROTEIN DISORDERS

A. Type I Familial Chylomicronemia

► H&P Keys

Childhood presentation with abdominal pain or acute pancreatitis, eruptive xanthoma, hepatosplenomegaly.

► Diagnosis

Increased triglycerides (> 1,000), cloudy plasma, lipoprotein electrophoresis.

► Disease Severity

Development of diabetes mellitus, pancreatitis.

► Concept and Application

Deficiency of lipoprotein lipase or its cofactor (apo C-II).

► Treatment Steps
1. Very low fat diet (< 20 g/day).
2. Supplemental medium-chain triglycerides.
3. Avoidance of alcohol.

B. Type II Hyperlipoproteinemia

► H&P Keys

Premature coronary artery disease (CAD), tuberous and tendinous xanthomas, corneal arcus.

► Diagnosis

Lipoprotein measurements with elevated low-density lipoprotein (LDL) alone (type IIa pattern) or elevated LDL and triglycerides (type II b).

► Disease Severity

Family history, age of onset of CAD, degree of lipid elevation.

► Concept and Application

Three distinct diseases: familial hypercholesterolemia (defect in LDL receptor), familial combined hyperlipidemia (overproduction of apoprotein B100), polygenic hypercholesterolemia.

► Treatment Steps
1. Low-fat and low-cholesterol diet.
2. Cholestyramine will lower LDL (nonabsorbed bile acid sequesterant, not to be used with untreated hypertriglyceridemia).
3. Niacin: will lower both LDL and triglycerides.
4. Hydroxymethylglutaryl coenzyme A (HMG CoA) reductase inhibitors to lower LDL cholesterol.
5. Gemfibrozil will lower triglycerides primarily (should not be used with HMG CoA reductase inhibitors).

C. Type III Dysbetalipoproteinemia

► H&P Keys
Obesity, palmar xanthomas, premature CAD.

► Diagnosis
Elevated cholesterol and triglycerides; lipoprotein analysis shows elevated very-low-density lipoprotein (VLDL) and intermediate-density lipoprotein (IDL), VLDL-cholesterol and plasma triglyceride ratio below 0.30.

► Disease Severity
Presence of premature CAD.

► Concept and Application
Abnormality in apolipoprotein E.

► Treatment Steps
1. Weight loss.
2. Screen for hypothyroidism.
3. Niacin and/or gemfibrozil.
4. Alcohol avoidance.

D. Type IV Hyperlipoproteinemia

► H&P Keys
May be obese, presence of CAD, gallstones.

► Diagnosis
Elevated triglycerides, elevated VLDL, decreased high-density lipoproteins (HDL); rule out renal disease and diabetes with appropriate tests.

► Disease Severity
Premature CAD.

► Concept and Application
Autosomal dominant inheritance as familial hypertriglyceridemia or familial combined hyperlipidemia.

► Treatment Steps
1. Low cholesterol, low saturated fat diet.
2. Weight loss.
3. Alcohol and estrogen avoidance.
4. Gemfibrozil or fenofibrate, niacin.

E. Type V Hyperlipoproteinemia

► H&P Keys
Obesity, history of pancreatitis, eruptive xanthomas (Fig. 3–5), hepatosplenomegaly.

Figure 3–5. Eruptive xanthomas on the arms of a patient with severe hyper-triglyceridemia and phenotypic type V hyperlipoproteinemia. (Reproduced, with permission, from Felig P. *Endocrinology and Metabolism,* 4th ed. New York: McGraw-Hill, 2001.)

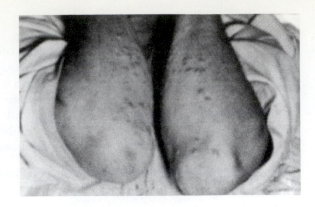

► **Diagnosis**

Elevated triglycerides, cloudy plasma, increased chylomicrons, and VLDL.

► **Disease Severity**

History of recurrent pancreatitis and/or diabetes.

► **Concept and Application**

Multiple molecular defects.

► **Treatment Steps**

1. Low-fat diet.
2. Weight loss.
3. Gemfibrozil or fenofibrate, niacin.

F. Decreased High-Density Lipoprotein

► **H&P Keys**

Often associated with states of increased triglycerides.

► **Diagnosis**

Lipid profile, electrophoresis with low α region.

► **Disease Severity**

Presence of premature CAD.

► **Concept and Application**

Multiple defects.

► **Treatment Steps**

1. Coronary risk factor modification.
2. Niacin or gemfibrozil may have some benefit.

G. Elevated Lp(a) Lipoprotein

► **H&P Keys**

None.

► **Diagnosis**

Electrophoresis.

► **Disease Severity**

Premature CAD, stroke.

► **Concept and Application**

LDL-like particle but with apo B-100 linked to a glycoprotein (apo [a]), which is structurally similar to plasminogen; may be prothrombotic.

► Treatment Steps

1. Coronary risk factor modification.
2. High-dose niacin. (Efficacy of drug therapy undetermined.)

VI. DIABETES MELLITUS

A. Type 1

Insulin dependent, juvenile onset, ketosis prone. Ten percent of all diabetics are type 1.

► H&P Keys

Usually younger patients, before age 20. Weight loss, polyphagia, polydipsia, polyuria, nausea, abdominal pain, and recent infection. Diabetic ketoacidosis (DKA). Thirty percent to fifty percent concordance rate in identical twins.

► Diagnosis

Usually acute or subacute presentation. Blood sugar > 200 md/dL with symptoms. Glucosuria and ketoneuria. Diabetic ketoacidosis (glucose > 300 mg/dL, low bicarbonate, low P_{CO_2}, K^+ may be high). Serum and urine ketones are elevated. Increased HbA_{1c}.

► Disease Severity

DKA, tachycardia, fever, poor skin turgor, lethargy, Kussmaul's respirations (deep, regular, frequent), stupor, coma. Long-term complications of retinopathy, nephropathy, neuropathy, cardiovascular disease, or peripheral vascular disease.

► Concept and Application

Insulin deficiency leading to increased lipolysis, free fatty acid formation, and ketosis. Glucagon excess, decreased malonyl CoA, and increased ketones. Human leukocyte antigen (HLA) types on chromosome 6 increase risk (HLA-DR3 and HLA-DR4). Viral infection of the pancreas with mumps, coxsackie, rubella may contribute. Autoimmune destruction of the β cells with lymphocytic infiltration. Antibodies to the islet cells are found. Can be associated with other autoimmune disease such as Hashimoto's thyroiditis.

► Treatment Steps

Diabetic Ketoacidosis

1. Respiratory support.
2. Intravenous NSS 1–2 L first 1–2 hours, then 150–500 mL/hour until hemodynamically stabilized.
3. K^+ replacement if serum K^+ normal or low.
4. IV insulin by continuous infusion, initial bolus 10 units followed by 10 units/hour.
5. Monitor blood glucose levels every hour and adjust insulin drip to maintain decrease of 75–100 mg/dL per hour.
6. Change fluids to D_5NSS when serum glucose 250.
7. Continue drip until anion gap normalized.

Maintenance

1. Insulin: split mixed regimen (NPH/Regular, lispro, or insulin aspart) before breakfast (two-thirds of total daily dose) and dinner (one-third of total daily dose). Also can use intermediate-acting or long-acting insulin 1–2 times daily with lispro or insulin aspart before each meal. Some patients prefer insulin pump.

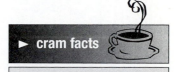

► **cram facts**

INSULIN TYPES

Rapid Acting
Humalog (lispro): Onset 15 minutes, peak 1–2 hours, lasts 3–5 hours
Novolog (aspart): Same as above

Short Acting
Regular insulin: Onset ½ to 1 hour, peak 2–4 hours, lasts 4–8 hours

Intermediate
NPH: Onset 1–3 hours, peak 4–10 hours, lasts 10–18 hours
Lente: Onset 2–4 hours, peak 4–12 hours, lasts 12–20 hours

Long Acting
Ultralente: Onset 6–8 hours, lasts 18–30 hours (no peak)
Lantus: Onset 2–3 hours, lasts > 24 hours (no peak)

2. American Diabetes Association (ADA) diet: carbohydrates, 55–60%; protein, 15–20%; fat < 30%. Regular exercise, weight reduction.

3. Monitor blood sugars goal (80–120 before meals, < 180 post-prandial). HbA$_{1c}$ goal 7%. (The Diabetes Control and Complications Trial [DCCT] has shown that near normalization of blood sugar helps prevent the retinopathy, nephropathy, and neuropathy.)

B. Type 2

Adult/maturity onset, noninsulin dependent, nonketosis prone. Accounts for 90% of diabetes cases.

► H&P Keys

Family history, obesity, limited exercise, polyuria, polyphagia, polydipsia, blurry vision, weakness, confusion, coma. Usually occurs over age of 40; rapidly increasing prevalence in children and teenagers.

► Diagnosis

Fasting blood sugar ≥ 126 mg/dL on two occasions; 2-hour post-prandial blood sugar 200 mg/dL; random glucose 200 mg/dL with symptoms. Exclude secondary causes, e.g., Cushing's syndrome, hyperthyroidism, growth hormone excess, steroid use, medications, pancreatitis, cystic fibrosis, and pregnancy. HbA$_{1c}$ > 7% consistent with diagnosis.

► Disease Severity

Retinopathy, neuropathy, nephropathy/end-stage renal disease, peripheral vascular disease, coronary artery disease. Hyperosmolar hyperglycemic nonketotic coma (HHNK).

► Concept and Application

Multiple defects. Patients typically overweight; impaired insulin secretion and peripheral insulin resistance; increased glucose production in the liver and decreased glucose uptake in muscle and adipose tissue.

► Treatment Steps

1. ADA diet. Weight reduction as needed. Regular exercise.
2. Diabetes education.
3. Insulin secretagogues (glipizide, glyburide, repaglinide, etc.); insulin sensitizers (metformin, pioglitazone, rosiglitazone); acarbose anhydrase inhibitors; insulin.
4. Control of lipid abnormalities: LDL goal < 100.
5. Angiotensin-converting enzyme (ACE) inhibitors for hypertension control or if micro/macro proteinuria present.
6. Yearly dilated ophthalmologic exam.

C. Hyperosmolar Hyperglycemic Nonketotic Coma (HHNK)

► H&P Keys

Usually an elderly patient with infection, myocardial infarction (MI), or cerebrovascular accident (CVA). Lethargy, confusion, coma.

► Diagnosis

Blood sugars often > 1,000 mg/dL. Low bicarbonate due to lactic acidosis; ketones normal to minimally elevated. Serum osmolality high. Average fluid deficit is 10 L.

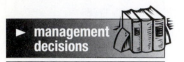

► **management decisions**

NEW-ONSET DIABETES MELLITUS

DKA
IV hydration; IV insulin continuous infusion; electrolyte management; search for precipitating event.

HHNK
IV hydration; search for precipitating event; IV insulin not necessary.

Type 2, symptomatic, blood sugars > 250–300 mg/dL
Subcutaneous insulin; meal planning and exercise. Consider switch to oral agents if blood sugar control improves in few months.

Type 2, symptomatic, blood sugars < 250
Meal planning and exercise; sulfonylurea or metformin, consider combination therapy if goals not met.

Type 2, asymptomatic, blood sugars < 200
Meal planning and exercise. Consider addition of oral agent if blood sugar goals not met.

► Concept and Application

Decrease water intake/inhibition of thirst mechanism or inability to consume more than deficits. Severe dehydration from osmotic diuresis causing further hyperglycemia and prerenal azotemia. Other causes high-protein tube feedings, peritoneal dialysis, high carbohydrate intake.

► Treatment Steps

1. Intravenous hydration with normal saline solution until hemodynamically stable.
2. Evaluate for inciting event (infection, MI, CVA).
3. Decrease to 1/2 NSS or D_5 1/2 NSS as glucose normalizes.
4. Low-dose insulin to control hyperglycema.

D. Hypoglycemia

► H&P Keys

Anxiety, sweating, intense hunger, headache, palpitations, blurred vision, irritability, pallor, nausea, diminished mental acuity, convulsions, syncope. Can occur fasting or after eating (reactive). Past history of gastrointestinal surgery, malabsorbtion, hyperparathyroidism, or pituitary tumor. Medications (insulin, sulfonylureas, pentamidine, etc.), alcohol consumption. Liver or renal disease.

► Diagnosis

Blood sugars < 45 mg/dL in men and < 35 in women with symptoms that improve with increase in plasma glucose.

Simultaneous measurement of glucose, insulin, C-peptide, and urine sulfonylurea metabolites during an episode of hypoglycemia; may need hospitalization for a 72-hour fast. Insulin antibodies can be determined.

► Disease Severity

Lethargy, coma, seizures, syncope, and death. In diabetes, symptoms may be masked if autonomic neuropathy is present or if the patient is on β-blockers.

► Concept and Application

Imbalances between hepatic production and glucose utilization. Increased utilization (insulinoma, exogenous insulin, sulfonylureas). Glucose overutilization by other tumors (sarcoma, fibroma, hepatoma, etc.). Diminished glucose production from alcoholism, liver disease, adrenal or pituitary deficiency.

► Treatment Steps

1. Identification and treatment of underlying cause. If decreased production, frequent meals and snacks. Decrease insulin or sulfonylurea dose.
2. If severe (coma, stupor), IV dextrose 50 mL of 50%, the infusion of 10% glucose to keep plasma glucose > 100 mg/dL.
3. Glucagon injection (1 mg), not effective if hepatic glycogen stores are depleted.
4. Surgery for insulinoma or nonpancreatic carcinoma.
5. Diazoxide and octreotide in refractory cases.

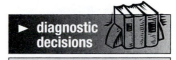

► **diagnostic decisions**

HYPOGLYCEMIA

Insulinoma
Whipple's triad, blood glucose < 50 mg/dL, elevated C-peptide and insulin levels, negative screen for sulfonylureas.

Insulin Overdose
Whipple's triad, blood glucose < 50 mg/dL, suppressed C-peptide level, elevated insulin level.

Sulfonylurea Induced
Whipple's triad, blood glucose < 50 mg/dL, elevated C-peptide and insulin levels, positive screen for sulfonylureas.

BIBLIOGRAPHY

Bardin CW. *Current Therapy in Endocrinology and Metabolism*, 6th ed. Philadelphia: Mosby-Year Book, 1997.

Braverman LE, Utiger RD (eds.). *Werner and Ingbar's The Thyroid: A Fundamental and Clinical Text*, 8th ed. Philadelphia: Lippincott, 2000.

DeFronzo RA. Pharmacologic therapy for Type 2 diabetes mellitus. *Ann Intern Med* 1999;131:281–303.

Degroot LJ. *Endocrinology*, 4th ed. Philadelphia: Saunders, 2000; 1, 2, 3.

Felig P. *Endocrinology and Metabolism*, 4th ed. New York: McGraw-Hill, 2001.

Greenspan FS, Gardner DG. *Basic & Clinical Endocrinology*, 7th ed. New York: McGraw-Hill, 2004.

Layon JA. Fluids and electrolytes. In: *Critical Care*. Philadelphia: Lippincott, 1988.

Lebovitz H. *Therapy for Diabetes Mellitus and Related Disorders*, 2nd ed. Alexandria, VA: American Diabetes Association Inc.,1994.

Mahley RW, Weisgraber KH, Innerarity TL, et al. Genetic defects in lipoprotein metabolism. *JAMA* 1991;265:78–83.

Scanu AM, Lawn RM, Berg K. Lipoprotein (a) and atherosclerosis. *Ann Intern Med* 1991;115:209–218.

Scriver CR. *The Metabolic Basis of Inherited Disease*, 8th ed. New York: McGraw-Hill, 2000.

Speroff L. *Clinical Gynecologic Endocrinology and Infertility*, 5th ed. Baltimore: Williams & Wilkins, 1995.

Thompson JS. *Genectics in Medicine*. Philadelphia: W.B. Saunders, 1986.

Wilson J, Foster D, Kronenberg H, Larsen PR (eds.). *Williams Textbook of Endocrinology*, 10th ed. Philadelphia: W.B. Saunders, 2002.

Diseases and Disorders of the Digestive System

4

I. ESOPHAGUS

A. Malignant Neoplasms

▶ **H&P Keys**

Symptoms that imply advanced disease include dysphagia, chest pain, weight loss, regurgitation, pulmonary symptoms, and iron-deficiency anemia. Endoscopy with biopsy is almost always diagnostic.

▶ **Disease Severity (Staging Techniques)**

1. Endoscopic ultrasonography (EUS).
2. Chest and abdominal computed tomography (CT) to assess distant organ involvement.

▶ **Concept and Application**

Epidemiology—The incidence is increasing. Mean age of diagnosis is 65 years. Ratio of men to women: 3:1. African-American men and women have an incidence three times greater than Caucasians. Certain countries (China, Iran, and South Africa) have a much higher incidence. Outcome is poor with a 10% 5-year survival.

Etiology—Squamous cell and adenocarcinoma are the two cell types. Adenocarcinomas are increasing. Among Caucasian males the incidence of adenocarcinoma rose > 350% over the last 20 years.

Risk Factors

1. Squamous cell carcinoma
   a. Major risk factors:
      - Alcohol and tobacco
   b. Other risks include:
      - Corrosive injury
      - Chronic vitamin deficiencies (vitamins A and C, iron, riboflavin)
      - Esophageal webs (Plummer–Vinson syndrome)
      - Achalasia
      - Human papillomavirus
      - Rubber and asbestosis exposure
      - Tylosis (palmoplantar ketoderma)
2. Adenocarcinoma
   a. Major risk factors:
      - Alcohol and tobacco
      - Barrett's esophagus: Barrett's, an intermediate stage between gastroesophageal reflux and esophageal adenocarcinoma, confers a 40 times greater risk of esophageal adenocarcinoma over the general population; median incidence is 1 cancer per 100 years of follow-up and increasing.
   b. The newest data imply *Helicobacter pylori* as a cofactor in the etiology of adenocarcinoma of the stomach.

▶ **Treatment Steps**

1. Primary surgical therapy for all with the possibility of cure. Survival correlates with TNM (tumor, node, metastasis) staging. Surgery is offered to < 40%, and among 85% of these, tumor is found to be at a more advanced stage.
2. Palliation is indicated in most cases to relieve dysphagia, control pain, and assist in nutrition. Expandable metal stents are some-

times needed in relieving dysphagia. Debulking therapies include electrocoagulation, laser photodestruction, laser photodynamic therapy, intra- and extraesophageal radiation, and endoscopic intramural injections of either toxins or chemotherapeutic agents. Chemotherapy includes fluorouracil, cisplatin, and paclitaxel. Combined modalities, including radiation and chemotherapy, have shown better results than chemotherapy alone. Chemoradiotherapy followed by surgery provides superior response to surgery alone.

3. Surveillance: Barrett's epithelium longer than 2–3 cm (confirmed by histologic identification of intestinal metaplasia) warrants surveillance if there is a potential to prolong life expectancy and treat an early cancer. Surveillance intervals are guided by the degree of dysplasia.

B. Gastroesophageal Reflux Disease (GERD)

▶ H&P Keys

Classic symptoms: heartburn and regurgitation. Heartburn: brought on or made worse by bending, lying flat, stooping, straining, heavy meals, particularly with high fat content, relieved by antacids or acid-suppressing drugs. Other symptoms include upper abdominal pain, bloating, "indigestion" and noncardiac chest pain, sore throat, hoarseness, asthma, dysphonia, chronic cough, globus, and burning tongue. Alarm symptoms: dysphagia, weight loss, iron deficiency anemia, and bleeding suggest severe disease, stricture, or cancer.

▶ Diagnosis

Patients with typical symptoms of GERD (without alarm symptoms) do not require any specific tests initially. In mild cases, simply giving a trial of a proton pump inhibitor (PPI) is diagnostic of GERD. Endoscopy reliably demonstrates the presence or absence of erosive esophagitis. However, severity of heartburn correlates poorly with presence or degree of erosive esophagitis. Endoscopy is useful in determining the presence or absence of Barrett's esophagus. A 24-hour pH probe and manometry are used if treatment is refractory to pharmacology or if surgery is contemplated.

▶ Pathophysiology

Incompetence of the lower esophageal sphincter (LES) through inappropriate or transient relaxations or through fixed low LES pressure (hypotensive LES). Anatomic disruption of the LES and the crural diaphragm, as occurs with hiatus hernia where two high pressure areas, the LES and the crural diaphragm with an intervening low-pressure area, the intrathoracic hiatal hernia, leads to impaired clearance of gastric acid.

▶ Treatment Steps

1. Initial goals are to relieve symptoms and heal esophagitis. Lifestyle modifications include reduction of dietary fat, weight reduction, smoking cessation, avoidance of large-volume meals and alcohol, avoidance of tight-fitting clothes, elevation of the head of bed, remaining upright for 2–3 hours after eating, and avoidance of reflux-promoting medications.

2. Medications include antacids and antacid/alginate combinations used for short-term symptom relief; and histamine$_2$ receptor antagonists (H$_2$RAs): cimetidine, ranitidine, famotidine, nizatidine, available over the counter, are useful for controlling symptoms in mild grades of GERD. PPIs are effective in relieving symptoms

and healing erosive esophagitis and clearly superior to H$_2$RAs. Low-dose PPI is now available over the counter. Some patients require twice-daily dosing of PPIs. Long-term maintenance treatment is necessary in most patients. There is no evidence that tolerance develops to PPIs. Laparoscopic antireflux surgery is an alternative for effective long-term management of GERD; however, recent 5-year follow-up postop data has not been encouraging for antireflux surgery.

C. Motor Disorders of the Esophagus

▶ H&P Keys

Dysphagia, chest pain, and reflux symptoms. Ascertain the level of dysphagia:

1. Oropharyngeal dysphagia patients describe food getting stuck in the back of the throat, often with coughing or choking, or nasal aspiration with attempted swallowing.
2. Esophageal dysphagia: patients have difficulty with food getting stuck in the substernal or subxiphoid level, often with odynophagia.

Progressive or intermittent dysphagia evaluation:

1. Progressive implies mechanical obstruction.
2. Intermittent suggests either a motility disorder or a Schatzki ring, which is also referred to as the "steakhouse syndrome," i.e., sudden difficulty swallowing a piece of meat with dysphagia relieved either spontaneously or with endoscopic removal.

Foods that trigger dysphagia:

1. Progressive obstructive lesions cause progressive dysphagia from large solid foods to soft foods to liquids.
2. Motility disorders have a less predictable progression and may occur with either liquids or solids.

▶ Diagnosis

If symptoms suggest oropharyngeal disorder, video esophagram. Alternatively, a barium swallow can be done.

Esophageal dysphagia: endoscopy to visualize any mucosal or structural abnormality, define strictures, and obtain biopsies. If no obstructive lesions are detected, motility disorders enter the differential diagnosis and esophageal manometry may be helpful (Fig. 4–1).

▶ Concept and Application

Three distinctive disorders of esophageal motor function:

1. Achalasia

Selective loss of inhibitory vasoactive intestinal peptide (VIP) and nitric oxide (NO) neurons within the LES leads to failure of sphincter relaxation after swallowing.

Manometric features of achalasia:

1. Absent or incomplete or inappropriately timed relaxation of the LES upon swallowing.
2. Simultaneous, low amplitude, nonpropagated contractions in the body of the esophagus.

Primary achalasia is differentiated from secondary, or carcinoma-related achalasia by endoscopy. Secondary achalasia is caused by car-

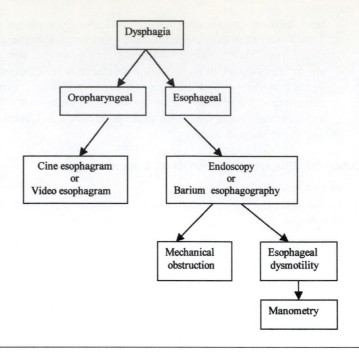

Figure 4–1. Dysphagia.

cinoma that infiltrates the LES, typically gastric cardia (most common), breast, prostate, and pancreas.

► Treatment Steps
1. Pharmacological approaches include calcium channel blockers and nitrates, which provide transient, short-term relief.
2. Botulinum toxin injected directly into the LES at endoscopy provides symptomatic improvement, but long-term studies indicate relapse of symptoms and no improvement in esophageal emptying.
3. Pneumatic dilatation and surgical myotomy are the main therapeutic options and are equally effective. A major advance in therapy is thoracoscopic and laparoscopic approaches to myotomy allowing for minimally invasive Heller myotomy.

2. Diffuse Esophageal Spasm (DES)
Patients present with intermittent episodes of chest pain and dysphagia.

Manometric features include episodic or intermittent simultaneous, nonpropagated, and high-amplitude contractions separated by periods of normal esophageal peristalsis. Radiographic features may be absent, but a "corkscrew" appearance of the esophagus indicates multiple simultaneous contractions. Radiographic and manometric features can be simulated by gastroesophageal reflux. Therefore, reflux can be considered as one of the causes of "spasm."

► Treatment Steps
Symptomatic: nitrates and calcium channel blockers via sublingual administration prior to meals.

3. Scleroderma
Esophageal manometry is a useful screening test for detection of visceral involvement of scleroderma and mixed connective tissue disorders. Visceral and systemic manifestations may not parallel; severe vis-

ceral involvement may occur in patients with relatively minor skin, vasomotor, or connective tissue manifestations.

Manometric features include low-amplitude aperistaltic contractions and a hypotensive LES. Scleroderma is associated with severe GERD, with progression to advanced esophagitis, stricture, and Barrett's esophagus. These conditions may also develop rapidly with minimal symptoms.

▶ Treatment Steps
1. Aggressive reduction of gastric acid with PPIs.
2. Surgery is rarely helpful.

II. STOMACH

A. Gastric Cancer

▶ H&P Keys

Early symptoms are nonspecific: abdominal pain, dyspepsia, weight loss, early satiety, and anemia. Systemic symptoms suggest advanced disease.

▶ Diagnosis

Endoscopy with biopsy and cytology. Tumor cells spread through lymphatic and along vascular pathways to liver, lung, bone, and brain. Some gastric tumors in women spread intraperitoneally to involve both ovaries (Krukenberg tumors).

▶ Disease Severity (Staging Techniques)

Endoscopic ultrasound is superior to CT for defining the depth of penetration (T-stage) and perigastric lymph nodes, with a limited view of the liver. Abdominal CT +/− laparoscopy to evaluate visceral, peritoneal, liver, and regional and distant lymph nodes (Virchow's node, Sister Mary Joseph's node).

▶ Concepts and Applications

Epidemiology—Gastric cancer was the most prevalent cause of cancer mortality in the United States prior to 1930. Incidence is steadily declining. It remains the second most common cancer in the world and continues in epidemic proportions in Japan, certain parts of Southeast Asia, China, San Marino, and Costa Rica. Overall, 5-year survival is 21%.

Pathogenesis—Genetic and environmental factors affect normal gastric mucosa to develop chronic gastritis, gastric atrophy, intestinal metaplasia, dysplasia, and cancer. *H. pylori* may have a causal role in gastric cancer.

Risk Factors—Environmental (Table 4–1): Postgastrectomy state (twofold increased risk at 10–20 years), gastric adenomas, and type A gastritis associated with pernicious anemia (characteristically seen in persons of Scandinavian and Northern European descent).

1. Other Types of Gastric Cancer

a. Gastric Lymphomas—These account for 3–5% of gastric cancers and are a common site for extranodal non-Hodgkin's lymphoma. Low-grade gastric mucosa–associated lymphoid tissue

4-1

ENVIRONMENTAL FACTORS ASSOCIATED WITH GASTRIC CANCER

Diet
  Nitrites derived from nitrates
  Smoked foods
  Pickled vegetables
  Excessive salt intake
  Decreased fresh vegetables and fruits
Infection with *H. pylori*
  Chronic gastritis with intestinal metaplasia
Pernicious anemia
  Chronic gastritis with intestinal metaplasia
Subtotal distal gastrectomy (Billroth I, II)

(MALT) lymphomas are associated with *H. pylori* infection. These may regress with eradication of *H. pylori* infection.

b. Kaposi's Sarcoma—Homosexual men with acquired immune deficiency syndrome (AIDS) are affected. It is caused by infection with Kaposi's sarcoma–associated human herpesvirus 8 (HHV-8).

c. Carcinoid Tumors of the Stomach—These may be induced by persistent hypergastrinemia associated with chronic gastritis or Zollinger–Ellison syndrome patients with multiple endocrine neoplasia type 1.

► Treatment Steps
1. Early detection and surgical removal for both cure and palliation.
2. Chemotherapy is applied for palliation of metastatic disease and as adjuvant therapy to surgery.
3. New approaches including postoperative intraperitoneal chemotherapy and neoadjuvant protocols designed to downstage tumors preoperatively.

► Screening
No guidelines exist for screening those at risk in the United States. Endoscopic screening is recommended for some patients who have undergone a partial gastrectomy ≥ 15 years prior.

B. Acid-Related Disorders of the Stomach

► H&P Keys
Periodic epigastric abdominal pain with characteristic pain-free periods lasting days or weeks. Pain is typically intermittent, relieved by antacids or eating. It may awaken a patient from sleep. In the elderly or in patients taking nonsteroidal anti-inflammatory drugs (NSAIDs), it may be asymptomatic, or the first presenting sign may be bleeding or perforation.

► Diagnosis

Endoscopy and Biopsy or Upper Gastrointestinal (UGI) Radiography—If the diagnosis of gastric ulcer is made radiographically, endoscopy and biopsy are needed to exclude malignancy.

H. pylori–*Infected Individuals with Asymptomatic Persistent Infections of* **H. pylori**—Only about 15% will develop gastric or duodenal ulcer.

► Diagnosis of *H. pylori* (See Table 4–2)
Patients should not receive PPIs (omeprazole, lansoprazole, pantoprazole) or antibiotics for 2 weeks prior to testing.

4-2

DIAGNOSTIC TESTS FOR *H. PYLORI* INFECTION

Test		Sensitivity	Specificity	Indications
Nonendoscopic				
In-office Ab test	Whole blood	67–88%	74–91%	Initial diagnosis
In-office Ab test	Serum	86–94%	75–88%	Initial diagnosis
Lab Ab test	ELISA	86–94%	78–95%	Initial diagnosis
Stool antigen		88–94%	89–92%	Initial diagnosis and follow-up
Urea breath		90–96%	88–98%	Initial diagnosis and follow-up
Endoscopic				
Biopsy urease		88–95%	95–100%	Initial diagnosis and follow-up
Histology		90–95%	98–99%	Initial diagnosis and follow-up
Culture		60–95%	100%	Initial diagnosis and follow-up

Ab, antibody; ELISA, enzyme-linked immunosorbent assay.

► Concept and Application

H. pylori and NSAIDs are the major etiologic factors. Eradication of *H. pylori* infection in ulcer patients can provide a permanent cure of the ulcer diathesis.

► Treatment Steps

1. Ulcers unrelated to *H. pylori:*
   - Long-term acid suppression.
   - Search for a cause (e.g., NSAIDs, Crohn's disease, Zollinger–Ellison syndrome) (Table 4–3).
2. Ulcers related to *H. pylori* (most ulcer patients have *H. pylori* infection):
   - All ulcer patients with *H. pylori* should receive treatment for *H. pylori* regardless of whether the ulcer was newly diagnosed or recurrent.
   - *H. pylori*–infected patients taking NSAIDs should also receive treatment for *H. pylori* and, if possible, the NSAIDs are stopped.
   - *H. pylori* treatment is indicated for all infected patients with a history of duodenal or gastric ulcer, including those with a history of ulcer complication (bleeding, perforation, obstruction).
3. *H. pylori* treatment regimes: See Table 4–4.

4-3

ETIOLOGIES OF GASTRIC AND DUODENAL ULCERS

Most common
  H. pylori
  NSAIDs
Less common
  Gastric malignancy
  Stress ulceration
  Viral infections (HSV-1, CMV)
Uncommon
  Zollinger–Ellison syndrome
  Drug-induced
  Crohn's disease
  Treponema pallidum
  Systemic mastocytosis
  Idiopathic (non–*H. pylori*) hypersecretory duodenal ulcer

CMV, cytomegalovirus; HSV-1, herpes simplex virus type 1; NSAIDs, nonsteroidal anti-inflammatory drugs.

4-4

FDA-APPROVED COMBINATION REGIMENS FOR *H. PYLORI* INFECTION IN PATIENTS WITH PEPTIC ULCER

Regimen	*H. pylori* Eradication Rate (intent to treat analysis)
Omeprazole 40 mg or esomeprazole 40 mg q day + clarithromycin 500 mg tid for 2 weeks, followed by omeprazole 20 mg q day (on esomeprazole 40 mg q day alone for a further 2 weeks)	64–74%
Ranitidine bismuth citrate (RBC) 400 mg bid + clarithromycin 500 mg tid for 2 weeks, followed by RBC 400 mg bid alone for a further 2 weeks	73–84%
Bismuth subsalicylate 525 mg qid + metronidazole 250 mg qid + tetracycline 500 mg qid for 2 weeks; H2-receptor antagonist in standard dose should be started at the same time and continued for a total of 4 weeks	77–82%
Lansoprazole 30 mg bid + clarithromycin 500 mg bid + amoxicillin 1,000 mg bid for 2 weeks	86%
Lansoprazole 30 mg tid + amoxicillin 1,000 mg tid for 2 weeks	70%

► Outcomes

H. pylori–*positive Patients*—Curing the infection eliminates recurrence of duodenal or gastric ulcers. Reinfection following cure of *H. pylori* is reported in < 2% of adults. True reinfection may be more frequent in underdeveloped countries and among very young children.

H. pylori–*negative Peptic Ulcer Patients*—May have a high risk of recurrence and complications.

C. Disorders of Gastric Motility

► H&P Keys

Accelerated emptying of liquids and solids is associated with dumping syndrome. Delayed gastric emptying is associated with postprandial fullness, early satiety, nausea, epigastric discomfort, and vomiting. These symptoms are nonspecific and may also be associated with peptic ulcer disease, mechanical obstruction, nonulcer dyspepsia, systemic illnesses, and certain medications.

► Diagnosis

Exclude mechanical obstruction with endoscopy or barium radiography (UGI). Scintigraphic assessment of gastric emptying is a reliable noninvasive study. Solid-phase emptying ^{99}mTc-labeled scrambled eggs is sensitive and specific. ^{13}C octanoic and ^{13}C acetate breath tests show reproducibility comparable to scintigraphy.

► Concept and Application

Normal gastric motility ensures trituration of ingested foodstuffs and coordinated delivery of chyme to the small intestine. Disordered gastric motility may result in accelerated or delayed gastric emptying. If gastroparesis is documented, a cause is looked for with the hope of providing specific therapy. Many medications can delay gastric emptying (e.g., narcotics, tricyclic antidepressants). Metabolic disorders (diabetes mellitus, hypokalemia, hypothyroidism, hypocalcemia, adrenal insufficiency, uremia) need to be considered. Systemic disorders include scleroderma and hollow visceral myopathy (Table 4–5).

4-5

CAUSES OF DELAYED GASTRIC EMPTYING

Mechanical obstruction
    Pylorus
    Duodenum
    Small intestine
Post gastric surgery
    Vagotomy/antrectomy
    Roux-en-Y
    Fundoplication
Metabolic/endocrine
    Diabetes mellitus
    Hypothyroidism
    Hyperthyroidism
    Adrenal insufficiency
Smooth muscle disorders
    Scleroderma
    Hollow visceral myopathy
Post viral gastroparesis
Medications
    Anticholinergics
    Narcotics
    L-Dopa
    Progesterone, estrogen
    Calcium channel blockers
Chronic mesenteric ischemia
Naturopathic disorders
    Parkinson's disease
    Paraneoplastic syndrome
    Shy–Drager syndrome
    Hollow visceral neuropathy
Idiopathic

► **Treatment Steps**
1. The goal of treatment is to correct the underlying motility disorder and provide symptomatic relief. For diabetics, optimize glucose control and correct ketoacidosis and dehydration. In all patients:
   - Avoid medications and dietary factors that may delay gastric emptying.
   - Avoid indigestible solids and fats.
   - Gastroparesis diet (Table 4–6).
   - If dumping is present, separate liquids and solids.

4-6

NUTRITIONAL MAINTENANCE OF GASTROPARESIS AND CHRONIC INTESTINAL PSEUDOOBSTRUCTION

Eat small frequent meals (six to eight) throughout the day
Choose foods that are
    Low-fiber
    Low-residue (avoid whole grain, raw vegetables, fatty foods)
    Lactose-free
Encourage sitting upright or walking after a meal
Avoid use of straws and carbonated beverages
Encourage blenderized pureed foods and commercial liquid formulas
Avoid eating fast to minimize air swallowing
Avoid opioids and anticholinergics

2. Pharmacological: established prokinetic agents include metoclopramide, domperidone, and erythromycin. Metoclopramide use is limited by side effects (dystonia, akathisia, tremor, depression, and extrapyramidal effects). Domperidone is not yet available in the United States. Erythromycin, a motilin agonist, is a potential prokinetic when administered orally as an elixir or intravenously. Its use is limited by tachyphylaxis but is useful for short-term, low-dose therapy.

3. For severe, nonresponsive symptoms that compromise nutrition and hydration, enteral formulation is given via percutaneous endoscopic gastrostomy (PEG). Enteral feedings are also provided via gastrojejunostomy. Enteral tubes can now be placed by interventional radiologists.

III. SMALL INTESTINE

A. Acute Enteric Infections

▶ H&P Keys

History—Define onset: abrupt or gradual? Duration: weeks, months, years, or lifelong? Define the pattern and character: loose, watery, large volume, small volume, foul smelling, continuous or intermittent? Is there fecal incontinence? Some individuals complain of diarrhea when their major difficulty is disordered continence. Abdominal pain: presence and character: mild, crampy, diffuse, or localized. Identify associated symptoms: nausea, vomiting, headache, fatigue, malaise, anorexia, arthralgias, myalgias, chills, and low-grade fever. Ask specific questions regarding:

- Presence of blood
- Weight loss
- Travel
- Food/milk intolerance
- History of gastrointestinal (GI) diseases
- Prior evaluations: Review previous evaluations whenever possible
- Abdominal surgery
- Radiation and chemotherapy
- Drug and alcohol use

Identify epidemiological factors, such as travel before the onset of illness, exposure to potentially contaminated food or water, and illness in other family members. Identify aggravating and mitigating factors, such as diet and stress. Consider factitious diarrhea in every patient with chronic diarrhea. Markers of factitious diarrhea include a history of eating disorders, secondary gain, or a history of malingering. Perform a careful review of systems to look for systemic diseases, such as hyperthyroidism, diabetes mellitus, collagen vascular diseases and other inflammatory conditions, tumor syndromes, AIDS.

▶ Diagnosis

Most acute diarrheal disorders resolve spontaneously and therefore do not need investigation. Get stool culture, ova and parasites (O&P), and *Clostridium difficile* toxin when suspicion of bacterial enteritis or parasitic is high. Note the signs of volume depletion, presence of blood, impaired host, and comorbid disease; and/or diarrhea lasting > 14 days (Table 4–7).

4-7

TESTS FOR DIARRHEA

Test	Comments
Stool culture	Not needed in 90% of acute diarrheal illnesses. Although bacterial infection rarely causes chronic diarrhea, it can be excluded by stool culture, including culture on special media for *Aeromonas* and *Pleisiomonas, Yersinia,* and *Campylobacter. Candida* in stool may cause acute or chronic diarrhea, both nosocomial and community acquired, even in immunocompetent individuals.
Fecal leukocytes	The presence of white blood cells in the stool suggests an inflammatory diarrhea. This is assessed by Wright's stain or during a stool ova and parasite examination. A latex agglutination test for the neutrophil granule protein lactoferrin may also be useful.
Stool lactoferrin	A recently developed latex agglutination test for the neutrophil product lactoferrin is highly sensitive and specific for the detection of neutrophils in stool.
Stool ova and parasites	Positive and negative predictive value is dependent on observer skill. Biopsy may be needed. Special techniques required to detect cryptosporidia and microporidia.
Fecal ELISA for *Giardia*-specific antigen	More sensitive and specific for the detection of *Giardia*.
Normalization of stool weight with fasting	Common with osmotic diarrhea.
Stool weight (g/24 hr)	Provides objective data on severity > 500 common with secretory diarrhea < 500 common with osmotic diarrhea
Stool electrolytes	Use with plasma osmolality to calculate stool osmotic gap[a] $2(\text{stool } [Na^+] + [K^+]) = P_{osm}$ common with secretory diarrhea $2(\text{stool } [Na^+] + [K^+]) < P_{osm}$ common with osmotic diarrhea
Osmotic gap (mOsm/kg) $290 - \{[Na] + [K] \times 2\}$	Large (> 125 mOsm/kg) in osmotic diarrhea in which nonelectrolytes account for most of the osmolality of stool water.[b] Small (< 50 mOsm/Kg) in secretory diarrhea in which electrolytes account for most of the stool osmolality.
Stool *C. difficile* toxin	Toxin B assay is gold standard, requires tissue culture ELISA-based tests detect toxin A, B, or, occasionally, both. For highest sensitivity, send three stool samples.
Sigmoidoscopy, or colonoscopy with mucosal biopsy	When the differential diagnosis includes ulceration, polyps, tumors, Crohn's disease, ulcerative colitis, amebiasis, microscopic colitis, amyloidosis, granulomatous infections, and chronic schistosomiasis and endoscopic biopsy of the proximal small bowel mucosa. A small bowel follow-through examination is preferable to an enteroclysis study for the radiographic evaluation of patients with chronic diarrhea.
Upper endoscopy with mucosal biopsy	Useful if small intestinal malabsorptive disorder, such as Whipple's disease, intestinal lymphoma, eosinophilic gastroenteritis, and celiac disease. Aspirate of small intestinal contents for quantitative aerobic and anaerobic bacterial culture is useful if small bowel bacterial overgrowth is suspected.
Computerized tomography	Useful in patients with chronic diarrhea when the differential diagnosis includes: chronic pancreatitis or pancreatic cancer, inflammatory bowel disease, chronic infections, intestinal lymphoma, carcinoid syndrome.
Stool pH	Values of < 5.6 are consistent with carbohydrate malabsorption.
Stool test for cathartics	A panel of tests to detect laxative abuse. Usually includes a test for phenolphthalein (pink color upon alkalization), Mg^{+2}, SO_4, and PO_4.
Stool for fat	Performed during the ingestion of a high-fat diet. The presence of excess stool fat should be evaluated by means of a Sudan stain or by direct measurement. The presence of excessively large and numerous fat globules by stain or measured stool fat excretion > 14 g/24 hr suggests malabsorption or maldigestion. Stool fat concentration of > 8% strongly suggests pancreatic exocrine insufficiency.
Fecal occult blood testing	A positive test result suggests the presence of inflammatory bowel disease, neoplastic diseases, or celiac sprue or other spruelike syndromes.

ELISA, enzyme-linked immunosorbent assay.

[a]Na and K are the major cations in fecal fluid. To simplify calculation of the contribution of electrolytes to stool amorality, anions are not directly measured, but assumed to equal the measured cations, hence the doubling of the cation concentration.

[b]Osmolality (mOsm/kg): Measured osmolality of stool water can vary widely and is generally an artifact of the collection process. Because the gut epithelium cannot maintain an osmotic gradient, in vivo stool water amorality is arbitrarily defined as 290–300.

▶ Concept and Application

Infectious agents are a major cause of diarrhea and may cause life-threatening infections in infants, elderly and immunocompromised patients, and patients with comorbid disease.

Bacterial Pathogens

- Enterotoxigenic diarrheal pathogens such as *Vibrio cholerae* and enterotoxigenic *Escherichia coli* (ETEC) colonize the gut, producing toxins that disturb water and electrolyte transport, causing high-volume, sometimes life-threatening diarrhea not associated with fever, vomiting, fecal leukocytes, or blood. Acidosis and hyopokalemia may develop.

- Other communicable bacterial pathogens such as *Campylobacter, Salmonella, Shigella,* and enteroinvasive *E. coli* (EIEC) cause diarrhea by invading and injuring the mucosa. These diarrheal illnesses are associated with high fever, abdominal cramping, bloating, vomiting, and bloody diarrhea. Almost all of these are self-limiting, except *Campylobacter,* which may have a relapsing course.
- Hemorrhagic *E. coli* (EHEC) (*E. coli* O157:H7) can also cause diarrhea by producing *Shigella*-like toxins, often in food-borne outbreaks of bloody diarrhea associated with undercooked meats and raw milk.
- Enteroadherent *E. coli* (EAEC) infection is a cause of infantile diarrhea.
- Brainerd diarrhea, a chronic idiopathic diarrhea caused by an unknown infectious agent first described in Brainerd County, Minnesota, is also found in travelers.
- Other food-borne bacterial pathogens cause diarrhea via enterotoxin production or by direct cytotoxic effect on the gut. *Staphylococcus aureus,* the most common cause of food poisoning, produces toxins that stimulate intestinal secretion and cause headache, nausea and vomiting. *Bacillus cereus,* from contaminated fried rice, causes severe vomiting and diarrhea. *Bacillus* spp., from contaminated meats, baked goods, and salads, produces predominantly diarrhea. *Clostridium perfringens* causes food poisoning primarily in outbreaks in the fall and winter. *Vibrio parahaemolyticus* is associated with raw or spoiled shellfish and can have a varying presentation of watery diarrhea or dysentery.

Viral Pathogens—Rotaviruses and Norwalk virus are major causes of self-limited diarrhea. Both cause watery stools (without fecal leukocytes), with vomiting, abdominal cramps, bloating, low-grade fever, and headache. Rotavirus affects children under the age of 2. Norwalk infects older children and adults in epidemic outbreaks of gastroenteritis.

Parasitic Pathogens—Helminths and protozoa may cause chronic diarrheal illness, particularly in areas with poor sanitation. Helminths that colonize the small bowel and could produce diarrhea and nutrient malabsorption include: *Capillaria philippinensis, Ascaris lumbricoides, Trichinella spiralis, Ancylostoma* (hookworms), and *Strongyloides stercoralis.* Trematodes: Schistosomiasis may cause diarrhea from the inflammatory response to schistosome eggs deposited in the intestine. Protozoa causing diarrhea include: *Cryptosporidium, Entamoeba,* and *Giardia lamblia.*

1. *Cryptosporidium* produces acute, often severe, crampy, watery diarrhea. Fever is uncommon.
2. *Entamoeba histolytica* is the only amoebic parasite that causes human disease. Diarrhea is typically mild to moderate, characterized by loose, intermittent stools, occasional blood or mucus, flatulence, and abdominal cramping.
3. *Giardia lamblia* is a major cause of water-borne diarrhea and traveler's diarrhea. Clinical presentation is variable, ranging from asymptomatic carrier to acute illness (explosive diar-

rhea, cramps, flatulence, nausea and vomiting) and chronic diarrhea. In children, chronic infection may cause growth retardation.

Yeast and fungi, primarily *Candida albicans* can cause both nosocomial and community-acquired chronic diarrhea in immunocompromised as well as immunocompetent individuals.

Diarrhea in Immunocompromised Patients—*G. lamblia* is important in patients with common variable immunodeficiency, AIDS, and immunoglobulin A (IgA) deficiency. *Salmonella* and *Shigella* are more frequent and severe in immunocompromised patients. *Legionella* and *C. albicans* may cause diarrhea in immunocompromised patients. AIDS patients are at particular risk for *Cryptosporidium, Isospora belli, Mycobacterium avium-intracellulare, Microsporidium,* and cytomegalovirus (CMV).

Noninfectious Diarrheas—Osmotic diarrhea results from poorly absorbed solutes within the intestinal lumen. Secretory diarrhea is the product of intestinal transport of ions from the epithelial cell into the lumen of the gut, resulting from the interplay among paracrine, immune, neural, and endocrine systems (PINES). "Pure" chronic secretory diarrheas, such as carcinoid and VIPoma (watery diarrhea, hypokalemia, and achlorhydria [WDHA], or gastrinoma and medullary carcinoma of the thyroid) are rare.

► Treatment Steps
1. Correct the underlying condition.
2. Control diarrhea.
3. Replacing fluid and electrolytes, nutrients, vitamins, and minerals. Fluid and electrolyte losses are best replaced with oral rehydration solutions to replace intestinal fluid losses (Table 4–8).
4. Antimotility agents are useful in all except those with dysentery or *C. difficile* infection where risk of mucosal invasion may lead to toxic megacolon.
5. Antibiotic therapy indications: traveler's diarrhea, cholera, pseudomembranous colitis, parasites, and sexually transmitted infections; and in immunosuppressed patients, debilitated patients with malignancy, patients with valvular or vascular prostheses, hemolytic anemia, and those with prolonged or relapsing course.

B. Celiac Sprue

► H&P Keys
Common in persons of western European heritage, where prevalence is 1 in 250. Prevalence in relatives of celiac patients is 15%. Certain disorders are associated with increased prevalence of celiac

4-8

REPLACEMENT OF DIARRHEAL FLUID LOSS

• Replace diarrheal fluid loss with oral standard solutions containing balanced electrolytes, minerals, and nutrients.
• Several are available on the market.

disease: diabetes mellitus type 1, autoimmune thyroid disease, Sjögren's syndrome, microscopic colitis, isolated IgA deficiency, epilepsy, Down syndrome, and dermatitis.

► Clinical Presentation

Vague ill health, osteopenia, nonspecific gastrointestinal symptoms such as bloating and indigestion, diarrhea, steatorrhea, weight loss, chronic iron deficiency anemia, osteopenia, hyposplenism with associated red cell abnormalities (Howell–Jolly bodies), and chronic neurologic syndromes including seizures.

► Diagnosis and Evaluation

In patients with overt generalized malabsorption without obvious cause, small bowel biopsy is the first diagnostic test. In patients without overt malabsorption, antibody screening tests are done first. Obtain a panel of IgA and IgG antigliadin (AGA) and IgA endomysial antibodies (EMAs). IgG AGA is not highly specific, but is important in the 5% of patients with celiac disease and IgA deficiency. EMAs are directed to tissue transglutaminase (TTG). TTG antibody enzyme-linked immunosorbent assay (ELISA) may replace EMA testing.

1. A positive antibody screen should be followed up with small bowel biopsy.
2. Consider screening for celiac disease in patients with iron deficiency anemia or osteopenia of uncertain cause and in populations with high prevalence, such as relatives of celiac patients.

► Disease Severity

Complications include chronic ulcerative jejunitis, enteropathy-associated T-cell lymphoma, and refractory sprue.

► Concept and Application

Ingested gliadins (components of gluten present in wheat, rye, barley, and oats) lead to an immunologic reaction in the small bowel mucosa. Most celiac patients have an HLA-DQ2 subtype or a closely related subtype. These human leukocyte antigen (HLA) molecules coded by these subtypes elicit a T-cell–mediated immunologic reaction in small bowel mucosa. This leads to mucosal infiltration by chronic inflammatory cells, epithelial cell damage, villous atrophy, and crypt hypertrophy. Damage to the small intestinal mucosa causes a variable degree of malabsorption. Patients can be asymptomatic or have selective nutrient malabsorption (such as iron and calcium) or have severe diarrhea and malnutrition.

► Treatment Steps

1. Patient education is important, as celiac disease is a lifelong disorder.
2. Every patient needs education about the physiology of the disease and the importance of diet and potential consequences, including anemia, osteopenia, and enteropathy-associated T-cell lymphoma (EATCL).
3. Refer every celiac patient to a dietitian and to a patient support group.
4. Primary treatment is a gluten-free diet.
5. Clinical response to gluten-free diet should be apparent within weeks.
6. EMA levels should fall if gluten is being avoided.

7. Lack of response should prompt a search for inadvertent ingestion of gluten or incorrect diagnosis, celiac-related pancreatic insufficiency, celiac-related bacterial overgrowth, other dietary intolerances (lactose, fructose, soya, milk protein), and development of small bowel lymphoma (EATCL) or ulcerative jejunoileitis (UJI).
8. Supplemental iron, folate, zinc, vitamin D, calcium.

IV. COLON

A. Invasive Diarrhea

▶ **H&P Keys**

Crampy lower abdominal pain, tenesmus, stool bloody or mucoid, volume < 1 L/day; fecal leukocytes are usually seen. History of prior administration of antibiotics suggests *C. difficile* as causative agent. Systemic symptoms may provide a clue to the diagnosis: Hemolytic uremic syndrome (hemolytic anemia, uremia, renal failure, and disseminated intravascular coagulation [DIC]) occurs with both *Shigella* and enterohemorrhagic *E. coli.* Reiter's syndrome (arthritis, urethritis, and uveitis) occurs after *Salmonella, Shigella, Campylobacter,* and *Yersinia* infections.

▶ **Diagnosis**

Stool studies for bacterial pathogens, ova, and parasites; stool cytotoxin assay for *C. difficile.* Proctosigmoidoscopy may show erythema, ulceration, hemorrhage, or pseudomembranes, yellow-white, raised plaques characteristic of pseudomembranous colitis associated with *C. difficile.*

▶ **Disease Severity**

Fever, tachycardia, volume depletion, leukocytosis, abdominal distention, guarding, tenderness, decreased bowel signs, signs of toxemia; development of peritoneal signs suggests toxic megacolon.

▶ **Concept and Application**

Invasive organisms cause histologic damage and may also produce signs and symptoms of systemic infection. Species of *Shigella, Salmonella, Campylobacter, Yersinia, Clostridium,* and *E. histolytica* produce invasive diarrhea.

▶ **Treatment Steps**

1. Avoid barium enema (could increase morbidity).
2. Oral rehydration in mild disease or intravenous hydration for the more severely ill.
3. Antibiotic therapy with vancomycin or metronidazole for *C. difficile,* ciprofloxacin or trimethoprim–sulfamethoxazole for *Shigella.*
4. Other enteric infections, such as *Campylobacter* and intestinal *Salmonella,* are self-limited and usually don't require antibiotics.
5. Antidiarrheals, which may delay clearance of the pathogen, should be avoided.

B. Irritable Bowel Syndrome (IBS)

▶ **H&P Keys**

Clinical features are formalized in the "Rome I criteria" (Table 4–9).

4-9

ROME CRITERIA FOR DEFINING IRRITABLE BOWEL SYNDROME

At least 3 months' continuous or recurrent symptoms:
>   Abdominal pain or discomfort that is either relieved with defecation *or* associated with
>   a change in frequency of stool *or* associated with a change in consistency of stool *and*

Two or more of the following on at least one-quarter of occasions or days:
>   Altered stool frequency
>   Altered stool form (lumpy and hard or loose and watery)
>   Altered stool passage (straining, urgency)
>   Feeling of incomplete evacuation
>   Passage of mucus
>   Bloating or feeling of abdominal distention

► Diagnosis

Identify symptoms complex and the compatible with IBS, associations of symptoms with factors that produce gut hyperactivity, and exclusion of organic cause of symptoms.

► Evaluation

Use diagnostic tests based on presenting symptoms (diarrhea or constipation). Colonoscopy with mucosal biopsy is used to exclude microscopic or collagenous colitis on histologic examination. Complete blood count (CBC), laxative screening, stool O&P, and small bowel radiography. Obtain a detailed dietary history to identify factors that may aggravate or cause symptoms, especially diarrhea, gas bloating, or constipation. Dietary factors include lactose, fructose, sorbitol, carbonated beverages, legumes, other gas-producing foods, and caffeinated beverages.

► Concept and Application

Almost 50% of patients who see American physicians in the United States for bowel symptoms do not have any organic cause for their symptoms. A chronic functional gastrointestinal disorder manifested by abdominal pain and altered bowel habits, which occurs chronically or recurrently at times of life stress, change in diet, menses, and emotional tension.

► Treatment Steps

1. Establish a good physician–patient relationship.
2. Educate patients about their condition.
3. Emphasize the excellent prognosis and benign nature of the illness.
4. Employ therapeutic interventions centering on dietary modifications, pharmacotherapy, and behavioral intervention.
5. Dietary fiber increases stool bulk, either by water retention or by serving as a substrate for microbial growth in the large intestine.
6. Pharmacological treatment:
   - Synthetic opioids such as loperamine and diphenoxylate are effective in those with diarrhea.
   - Smooth-muscle relaxants (anticholinergics and calcium channel blockers) relieve GI symptoms by inhibiting smooth muscle contractions.
   - Tegaserod is engineered specifically for women with constipation-component IBS refractory to standard treatment.
   - Tricyclic antidepressants in low doses are advocated for chronic somatic or visceral pain.

- Selective serotonin reuptake inhibitors (SSRIs) are helpful in patients with a diagnosis of depression, obsessive–compulsive disorder, or phobias.
7. Psychological and behavioral therapies: hypnotherapy and psychotherapy are the most effective, cognitive and cognitive–behavioral therapy; relaxation, biofeedback, and combinations of the above may be helpful.

C. Colorectal Carcinoma (CRC)

The most common GI malignancy in the United States and more common than all others combined. CRC affects women and men equally. The lifetime risk is about 6%. Both incidence and mortality are higher among African-Americans than Caucasians.

▶ H&P Keys

Colorectal cancer is considered to arise by a combination of genetic and environmental risk factors with inheritance determining the individual susceptibility. Environmental factors interact with the susceptibility to give rise to the development of small adenomatous polyps, larger adenomatous polyps, and finally cancer. Environmental factors play an important role in CRC (Table 4–10). Inherited factors are important to the pathogenesis of CRC. Specific genetic syndromes are associated with increases of the following hereditary colorectal cancer syndromes:

Familial Adenomatosis Polyposis (FAP)—Characterized by hundreds to thousands of adenomatous polyps, which appear at an average age of 16 years, with cancer inevitable at an average age of 39 years. There is the frequent occurrence of polyps in the UGI tract and specific extraintestinal manifestations including desmoid tumors, osteomas of the mandible and long bones, congenital hypertrophy of the retinal pigment epithelium, and soft tissue tumors.

Hereditary Nonpolyposis Colorectal Cancer (HNPCC)—Previously known as Lynch syndrome or cancer family syndrome, characterized by the development of adenomatous polyps that occur at a younger age and often more advanced pathologic characteristics com-

4-10

ENVIRONMENTAL FACTORS THAT MAY INFLUENCE COLORECTAL CARCINOGENESIS[1]

Probably related	Possibly protective[4]
High dietary fat consumption[2]	Yellow-green cruciferous vegetables
Low dietary fat consumption[2]	Foods rich in carotene (vitamin A)
Possibly related	Vitamins C and E
Environmental carcinogens and mutagens	Selenium
Heterocyclic amines (from charbroiled or fried foods)	Folic acid
Products of bacterial metabolism	Cyclooxygenase-2 (COX-2) inhibitors
Beer and ale consumption (rectal cancer)	Hormone replacement therapy (estrogen)
Low dietary selenium	
Probably protective	
Dietary fiber consumption (wheat bran, cellulose, lignin)	
Dietary calcium	
Aspirin and NSAIDs[3]	
Physical activity/low body mass	

[1]Based on epidemiologic observations.

[2]Dietary fats and fibers are heterogeneous in composition and which individual components are causative or protective remains to be determined.

[3]NSAIDs, nonsteroidal antiinflammatory drugs.

[4]Data are limited.

Used by permission from Friedman SL, McQuaid KR, Grendell JH. *Current Diagnosis & Treatment in Gastroenterology*, 2nd ed. New York: McGraw-Hill, 2003.

pared to the general population. HNPCC kindreds are recognized by three features:

1. At least three first-degree relatives with cancer of the colorectum, endometrium, small bowel, ureter, or renal pelvis, and one should be a first-degree relative of the other two.
2. At least two successive generations affected.
3. At least one case diagnosed before the age of 50.

Individuals in the general population may carry familial risk of CRC. Genetic testing is available for identifying affected individuals in families clinically known to have FAP or HNPCC, but formal genetic counseling is important before testing is considered (Table 4–11).

Prevention—Primary prevention entails lifestyle, dietary, or chemopreventive measures to prevent adenomas and carcinomas from developing. Diet and lifestyle recommendations published by the American Cancer Society and generally endorsed by the National Cancer Institute aim to decrease not just the risk of colorectal cancer but cancer in general. They include:

- Increase daily fiber intake approximately threefold from the present average of 7 grams a day.
- Decrease fat intake to 30% of calories.
- Moderate intake of red meats and salt-cured and smoke-cured meats.
- Five to seven portions of fruits and vegetables a day.
- Eliminate tobacco.
- Moderate alcohol.
- Regular exercise and weight control.

Daily aspirin may be associated with a decreased incidence and mortality from sporadic colorectal cancer.

Secondary prevention includes discovering adenomas or early-stage carcinomas and removing them to avert the development of advanced carcinoma. Studies demonstrate that the successful detection of earlier-stage tumors by screening decreases colorectal cancer mortality. Rationale for colorectal screening: Colon cancer is common, curable in its early stages, and asymptomatic in its early stages. Average-risk screening: fecal occult blood testing (FOBT) annually and sigmoidoscopy every 5 years, *or* colonoscopy every 10 years or barium enema every 5–10 years (Table 4–12). Screening in higher-

4-11

HEREDITARY NONPOLYPOSIS COLORECTAL CANCER

Three or more relatives with colorectal cancer (one must be a first-degree relative of the other two)
Colorectal cancer involving at least two generations
One or more colorectal cancer cases before age 50 years

Used by permission from Friedman SL, McQuaid KR, Grendell JH. *Current Diagnosis & Treatment in Gastroenterology*, 2nd ed. New York: McGraw-Hill, 2003.

4-12

COLORECTAL CANCER SCREENING GUIDELINES BASED ON FAMILIAL RISK

Setting	Age to Begin	Test	Interval
General population	50	FOBT	Annual
		Sigmoidoscopy *or*	Every 5 years
		Colonoscopy *or*	Every 10 years
		Barium enema	Every 5–10 years
First-degree relative with CRC	40	Same as general population	Same as general population
Two first-degree relatives with CRC or CRC in first-degree relative before age 50	40	Colonoscopy	Every 3–5 years
At risk for HNPCC	25	Colonoscopy	Every 2 years;
		Genetic counseling/testing	annual > 40
At risk for FAP	10–12	Sigmoidoscopy	Every 1–2 years
		Genetic counseling/testing	

risk populations includes screening/surveillance recommendations for the familial categories detailed in Table 4–12. Other high-risk individuals include patients with inflammatory bowel disease and those with a history of a colonic hamartomatous polyposis syndrome (juvenile polyposis, Peutz–Jeghers syndrome, serrated polyposis syndrome, and other rare syndromes).

▶ Diagnosis

Colonoscopy is the preferred examination for patients with positive screening tests (FOBT, sigmoidoscopy), asymptomatic iron deficiency anemia, or colonic symptoms. The goal of colonoscopy is to detect cancer, remove adenomas, and, in the case of ulcerative colitis, to search for dysplastic lesions that might indicate a higher risk.

▶ Disease Severity

Tumor stage is the most important prognostic factor. Determinants of stage are the depth of penetration through the bowel wall and the presence and number of lymph nodes pathologically. Method of staging includes endoscopic ultrasound. It is the staging procedure of choice for rectal cancers to assess depth of invasion and lymph node metastasis. Surgical staging correlates with 5-year survival (Table 4–13). Five-year survival for node-negative patients varies from 85–95% if the tumor has not penetrated the muscularis propria; and 60–80% if the tumor has penetrated the muscularis propria. With positive nodes, 5-year survival is < 60%.

4-13

SURGICAL STAGE AND SURVIVAL

TNM Stage	AJCC Stage	Dukes' Stage	Survival (%) Five-Year
I	T1–2, N0, M0	A, B1	85–95
II	T3–4, N0, M0	B2, B3	60–80
III	Any T, N1–3, M0	C	30–60
IV	Any T, any N, M1	D	5

▶ Concept and Application

Biologic basis for CRC prevention:

- Most CRC arises from adenomatous polyps.
- Adenomatous polyps are found in 25% of people by age 50, and the prevalence increases to about 50% by age 75.
- CRC arises from a series of specific mutations in tumor suppressor genes, oncogenes, and DNA mismatch repair genes. The earliest mutation in the progression is in the adenomatous polyposis coli gene (APC—a tumor suppressor gene). Many, if not all, adenomas begin with a mutation of the APC gene. After the APC "gate-keeper" gene is lost, other mutations in colon cancer include K-raps, p53, and DCC (deleted in colon cancer) and DNA mismatch repair (MMR) genes.

▶ Treatment Steps

1. Surgery is the mainstay of curative therapy. Surgical therapy is applied to most colorectal cancers, even when metastasis is present, to prevent obstruction or hemorrhage.
2. The value of preoperative CT scans is debated.
3. Chemotherapy plays an adjuvant and palliative role.
4. Radiation therapy improves outcome of some rectal cancers and is standard therapy for stage II and III rectal carcinomas.
5. Carcinoembryonic antigen (CEA) is obtained preoperatively for follow-up purposes.
6. Follow-up after resection:
    - Goals include detection of recurrence of the original malignancy and detection of metachronous polyps and cancers.
    - The rationale is that almost all CRC recurrences will occur within 5 years and most will recur within 2 years.
    - The approach is to perform history, physical examination, and CEA every 3–6 months for 2–3 years, then annually. Colonoscopic surveillance recommendations are identical to those for adenoma follow-up.

D. Appendicitis

▶ H&P Keys

Typically, the first symptom is upper midline or perimbilical pain. Discomfort develops over several hours and is followed by anorexia, nausea, and vomiting. Once the serosal surface of the appendix becomes inflamed, the pain and tenderness shifts to McBurney's point. The usual presentation of periumbilical pain shifting to the right lower quadrant (RLQ) is seen less frequently in older patients, in whom diffuse pain and nonlocalized tenderness are more common. Perforation is suspected if the temperature is > 38°C or if the leukocyte count is > 15,000 cells/mm.

▶ Diagnosis

Appendicitis is a clinical diagnosis, supported by carefully selected laboratory studies. Patients with historical features and physical examinations do not need additional diagnostic studies. Immediate surgical exploration is indicated for the following:

- Abnormal gas pattern on abdominal radiographs: RLQ ileus or diffuse small bowel air–fluid levels are seen in 62% of patients with uncomplicated appendicitis, 71% of those with periappendiceal phlegmon, and 97% of those with gangrenous appendicitis or perforation.

- In patients in whom the diagnosis is ambiguous, CT is a reliable method for differentiating periappendiceal phlegmon from abscess.

► Concept and Application

Most common cause of acute abdomen in the United States. About 250,000 appendectomies are performed in the United States annually, with 2,000 deaths resulting from complications of the disease. One in 15 develops appendicitis during his or her lifetime. Appendicitis develops as a result of obstruction of the appendiceal lumen by fecalith or appendiceal. Overall perioperative mortality is 0.5%. Fewer than 0.2% of nonperforated patients die. Mortality rises tenfold with perforation. Mortality rises steeply with advancing age. The rate is < 1% for patients < 50, and > 15% for patients > 71 years of age. Septic complications occur with increased frequency in the presence of perforation.

► Treatment Steps

1. Emergency appendectomy.
2. In 10–20% of patients explored for presumed appendicitis, a normal appendix is found. Mesenteric lymphadenitis, Meckel's diverticulum, cecal diverticulitis, pelvic inflammatory disease, ectopic pregnancy, and ileitis mimic appendicitis.

E. Inflammatory Bowel Disease (IBD)

1. Ulcerative Colitis (UC)

► H&P Keys

Classic symptoms: bloody diarrhea, rectal urgency tenesmus, extracolonic manifestations (uveitis, episcleritis, scleritis, primary sclerosing cholangitis, pyoderma gangrenosum). Among precipitating factors consider NSAIDs, antibiotics, estrogens, smoking.

► Diagnosis (Fig. 4–2)

Exclude self-limited colitis:

- Sigmoidoscopy/colonoscopy and biopsy.
- Stool exam for culture/O&P.
- Serologic studies—ameba.
- Stool *C. difficile* toxin.

Consider sexually transmitted diseases/AIDS, radiation, ischemia, drugs, gold cleansing agents, "crack," cocaine.

► Assessment of Disease Severity

Severity:

- Mild: < 4 bowel movements (BMs)/day, with or without blood; no toxicity; CBC, erythrocyte sedimentation rate (ESR).
- Moderate: > 4 BMs/day without toxicity.
- Severe: > 6 bloody BMs/day, toxicity, fever, tachycardia, anemia, leukocytosis, thrombocytosis, elevated ESR.

Extent:

- Proctitis.
- Proctosigmoiditis.
- Left colon involvement.
- "Pancolitis" extending proximal to the hepatic flexure.

► Concept and Application

Remission can be predicted by the natural history of the individual patient. The longer the remission, the higher likelihood that remis-

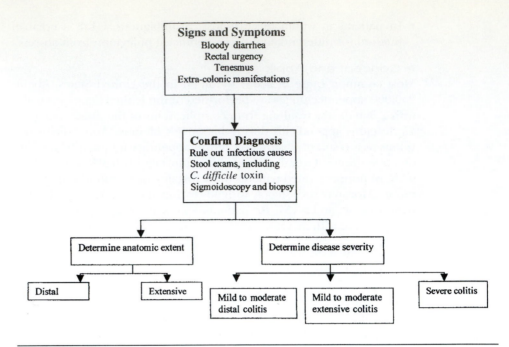

Figure 4–2. Ulcerative colitis: diagnosis. (Adapted, with permission, from Hanauer SB, Meyers S. Management of Crohn's Disease in Adults. ACG Practice Parameters. *Am J Gastroenterol* 1997;92:559–566.)

sion will be sustained. Surveillance colonoscopy at 1- to 2- year intervals after 7 years in patients with extensive disease and after 13 years in patients with left-sided disease.

▶ **Treatment Steps**

1. Medical therapy goals: induction of remission: defined by (clinical) absence of inflammatory symptoms (e.g., no diarrhea, mucoid bloody stool, or urgency); (endoscopic) regression of findings consistent with regenerated intact mucosa (e.g., absence of ulcers, granularity, or friability); (histologic) absence of inflammatory infiltrate or crypt abscesses.

2. Maintenance of remission.

3. Choice of therapy: Mild to moderate distal colitis: combined oral and topical therapy often achieves prompt response. Oral aminosalicylates sulfasalazine, 5-ASA (Dipentum, Asacol, Pentasa) *and* topical aminosalicylates: mesalamine suppositories, mesalamine enemas, or corticosteroids: hydrocortisone enemas.

4. Extensive colitis: oral aminosalicylates, 5-ASA, oral prednisone: taper once improvement occurs, azathioprine/6-mercaptopurine (6-MP).

5. Severe colitis: toxic patient refractory to oral medication. Hospital admission for IV corticosteroids—300 mg hydrocortisone or 60 mg methylprednisolone/day, maximum 7–10 days. Failure to improve: surgery. Total parenteral nutrition (TPN) is sometimes needed but not effective in forestalling surgery. Avoid narcotics, antidiarrheals, anticholinergics, and antidepressants.

6. Urgent indications for surgery include massive hemorrhage, perforation, toxic megacolon, and failure of maximal medical therapy.

Nonemergent indications are suspected carcinoma or confirmed dysplasia, growth failure in children, debility and intolerance of side effects of corticosteroids, distal colitis with poor quality of life, intractable extraintestinal complications such as hemolytic anemia and pyoderma gangrenosum.

7. Urgent surgical procedures include subtotal colectomy with Brook ileostomy and Hartmann pouch or mucous fistula.

Elective procedures are complete proctoctomy (abdominoperineal resection), or ileal pouch–anal anastomosis with rectal mucosal stripping or stapled anastomosis.

2. Crohn's Disease

▶ H&P Keys

Vague and variable manifestations: chronic diarrhea, abdominal pain, weight loss, anorexia, weight loss, fever, recurrent oral aphthous ulcerations, pallor, cachexia, abdominal mass or tenderness or history of intestinal obstruction, history of perianal fissures, fistulae, abscesses; extraintestinal manifestations affecting the skin, eyes, joints, growth retardation amount children. Exacerbating factors: infection (respiratory or enteric), cigarette smoking, NSAIDs.

▶ Diagnosis

Exclude ischemia, neoplasm, infection, drugs, and AIDS-related illness.

Workup: laboratory tests that include CBC, red blood cell (RBC) indices, ferritin, B_{12}, folate, ESR, electrolytes, calcium, magnesium, albumin, prothrombin time, vitamin D, liver chemistries, stool O&P, culture, *C. difficile* toxin.

Depending on the site and suspected complication: x-ray of small-bowel series, barium enema, CT scan, colonoscopy to evaluate colonic or anastomotic strictures, monitor recurrences at anastomoses, and surveillance for dysplasia.

▶ Disease Severity

Clinical patterns include inflammatory, stenosing/obstructive, or fistulizing. Systemic manifestations are:

- Mild to moderate: ambulatory, tolerating symptoms.
- Moderate to severe: fever, weight loss > 10% of total body weight, pain and tenderness, nausea, emesis, anemia.
- Severe to fulminant: despite corticosteroids, development of high fever, persistent emesis, signs of obstruction, peritoneal inflammation, cachexia, abscess.

▶ Concept and Application

Entire GI tract is susceptible. Onset is most common among teenagers and young adults with a second peak in the 60s and 70s (usually segmental colonic). Management varies with disease location, severity, and presence of complications.

▶ Treatment Steps

Goal: symptomatic improvement with tolerance of medical therapy. See Figure 4–3.

1. Mild to moderate disease: Anticipate 50% response. Oral aminosalicylates: sulfasalazine 3–6 g/day or mesalamine 3.2–4.8 g/day. Antibiotics: metronidazole 10–20 mg/kg/day, ciprofloxacin 500 mg bid. Add PPI for gastroduodenal Crohn's disease. Use topical mesalamine or corticosteroids for distal colonic disease.
2. Moderate to severe disease: Prednisone, 40–60 mg/day until improvement, then taper; treat concomitant infection; nutritional support; azathioprine/6-MP.
3. Severe/fulminant disease: hospitalization; IV corticosteroids; antibiotics; surgical consultation for obstruction or progression to

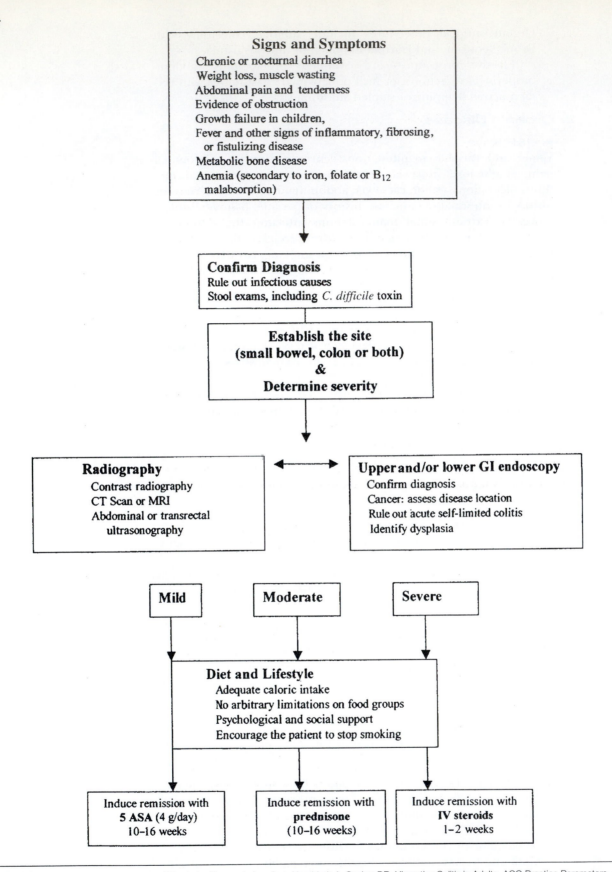

Figure 4–3. Crohn's disease management. (Adapted, with permission, from Kornbluth A, Sachar DB. Ulcerative Colitis in Adults. ACG Practice Parameters. *Am J Gastroenterol* 1997;92:204–211.)

abscess, dysplasia, or peritoneal inflammatory findings; tumor necrosis factor-α (TNF-α) for closing enterocutaneous and perianal fistulas, refractory active disease, and maintenance of remission.

F. Ischemic Bowel Disease

▶ H&P Keys

Typically seen in patients over age 60 with significant cardiac disease; may have history of "intestinal angina," arrhythmias, recent myocardial infarction, previous arterial emboli. Rheumatic heart disease and atherosclerotic heart disease have high risk for ischemic bowel disease. In early occlusive mesenteric ischemia, acute crampy abdominal pain out of proportion to physical findings with spontaneous evacuation and pain with absence of defecatory urge in nonocclusive ischemia. Other signs: vomiting, diarrhea, abdominal distention, hyperperistalsis, tenderness, hematochezia. For thrombotic disease of mesenteric veins, predisposing conditions include peritonitis, abdominal inflammation, trauma, portal hypertension, intra-abdominal tumors, coagulopathy, oral contraceptives.

▶ Diagnosis

Hemoconcentration, leukocytosis, elevated amylase levels; abdominal x-rays may show "thumbprinting" caused by submucosal hemorrhage and edema; visceral arteriography to exclude acute thromboses.

▶ Disease Severity

Abdominal tenderness, distention, leukocytosis, hemoconcentration, bloody peritoneal transudate, metabolic acidosis (late).

▶ Concept and Application

Four syndromes: acute mesenteric infarctions, ischemic colitis, focal ischemia, and intestinal angina. Infarction results from abrupt arterial occlusion. Nonocclusive ischemia results from poor perfusion. Venous thrombosis has a more insidious course.

▶ Treatment Steps

1. Early intervention for acute occlusive disease of arteries or veins.
2. Treatment for nonocclusive ischemia: bowel rest, fluids, antibiotic therapy resulting in complete resolution in 50%, healing with stricture in 30%, and gangrenous gut requiring resection in 20%.

G. Intestinal Obstruction

▶ H&P Keys

Crampy, spasmodic abdominal pain, vomiting, borborygmi, abdominal distention, obstipation; can develop slowly (months or years) or acutely (over hours). With mechanical obstruction, distress is apparent by extreme restlessness. With ileus, pain is usually less severe. Careful inspection of skin; palpation of umbilicus, lower-trunk inguinal, and femoral areas to detect hernias, intra-abdominal masses, hepatosplenomegaly; rectal and vaginal exam for masses and occult blood. Bowel sounds are infrequent and hypoactive in ileus. In obstruction, bowel sounds become loud, high-pitched, and hyperactive.

▶ Diagnosis

Biochemical and hematologic tests including: CBC, levels of amylase, alkaline phosphatase, aspartate aminotransferase, alanine aminotransferase, lactate dehydrogenase; acid–base balance;

roentgenographic obstruction series, including plain films of the abdomen to localize the level of obstruction, upright chest film in the lateral and posteroanterior views to detect pneumonia, free air, air–fluid levels. Use barium for retrograde studies but avoid barium if perforation is a possibility. CT scan may be helpful. Endoscopy to visualize and obtain tissue for biopsy from obstructing lesions in the esophagus, stomach, duodenum, rectum, and large intestine.

▶ Disease Severity

Fever, rebound tenderness, leukocytosis, unexplained hyperamylasemia.

▶ Concept and Application

Most common causes of obstruction in adults are adhesions and hernias in the small bowel and cancer in the colon.

▶ Treatment Steps

1. Decompression via nasogastric tube for either obstruction or ileus.
2. Complete obstruction requires urgent surgery to detect strangulation, resect necrotic bowel, and preserve viability of adjacent bowel as soon as preoperative fluid and electrolyte resuscitation and nasogastric decompression are established.

H. Diverticulitis

▶ H&P Keys

Acute diverticulitis commonly manifests with fever, localized left lower quadrant abdominal pain, leukocytosis, and a palpable mass seen, typically, in American patients above the age of 35.

▶ Diagnosis

Leukocytosis, roentgenographic obstruction series, ultrasonographic or CT imaging. As the process resolves, colonic evaluation (either colonoscopy or flexible sigmoidoscopy and barium enema) to confirm the diagnosis and exclude other colonic pathology (e.g., Crohn's disease, carcinoma). The risk of perforation in colonoscopy is higher within 4 weeks of resolved diverticulitis.

▶ Disease Severity

Complications include gross perforation and peritonitis: a surgical emergency requiring aggressive resuscitation, broad-spectrum antibiotics, laparotomy, and colonic resection with fecal diversion. Elective resection is indicated after two documented episodes of acute diverticulitis, depending on age, operative risk, and severity. Immunocompromised patients should be treated surgically after one attack due to the higher risks and higher mortality. Chronic diverticulitis is acute diverticulitis complicated by colonic fistula, large-bowel obstruction, or stricture. Colovesical fistula is the most common fistula. All symptomatic manifestations of chronic diverticulitis are treated surgically by resection and primary anastomosis after resolution.

▶ Treatment Steps

1. Diet and lifestyle: acute uncomplicated diverticulitis—bowel rest and antibiotic therapy. Outpatient treatment: clear liquids until symptoms resolve. Inpatient: clear liquids until symptoms resolve; NPO, IV hydration.
2. Antibiotic outpatient regime includes: ciprofloxacin and met-

ronidazole; or trimethoprim–sulfamethoxazole and metronidazole; or trovofloxicin 200 mg/day for 7–10 days.

Inpatient antibiotic regimen includes imipenem 500 mg q6h, ticarcillin/clavulinic acid 3.1 g IV q6h, piperacillin/tazobactam 3.375 mg IV q6h; or trovafloxacin 300 mg IV day, then 200 mg PO q day.

I. Constipation

▶ H&P Keys

Onset and duration of complaint: constipation present from birth or neonatal period suggests congenital disorder; recent onset demands a workup for organic disorders. Frequency of defecation, defecatory difficulties such as excessive straining, discomfort, sense of incomplete evacuation. Drug history. Careful physical examination with abdominal palpation for distention, retained stool, prior surgical procedures, autonomic dysfunction; anorectal and perineal examination.

▶ Diagnosis

Flexible sigmoidoscopy and barium enema; exclude metabolic and endocrine disorders such as diabetes mellitus, hypothyroidism, hypercalcemia, hypokalemia; exclude muscular collagen vascular and neurogenic disorders. Anal manometry and full-thickness rectal biopsies when Hirschsprung's disease is suspected.

▶ Disease Severity

Colonic transit studies, defecography, and anal manometry for patients with severe constipation who have not responded to simple dietary measures.

▶ Concept and Application

Impairment in large-bowel transit can be a primary motor disorder, in association with a large number of diseases, and a side effect of many drugs.

▶ Treatment Steps

1. Adequate dietary fiber.
2. Behavioral approaches; biofeedback.
3. Discouragement of routine use of laxatives except bulk-forming agents.

J. Peritonitis

▶ H&P Keys

Severe abdominal pain and rigidity, intercostal breathing, fever, tachycardia, hypovolemia, tenderness on direct and referred palpation, voluntary guarding, tenderness on rectal and pelvic exams, tenderness on percussion, loss of liver dullness, decrease or absence of bowel sounds.

▶ Diagnosis

Leukocytosis with left shift or leukopenia, hemoconcentration, metabolic acidosis, hyperkalemia, paralytic ileus, or free air.

▶ Disease Severity

Suppurative peritonitis has abrupt onset and relatively short course with rapid progression. Mortality from fluid shifts, hypovolemia, and septic shock with resultant renal, respiratory, cardiac, and hepatic failure.

► Concept and Application

Common causes are intra-abdominal organ disease such as appendicitis, diverticulitis, perforating carcinoma, perforating ulcer, and trauma. Mortality results from fluid shifts and endotoxin that may cause hypovolemia and septic shock.

► Treatment Steps

1. Fluid and electrolyte resuscitation.
2. Surgical repair of primary process and removal of debris.
3. Systemic antibiotics with careful monitoring of cardiac reserve via Swan–Ganz catheter, blood pressure, arterial blood gas determination, Foley catheter for recording urine volume, nasogastric intubation to decompress stomach, supplemental oxygen.

K. Familial Mediterranean Fever (Recurrent Polyserositis)

► H&P Keys

Autosomal recessive genetic disorder affects Armenians, Arabs, and Sephardic Jews. Most common manifestation is peritonitis. In 90% the first manifestation occurs at the end of the second decade.

► Diagnosis

No specific test. However, a high sedimentation rate could be present. Six diagnostic features: fever, serositis, amyloidosis, ethnic background, family history, and exclusion of other causes. Unless a strong family history is obtained, the diagnosis is often made at laparotomy, where diffuse inflammation of serosal surfaces without other intra-abdominal pathology is seen. No bacteria are cultured. Appendectomy is indicated so that future episodes can be differentiated from acute appendicitis.

► Disease Severity

In most patients, the disease is relatively benign. Attacks precipitated by a variety of factors. Complications include amyloidosis, degenerative arthritis, renal vein thrombosis, narcotic addiction.

► Concept and Application

Recurring inflammation of any serosal surface including peritoneum, pleura, pericardium, meninges, and synovial membranes.

► Treatment Steps

Colchicine treatment may prevent and ameliorate acute attacks and prevent amyloidosis.

V. RECTUM

A. Malignant Neoplasm of Rectum

See Colorectal Carcinoma.

B. Hemorrhoids

► H&P Keys

Anal discomfort, pruritus ani, fecal soiling, prolapse, bleeding, pain.

► Diagnosis

Flexible sigmoidoscopy or anoscopy. Occult bleeding in the stool requires a complete colonic evaluation, regardless of the presence of hemorrhoids. Hemorrhoids are classified according to their degree of protrusion or prolapse. First-degree bulge into the lumen of the anorectal canal on anoscopy but do not protrude out of the anus. Second-degree hemorrhoids prolapse out of the anus with defecation or straining but reduce to normal anatomic position spontaneously. Third-degree hemorrhoids prolapse out of the anus with defecation or straining and require digital reduction. Fourth-degree are irreducible and are at risk for strangulation.

► Disease Severity

Acute, severe bleeding may require transfusion. Chronic bleeding can cause iron deficiency anemia. External hemorrhoid thrombosis can be extremely painful and must be distinguished from strangulated hemorrhoids, which are larger and more circumferential. Strangulated hemorrhoids cause significant pain and usually have an external and internal component and occur secondary to prolapse, with subsequent lack of blood supply. Progression to gangrene with resultant infection is life threatening.

► Concept and Application

Hemorrhoids result from dilatation of the superior and inferior hemorrhoidal veins. Internal hemorrhoids are lined with rectal mucosa and arise from the superior hemorrhoidal cushion above the mucocutaneous junction (dentate line). External hemorrhoids arise from the inferior hemorrhoidal venous plexus below the mucocutaneous junction and are lined by perianal squamous epithelium.

► Treatment Steps

1. Thrombosis of external hemorrhoids and mild bleeding of internal hemorrhoids: treat with sitz baths, two to three per day; bed rest to minimize additional thrombosis and swelling; stool-softening agents; topical therapy with anesthetic ointments and witch hazel–impregnated pads.
2. Strangulated hemorrhoids require immediate surgical therapy.
3. Other treatment options include rubber band ligation for third- and fourth-degree hemorrhoids and hemorrhoidectomy for strangulated hemorrhoids.

C. Anal Fissure

► H&P Keys

Severe pain during or after defecation associated with scant, bright red rectal bleeding. Most commonly found in young and middle-aged adults.

► Diagnosis

Inspection after spreading the buttocks. Anoscopy is difficult without topical anesthesia. Linear tears are perpendicular to the dentate line.

► Disease Severity

Can progress to chronic fissure.

► Concept and Application

Because elliptical anal sphincteric fibers offer less muscular support posteriorly, 90% occur posterior midline. Lateral tears suggest underlying disease (IBD, proctitis, leukemia, carcinoma).

► Treatment Steps

1. High-fiber diet and adequate fluid intake.
2. Topical anesthetic preparations for symptomatic relief.

3. Warm sitz baths to relax the anal sphincter.

4. Chronic fissures (> 6 weeks) usually require surgical therapy.

D. Anorectal Abscess

▶ H&P Keys

Acute pain and swelling. Pain in absence of swelling with small intersphincteric or pelvorectal abscesses. Sitting, movement, defecation increase pain. Antecedent history of constipation, diarrhea, trauma. Fever, malaise, and purulent foul-smelling drainage are common. Associated medical diseases include diabetes, hypertension, heart disease, IBD, and a neutropenic state as a result of hematologic malignancy.

▶ Diagnosis

Inspection of the perineum reveals redness, heat, swelling and tenderness, drainage from infected crypt orifice. Rectal examination is difficult without anesthesia.

▶ Disease Severity

Delay in making the diagnosis can lead to necrotizing anorectal infection and increases risk of overwhelming sepsis.

▶ Concept and Application

Obstruction, stasis, and infection of anal glands is most common cause. Obstruction may occur as a result of trauma, eroticism, diarrhea, hard stools, and foreign bodies.

▶ Treatment Steps

1. Abscesses require drainage. Superficial abscesses can be drained under local anesthetic in outpatient setting. All others require drainage in the operating room with anesthesia and surgical instrumentation.

2. Antibiotics are not necessary for otherwise healthy patients. Perioperative antibiotics are used for patients with underlying disease such as acute leukemia, valvular heart disease, diabetes.

3. Postoperative management: inspection to ensure proper healing, sitz baths, analgesia, bulk-forming agents to soften stool.

E. Anorectal Fistula

▶ H&P Keys

Chronic purulent drainage. Prior history of anorectal abscess. Pain with defecation but not as severe as with anorectal abscess or anal fissure. Perianal skin may be excoriated.

▶ Diagnosis

Inspection of the perineum usually reveals a red, granular papule from which pus is expressed. Anoscopy and sigmoidoscopy to identify primary orifice and proctocolitis.

▶ Disease Severity

Multiple secondary openings suggest either Crohn's disease or hidradenitis suppurativa.

▶ Concept and Application

Primary orifice is at level of dentate line. Secondary orifice is anywhere else on the perineum.

▶ Treatment Steps

1. Anorectal fistula is approached surgically, with postoperative care similar to anorectal abscess.

2. Anorectal disease as a manifestation of Crohn's disease requires special consideration. Metronidazole will heal perineal Crohn's disease. Discontinuation of therapy is associated with flaring of disease. Remicade may enhance the healing rate of perineal Crohn's and fistulae.

F. Pilonidal Disease

► H&P Keys
Pain, swelling, drainage midline skin lesion of internatal or gluteal cleft seen most commonly in young men.

► Diagnosis
Inspection: characteristic midline location. Appearance and lack of communication with anorectum distinguish pilonidal disease from anorectal fistula and hidradenitis suppurativa.

► Disease Severity
Acute abscess versus chronic drainage.

► Concept and Application
Common acquired lesion of coccygeal skin, possibly induced by local stretching forces. Small skin pits secondarily invaded by hair precede development of draining sinus or abscess.

► Treatment Steps
1. Acute pilonidal abscess requires incision, drainage, and hair removal.
2. Chronic draining pilonidal lesions require surgical closure.

VI. GALLBLADDER

A. Acute Cholecystitis

► H&P Keys
Acute onset of right upper quadrant (RUQ) pain (typically radiating to the right shoulder blade), nausea, vomiting, and fever. Murphy's sign: inspiratory arrest elicited when palpating under the liver.

► Diagnosis
Laboratory leukocytosis with preponderance of polys and bands. Minor elevations in aminotransferase levels and bilirubin. Ultrasound is the preferred initial screening study. Cholescintigraphy (hepato-iminodiacetic acid [HIDA], diisopropyl iminodiacetic acid [DISIDA]) when clinical suspicion is high but ultrasound is normal.

► Disease Severity
Secondary bacterial infection can progress to empyema, gangrene, and perforation.

► Concept and Application
Most common cause of acute cholecystitis is obstruction of a distended gallbladder with concentrated bile. Acalculus (5–10%) occurs in setting of major surgery, critical illness, extensive trauma, and burns.

► Treatment Steps
1. Initial: hospitalization, NPO, intravenous hydration, and intravenous antibiotics to cover enteric organisms.

2. Definitive: surgical laparoscopic cholecystectomy is the standard approach. Open cholecystectomy done in cases of generalized peritonitis, septic shock, severe coagulopathy, known cancer of the gallbladder, and patients in the third trimester of pregnancy.

B. Cholelithiasis

▶ H&P Keys

Biliary pain, nausea, and vomiting. Predisposing factors include obesity, oral contraceptives, pregnancy, clofibrate, ileal disease or resection, and genetic factors.

▶ Diagnosis

Ultrasonography has > 90% sensitivity in diagnosing gallstones.

▶ Disease Severity

Biliary pain lasting for more than 3 hours indicates progression to cholecystitis.

▶ Concept and Application

Cholesterol gallstones constitute 85% of all gallstones. Bile that is supersaturated with cholesterol can lead to formation of cholesterol gallstones.

▶ Treatment Steps

1. Asymptomatic stones require no treatment.
2. Symptomatic gallbladder stones are treated with cholecystectomy.
3. Oral bile acid therapy (Ursodiol) is a treatment option for mildly symptomatic patients with small (< 10 mm) cholesterol stones within a functioning gallbladder.
4. Common bile duct stones, particularly in the elderly and those with comorbid disease are best treated with endoscopic retrograde cholangiopancreatography (ERCP).

C. Choledocholithiasis and Acute Suppurative Cholangitis

▶ H&P Keys

Biliary pain, involving the central upper abdomen, jaundice, chills and rigors (Charcot's triad), mild hepatomegaly, occasional rebound.

▶ Diagnosis

Leukocytosis with a left shift, mild elevation of serum transaminases and alkaline phosphatase, hyperbilirubinemia, serum amylase level. Ductal dilatation documented by ultrasonography or CT. Lack of dilatation does not exclude obstruction. Gold standard is ERCP for diagnosis and management. Magnetic resonance cholangiopancreatogram (MRCP) and spiral CT provide excellent images of common duct stones and are among available noninvasive alternatives to diagnostic ERCP.

▶ Disease Severity

Progression leads to ascending cholangitis and endotoxemia with shock and liver abscess.

▶ Concept and Application

Gallstones passing into the common duct can lead to acute obstruction, bile stasis, bacterial infection.

► Management

Initial resuscitation and stabilization, systemic antibiotics to cover *E. coli, Klebsiella, Pseudomonas,* and enterococci. Removal of obstruction via ERCP, and possible papillotomy, followed by active instrumentation for ductal clearance. If multiple large common-duct stones cannot be removed in one session, temporary drainage must be established via placement of stent or nasobiliary catheter to control biliary sepsis.

VII. LIVER

A. Hepatitis

► H&P Keys

Pertinent information: age, gender, race, preceding episodes, history of chronic liver disease or cirrhosis, alcohol consumption (Table 4–14), drug and toxin exposure (include herbal as well as "traditional" medications), occupation and work environment, sexual history, immunologic and nutritional status, immunizations, travel history, and family history.

Hepatitis may present with a flulike or serum sickness syndrome, anorexia, malaise, fever, arthralgia, arthritis, rash, and/or angionecrotic edema, with or without jaundice, dark urine, light stools, abdominal discomfort. Nonspecific constitutional symptoms may be present for a short or protracted time.

Physical findings may be subtle or nonexistent. Findings are often reflective of the duration and severity of liver disease and are common to all forms of hepatitis and include jaundice, hepatomegaly (typically mild), lymphadenopathy, ascites, splenomegaly, encephalopathy. Some findings are typically associated with alcoholic liver disease: palmar erythema, Muehrcke's lines and white nails, Dupuytren's contracture, parotid and lacrimal gland enlargement.

1. Viral Hepatitis

► Diagnosis

Use specific tests for viral antigens, viral antibodies, and/or nucleic acids.

- Acute hepatitis A, B, C (see Tables 4–15, 4–16, and 4–17).
- Acute δ coinfection: presence of IgM anti-HBc and IgM anti–hepatitis D virus (HDV) or HDV RNA.
- Acute δ superinfection: presence of IgM anti-HDV or HDV RNA.
- Acute hepatitis E: IgM anti–hepatitis C virus (HCV) and compatible clinical features.

4-14

CAGE QUESTIONNAIRE

1. Have you tried to **C**ut down on your drinking?
2. Are you **A**nnoyed by criticism of your drinking?
3. Do you feel **G**uilty about your drinking?
4. Do you need an **E**ye opener each morning?

Scoring: 1 point for each yes answer. A total of 2 or more indicates a likelihood of underlying alcoholism.

4-15

DIAGNOSTIC SEROLOGY FOR ACUTE VIRAL HEPATITIS

Serology

Preliminary	Confirmatory	Diagnosis
+Anti-HAV	+IgM anti-HAV	Acute hepatitis A
+HbsAg	+IgM anti-HBc	Acute hepatitis B[a]
+Anti-HCV	+RIBA, HCV RNA	Hepatitis C (acute or chronic)

[a]Get anti-HDV if risk factors.

2. **Chronic Hepatitis**
   - Hepatitis A: no chronic state.
   - Hepatitis B: presence of hepatitis B surface antigen (HBsAg), hepatitis Be antigen (HBeAg), HBV DNA, IgG anti-HBc.
   - Chronic C: presence of anti-HCV ELISA. False positives may be seen in low-risk populations. Confirm with anti-HCV RIBA or HCV RNA.
   - Chronic D: HBsAg and HDV RNA.

3. **Alcoholic Hepatitis**

4. **Drug-Induced Hepatotoxicity (See Table 4–18)**

5. **Autoimmune Hepatitis**
   Suspect among women ages 15–35 and again at menopause: 40% present with the abrupt onset of illness that can resemble acute viral or toxic hepatitis; 25% have cirrhosis at the time of presentation. The disease is fatal without treatment. History of concurrent autoimmune disease: autoimmune thyroiditis, vasculitis, ulcerative colitis, Graves' disease, vitiligo, insulin-dependent diabetes. Symptoms: fatigue, jaundice, bleeding, easy bruisibility, RUQ pain. Transaminases range from 200 to 1,000 U/dL; total serum globulin, γ-globulin, or immunoglobulin G level ≥ 1.5 normal; antinuclear antibodies (ANAs), smooth muscle antibodies (SMAs), antibodies to liver/kidney microsome type 1 (anti-LKM1) titers $\geq 1:80$ in adults or $\geq 1:20$ in children, antibodies to soluble liver antigen (anti-SLA), antimitochondrial antibodies (AMAs).

▶ **Concept and Application**

Hepatitis, a necroinflammatory process of the liver parenchyma, can be either acute (< 6-month duration) or chronic (> 6-month duration). Acute hepatitis can resolve, progress to hepatic failure, or continue as chronic hepatitis leading to cirrhosis and hepatocellular carcinoma.

4-16

CLINICAL SITUATIONS/SYNDROMES ASSOCIATED WITH HBV INFECTION

	HBs Ag	Anti-HBs	Anti-HBc	IgM anti-HBC	HBe Ag	HBV DNA	Anti-HDV
Acute hepatitis B	+	–	+	+	+	+	–
Chronic hepatitis B	+	+/–	+	–+/–	+	–	
Healthy carrier	+	+/–	+	–	–	–	–
Vaccinated	–	+	–	–	–	–	–
Recovered HVB	–	+	+	–	–	–	–
Acute hepatitis D	+	–	+	+	+/–	+/–	+
Chronic hepatitis D	+	–	+	–	+/–	+/–	+

4-17

CLINICAL SITUATION/SYNDROMES ASSOCIATED WITH HCV INFECTION

	Anti-HCV (ELISA)	Anti-HCV (RIBA)	ALT	HCV RNA
Acute hepatitis C	=/–	+	Raised	+
Chronic hepatitis C	+	+	Raised	+
HCV carrier	+	+	Normal	+
Recovered HCV	+	+	Normal	–
False positive	+	–	Normal	–

A variety of pathogenic mechanisms may cause hepatitis, including viral infection, toxic injury, autoimmune and hereditary disorders.

Viral Hepatitis—Can be caused by infection with the hepatotropic hepatitis viruses A–E (HAV, HBV, HCV, HDV, HEV) and the non-A–E viruses. HAV and HEV can cause only acute viral hepatitis. HBV, HCV, HDV causes both acute and chronic viral hepatitis, cirrhosis, and hepatocellular cancer. HDV is dependent on HBV for both survival and replication. HDV induces illness only in the presence of HBV, either by coinfection or superinfection. HEV, an RNA virus, reported in developing nations in areas of poor sanitation after flooding, is similar to HAV but carries a higher mortality, particularly in pregnant women. Non-A–E viral hepatitis has two distinct profiles: (1) a parenteral or community-acquired hepatitis with a benign course and (2) a persistent viral infection that may have a fulminant course.

Alcohol-Induced Liver Injury—No particular quantity of alcohol is predictive of alcoholic liver disease. The incidence of serious liver disease begins to rise when the daily consumption of alcohol exceeds 60 g/day for men and 20 g/day for women. In addition to habitual alcohol consumption, other factors that predispose to alcohol-induced liver disease include: female gender, race, coexposure to other drugs, coinfection with the hepatotrophic viruses HBV and HCV, nutritional status, and immune dysfunction.

Drugs—Drugs causing liver injury can be "predictable," or "direct," hepatotoxins and "unpredictable," or "idiosyncratic," hepatotoxins. Direct hepatotoxins produce injury in a predictable, dose-dependent fashion. Characteristically, direct hepatotoxins produce liver cell necrosis in a predictable region of the hepatic lobule. Idiosyncractic hepatotoxins produce liver injury in an unpredictable manner. The pattern of injury is diffuse and consists of hepatocellular necrosis and/or cholestasis. Some idiosyncratic hepatotoxins are associated with fever, rash, eosinophilia, and au-

4-18

PATTERNS OF HEPATOTOXICITY

Type of Reaction	Examples
Direct reaction	Acetaminophen, carbon tetrachloride, mushrooms, phosphorus
Idiosyncratic reaction	Isoniazid, disulfiram, propylthiouracil
Toxic-allergic reaction	Halothane, isoflurane, ticrynafen
Allergic hepatitis	Phenytoin, amoxicillin–clavulanate, sulfonamides
Chronic hepatitis	Nitrofurantoin, methyldopa
Alcoholic hepatitis-like	Amiodarone, valproic acid

toantibody production. Examples of direct hepatotoxins include acetaminophen and carbon tetrachloride (see Table 4–19). Idiosyncratic hepatotoxins can be produced by isoniazid and chloropromazine.

Autoimmune Hepatitis—Inflammation of the liver of unknown cause that is characterized by interface hepatitis (piecemeal necrosis), hypergammaglobulinemia, and autoantibodies in serum.

Hereditary Disorders

- *Hemochromatosis (HCC),* an HLA-linked autosomal recessive disorder of iron absorption, has a disease prevalence of 1 in 250. Symptomatic HCC presents with hepatomegaly, well-established hepatic fibrosis and cirrhosis, diabetes mellitus, and hyperpigmentation. Aspartate transaminase (AST) and alanine transaminase (ALT) may be slightly elevated.
- *Wilson's disease,* an HLA-linked autosomal recessive disorder of copper metabolism, has a disease prevalence of 1 in 30,000. Young patients (mean age 8–12 years) may present with hepatitis and fulminant hepatic failure.
- α_1-*Antitrypsin deficiency* is an important cause of neonatal hepatitis and cirrhosis in children and early emphysema in young adults. Fifteen percent to thirty percent of neonates with conjugated hyperbilirubinemia have α_1-antitrypsin deficiencies.

▶ Treatment Steps

Treatment for acute hepatitis is primarily supportive care. Basic principles include:

1. Avoidance of potentially liver-damaging circumstances, fluid and electrolyte replacement, ambulation within the bounds of fatigue, a regular or high-protein diet (in the absence of encephalopathy).
2. Follow physical exam and biochemical tests: prothrombin time is the best biochemical indicator of prognosis; also follow bilirubin, ALT, AST twice weekly while values are rising, weekly during the plateau, then at lesser intervals until normalized.
3. Consideration for hospitalization is indicated for severe anorexia, vomiting, changes in mentation and biochemical changes, including a bilirubin value > 15 or 20 mg/dL, persistence hyperbilirubinemia, rapidly falling aminotransferase activity with a rising bilirubin, increasing protrombin time, and other evidence of hepatic failure.
4. *Acute viral hepatitis.* Most individuals with adequate family and medical support are treated in the outpatient setting. Hospital-

4-19

SOME IMPORTANT INDUSTRIAL AND ENVIRONMENTAL TOXIC CAUSES OF HEPATITIS	
Chemical	Uses
Arsenic	Pesticides and in production of ceramics, drugs, dyes, fireworks, paint, petroleum, ink, and semiconductors
Carbon tetrachloride	Degreasers, fat processors, fire extinguishers, fumigants, insecticides, refrigerants, lacquer, ink propellants, rubber, and wax
Tetrachloroethylene	Dry-cleaning agents, fumigants, solvent, degreasers
Yellow phosphorus	Munitions, explosives, fertilizers, rodenticides, semiconductors, luminescent coatings

4-20

INDICATIONS FOR HEPATITIS A VACCINATION

Travelers to endemic areas
Military personnel
Special populations where cyclic HAV epidemics occur
Homosexual males
Users of illicit intravenous drugs
Caretakers of the developmentally challenged
Employees of child day care centers
Laboratory personnel handling live HAV
Handlers of primates that may be handling HAV

ization for isolation is not required (the period of infectivity precedes symptoms). Immunoprophylaxis (Tables 4–20 and 4–21).

5. *Chronic viral hepatitis B.* Patients with chronic hepatitis B are candidates for therapy if they have evidence of active viral replication (HBeAg or HBV DNA in serum) and raised serum aminotransferases. Patients with decompensated cirrhosis should be treated with extreme caution. The mainstay of therapy of chronic hepatitis B is α-interferon (Table 4–22). Because of the side effects associated with interferon (Table 4–23) and relatively low response rates, alternative therapies are emerging. Second-generation nucleoside analog, lamivudine is Food and Drug Administration (FDA)-approved for hepatitis B.

6. *Chronic viral hepatitis C.* Current standard therapy for chronic hepatitis C is α-interferon with ribavirin. Ribavirin, a nucleoside analog, is administered orally. Ribavirin is teratogenic; therefore, it should not be used during conception and pregnancy. There are multiple interferon-specific agents available for hepatitis C with once-weekly SQ interferon in combination with daily PO ribavirin.

7. *Drug-induced liver disease.* Discontinue the implicated agent.

4-21

PERSONS RECOMMENDED FOR HBV PROPHYLAXIS (VACCINE OR HBIG OR BOTH)

Preexposure prophylaxis
    Persons with occupational risk, including clients and staff of institutions
    Clients/staff of institutions for developmentally disabled
    Patients on hemodialysis
    Sexually active homosexual men
    Sexually active heterosexual men and women
    Users of illicit injectable drugs
    Recipients of certain blood products, e.g., clotting factors
    Household and sexual contacts of HBV carriers
    Adoptees from countries of high HBV endemicity
    Populations with high endemicity
    Inmates of long-term correctional facilities
    International travelers to HBV-endemic areas for > 6 months
Postexposure immunoprophylaxis for hepatitis B

Type of Exposure	Immunoprophylaxis
Perinatal exposure	Vaccination + HBIG
Sexual, acute infection	HBIG ± vaccination
Sexual, carrier	Vaccination
Household contact, carrier	Vaccination
Household contact, known exposure	HBIG ± vaccination
Infant < 12 months, acute case, primary caregiver	HBIG ± vaccination
Inadvertent percutaneous or permucosal	Vaccination + HBIG

4-22

ALGORITHM FOR THERAPY OF HEPATITIS B

Initial evaluation
- Serial ALT, HBsAg, HBeAg, HBV DNA
- Liver biopsy
- Review side effects and expected results
- Verify lack of contraindications

Initial therapy
- α-interferon, 5 μ daily or 10 μ three times weekly for 16–24 weeks

Monitor during therapy
- Every 2–4 weeks:
  Signs and symptoms
  ALT, AST, bili, albumin, CBC + differential
- At 2 and 4 months
  HBeAg, HBsAg, protime, TSH
- Follow up after therapy
- Every 2–3 months
  Signs and symptoms
  ALT, AST, bili, albumin, CBC
- At 6 months
  HBsAg, protime, TSH

8. *Alcoholic liver disease.* Withdrawal of alcohol and substitution of a nutritious diet. Consider hospitalization for individuals with extrahepatic complications of alcohol ingestion (GI bleeding, coexistent infections, fluid and electrolyte abnormalities, pancreatitis, alcohol withdrawal syndromes).

9. *Autoimmune hepatitis.* Responds to prednisone and/or azathioprine. Remission can be induced within 2 years of treatment in > 70%. Relapse is common after withdrawal of drug therapy.

10. *Hemachromatosis.* Requires long-term phlebotomy and chelation therapy.

11. *Wilson's disease.* Requires lifelong copper chelation therapy.

Prevention—The health consequences of acute viral hepatitis are reduced by public health measures and immunization.

HAV—As the principal mode of transmission is person-to-person, prevention efforts are aimed at sanitation, chlorination, and proper handling of sewage and identification of individuals at risk. The hepatitis A vaccine, used in Europe since 1991, is now

4-23

SIDE EFFECTS OF INTERFERON

Side Effects of Interferon

Early
  Severe/life-threatening syndrome
    None
  Mild:
    Influenza-like
Late
  Severe/life-threatening
    Severe depression/suicide
    Acute renal failure
    Cardiotoxicity
    Seizures
    Exacerbation of preexisting autoimmune disease
      (e.g., inflammatory bowel disease)
  Mild
    Fatigue
    Emotional lability
    Bone marrow suppression

approved by the FDA for use in the United States. It is indicated for persons traveling to or working in countries with intermediate or high HAV endemicity (countries other than Australia, Canada, Japan, New Zealand and in Western Europe and Scandinavia), military personnel, native peoples of Alaska and areas of the Americas where cyclic HAV epidemics occur: homosexual males; users of illicit intravenous drugs; employees of child day care centers; laboratory workers who handle live HAV; and handlers of primates known to harbor the HAV virus (see Table 4–20). Immune globulin (IG) is recommended for children under the age of 2 who are traveling to endemic areas (Havrix is not approved for children of < 2 years of age) and postexposure, preferably within 2 weeks, for contacts of person with acute hepatitis A.

HBV—Despite the development and introduction of the hepatitis B vaccine in the 1980s, the incidence of hepatitis B has actually increased in the United States since 1980. One important reason for the failure of the vaccine has been an inability to reach an estimated 22 million people who are at highest risk. As a result, an expanded vaccination strategy focuses on the universal hepatitis B immunization for newborns, children, and adolescents, including infants born to HBeAg-positive mothers by vaccine plus HBIG within 12 hours of birth.

HCV—Development of specific serologic assays has dramatically decreased the dissemination of transfusion-related hepatitis. The residual risk is estimated to be 0.03%. The use of IG for percutaneous exposure to HCV-positive material is not recommended. No vaccine for hepatitis C is available.

HDV—No effective vaccine. However, transmission of HDV can be avoided with the hepatitis B vaccine. Carriers of HBsAg are at risk from continued IV drug abuse or sexual promiscuity.

B. Hepatocellular Carcinoma

► H&P Keys

Hepatocellular carcinoma (HCC) has a specific geographic distribution. HCC is common in sub-Sahara Africa, China, Japan, and the Southeast, where it is strongly associated with chronic hepatitis HBV infection and repeated heavy exposure to the mycotoxin aflatoxin B. Intermediate risk for HCC in areas of southern Europe and Japan is associated with HCV infection. In other parts of the world, HCC occurs as a late complication of cirrhosis (particularly alcoholic liver disease and hemachromatosis).

Clinical Presentation—Among southern black Africans and Chinese patients, HCC occurs in relatively young (mean age 33 years) and apparently healthy individuals. Typically, the disease is silent in its early stages. Onset of symptoms: abdominal pain, fullness, early satiety, anorexia, and weight loss corresponds to advanced disease. Physical findings include hepatomegaly, hepatic arterial bruit, ascites, splenomegaly, jaundice, fever. Among individuals with cirrhosis, an unexplained deterioration in liver function may be the only clue.

► Diagnosis

Tumor Markers—In high-incidence geographic regions, serum α-fetoprotein (AFP) is the most useful diagnostic test. Most symptomatic individuals (> 75%) from these regions which will have a diagnostic level (> 500 ng/mL) at presentation. In low-incidence regions, the AFP test is far less useful as a single tumor marker. A combination of tumor markers: tumor-associated isoenzymes of γ-glutamyl transferase (elevated total GGT leads to isoenzyme fractionation) and the abnormal prothrombin, des-γ-carboxy prothrombin may be abnormal when the AFP is nondiagnostic.

Newer molecular techniques amplify small amounts of tumor-specific gene-transcripts for albumin and α-fetoprotein mRNA promise to enhance detection of malignant hepatocytes in circulation.

Imaging—In patients with suspected HCC, the combination of arterial phase and portal venous phase CT imaging will detect the majority of tumors. Magnetic resonance (MR) is useful for detecting small (< 5 cm) HCC, differentiating HCC from hemangiomas and evaluating the proximity of HCC to adjacent blood vessels. Dynamic MR is superior to hepatic arteriography. Ultrasound is less useful. Hepatic scintigraphy has surpassed other imaging modalities.

Pathology—A definitive diagnosis depends on histologic appearance. Ultrasound or CT-guided percutaneous biopsy carries the risk of systemic dissemination or seeding of the tumor but is often necessary.

► Disease Severity

Symptomatic HCC carries a poor prognosis. In Africa and China, average survival is less than 4 months from the onset of symptoms. In other geographic regions the course may be somewhat more indolent. Prognosis is more favorable when tumors are detected prior to the onset of symptoms. A high incidence of extrahepatic recurrence and reappearance of tumor in the donor liver after transplantation reflects early hematogenous spread of micrometastases. The use of reverse transcriptase polymerase chain reactions to amplify small amounts of tumor-specific gene transcripts offer promising results to detect small numbers of malignant hepatocytes in peripheral blood.

► Concept and Application

HBV and HCV promote mutagenesis indirectly by stimulating necroinflammatory activity in the liver. Emerging evidence indicates that both viruses also have direct oncogenic potential. Geographic differences in the incidence of HCC among populations with comparable dietary aflatoxin B1 exposure may be due to individuals' capacity to detoxify mutagenic metabolites.

► Treatment Steps

1. In areas where HBV-related HCC is common, there is some hope that early vaccination will decrease the incidence of HCC. For HCV-related HCC, vaccination remains a distant goal. Parenteral drug abuse and the high incidence of sporadic HCV infection in countries at intermediate risk for HCC offer little hope for reducing the incidence of HCV-related HCC.

2. Dismal results are obtained with all forms of treatment for symptomatic tumors. Newer molecular markers and imaging modalities may increase the detection of small, asymptomatic and potentially resectable HCC in high-risk individuals or populations. Small (< 5 cm) lesions may be resectable when the tumor appears

to be confined to one lobe and the remaining liver is noncirrhotic.

3. Liver transplantation is considered for individuals with end-stage liver failure who coincidentally have a small single tumor without vascular invasion or extrahepatic spread.

4. When operative treatment is not an option, dearterialization, embolization, and chemoembolization or injection of alcohol directly into the lesion may reduce the intrahepatic tumor burden.

C. Hepatic Fibrosis and Cirrhosis

▶ H&P Keys

In its early stages, the process may reverse on withdrawl of the injurious agent (early fibrosis). Persistent injury leads to irreversible scar tissue deposition, increased resistence to blood flow, impaired exchange of nutrients and metabolites, and failure of synthetic function. A gradual and tedious clinical course is typically interrupted by life-threatening complications: bleeding varices, decompensated ascites, peritonitis, or encephalopathy. Alcohol and chronic viral hepatitis B and C are the most common causes. Other etiologies include drugs and toxins, autoimmune hepatitis, primary biliary cirrhosis, biliary obstruction, heart failure, metabolic and hereditary disorders (hemochromatosis, Wilson's disease, and α_1-antitrypsin deficiency). Pertinent history includes alcohol use, risk factors for viral hepatitis, drug and toxin exposure, and family history.

Stigmata suggestive but not necessarily diagnostic of cirrhosis include jaundice, spider angiomata, palmar erythema, Dupuytren's contracture, digital clubbing, easy bruising, loss of secondary sexual characteristics, skeletal muscle wasting, abdominal hernias, and caput medusae.

▶ Diagnosis

Laboratory tests, imaging studies, and liver biopsy screen for the presence, severity, potential causes, and prognosis of liver disease. No single battery of tests is applicable to all patients. The initial battery of biochemical tests, the so-called liver function tests reflect the following:

- *Synthetic function:* albumin, prothrombin time, coagulation factor levels, lipoproteins.
- *Hepatocellular injury:* aminotransferases (ALT, AST).
- *Cholestasis:* alkaline phosphatase.
- *Excretory function and anion transport:* bilirubin.

Obtain additional tests when specific diagnoses are suspected:

- *Chronic viral hepatitis B and C:* HBsAg, anti-HCV.
- *Autoimmune hepatitis:* ANA, SMA, serum globulins.
- *Primary biliary cirrhosis:* antimitochondrial antibody.
- *Hemachromatosis:* iron, transferrin, ferritin.

Ultrasonography is the noninvasive imaging study of the liver for jaundice, suspected biliary obstruction, and mass lesion. The presence of cirrhosis is suggested by signs of portal hypertension: splenomegaly, ascites, decreased or reversed portal flow (via Doppler measurements). Supplemental diagnostic studies: ERCP, CT, and MR have value for specific situations:

- *Mass lesion:* MR, CT portography.
- *Iron overload and fatty infiltration:* MR.

- *Extrahepatic bile duct obstruction:* ERCP.
- *Bleeding varices:* upper endoscopy, ligation, and/or sclerosis.
- *New-onset or decompensated ascites:* diagnostic paracentesis.

Liver biopsy plays a central role in the diagnosis of all stages of fibrosis and cirrhosis. Other indications for liver biopsy include otherwise unexplained hepatomegaly and/or liver biochemical abnormalities, documentation of neoplastic disease, assessment of chronic hepatitis, assessment of veno-occlusive disease, and rejection after transplantation.

► Disease Severity

Severity of cirrhosis is manifested by its clinical consequences: episodes of variceal bleeding, spontaneous bacterial peritonitis, intractable ascites, and poorly controlled encephalopathy. The Child–Turcotte–Pugh scale (Table 4–24) provides a rough measure of prognosis. Potential candidates for liver transplantation need referral to the liver transplantation center well before they develop the following signs of decompensation: uncontrolled variceal bleeding, intractable ascites, poorly controlled encephalopathy, and fulminant hepatic failure.

► Concept and Application

Fibrosis and *cirrhosis* are histologic terms that refer to the accumulation of excess extracellular matrix (ECM) within the liver with or without an accompanying inflammatory response. Recent evidence indicates that the ECM has important biologic effects of liver cell function in addition to its well-characterized effects on blood flow.

► Treatment Steps

1. *Cirrhotic ascites:* dietary salt restriction, diuretic therapy. Consider large-volume paracentesis, peritoneovenous shunting, transjugular intrahepatic portosystemic shunting (TIPS), and liver transplantation for refractory ascites.
2. *Spontaneous bacterial peritonitis (SBP):* cefotaxime is effective for initial therapy.
3. *Encephalopathy:* correction of any precipitant factors (GI bleeding, infection, electrolyte imbalance), reduction of dietary protein, and decrease in intestinal ammonia absorption of nonabsorbable carbohydrates, especially lactulose.
4. *Acute variceal bleeding:* variceal band ligation, sclerotherapy, and/or pharmacologic therapy: somatostatin, octreotide, vaso-

4-24

CHILD–TURCOTTE–PUGH SCALE

	Child–Turcotte–Pugh Score		
	1	2	3
Encephalopathy	None	1, 2	3, 4
Ascites	Absent	Slight	Moderate
Bilirubin (mg/dL)	1–2	2–3	> 3
Albumin (g/dL)	> 3.5	2.8–3.5	< 2.8
Prothrombin time (s. prolonged)	1–4	4–6	> 6

Total score
  1–6 =   A
  7–9 =   B
  10–15 = C

pressin, vasopressin/nitroglycerin. Consider TIPS for failure of urgent endoscopic and pharmacologic therapy.

5. *Prevention of rebleeding:* variceal band ligation, sclerotherapy, non-selective β-blockade (nadolol, propranolol). Consider TIPS for endoscopic and pharmacologic failures.

6. *Liver transplantation:* for all forms of cirrhosis, primary biliary cirrhosis, primary sclerosing cholangitis, biliary atresia, and fulminant hepatic failure.

VIII. PANCREAS

A. Pancreatic Carcinoma

► H&P Keys

Risk factors for the development of pancreatic cancer include: chronic pancreatitis, hereditary pancreatitis, smoking, a diet high in fat content, and exposure to various chemicals including β-naphthylamine. Earlier studies that reported an association with caffeine appear unfounded.

Most common presenting features are abdominal pain, weight loss, jaundice, and anorexia. With pancreatic head tumors, distended gallbladder (Courvoisier gallbladder) may be palpable. Occasionally, acute pancreatitis or hypergylcemia may be the presenting features. Thromboembolic phenomena occur in 10% of patients with pancreatic adenocarcinoma.

Tumor markers: CEA, CA 19-9 can be helpful (although not diagnostic) when very high.

► Diagnosis

In patients with suspected pancreatic cancer the goals of the evaluation are (1) to establish the diagnosis and (2) to determine resectability. Several imaging modalities are useful.

- Biphasic helical CT with thin cuts through the pancreas is the best imaging study for both diagnosis and staging.
- ERCP: useful for evaluating biliary or pancreatic duct obstruction in the absence of a suspicious mass on CT. ERCP and brush cytology may support a diagnosis of malignancy.
- Transabdominal ultrasound provides little in the evaluation of the pancreas. It is useful in the evaluation of obstructive jaundice when there is a strong suspicion of choledocholithiasis.
- Endoscopic ultrasonography (EUS) with fine-needle aspiration biopsy is the most accurate test to assess resectability.
- MR cholangiopancreatography is less sentitive than ERCP. However, because of its noninvasive nature, it may be useful for patients requiring repeat imaging of the pancreatic duct.
- Biopsy: limited indications.

A confirming biopsy prior to resection is unnecessary when:

- Clinical suspicion of pancreatic cancer is high.
- The cancer is surgically resectable.
- The patient is a satisfactory candidate for surgical resection.

A confirming biopsy may be needed prior to treatment when:

- The diagnosis of pancreatic cancer is doubtful.
- The cancer is not surgically resectable.
- The patient is a poor operative candidate.

- When tissue diagnosis is needed prior to initiating chemotherapy or radiation therapy.

► Concept and Application

Tenth most common type of new cancer. Frequency is increasing. Pancreatic cancer accounts of 5–6% of the cancer deaths among men and women, making it the fourth leading cause of cancer deaths. Five-year survival overall remains 4%. It is the lowest survival rate among all reported sites.

► Treatment Steps

Treatment options remain limited. Stage of disease at the time of diagnosis determines optimal treatment.

1. Surgical resection: in the absence of locally advanced or metastasis disease. Adjuvant or neoadjuvant therapy may improve survival.
2. Unresectable disease: > 75% of pancreatic cancers are unresectable at the time of diagnosis, either because of locally advanced disease or metastatic disease. Treatment goals are palliation of symptoms and treatment of unresected malignancy. Symptoms to be palliated include: jaundice, gastric or duodenal obstruction, and pain.
3. Obstructive jaundice may be palliated endoscopically, radiologically, or surgically. Endoscopic or radiologic decompression methods are associated with lower early complications and shorter hospital stay.
4. Gastric outlet obstruction occurs in 10–15% of cases and can be palliated by surgical gastrojejunostomy or the placement of self-expanding metallic stents such as those used for biliary decompression.
5. Pain is a major concern among patients and is present in 90% of those with advanced disease.
6. Transdermal or long-acting narcotics supplemented with shorter-acting agents are used for breakthrough pain. External beam radiation may provide relief. Pain due to obstruction of the pancreatic duct can sometimes be alleviated by endoscopic pancreatic duct stenting. Celiac nerve block provides pain relief in 80–90%. Benefit is limited to about 6 months. For many pancreatic cancer patients who are not likely to survive for > 6 months, the benefit is lasting.
7. Chemotherapy radiation: gemcitabine is the standard treatment for patients with locally advanced or metastatic pancreatic cancer. Patients may also benefit from radiation therapy given with a radiosensitizing agent such as 5-FU.

B. Acute Pancreatitis

► H&P Keys

Abdominal pain, nausea, vomiting. Patients appear ill, anxious, and restless. Hypotension, tachypnea, tachycardia, hyperthermia or hypothermia, jaundice, mild distention, involuntary guarding in upper abdomen, generalized abdominal tenderness, bowel sounds diminished, basilar atelectasis, pleural effusions, flank and periumbilical ecchymosis (Grey Turner's and Cullen's signs).

► Diagnosis

Elevated serum amylase (within 2–12 hours, declining over the next 3–5 days), elevated lipase (persists 5–7 days, can be detected after amylase normalizes), elevated hematocrit, leukocytosis with a leftward shift of the differential, hyperglycemia, hypoalbuminemia, hypocalcemia, prerenal azotemia with elevated blood urea nitrogen and serum creatinine, hyperbilirubinemia, and hypertriglyceridemia. Routine roentgenography, ultrasonography, and CT scanning.

► **Disease Severity**

Ranson's criteria for prognosis on admission and during initial 48 hours do not predict course or outcome for individual patients.

► **Concept and Application**

Biliary tract stone disease and alcohol abuse account for 60–80% of cases. Other causes: infections (*Mycoplasma pneumoniae*, mumps, coxsackie, *Ascaris*, *Opisthorchis*), drugs (azathioprine, thiazide diuretics, sulfonamides), lipid abnormalities, trauma, and ERCP. Most attacks of acute pancreatitis result from injury to the pancreas by digestive enzymes.

► **cram facts**

CAUSES OF ACUTE PANCREATITIS

Obstruction of pancreatic duct
Choledocholithiasis and microlithiasis
Pancreas divisum with pathologically stenotic
   minor papilla
Choledochocele
Sphincter of Oddi dysfunction
Pancreatic duct stricture
Ascariasis or clonorchiasis
Pancreatic or ampullary carcinoma

Toxins
Ethyl alcohol
Methyl alcohol
Organophosphate insecticides
Scorpion venom

Drugs
Antineoplastic
   Azathioprine, 6-mercaptopurine
Antibiotics and antivirals
   Didanosine (DDI)
   Pentamidine
   Sulfonamides
   Tetracycline
   Metronidazole
   Nitrofurantoin
   Erythromycin
Others
   Estrogens (due to hyperlipidemia)
   Furosemide
   5-aminosalicylates
   Sulindac
   Methyldopa
   Cimetidine and ranitidine
   Salicylates

Metabolic
Hyperlipidemia
Hypercalcemia

Infections
Viral
   CMV
   Mumps
   Hepatitis A, B, C
   Coxsackie B
   Adenovirus
   Epstein–Barr virus
   HIV
Bacterial
   Mycobacterium (tuberculosis and MAC)
   Legionella
   Leptospirosis
   Mycoplasma
Parasite
   Ascaris
   Clonorchis
   Cryptosporidium
Trauma (including ERCP)
Ischemia
   Postoperative (especially after heart–lung
     bypass)
   Hypotension
   Vasculitis
Idiopathic
Other
   Posterior penetrating duodenal ulcer
   Cystic fibrosis (usually presents as chronic
     pancreatitis)

► Treatment Steps
1. General supportive measures, with meticulous management of fluid, electrolyte, ventilatory and hemodynamic alterations, and parenteral alimentation.
2. Early (within 72 hours) intervention (ERCP) to remove stones from the ductal system improves outcome.
3. Anticipate possible local complications: pseudocyst infection, pancreatic ascites, abscess, blood vessel with or without rupture or thrombosis, bowel necrosis or stricture, esophageal varices, and fistulas.

C. Chronic Pancreatitis

► H&P Keys
Recurrent or persistent abdominal pain, weight loss, steatorrhea, glucose intolerance, epigastric tenderness.

► Diagnosis
Plain x-ray of the abdomen may show pancreatic calcification. Ultrasonography or CT scan may show enlarged gland, dilated pancreatic duct, or calculi. ERCP is most sensitive and specific test for chronic pancreatitis. ERCP can differentiate chronic pancreatitis from pancreatic carcinoma. Tests of pancreatic exocrine function (secretin, cholecystokinin [CCK], or bentiromide test) for the rare patient with relatively minor ductal changes on ERCP in whom the diagnosis remains in doubt.

► Disease Severity
Complications include pseudocyst, pancreatic ascites, fistula, and splenic vein thrombosis. Suspect pseudocyst when a stable chronic pancreatitis patient experiences worsening of abdominal pain.

► Concept and Application
Alcohol in Western societies (70–80%) and malnutrition worldwide represent major etiologies.

► Treatment Steps
1. Avoidance of alcohol, analgesia, enzyme therapy for malabsorption and pain control, especially for patients with non–alcohol-induced chronic pancreatitis.
2. Celiac plexus block.
3. Surgery if all other measures have failed.

D. Cystic Fibrosis

► H&P Keys
Infants fail to gain weight despite vigorous appetite; watery stools. Eighty percent have pancreatic exocrine insufficiency at diagnosis, hypoproteinemia with edema, and "pot belly" on physical examination.

► Diagnosis
Sweat electrolytes: sodium and chloride are elevated in sweat in 99%; pancreatic stimulation test with CCK and secretin may confirm diagnosis when sweat test is equivocal; fetal screening and chromosomal analysis to diagnose cystic fibrosis by DNA analysis in the future.

► Disease Severity
Malnutrition and recurrent pulmonary infections are major concerns. Associated conditions include chronic meconium ileus in

15%, distal small-bowel obstruction (meconium ileus equivalent) in older patients, rectal prolapse, intussusception, diabetes mellitus, chronic liver disease, abdominal pain, and recurrent episodes of pancreatitis.

► Concept and Application

Increased viscosity of exocrine secretions leads to precipitation of exocrine secretions in all exocrine glands (pancreatic acini, intestinal glands, intrahepatic bile ducts, gallbladder, prostate, salivary glands) resulting in impaired pancreatic exocrine secretion, intestinal obstruction, focal biliary cirrhosis, obstructive pulmonary disease, and obstructive lesions of the male genital tract.

► Treatment Steps

Treatment of malnutrition with adequate caloric intake, balanced diet with vitamin supplementation (vitamins A, D, E, and K), pancreatic enzyme replacement, and H_2 blockers to improve maldigestion.

IX. ABDOMINAL AORTIC ANEURYSM

► H&P Keys

Usually asymptomatic until rupture. Physical examination may reveal a tender, pulsatile mass. Abdominal discomfort, tenderness, ureteral obstruction suggest inflammatory aneurysms. Mycotic aneurysms present as tender enlarging masses.

► Diagnosis

Ultrasonography has a sensitivity approaching 100% and is cost-effective for aneurysm detection and sequential follow-up. CT scan is equally effective and should be used when ultrasonography is not possible and precise sizing is required. MRI may be better than either ultrasonography or CT, both for accurate aneurysm measurement and views of relevant vascular anatomy. Chest x-rays are done to exclude thoracic aortic aneurysm. Preoperative aortography if visceral, renal, or peripheral vascular disease is suspected. Selective screening of high-risk patients between the ages of 55 and 80: hypertension, aneurysms of femoral or popliteal artery, and family history of abdominal aortic aneurysm.

► Disease Severity

Most abdominal aneurysms remain asymptomatic until rupture. Symptoms and complications are related to aneurysm size and expansion rate. Aneurysms smaller than 4 cm have a risk of rupture of about 2%; 25–41% of aneurysms larger than 5 cm rupture within 5 years. Risk factors for rupture include initial diameter of the aneurysm, elevated blood pressure, and presence of chronic obstructive pulmonary disease.

► Concept and Application

Pathogenesis is multifactorial: genetic predisposition, biochemical alterations of aortic wall, and hemodynamic mechanical factors contributing. Inflammatory reaction can develop around the external calcified layer (inflammatory aneurysms). Mycotic aneurysms can be caused by bacterial or fungal infection and are rare.

► Treatment Steps

1. Repair of symptomatic or ruptured abdominal aortic aneurysms and of all symptomatic aneurysms larger than 5 cm.

2. Contraindications to elective aortic reconstruction: myocardial infarction (within 6 months), intractable angina pectoris, severe pulmonary insufficiency with dyspnea at rest, severe chronic renal insufficiency, incapacitating stroke, and life expectancy of < 2 years.

BIBLIOGRAPHY

Agrawal NM, Van Kerckhove HEJM, et al. Misoprostol coadministered with diclofenac for prevention of gastroduodenal ulcers: a one-year study. *Dig Dis Sci* 1995;40:1125–1131.

Alter HJ, Bradley DW. Non-A, non-B, hepatitis unrelated to the hepatitis C virus (non-ABC). *Sem Liver Dis* 1995;15,1, 110–120.

Baaer DM, Simons JL, et al. Hemachromatosis screening asymptomatic ambulatory men 30 years of age and older. *Am J Med* 1995;98:464–468.

Balthazar EJ, Freeny PC, VanSonnenberg E. Imaging and intervention in acute pancreatitis. *Radiology* 1994;193:297–306.

Batey RG, Burns T, et al. Alcohol consumption and the risk of cirrhosis. *Med J Aust* 1992;156:413–416.

Bazzoli F, Fossi S, et al. The risk of adenomatous polyps in asymptomatic first-degree relatives of persons with colon cancer. *Gastroenterology* 1995;109:783–788.

Bond JH, for the Practice Parameters Committee of the ACG. Polyp guideline: Diagnosis, treatment, and surveillance for patients with nonfamilial colorectal polyps. *Ann Int Med* 1993;199:836–843.

Cameron AJ, Lomboy CT, et al. Adenocarcinoma of the esophagogastric junction and Barrett's esophagus. *Gastroenterology* 1995;109:1541–1546.

Cutler AF, Prasad VM. Long-term follow-up of *Helicobacter pylori* serology after successful eradication. *Am J Gastroenterol* 1996;91:85–87.

deBoer W, Driessen W, et al. Effect of acid suppression on efficacy of treatment for *Helicobacter pylori* infection. *Lancet* 1995;345:817–820.

Desmet VJ, Gerber M, et al. Classification of chronic hepatitis: Diagnosis, grading and staging. *Hepatology* 1994;19:1513–1516.

DeVault KR, Castell DO, et al. Guidelines for the diagnosis and treatment of gastroesophageal reflux disease. *Arch Int Med* 1995;155:2165–2173.

Elton E, Hanauer SB. Review article: the medical management of Crohn's disease. *Aliment Pharmacol Ther* 1996;10:1–22.

Ernst CB. Abdominal aorta in aneurysm. *New Eng J Med* 1993;328:1167–1172.

Gallstones and laparoscopic cholecystectomy. *NIH Consensus Statement online* 1992;10(3):1–20.

Hanauer SB. Medical therapy for ulcerative colitis. *Ann Int Med* 1993;118:540–549.

Isaacson PG. Gastrointestinal lymphoma. *Hum Pathol* 1994;25:1020–1029.

Lee WM. Drug-induced hepatotoxicity. *N Engl J Med* 1995;333:1118–1127.

Liskow B, Campbell J, Nickel EJ. Validity of the CAGE questionnaire in screening for alcohol dependence in a walk-in (triage) clinic. *J Stud Alcohol* 1995;56:277–281.

Masuko K, Mitsui T, et al. Infection with hepatitis GB virus C in patients on maintenance hemodialysis. *N Engl J Med* 1996;334;23:1485–1489.

MMWR Morbid Mortal Wkly Rep 1991.40:I.

Ottinger LW. Current concepts: mesenteric ischemia. *New Eng J Med* 1982;307:535–537.

Owens DM, Nelson DK, Talley NJ. The irritable bowel syndrome: long-term prognosis and the physician–patient interaction. 1995;122:107–112.

Pasricha PJ, Ravich WJ, et al. Intrasphincteric botulinum toxin for the treatment of achalasia. *N Engl J Med* 1995;322:774–778.

Rao SSC, Gregersen H, et al. Unexplained chest pain: The hypersensitive, hyperreactive and poorly compliant esophagus. *Ann Intern Med* 1996;124:950–958.

Rees JH, Soudain SE, et al. *Campylobacter jejuni* infection and Guillain-Barré syndrome. *N Engl J Med* 1995;333:1374–1379.

Rosch T, Braig C, et al. Staging of pancreatic and ampullary carcinoma by endoscopic ultrasonography: comparison with conventional sonography, computed tomography, and angiography. *Gastroenterology* 1992;102:188.

Salam I, Katelaris P, et al. Randomised trial of single-dose ciprofloxacin for travellers' diarrhea. *Lancet* 1994;344:1537–1539.

Soll AH, for the Practice Parameters Committee of the ACG. NIH consensus conference: medical treatment of peptic ulcer disease. *JAMA* 1996;275:622–629.

Terrault N, Wright T. Interferon and hepatitis C. *N Engl J Med* 1995;332:1509–1511.

Toribara NW, Sleisenger MH. Screening for colorectal cancer. *N Engl J Med* 1995;332:861–866.

Valdimarsson T, Franzen L, et al. Is small bowel biopsy necessary in adults with suspected celiac disease and IgA antiendomysium antibodies? 100% positive predictive value for celiac disease in adults. *Dig Dis Sci* 1996;41:83–87.

Warshaw AL, Gu Z, et al. Preoperative staging and assessment of resectability of pancreatic cancer. *Arch Surg* 1990;125:230.

Winawer BJ, Zauber AG, et al. Risk of colorectal cancer in families of patients with adenomatous polyps. *N Engl J Med* 1996;334:82–87.

Wright TL, Perreira B. Liver transplantation for chronic viral hepatitis. *Liver Transplant Surg* 1995;10:471–480.

Hematology and Oncology | 5

I. ANEMIA

A. Iron Deficiency Anemia

► H&P Keys

Etiology—Menstrual and pregnancy-related losses, iron-deficient diet, chronic gastrointestinal (GI) bleeding, chronic alcohol, aspirin, steroid, or nonsteroidal anti-inflammatory drug (NSAID) use.

Signs and Symptoms—Glossitis, spooning of nails, fatigue, weakness, dyspnea, pallor, pagophagia (ingestion of ice).

► Diagnosis

Hypochromic, microcytic cells on peripheral smear. Mean corpuscular volume (MCV) and mean corpuscular hemoglobin (MCH) are low; low serum ferritin, low serum iron, increased total iron-binding capacity (TIBC), low percentage of saturation, increased red cell distribution width (RDW), thrombocytosis, and low reticulocyte count.

► Disease Severity

Absence of iron on bone marrow aspiration (Prussian blue staining).

► Concept and Application

Underproduction anemia caused by inability to synthesize heme, which requires iron. May be the result of impaired iron absorption, deficient dietary intake, chronic blood loss, chronic intravascular hemolysis.

► Treatment Steps

1. Determine etiology.
2. Begin supplemental oral iron if patient is mildly to moderately symptomatic.
3. Transfuse if patient has any sign of cardiac compromise or is severely symptomatic.
4. Reassess oral replacement in 14–21 days expecting to see a significant reticulocytosis and the hemoglobin corrected by at least half. If it has not, assess compliance and absorption issues.
5. Some patients do not absorb or cannot tolerate oral iron and must receive either transfusion or intravenous supplementation.

B. Folic Acid Deficiency

► H&P Keys

Symptoms of anemia. No neurologic sequelae as in B_{12} deficiency. Nutritional deficiency (lack of green, leafy vegetables, fruit); chronic alcohol use; patients with malabsorption syndromes. Increased losses or increased utilization (dialysis, pregnancy). Chronic hemolytic anemias (i.e., sickle cell disease).

► Diagnosis

Low serum and red blood cell (RBC) folate levels (serum folate levels quickly correct following one hospital meal; therefore, RBC folate levels are more accurate). Macrocytic anemia and hypersegmented neutrophils on peripheral smear. Megaloblastic bone marrow cells. Normal B_{12} level. Increased lactic dehydrogenase (LDH). Increased bilirubin.

► **Disease Severity**

Pancytopenia; infertility, skin pigmentation abnormalities. Severe malabsorption syndromes diagnosed by jejunal biopsy. Neural tube defects if folate deficiency present during pregnancy.

► **Concept and Application**

Folic acid absorbed in the proximal jejunum. Folate deficiency leads to diminished thymidylate synthesis and abnormal DNA replication.

► **Treatment Steps**

1. Determine etiology.
2. Replace with oral folic acid 1 mg/day.

C. α-Thalassemia

► **H&P Keys**

An inherited disorder seen in American blacks and people of Mediterranean or Southeast Asian background. Carrier state (lack of one normal allele) is undetectable and very common. Patients who lack two alleles (called α-thalassemia trait) are usually asymptomatic, although they may have a mild microcytic anemia. Patients with deletion of three alleles (hemoglobin [HbH]) have moderately severe hemolytic anemia. Absence of α chains is incompatible with life.

► **Diagnosis**

Microcytosis on peripheral smear in patients with α-thalassemia trait. Normal iron studies. Elevated RBC count. RBC inclusions in patients with HbH and evidence of hemolysis (elevated LDH and bilirubin). Coombs' test is negative. Molecular studies can quantitate number of copies.

► **Disease Severity**

Hemolytic anemia and splenomegaly in patients with HbH. Hydrops fetalis occurs in homozygotes, in whom no α-globin is produced. Affected fetuses are either stillborn or die shortly after birth.

► **Concept and Application**

Caused by deletion of one or more α-globin genes. Presence or absence of symptoms depends on number of alleles deleted (or mutated). Inadequate production of α-globin leads to precipitation of β-globin (in HbH) or to β4 (β chain tetramer) formation, which is incompatible with life.

► **Treatment Steps**

1. Establish diagnosis by molecular studies or staining of peripheral blood smear with cresyl blue.
2. Rule out underlying iron deficiency.
3. Symptomatic patients may need periodic transfusions.
4. Prenatal diagnosis can identify fetus at risk for hydrops fetalis.
5. Splenectomy can be beneficial in patients with HbH.

D. β-Thalassemia

► **H&P Keys**

Most common in patients of Mediterranean background or from equatorial regions of Asia and Africa. Thalassemia minor (heterozygotes) patients usually have asymptomatic mild anemia. Thalassemia major (homozygotes) presents in childhood with symptoms of anemia. Splenomegaly occurs in thalassemia major. Frontal bossing from expansion of marrow cavity and bilirubin gallstones also seen.

▶ Diagnosis

Basophilic stippling and target cells on peripheral smear. Microcytic, hypochromic anemia, elevated RBC count. MCV usually < 75. Hb electrophoresis.

▶ Disease Severity

Severity of disease depends on type of genetic abnormality and amount of HbF present. Some defects result in no β chain production, others produce a decreased amount of β chain. Thalassemia minor results in a mild hypochromic microcytic anemia. Elevated hemoglobin A_2 (HbA_2) on Hb electrophoresis is diagnostic. In thalassemia major, splenomegaly results in shortened RBC survival and at times thrombocytopenia or neutropenia. Serum ferritin to detect iron overload in transfused patients.

▶ Concept and Application

Hereditary anemia resulting from deletion or defective transcription of β-globin genes. Excess α chains precipitate, causing rapid splenic clearing of RBCs. Frequent transfusions lead to iron overload.

▶ Treatment Steps

1. Transfusions required on a regular basis.
2. Start iron chelation with desferoxamine early to minimize complications of iron overload.
3. Bone marrow transplantation beneficial in thalassemia major.
4. Genetic counseling.

E. Vitamin B_{12} Deficiency

▶ H&P Keys

Symptoms of anemia (pallor, fatigue, weakness, dyspnea). Neurologic symptoms such as paresthesias, abnormal mental status, ataxia, and premature graying. History of autoimmune or intestinal diseases, such as atrophic gastritis, gastrectomy, sprue, and blind loop syndrome. Dietary deficiency rare.

▶ Diagnosis

Hypersegmented neutrophils (Fig. 5–1), macrocytic, hyperchromic anemia (high MCV). Increased LDH, low serum B_{12} level. Document achlorhydria. Schilling test done in the past. Intrinsic factor antibody analysis is now test of choice. Bone marrow, which is not required for diagnosis, shows megaloblastic hematopoiesis with immature nuclei compared to cytoplasm (nuclear cytoplasmic dissociation). Complete neurologic exam.

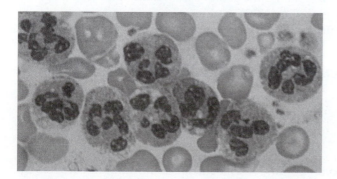

Figure 5–1. Hypersegmented neutrophils associated with vitamin B_{12} deficiency.

► **Disease Severity**

Serum B_{12} level is low. Neurologic symptoms consistent with long-tract disease, then cerebral dysfunction. No correlation between anemia and neurologic symptoms.

► **Concept and Application**

Body stores of B_{12} last 3–4 years. B_{12} present in animal protein (meats, eggs, milk products). Impaired DNA synthesis, but normal RNA synthesis, induces ineffective erythropoiesis. Defective conversion of propionate to succinyl coenzyme A (CoA) may lead to defective myelin synthesis and patchy demyelination. Absorption of vitamin B_{12} requires secretion of intrinsic factor by the stomach and occurs in the terminal ileum.

► **Treatment Steps**

B_{12} 1,000 μg given parenterally as a loading dose daily for 5 days, then 1,000 μg/month for life.

F. Aplastic Anemia

► **H&P Keys**

Weakness, fatigue, pallor, petechiae, bleeding, and evidence of infection. Etiology may be idiopathic, familial (e.g., Fanconi's syndrome), or acquired (e.g., secondary to radiation, drugs, hepatitis, or autoimmune mechanisms).

► **Diagnosis**

Hypocellular bone marrow. Normal cytogenetics. Decreased reticulocyte count (< 5%). Normochromic and normocytic RBCs. Rule out paroxysmal nocturnal hemoglobinuria with a Ham test (sucrose hemolysis test).

► **Disease Severity**

Severe aplastic anemia defined as two or more of the following: absolute neutrophil count < 500, reticulocyte count < 1%, and platelets < 20,000. Percentage of bone marrow cellularity < 25%.

► **Concept and Application**

Immune suppression of hematopoiesis in most. Some patients have stem cell defect. Associated with benzene, chloramphenicol, parvovirus B19, as well as other drugs and viral infections.

► **Treatment Steps**

1. Determine etiology if possible.
2. Human lymphocyte antigen (HLA)-matched bone marrow transplant if patient has a donor.
3. If transplant is not an option, other treatment options include antithymocyte globulin (ATG), cyclosporine, and corticosteroids.
4. Avoid transfusions as much as possible if bone marrow transplant is planned.

G. Anemia of Chronic Renal Disease

► **H&P Keys**

Pallor and fatigue. Renal failure patients (not necessarily dialysis dependent).

► **Diagnosis**

Low reticulocyte count. Normochromic, normocytic RBCs. Increased serum creatinine. Serum erythropoietin level decreased.

Iron deficiency, folate deficiency, and blood loss can complicate this disorder.

► Disease Severity

Development of transfusion dependency.

► Concept and Application

Decreased erythropoietin production. Iron and folate are lost during dialysis. Increased RBC loss and destruction; decreased RBC survival secondary to azotemia.

► Treatment Steps

1. Erythropoietin one to three times per week.
2. Iron and folate replacement.

H. Hemolytic Anemia

► H&P Keys

Hereditary intrinsic enzymatic defects, e.g., pyruvate kinase and hexokinase deficiencies. Drug history: glucose-6-phosphate dehydrogenase (G6PD) deficiency leads to episodic hemolysis, after exposure to oxidative stress. Chronic hemolysis can result in splenomegaly. Acquired secondary to lymphoid malignancies (chronic lymphocytic leukemia, lymphoma), systemic lupus erythematosus (SLE), bacterial (*Mycoplasma*) or viral (infectious mononucleosis) infections. Bilirubin gallstones with chronic hemolysis.

► Diagnosis

Elevated reticulocyte count. Coombs' test positive in immune process. Coombs' test detects immunoglobulin and/or complement on RBC surface. Elevated MCV, LDH, indirect bilirubin.

G6PD deficiency can detect Heinz bodies on peripheral smear, quantitate G6PD in nonacute setting.

Warm antibodies usually immunoglobulin G (IgG): microspherocytes. Cold antibodies usually immunoglobulin M (IgM): Coombs' positive for complement.

Microangiopathic hemolytic anemias (disseminated intravascular coagulation [DIC], thrombotic thrombocytopenic purpura [TTP], malfunctioning heart valve), RBC fragmentation (schistocytes, helmet cells). Intravascular hemolysis results in depletion of serum haptoglobin, urinary hemosiderin, and free urine hemoglobin.

► Disease Severity

Low Hb and haptoglobin. High LDH and indirect bilirubin levels.

► Concept and Application

May be immune (antibody-mediated) or nonimmune (unstable hemoglobin, deficiency of G6PD). Intravascular versus extravascular hemolysis.

► Treatment Steps

1. Determine etiology.
2. Transfuse least-incompatible blood if patient requires.
3. G6PD—the primary management is avoidance of oxidative stress, particularly known medications like quinine.
4. Warm antibodies are treated by corticosteroids, less often splenectomy or immunosuppression.
5. Cold antibodies are treated by keeping the patient, especially extremities, warm; steroids and occasionally cytotoxics.
6. Treat underlying disorder.

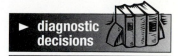

► diagnostic decisions

ANEMIA

Microcytic
Iron Deficiency
Menstruating females, chronic GI bleeding, low serum iron, low percent saturation, low ferritin, and high TIBC.

α- or β-Thalassemia
African, Mediterranean, or Southeast Asian ancestry, normal iron stores.

Anemia of Chronic Disease
Look for chronic inflammatory processes, usually normocytic; low TIBC; and elevated ferritin.

Macrocytic
B₁₂ Deficiency
Significant body stores, so rarely related to malnutrition. Neurologic changes can precede significant anemia, hypersegmented polys.

Folate Deficiency
No body stores, so develops more quickly. Replacement can improve anemia of combined B₁₂ deficiency but does not treat the neurologic sequelae. Serum levels inaccurate. If definite proof required, get RBC folate levels.

Normocytic
Acute Blood Loss
Should be obvious; transfuse as needed.

Aplastic Anemia
Fairly acute onset with no gross bleeding; look hard for possible drugs or treatable infections. Avoid transfusions if possible.

Anemia of Chronic Renal Disease
Often combined with iron-deficiency; patients don't have to be on dialysis.

I. Anemia of Chronic Disease

► H&P Keys
Symptoms of underlying disorder (weight loss, anorexia, myalgias, arthralgias).

► Diagnosis
- Hb rarely < 9 g/dL, normochromic normocytic.
- Normal or increased serum ferritin.
- Decreased reticulocyte count and TIBC.
- Bone marrow: adequate to increased iron stores.

► Disease Severity
Clinical signs of anemia.

► Concept and Application
Abnormal utilization of iron. Decreased RBC survival. Inadequate production of erythropoietin with respect to anemia.

► Treatment Steps
1. Treat underlying disease.
2. Subcutaneous erythropoietin, usually weekly.
3. Transfuse if necessary.

J. Sickle Cell Anemia

► H&P Keys
History of painful crises, leukocytosis, splenic infarctions, renal papillary necrosis, aseptic necrosis, cerebrovascular accident (CVA), priapism, bilirubin stones, infections with encapsulated microorganisms, osteomyelitis with *Staphylococcus* or *Salmonella*. Family history.

► Diagnosis
Peripheral smear reveals sickle-shaped cells, Howell–Jolly bodies, nucleated RBCs, reticulocytosis, thrombocytosis. HbS on electrophoresis. Prenatal diagnosis by amniotic fluid DNA analysis.

► Disease Severity
Heterozygous state (sickle cell trait) usually asymptomatic, but a frequent cause of hematuria secondary to papillary necrosis. Homozygous state results in severe hemolytic anemia (Fig. 5–2).

Factors that induce sickling: infection, dehydration, low oxygen tension, low pH. Microvascular occlusion can lead to ischemia and tissue infarction known as a *pain crisis*. Aplastic crisis (abrupt halt in erythropoiesis) caused by parvovirus B19 infection.

► Concept and Application
Point mutation at position 6 of β-globin chains (glutamic acid to valine) allows for polymerization. Amount of Hb in cell important; sickle trait plus thalassemia less severe than homozygous sickle cell anemia.

► Treatment Steps

Chronic
1. Folate 1–2 mg PO daily.
2. Pneumovax.
3. Antibiotic prophylaxis in childhood.
4. Genetic counseling.
5. Hydroxyurea helpful in some patients.
6. Hypertransfusion to suppress Hb S levels.

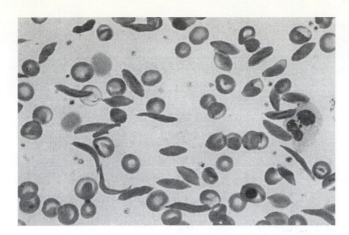

Figure 5–2. Homozygous sickle cell disease.

Acute

1. Treat pain crises with hydration, adequate analgesia, and treatment of inciting event if known.
2. Oxygen if patient is hypoxic.
3. Transfusion or exchange transfusion for CVA or acute chest syndrome.

II. MALIGNANT DISEASES

A. Acute Myelogenous Leukemia (AML)

▶ H&P Keys

Fatigue, bruising, petechiae, overt bleeding (e.g., menorrhagia), fever, or evidence of infection. In certain subtypes of AML gingival hypertrophy, skin lesions, or DIC; modest splenomegaly.

▶ Diagnosis

CBC reveals anemia and thrombocytopenia. White blood count (WBC) usually elevated with increased blasts or occasionally depressed. Auer rods in some subtypes. Bone marrow is usually hypercellular, positive peroxidase or Sudan black staining, negative periodic acid-Schiff (PAS) staining. Flow cytometry to determine cell surface markers. Cytogenetic abnormalities include: t(8;21) (M2), t(15;17) (M3), inv16 (M4 with eosinophils). Central nervous system (CNS) involvement can be seen in M4 and M5 subtypes. Spuriously low Po_2 and serum glucose can be seen with high WBC.

▶ Disease Severity

Very high WBC can cause leukostasis with CNS symptoms or pulmonary syndromes. AML in elderly patients, AML occurring after chemotherapy for other malignancies, and AML developing in a patient with myelodysplastic syndrome (MDS) has a very poor prognosis.

French–American–British (FAB) Classification—Still in common use but many modifications exist:

- M0: undifferentiated cells
- M1: minimal maturation
- M2: early differentiated cells, Auer rods, t(8;21)
- M3: acute promyelocytic leukemia (APL), large granules, Auer rods, t(15;17)

- M4: myelomonocytic leukemia, inv (16)
- M5: monocytic leukemia, 11q23 mutations
- M6: erythrocytic leukemia, 5 and 7 deletions
- M7: megakaryoblastic leukemia

▶ Concept and Application

Failure of myeloid stem cells to differentiate normally leads to progressive accumulation of leukemic blasts. Anemia and thrombocytopenia are due to lack of normal stem cells.

▶ Treatment Steps

1. Pathologic diagnosis based on bone marrow biopsy, cytogenetics, and cell typing.
2. Antibiotics if infected.
3. Transfusion of blood products as needed.
4. All-trans retinoic acid (ATRA) for acute promyelocytic leukemia (APML) (M3). Monitor for DIC. Conventional cytotoxics once induction is complete.
5. Allopurinol to prevent urate nephropathy.
6. Monitor for tumor lysis with serum K^+, creatinine, and PO_4.
7. Treatment usually includes an induction phase followed by 2–4 consolidation cycles.
8. Bone marrow transplant later in appropriate patients.

B. Acute Lymphocytic Leukemia (ALL)

▶ H&P Keys

Fatigue, anorexia, easy bruising or overt bleeding (petechiae), fever or evidence of infection, lymphadenopathy, splenomegaly, or mediastinal mass. Headache or stiff neck suggests CNS disease. Testicular mass can be seen occasionally.

▶ Diagnosis

Hypercellular bone marrow with > 30% blasts. Blasts are often positive for terminal deoxynucleotidyltransferase (TdT), common acute lymphoblastic leukemia antigen (CALLA) (CD10), and PAS; and negative for peroxidase and Sudan black. Flow cytometry to determine cell surface markers. Elevated WBC, anemia, thrombocytopenia. Lumbar puncture to rule out CNS involvement. Elevated creatinine, LDH, PO_4, K^+ predict for tumor lysis syndrome. Philadelphia (Ph) chromosome t(9;22), seen in 10% of children and 30% of adults, confers a poor prognosis. Burkitt's type of ALL accompanied by t(8;14), t(2;8), or t(8;22) involving c-myc oncogene.

▶ Disease Severity

Favorable Prognostic Factors—Young age, low WBC, Ph negative, no CNS disease, CALLA positive, rapid induction of remission.

Subclassifications—Significant revisions under way—expect more complex terminology soon.

- L1: small cells, scant cytoplasm, most common in children
- L2: large cells, moderate cytoplasm, most common in adults
- L3: vacuolated, abundant cytoplasm, Burkitt's type

▶ Concept and Application

Block in differentiation results in the accumulation of immature cells with abnormal function.

► Treatment Steps

1. Pathologic diagnosis based on bone marrow biopsy, cytogenetics, and cell typing.
2. Antiobiotics if infected.
3. Transfusion of blood products as needed.
4. Induction chemotherapy followed by maintenance for 2–3 years.
5. Monitor for tumor lysis.
6. CNS prophylaxis with intrathecal chemotherapy.
7. Maintenance chemotherapy for 2–3 years.
8. Bone marrow transplant in selected patients.

C. Chronic Myelogenous Leukemia (CML)

► H&P Keys

Nonspecific complaints most common; weakness, malaise, weight loss. Left upper quadrant fullness, early satiety and discomfort secondary to splenomegaly. In acute phase of disease, can present like acute leukemia.

► Diagnosis

Bone marrow is hypercellular with a marked proliferation of all granulocytic elements, increased eosinophils and basophils, and mild fibrosis. Ph chromosome t(9;22) positive, low leukocyte alkaline phosphatase (LAP) score. Increased WBC (50,000–300,000/μL), hyperuricemia, and increased serum B_{12}. Normal platelets and mild anemia in chronic phase.

► Disease Severity

Degree of splenomegaly, percentage of blasts, basophilia and eosinophilia can predict for survival. Presence of cytogenetic abnormalities in addition to Ph chromosome predicts for blastic transformation.

► Concept and Application

Myeloproliferative disorder characterized by an abnormal proliferation of myeloid cells without the loss of capacity to differentiate; bcr-abl rearrangement seen in nearly all patients.

► Treatment Steps

1. Gleevec should be started as soon as the diagnosis is confirmed.
2. Allopurinol to prevent urate nephropathy if WBC count high.
3. Bone marrow transplant is considered for some patients with HLA-matched donors.

D. Chronic Lymphocytic Leukemia (CLL)

► H&P Keys

Usually a disease of elderly patients. Often asymptomatic leukocytosis. Some patients present with lymphadenopathy, hepatosplenomegaly, anemia, or thrombocytopenia.

► Diagnosis

Elevated WBC (> 15,000 μL with lymphocytes > 60%). Look for κ/λ clonal excess or presence of CD5+ CD19+ cells to confirm diagnosis. Chromosomal abnormalities such as 14q+ and trisomy 12 can be seen (Fig. 5–3). Bone marrow is hypercellular and monotonous, with diffuse infiltration of small- and medium-size lymphocytes.

Observable autoimmune phenomena (e.g., Coombs' test positive, hemolytic anemia, immune thrombocytopenic purpura). Hypogammaglobulinemia.

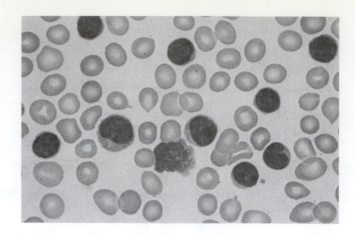

Figure 5–3. Chronic lymphocytic leukemia.

► **Disease Severity**

Several staging systems. Rai staging best known:

- Stage 0: lymphocytosis only
- Stage 1: lymphocytosis with lymphadenopathy
- Stage 2: lymphocytosis with splenomegaly
- Stage 3: lymphocytosis with anemia
- Stage 4: lymphocytosis with thrombocytopenia

Modified Rai staging:

- Low risk: stages 0 and 1
- Intermediate risk: stages 2 and 3
- High risk: stage 4

Aggressive transformation into large-cell lymphoma, Richter's transformation.

► **Concept and Application**

Monoclonal proliferation of dysfunctional mature β lymphocytes. More frequent infections due to lack of opsonization.

► **Treatment Steps**

1. Observation for low-risk patients.
2. Treat higher-risk or symptomatic patients with chlorambucil and prednisone or fludarabine.

E. Hodgkin's Disease

► **H&P Keys**

Frequently younger patients. Superficial, painless, enlarged "rubbery" lymph nodes (60–80% cervical or axillary, nontender), splenomegaly. "B" symptoms: fevers, night sweats, weight loss. Infections associated with depressed cell-mediated immunity. Bimodal peak incidence.

► **Diagnosis**

Lymph node biopsy reveals Reed–Sternberg cells with reactive lymphocytes (Fig. 5–4). Disease spread by contiguous lymph node chains. Initial staging tests include computed tomographic (CT) scans of the chest, abdomen, and pelvis, bone marrow aspiration and biopsy. Positron-emission tomography (PET) and gallium scans are useful in bulky disease. Laparotomy and lymphangiogram are rarely performed. Nodular sclerosing subtype most common. Lymphocyte-depleted histologic specimens associated with poor prognosis. Mixed cellularity and lymphocyte-predominant tissues offer better prognosis.

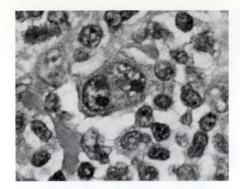

Figure 5–4. Reed–Sternberg cell of Hodgkin's disease.

► **Disease Severity**

Ann Arbor Staging
- Stage I: single lymph node group
- Stage II: multiple lymph node groups on the same side of the diaphragm
- Stage III: involved lymph node groups on both sides of the diaphragm
- Stage IV: extranodal disease (bone marrow involvement, liver involvement, lung or skin involvement)

"B" symptoms: fevers, night sweats, and 10% weight loss. Stage A: absence of B symptoms. B symptoms are a poor prognostic marker independent of stage.

► **Concept and Application**

Cell of origin is a centroblast (proliferating germinal center cell). Defective T-cell function.

► **Treatment Steps**

1. Staging as outlined previously is critical.
2. Treatment is stage related.
   - Stage IA–IIA: extended field radiation
   - Stage IB–IIB: extended field and chemotherapy
   - Stage IIIA/B and IVA/B: combination chemotherapy
   - Bulky disease: radiation and chemotherapy

Chemotherapy consists of mechlorethamine, Oncovin (vincristine), procarbazine, and prednisone (MOPP)/Adriamycin (doxorubicin), bleomycin, and vinblastine (ABV).

F. Low-Grade Lymphoma

► **H&P Keys**

Lymphadenopathy usually diffuse and not necessarily contiguous. Splenomegaly can be seen. Extranodal (e.g., bone marrow) disease common. Rarely, fever, weight loss, night sweats.

► **Diagnosis**

Lymph node biopsy. Bone marrow aspiration and biopsy (bone marrow involvement common). κ/λ clonal excess. Immunoglobulin gene rearrangement. Cytogenetic studies, e.g., t(14;18), associated with follicular lymphoma (Fig. 5–5).

► **Disease Severity**

Ann Arbor staging system (see Hodgkin's disease staging). Chest x-ray (CXR), CT scans of chest, abdomen, and pelvis. Often stage IV

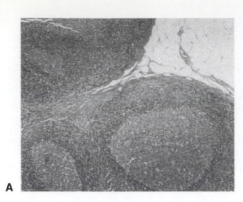
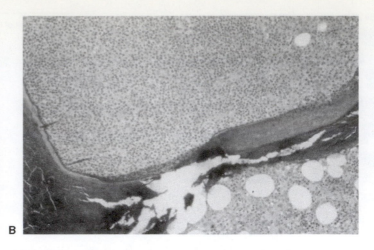

Figure 5–5. (A) A benign lymphoid follicle compared to (B) lymphoma involving the marrow.

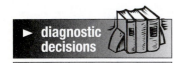

LYMPHOMAS

Low Grade
Patients are older, often with stage III or IV disease; disease is treatable and the life expectancy is usually many years. Types include: small lymphocytic (same as CLL), plasmacytoid, follicular small cell, and follicular mixed.

Intermediate Grade
Lots of variability; some behave in more indolent fashions and some are more aggressive. Individual type very important. Types include: follicular large cell, diffuse small cleaved, diffuse mixed, and maybe diffuse large cell.

High Grade
Often younger patients; aggressive therapy can result in cure. Types include: immunoblastic, lymphoblastic, and Burkitt's.

due to bone marrow infiltration. Presence of B symptoms, LDH, performance status.

▶ Concept and Application

Clonal proliferation of B-cell lymphocytes, rarely T cells. Can transform into more aggressive lymphoma.

▶ Treatment Steps
1. Watchful waiting acceptable if asymptomatic.
2. Treatment for bulky disease, obstruction of vital structures, cytopenias, or autoimmune complications.
3. Treatment options include alkylating agents plus corticosteroids, radiation, fludarabine, Rituxan. Occasional patients require aggressive cytotoxics.

G. Intermediate- or High-Grade Lymphoma

▶ H&P Keys

Lymphadenopathy, splenomegaly. Extranodal disease can be seen. Fatigue, malaise. Rapidly enlarging lymphadenopathy can occur (especially Burkitt's lymphoma). Mediastinal mass can cause symptoms.

▶ Diagnosis

Lymph node biopsy to make diagnosis. Needle biopsy not sufficient. Bone marrow aspiration and biopsy. Spinal tap to rule out meningeal spread especially in lymphoblastic lymphoma. Burkitt's lymphoma associated with Epstein–Barr virus (EBV) and translocation t(8;14), t(2;8) or t(8;22). Increased LDH in aggressive disease. CXR to evaluate mediastinum. CT scans of chest, abdomen, and pelvis. PET can be helpful. Testing for human immunodeficiency virus (HIV). Tumor lysis can be seen with rapidly growing lymphomas (e.g., Burkitt's).

▶ Disease Severity

Ann Arbor staging system. Bone marrow involvement or CNS involvement have worse prognosis. Evidence of tumor lysis. Poor prognosis, increased age, large tumor masses, B symptoms, bone marrow involvement, increased LDH, poor performance status, HIV associated.

▶ Concept and Application

Most commonly clonal proliferation of B cells. Lymphoblastic lymphoma and cutaneous lymphomas frequently of T-cell origin. Different histologies represent block at different stages of B-cell development.

▶ Treatment Steps

1. Staging as outlined previously.
2. Monitor LDH, PO_4, creatine for tumor lysis complications.
3. Allopurinol in acute treatment period to prevent urate nephropathy.
4. Intensive combination chemotherapy—CHOP (cytoxan, doxorubicin, Oncovin [vincristine], and prednisone) remains the standard. Add Rituxamab if CD20+.
5. If CNS is involved, intrathecal chemotherapy.
6. Relapsed but still responsive disease can be considered for dose-intense chemotherapy with marrow support.

H. Multiple Myeloma

▶ H&P Keys

Anemia, bone pain, increased susceptibility to infections, fatigue, weight loss, renal insufficiency, altered mental status.

▶ Diagnosis

Anemia, hypercalcemia, presence of a paraprotein (or M-component) on serum protein electrophoresis (SPEP), Bence Jones proteins on urine protein electrophoresis (UPEP), lytic bone lesions on skeletal survey, bone marrow with > 30% plasma cells. Measure β_2 microglobulin and serum creatinine. Quantitate amount of immunoglobulin present. Serum viscosity if altered mental status present.

▶ Disease Severity

• Stage I: Low tumor burden with Hb > 10 g/dL, normal calcium, IgG < 5 g/dL, IgA < 3 g/dL, urine light chains < 4 g/24 hours, and normal skeletal survey.
• Stage II: Intermediate tumor burden; patients who are neither stage I nor stage III.
• Stage III: High tumor burden and any one of the following: Hb < 8.5 g/dL, serum calcium > 12 mg/dL, IgG > 7 g/dL, IgA > 5 g/dL, urine light chains > 12 g/24 hours, or extensive lytic bone lesions. The following subclassification of stages is used:
  A. Creatinine level > 2 mg/dL
  B. Creatinine level ≥ 2 mg/dL

   Elevated β_2 microglobulin at diagnosis reflects a poor prognosis.

▶ Concept and Application

Monoclonal proliferation of plasma cells in the bone marrow. Osteoclastic activating factors (possibly interleukins [IL-1, IL-6], tumor necrosis factor [TNF]) responsible for bone lesions. Bone destruction leading to pathologic fractures, pain, hypercalcemia. Patients can develop amyloid deposition over time.

▶ Treatment Steps

1. Manage low stage disease conservatively.
2. Chemotherapy for symptomatic or more advanced disease—melphalan and prednisone or VAD (vincristine, adriamycin,

decadron) are common first-line approaches. Thalidomide has recently been approved.

3. Radiation for palliation of localized lesions causing pain.
4. High-dose chemotherapy with bone marrow transplant useful for certain patients.

I. Monoclonal Gammopathy of Undetermined Significance

▶ **H&P Keys**

Patients are generally asymptomatic.

▶ **Diagnosis**

Presence of a paraprotein on serum electrophoresis that is monoclonal, without suppression of the other immunoglobulins. No other evidence of disease.

▶ **Disease Severity**

Should be none.

▶ **Concept and Application**

Monoclonal proliferation of plasma cells in the bone marrow without evidence of organ damage. Paraprotein does not reach significant levels, and marrow function is not compromised. Thirty-three percent of patients will ultimately develop a clear-cut process in a 20-year follow-up period. Of those 33%, 66% will develop multiple myeloma, 12% macroglobulemia, 14% amyloidosis, and 8% another lymphoproliferative disorder.

▶ **Treatment Steps**

1. Follow the immunoglubulin levels, 3, 6, and 12 months. Yearly follow-up is probably adequate in a patient whose levels are not rising appreciably.
2. Intervene only if process progresses to a definable disease.

III. OTHER DISORDERS

A. Polycythemia (Erythrocytosis)

▶ **H&P Keys**

Often asymptomatic, diagnosed on routine lab tests. Splenomegaly, early satiety, hypertension, facial plethora, venous thromboses, hemorrhages. History of tobacco use, travel to high altitudes. Spurious erythrocytosis results from decreased plasma volume. If a true erythrocytosis, consider if physiologically appropriate: chronic obstructive pulmonary disease (COPD), right-to-left cardiac shunt, high-affinity Hb, carboxyhemoglobinemia. Physiologically inappropriate: tumors producing erythropoietin (renal cell, hepatocellular), renal disease, adrenal cortical hyperplasia, exogenous androgens.

▶ **Diagnosis**

Increased RBC mass with normal plasma volume key to diagnosis. In primary process, polycythemia rubra vera (PRV), erythropoietin levels are normal or low. Hypercellular bone marrow. WBC and platelet counts are normal or elevated, increased LAP, increased B_{12}, low or absent iron stores. Other causes (see above) must be ruled out.

► Disease Severity

Degree of hematocrit (Hct) elevation determines whole-blood viscosity. Decreased cerebral blood flow. Thromboembolism or life-threatening hemorrhage can occur. Can transform to myelofibrosis or acute leukemia but not secondary or spurious polycythemia.

► Concept and Application

PRV is an autonomous proliferation of erythroid progenitors resulting from clonal proliferation of the pluripotent hematopoietic stem cell. Secondary polycythemia is stimulation of red cell production either because of physiologically appropriate or inappropriate secretion of erythropoietin.

► Treatment Steps

1. Phlebotomy combined with hydroxyurea for PRV.
2. If secondary, balance phlebotomies with physiologic needs.
3. Optimal Hct is approximately 45%.
4. P32 used occasionally for elderly patients.

B. Transfusion Reactions

► H&P Keys

Occur minutes, hours, or days after transfusion. Most severe is immune-mediated hemolytic reaction: fever, chest or back pain, hypotension, dyspnea, hemoglobinuria, shock. Most common are febrile reactions caused by WBCs present in packed RBCs, now decreased secondary to common use of WBC filtering by blood banks. Rarely, febrile reactions are due to bacterial contamination.

Patients with IgA deficiency can have anaphylactic reaction: sudden onset; no fever; may have cough, respiratory distress, hypotension, nausea, vomiting, abdominal pain, loss of consciousness, and shock. Delayed hemolytic transfusion reaction results from minor antigen mismatch (not detected by indirect Coombs' test). Post-transfusion purpura results in moderate to severe thrombocytopenia 2–10 days following transfusion of packed RBCs.

► Diagnosis

Stop transfusion and return unit to blood bank. Monitor Hb and Hct, hemoglobinuria, unconjugated bilirubin, haptoglobin, LDH, coagulation profile, and renal profile. Repeat ABO, Rh, and compatibility screens. Direct antiglobulin test on posttransfusion blood sample from patient. Check IgA level if anaphylaxis. Culture remainder of blood product.

► Disease Severity

Most severe reactions are major hemolytic transfusion reaction and anaphylaxis.

► Concept and Application

Major hemolytic transfusion reaction caused by ABO incompatibility. Most often a result of clinical error.

► Treatment Steps

1. Stop transfusion.
2. Maintain blood pressure and urine output with IV fluids.
3. For anaphylaxis: epinephrine, diphenhydramine hydrochloride (Benadryl), and glucocorticoids.
4. Antibiotics if bacterial contamination suspected.
5. Premedicate with acetaminophen and use WBC filters to prevent febrile reactions.

C. Hemophilia A and B

▶ H&P Keys

Hereditary bleeding disorders. Hemophilia A most common. A and B are clinically indistinguishable. Frequent episodes of bleeding into joints, muscles, and skin with minimal or no trauma. Can result in chronic arthritis. Prolonged postoperative hemorrhage. Intracranial hemorrhage can occur.

▶ Diagnosis

Elevated partial thromboplastin time (PTT) and low factor VIII or IX level. Normal bleeding time, normal prothrombin time (PT), normal thromboplastin time (TT). Specific assays for factor VIII or IX. Polymerase chain reaction (PCR) analysis for prenatal detection.

▶ Disease Severity

Patients with < 1% factor VIII (or IX) level have severe disease; > 5% factor VIII (or IX) results in mild disease. Clinical history very important in predicting bleeding tendency.

▶ Concept and Application

X-linked recessive bleeding disorder resulting from deficiency of factor VIII (hemophilia A) or IX (hemophilia B).

▶ Treatment Steps

Mild Hemophilia A

1. First-line therapy is desmopressin (DDAVP) (stimulates immediate release of VIII:C and von Willebrand factor [vWF] from endothelial cell stores).
2. Second-line therapy is recombinant human factor VIII.

Severe Hemophilia A

Recombinant human factor VIII or factor VIII concentrate.

Hemophilia B

1. Desmopressin not effective.
2. Recombinant human factor IX.

D. von Willebrand Disease

▶ H&P Keys

Mucocutaneous bleeding, epistaxis, GI bleeding, menorrhagia. Joint and intramuscular bleeding rare. Posttraumatic, postsurgical, and dental bleeding may be severe.

▶ Diagnosis

(1) Prolonged bleeding time. PTT can be prolonged or normal. (2) Decreased factor VIII:C activity. (3) Decreased ristocetin cofactor on platelet aggregation studies. (4) Decreased vWF. (5) Multimeric analysis.

Type I—Generalized decrease in all multimeric forms of plasma vWF.

Type II—Selective deficiency of higher-molecular-weight forms. Normal or near-normal levels but dysfunctional.

Type III—Markedly decreased plasma and platelet levels of vWF. Autosomal recessive.

Pseudo von Willebrand Disease—Abnormal vWF platelet receptor.

► Disease Severity

Repeat testing may be necessary to make diagnosis. Hemorrhagic tendency widely variable. Clinical history very important.

► Concept and Application

Quantitative or qualitative abnormalities of the vWF protein, which is required for normal attachment of platelets to the endothelium. This interaction is critical for normal platelet function. vWF is also necessary for normal factor VIII coagulant activity. Autosomal dominant trait with variable presentation.

► Treatment Step

1. Establish form of von Willebrand disease.
2. DDAVP for patients with mild disease. This is not useful in most types of patients with type II or any type III.
3. Factor VIII concentrate for moderate to severe disease.
4. Platelets for pseudo von Willebrand disease.
5. Aminocaproic acid (Amicar) lessens mucosal bleeding.

E. Vitamin K Deficiency

► H&P Keys

Inadequate supply (dietary deficiency, antibiotic therapy). Surreptitious ingestion of warfarin anticoagulants. Prolonged hospitalization.

► Diagnosis

Elevated PT, normal PTT, and normal bleeding time. Mixing study corrects prolonged PT.

► Disease Severity

Bleeding.

► Concept and Application

Vitamin K essential for final posttranslational carboxylation of factors II, VII, IX, and X.

► Treatment Steps

Oral or subcutaneous vitamin K, rarely IV.

F. Hypercoagulable States

► H&P Keys

Patients may have recurrent thrombosis, emboli, or recurrent miscarriages. Lupus inhibitors are more common in patients with autoimmune diseases, malignancies, and HIV/AIDS. Family history of thrombosis, particularly at younger ages.

► Diagnosis

Lupus inhibitor, anticardiolipin antibodies, protein C activity, protein S activity, factor V Leiden mutation, prothrombin gene mutation, antithrombin III activity, homocysteine.

► Disease Severity

Thromboses such as deep vein thrombosis (DVT), pulmonary embolism, cerebrovascular accident (CVA), or recurrent miscarriages.

► Concept and Application

Abnormalities in the coagulation system that results in either increased clot formation or decreased clot-limiting factors.

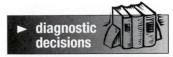

► diagnostic decisions

COAGULOPATHIES

Prolonged Prothrombin Time (PT)

1. Vitamin K deficiency: patients on antibiotics, prolonged hospitalizations, poor oral intake.
2. Warfarin (Coumadin): related also to a common rat poison.
3. Factor VII deficiency.

Prolonged Activated Partial Thromboplastin Time (aPTT)

1. Heparin: check the blood draw site—was it above the IV infusing the heparin; was the sample drawn from a heparinized port?
2. Factor VIII deficiency/inhibitor: deficiency is usually manifest from birth and there is usually a family history; the inhibitor is acquired and occurs later in life.
3. Factor IX deficiency/inhibitor: less common than VIII but the same issues apply.
4. XI, XII, and high-molecular-weight kininogen (HMWK) deficiency: very rare.

Combined

1. Hepatic dysfunction.
2. Very severe compromise of the vitamin K–dependent factors.
3. Factor V deficiency.
4. Factor X deficiency.
5. Abnormal thrombin.

► **Treatment Steps**
1. Therapy not required for asymptomatic patients.
2. Treat thromboses and emboli with heparin acutely.
3. Consider prophylactic anticoagulation during hypercoaguable periods (e.g., postop, pregnancy).
4. Consider chronic anticoagulation for repeated thrombotic events or a single life-threatening event. Choice of agent will vary depending on the underlying cause.

G. Disseminated Intravascular Coagulation (DIC)

► **H&P Keys**

Activation of coagulation pathways resulting in both clotting and bleeding tendencies. Diffuse bleeding (IV sites, etc.), petechiae, purpura; may also see evidence of thrombosis. Caused by sepsis, cancers (particularly associated with APML and adenocarcinomas), tissue damage, and amniotic fluid embolism.

► **Diagnosis**

PT and PTT elevated. Low fibrinogen, increased fibrin split products (FSPs), decreased factors V and VIII. Presence of D-dimers. Microangiopathic hemolytic anemia with schistocytes on peripheral smear; thrombocytopenia.

► **Disease Severity**

Degree of decrease in fibrinogen and platelet levels and PT prolongation. Degree of organ damage secondary to bleeding and clotting.

► **Concept and Application**

Pathologic activation of coagulation with resultant intravascular generation of excess thrombin. Thrombin stimulates platelet aggregation. Platelets become trapped in fibrin deposited in the microvasculature. Fibrin strands "clog" microvasculature and induce localized hemolysis.

► **Treatment Steps**
1. Treat underlying disease.
2. Carefully replace clotting factors and platelets as necessary.

H. Idiopathic Thrombocytopenic Purpura (ITP)

► **H&P Keys**

Mucosal and skin bleeding. ITP in children has acute onset and is often a self-limited disease that develops after a viral infection and lasts 5–6 months. Adults have a gradual onset, with only 10–15% developing spontaneous remissions. Often, ITP is associated with SLE, Hodgkin's disease, CLL, ulcerative colitis, and infection.

► **Diagnosis**

Decreased platelet count. Increased number of megakaryocytes in bone marrow. Peripheral smear often reveals large platelets.

► **Disease Severity**

Severity of thrombocytopenia (platelets < 20,000 associated with risk of spontaneous bleeding).

► **Concepts and Application**

Usually autoimmune. Accelerated platelet destruction in spleen after coating of platelets by IgG autoantibody. Extravascular platelet destruction.

▶ Treatment Steps
1. Corticosteroids are first-line therapy.
2. Second-line therapy is variable and includes immunoglobulin, splenectomy, Win RhoD, and danazol.
3. Treat associated disease process.

I. Thrombotic Thrombocytopenic Purpura (TTP)

▶ H&P Keys

Onset may be fulminant or subacute, single episode or recurring. Mental status changes result of intermittent ischemia. Classic pentad: fever, renal dysfunction, neurologic changes, thrombocytopenia, microangiopathic hemolytic anemia.

▶ Diagnosis

Low platelet count, normal or increased number of megakaryocytes in bone marrow, increased LDH, and schistocytes on smear. Elevated blood urea nitrogen (BUN), creatinine, and proteinuria reflect renal disease. DIC testing is negative.

▶ Disease Severity

Severity of neurologic symptoms (coma) and hemolysis.

▶ Concept and Application

Endothelial damage in microcirculation leads to platelet microthrombi, occlusion of small vessels, and ischemia in tissues. Abnormal vWf multimers.

▶ Treatment Steps
1. Plasmapheresis.
2. If plasmapheresis unavailable, infuse fresh frozen plasma.
3. Treat underlying condition.
4. Corticosteroids usually given unless contraindicated.

J. Essential Thrombocythemia

▶ H&P Keys

Usually asymptomatic. Neurologic symptoms most common: headache, visual changes. Episodes of thrombosis, embolism, or hemorrhage can occur.

▶ Diagnosis

Platelet count > 800,000. Bone marrow: increased number of megakaryocytes. Normal Hb level. Mildly increased WBC. Platelet function testing usually abnormal. Rule out chronic inflammation, iron deficiency.

▶ Disease Severity

Complications infrequent in younger patients. In elderly patients, transient ischemic attack (TIA) is the most common complication. CNS hemorrhage or CVA secondary to emboli.

▶ Concept and Application

Uncontrolled clonal proliferation of megakaryocytic precursors.

▶ Treatment Steps
1. Hydroxyurea.
2. Antiplatelet agents for ischemia.

K. Platelet Dysfunction

▶ H&P Keys

Intrinsic—Congenital defect, easy bruising, epistaxis, menorrhagia with normal platelet count.

Extrinsic—Acquired defect secondary to myeloproliferative disease, uremia, or drugs (aspirin, clopidrogel).

▶ Diagnosis

Increased bleeding time. Abnormal aggregation studies.

▶ Disease Severity

Spontaneous platelet-type bleeding.

▶ Concept and Application

Platelets fail to adhere to endothelium or to aggregate because of a deficiency of surface glycoproteins that bind fibrinogen or vWf. Failure to release platelet storage pool.

▶ Management

1. For congenital platelet dysfunction, trial of DDAVP.
2. For uremia, dialysis and DDAVP.
3. Discontinue offending drugs.
4. Transfuse platelets as necessary for bleeding.

L. Agnogenic Myeloid Metaplasia

▶ H&P Keys

Presents with symptoms of anemia or splenomegaly. Weight loss, fatigue, early satiety, lymphadenopathy. Older patients.

▶ Diagnosis

Anemia, nucleated RBCs, teardrop cells. Bone marrow biopsy shows increased fibrosis, increased megakaryocytes.

▶ Disease Severity

Extent of fibrosis in bone marrow and extramedullary hematopoiesis. Can evolve into acute leukemia.

▶ Concept and Application

Increased type III collagen production. Replacement of normal bone marrow with fibrosis.

▶ Treatment Steps

1. Transfuse as needed.
2. Colony stimulating factors (erythropoietin, granulocyte colony-stimulating factor [G-CSF], granulocyte macrophage colony-stimulating factor [GM-CSF].
3. Splenectomy rarely for painful enlargement or refractory cytopenias caused by splenic sequestration.

M. Neutropenia

▶ H&P Keys

Acquired or congenital. Autoimmune neutropenia (Felty's syndrome) is seen as an isolated event and in rheumatoid arthritis and other systemic autoimmune disorders. Cyclic neutropenia: fatigue, decreased appetite, mouth sores that occur every 3 weeks and last 3–4 days. Evidence of infection: mouth sores, sore throat, skin infections, pneumonia, urinary tract infection.

► Diagnosis

CBC, follow sequential absolute neutrophil counts (ANCs). Perform bone marrow study to rule out malignancy. If febrile and ANC < 500, obtain cultures.

► Disease Severity

Fungal infections or sepsis can develop. Agranulocytosis is very serious (ANC < 200).

► Concept and Application

Cyclic neutropenia results from stem cell defect. Neutrophil-specific antibodies of IgG and IgM subtypes are detected in Felty's syndrome. Drug-induced marrow suppression often reversible if neutropenia; if agranulocytosis, often irreversible.

► Treatment Steps

1. Chronic G-CSF.
2. If possible, treat underlying disorder.
3. If febrile, broad-spectrum antibiotics.

BIBLIOGRAPHY

Armitage J (ed.). *Atlas of Clinical Hematology.* Philadelphia: Lippincot Williams & Wilkins, 2004.

Lichtman MA, et al (eds.). *Williams Hematology,* 7th ed. New York: McGraw-Hill, 2006.

Colman RW (ed.). *Hemostasis and Thrombosis: Basic Principles and Clinical Practice.* Philadelphia: J.B. Lippincott, 2000.

DeVita V, Hellman S, Rosenberg S (eds.). *Cancer: Principles & Practice of Oncology,* 6th ed. Philadelphia: Lippincott-Raven, 2001.

Hoffman R, Benz E Jr., Shattil S, et al (eds.). *Hematology: Basic Principles and Practice,* 4th ed. New York: Churchill Livingstone, 2005.

Immunology and Allergy | 6

I. BRONCHIAL ASTHMA

▶ H&P Keys

Chronic or recurrent cough, dyspnea, or wheezing. Prolonged expiration and wheezing with or without use of accessory muscles. Affects > 5% of the population. Incidence, mortality, and hospitalization rates increasing. Allergic (extrinsic) asthma related to exposure to allergens (seasonal pollens such as grasses, trees, and weeds; animal dander, dust mites, and mold). Nonallergic asthma (intrinsic) associated with infection, stress, environmental pollution, exercise, cold air, and in a small percentage of patients, aspirin use.

▶ Diagnosis

Pulmonary function studies with a reversible obstructive pattern, positive methacholine challenge, sputum rich in eosinophils, and response to bronchodilator therapy. Chest x-ray (CXR), total eosinophil count, total immunoglobulin E (IgE), and allergy skin tests. Oximetry and arterial blood gases (ABGs) in acutely ill patients.

▶ Disease Severity

Mild Intermittent—Symptoms < 2/week, insomnia related to asthma < 3/month, forced expiratory volume (FEV) > 80% of predicted.

Mild Persistent—Symptoms > 2/week but < 1/day, insomnia > 2/month, FEV > 80% of predicted.

Moderate Persistent—Daily symptoms, symptoms affect activity, insomnia > 1/week, FEV > 60% but < 80% of predicted.

Severe Persistent—Continual symptoms, limited physical activity, frequent insomnia, FEV < 60% of predicted.

▶ management decisions

ASTHMA

Disease	Treatment
Exercise-induced asthma	Short-acting β_2-adrenergic (albuterol)—2 puffs 15 minutes prior to exercise. and/or Cromolyn (Intal)—2 puffs prior to exercise.
Mild intermittent asthma	Short-acting β_2-adrenergic (albuterol)—2 puffs qid, prn.
Mild persistent asthma	Add inhaled low- to medium-potency corticosteroid (Flovent 44 or 110—2 puffs bid).
Moderate persistent asthma	Add leukotriene modifier (Singulair, 10 mg qd) or long-acting β_2-adrenergic (Serevent—2 puffs bid). and/or Increase the inhaled corticosteroid dose.
Severe persistent asthma	Increase the inhaled corticosteroid dose (Flovent 220—2–4 puffs bid). Add theophylline, nedocromil (Tilade), leukotriene modifier, oral long-acting β_2-adrenergic or oral corticosteroids.

► Concept and Application

Mast cell mediator release causes inflammatory changes including denudation of airway epithelium, edema, collagen deposition beneath basement membrane, mucus hypersecretion, smooth muscle contraction, and infiltration of neutrophils, eosinophils, and T-helper lymphocytes type 2 (Th2). Mediators include eosinophil chemotactic factor of anaphylaxis (ECF-A), neutrophil chemotactic factor of anaphylaxis (NCF-A), histamine, leukotrienes, prostaglandins, and platelet activating factor (PAF). Mast cell mediator release involves IgE trigger only in allergic type of asthma.

► Treatment Steps

General

1. Avoidance of precipitating factors, patient education.
2. Use peak flow meters in moderate and severe persistent asthma.
3. Immunotherapy (allergy injections) can be added as an anti-inflammatory adjunct.
4. Quick-relief medicine is the first step.
5. Add a long-term controller if a quick-relief medicine is necessary more than twice weekly.

Quick-Relief Medicines

1. Inhaled short-acting β_2-adrenergic (Albuterol HFA or Xopenex via nebulizer).
2. Inhaled ipratropium bromide (Atrovent).
3. Subcutaneous epinephrine.
4. Oral corticosteroids.
5. Intravenous corticosteroids.
6. Intravenous aminophylline.
7. Oxygen.
8. Combination inhaled short-acting β_2-adrenergic and ipratropium bromide (Combivent).

Long-Term-Control Medicines

1. Inhaled corticosteroid (Flovent 44, 110, or 220).
2. Inhaled long-acting β_2-adrenergic (Serevent Diskus).
3. Inhaled cromolyn sodium (Intal).
4. Inhaled nedocromil sodium (Tilade).
5. Oral sustained-release theophylline (UniDur).
6. Oral long-acting β_2-adrenergic (Volmax).
7. Oral leukotriene modifiers (Singulair, Accolate, Zyflo).
8. Combination inhaled corticosteroid and long-acting β_2-adrenergic (Advair 100/50, 250/50, or 500/50).

Treatment of Mild Intermittent Asthma

1. Inhaled short-acting β_2-adrenergic (Albuterol HFA), 2 puffs qid, prn.
2. For exercise-induced asthma, treat with an inhaled short-acting β_2-adrenergic (as previously) 15–20 minutes prior to exercise and/or Intal, 2 puffs, also prior to exercise.

Treatment of Mild Persistent Asthma

1. See the treatment of mild intermittent asthma.
2. Add an inhaled corticosteroid (Flovent 44, 2 puffs bid), followed by rinsing of the mouth to decrease the incidence of thrush.

Treatment of Moderate Persistent Asthma

1. See the treatment of mild persistent asthma.
2. Increase the strength and/or dose of the inhaled corticosteroid (Flovent 110, 2 puffs bid), followed by rinsing of the mouth.
3. Add a leukotriene modifier (Singulair 10 mg qd) and/or a long-acting β₂-adrenergic (Serevent 2 puffs bid).

Treatment of Severe Persistent Asthma

1. See the treatment of moderate persistent asthma.
2. Increase the strength and/or the dose of the inhaled corticosteroid (Flovent 220, 2 to 4 puffs bid), followed by rinsing of the mouth.
3. Add an oral sustained-release theophylline (Uniphyl).
4. Use a home nebulizer to deliver short-acting β₂-adrenergic therapy (albuterol solution 0.5%, 0.5 cc in 3 cc saline) and/or ipratropium bromide (one vial of Atrovent qid).
5. Tilade 2 puffs qid tapered to bid or Intal 2 puffs tid–qid may be added in the effort to decrease the use of inhaled corticosteroids.
6. Add a short course of oral corticosteroids (prednisone, 20 mg bid for 5 days).
7. If short courses of oral corticosteroids are used frequently, then change to alternate-day oral corticosteroids (prednisone, 20 mg every other morning). Morning dosing is preferred to minimize side effects involving the hypothalamic–pituitary–adrenal axis.
8. If symptoms are still unstable, resort to oral corticosteroids temporarily on a daily basis (prednisone, 20 mg qd) and wean to every-other-morning dosing.

Acute Episodes with Respiratory Distress—Nebulized sympathomimetic (albuterol), oxygen, IV corticosteroids, and in respiratory failure, intubation and mechanical ventilation.

II. ALLERGIC RHINITIS AND CONJUNCTIVITIS

► H&P Keys

Affects 20% of the population. Frequently affects other family members. Itchy eyes, nose, paroxysms of sneezing, pruritus of palate and throat. Postnasal drip, rhinorrhea, anosmia. Associated with serous otitis media, otitis media, or sinusitis. Seasonal symptoms caused by pollen or mold. Perennial symptoms result from exposure to animal dander, house dust mites, mold, and occupational allergens (e.g., flour). More common in children than adults. Signs include swollen bluish turbinates, nasal crease, injected conjunctivae, allergic shiners, allergic salute, and mouth breathing.

► Diagnosis

Positive allergy skin tests (epicutaneous and/or intradermal tests) or radioallergosorbent test (RAST) to suspected allergens. Nasal or conjunctival smear filled with eosinophils. Elevated total IgE.

► Concept and Application

Patient develops specific IgE antibodies to offending allergens. IgE binds to mast cells of nasal and conjunctivae mucosa. Environmental allergens trigger mast cell mediator release, including ECF-A, NCF-A, histamine, leukotrienes, prostaglandins, and PAF. Eosinophils and

► **management decisions**

ALLERGIC RHINOCONJUNCTIVITIS

Severity	Treatment
Mild	Avoidance techniques.
	Oral antihistamine (Allegra, 180 mg qd) with or without a decongestant (Sudafed).
	Ocular antihistamines (Naphcon A) or ocular antihistamine/mast cell stabilizer (Optivar).
Moderate	Add nasal corticosteroids (Nasonex—2 sprays each nostril qd).
	Add immunotherapy (allergy injections).
Moderate to severe	Add nasal antihistamine (Astelin—2 sprays in each nostril bid prn)
	or
	Nasal ipratropium bromide (Atrovent 0.03%—2 sprays in each nostril bid prn).
Severe	Nasal decongestants (Afrin—1–2 sprays in each nostril bid for 2–3 days).
	Oral corticosteroids (prednisone—1–2 mg/kg/day for 5–7 days).

neutrophils are found at site of allergic reaction and participate in the inflammatory reaction.

► **Treatment Steps**

1. Avoidance by removal of offending allergen from home (dog, cat), use of an air cleaner, or dust-proofing home.
2. Medicines:
   a. Oral antihistamines (Benadryl or Zyrtec) may be added to oral decongestants (Sudafed).
   b. Oral antihistamine/decongestant combination preparations (Allegra D or Claritin D) may be used instead of individual antihistamines and decongestants.
   c. Nasal corticosteroids (Nasacort AQ).
   d. Nasal antihistamines (Astelin).
   e. Nasal ipratropium bromide (Atrovent 0.03%).
   f. Nasal cromolyn sodium (Nasalcrom).
   g. Nasal decongestants (Afrin) should be avoided for extended periods as they may cause rhinitis medicamentosa.
   h. Ocular antihistamines/decongestants (Naphcon A).
   i. Ocular mast cell stabilizers (Patanol).
   j. Ocular corticosteroids (FML).
   k. Oral corticosteroids (prednisone).
3. Desensitization, also known as immunotherapy, to inhaled allergens.

III. ANAPHYLAXIS OR ANAPHYLACTOID REACTIONS

► **H&P Keys**

Sudden onset of urticaria, angioedema, wheezing, dyspnea, or hypotension. Patients may also have gastrointestinal or uterine cramps. Severe reaction may lead to hypovolemic shock and hypoxemia. Symptoms occur soon after taking a medication (e.g., penicillin, aspirin, IV contrast medium), exposure to allergen (food), or following an insect sting. Signs include pallor; cyanosis; diaphoresis; impaired or loss of consciousness; tachycardia; weak or irregular pulse; cold, clammy extremities; tachypnea; and stridor.

► Diagnosis

Positive allergy skin tests or RAST to offending allergen. IgE-specific antibodies are not identified in anaphylactoid reactions. Other studies include complete blood count (CBC), total IgE, total eosinophil count, elevated serum tryptase, and urine histamine.

► Concept and Application

Mast cells and basophils rich in mediators (ECF-A, NCF-A, PAF, histamine, leukotriene, prostaglandins, etc.) suddenly undergo degranulation following exposure to an allergen as a result of specific IgE directed against that allergen, or, in the case of anaphylactic reactions, allergens cause mediator release through a non-IgE-mediated mechanism. Mast cell mediator release leads to shifting of intravascular fluid to interstitial tissues and hypotension, and may lead to hives and angioedema. Asthmatic patient will become dyspneic and wheeze.

► Treatment Steps

1. Oxygen if cyanosis, dyspnea, or wheezing is present.
2. Trendelenburg position if hypotensive.
3. Epinephrine (1:1,000 0.30–0.50 mL SQ or 0.1 mL/kg in children).
4. Tourniquet—place a tourniquet proximal to the site of injection or sting on an extremity, if applicable.
5. Antihistamines (Benadryl IV 1–2 mg/kg up to 100 mg).
6. H_2 blockers (famotidine 20 mg IV).
7. IV fluids through large-gauge line to maintain systolic blood pressure $\geq$ 100 mm Hg in adults, 50 mm Hg in children.
8. Nebulized β_2 agonist if there is bronchospasm (albuterol 0.5 cc in 3 cc saline).
9. Corticosteroids (hydrocortisone IV 7–10 mg/kg).
10. Vasopressors (dopamine IV 0.3–1.2 mg/kg/hr).
11. Shock trousers.
12. Intubation and ventilation.
13. Tracheostomy if airway obstruction secondary to airway edema.
14. Prevention of future reaction by avoidance, hyposensitization in cases of insect venom hypersensitivity.

IV. URTICARIA

► H&P Keys

Generalized pruritus; hives vary in size from 3–4 mm to giant lesion 10–15 cm in diameter. Usually have central clearing with peripheral erythema. Often associated with angioedema of soft tissues including eyes, lips, and tongue. Lesions leave no permanent changes in the skin and are transient. Acute urticaria: hives occur over a period of < 6 weeks. Chronic urticaria: hives persist for a period > 6 weeks. Hives may be induced by extrinsic agents (e.g., drugs such as antibiotics, nonsteroidal anti-inflammatory agents [NSAIDs], and opiates; radiocontrast media; and foods such as shrimp, peanuts, and strawberries), physical agents (e.g., light, heat friction, pressure, cold, and vibration), and underlying systemic disease (e.g., serum sickness, infection, autoimmunity, malignancy).

► Diagnosis

CBC, sedimentation rate, antinuclear antibodies (ANAs), serum protein electrophoresis (SPEP), urinalysis (UA), liver function tests

► **management decisions**

URTICARIA

Severity	Treatment
Mild	One or two antihistamines from different classes (Allegra, 180 mg in A.M., Zyrtec, 10 mg in P.M.)
Moderate	Add H_2 blocker (Zantac, 150 mg bid).
Moderate to severe	Add tricyclic antidepressant (Sinequan, 10 mg tid) and/or leukotriene modifier (Singulair).
Severe	Add oral β_2-adrenergic (Volmax, 4–8 mg bid) and/or
	Oral corticosteroids (prednisone, 1–2 mg/kg/day).

(LFTs), thyroid-stimulating hormone (TSH), thyroid autoantibodies, and skin biopsy. Total IgE, allergy tests for suspected allergens.

► **Disease Severity**

Mild disease includes intermittent hives responding to antihistamines. Moderate to severe disease includes persistent urticaria that requires corticosteroid treatment or is associated with angioedema of the respiratory or gastrointestinal tracts.

► **Treatment Steps**

1. Avoid provocative factors.
2. Antihistamine (hydroxyzine, 25–500 mg qid).
3. Additional antihistamine (Allegra, 180 mg qd).
4. H_2 blocker (Zantac, 150 mg bid).
5. Leukotriene modifier (Singulair, 10 mg qd).
6. Tricyclic antidepressants in low doses (Sinequan, 10–20 mg tid or 30–50 mg qhs).
7. Oral adrenergic (Volmax, 4–8 mg bid).
8. Oral corticosteroids (prednisone, 1–2 mg/kg/day).
9. Anabolic steroids (stanozolol, 1–2 mg bid).
10. Epinephrine (for emergency treatment 1:1,000, 0.2–0.3 mL SQ or 0.01 mL/kg in children, repeated in 20–30 minutes if needed).

V. IMMUNODEFICIENCY

A. Humoral Immunodeficiency

► **H&P Keys**

Recurrent infections including pneumonia, sinusitis, otitis media, and skin infections. Frequent complaints of diarrhea and arthralgia or arthritis. Children may suffer from failure to thrive. Young males may have X-linked agammaglobulinemia. Older children and adults often suffer common variable hypogammaglobulinemia. Patients may have absent lymph nodes, and the physical signs relate to the site of infection. Patients with recurrent bacterial infections usually lack immunoglobulins (humoral immunodeficiency); those with recurrent fungal or viral infection suffer from absent or defective T cells (cellular immunodeficiency).

► Diagnosis

CBC, quantitative immunoglobulins (IgG, IgG subclass levels, IgM, IgA), T- and B-cell enumeration, anergy panel, chest and sinus x-rays, sweat test, human immunodeficiency virus (HIV) testing.

► Concept and Application

Failure of B cells to differentiate into immunoglobulin-producing cells or other defect in immunoglobulin production or secretion. Patients with IgA deficiency often have few symptoms.

► Treatment Steps

1. IV γ globulin (IVIG), 300–400 mg/kg/month to maintain trough serum IgG levels 4 weeks after treatment at > 500 mg/dL.
2. Hyperimmune γ globulin preparations (e.g., zoster immune globulin obtained from immunized donors).
3. Early use of antibiotics in infections.
4. Prevent transfusion reactions. IgA-deficient patients may have anti-IgA antibodies and require blood products depleted of IgA. Similarly, IVIG may cause anaphylaxis and is not indicated in IgA-deficient patients.

B. Cellular (T-Cell) Immunodeficiency

► H&P Keys

Usually affects infants and young children. Patients often suffer from chronic diarrhea, failure to thrive, viral infections, or persistent fungal infections (*Candida*). Patients with combined immunodeficiency (loss of both T-cell and B-cell function) often fail to respond to therapy and die within the first year of life.

► Diagnosis

Absence or diminution of T cells or their subsets. Decreased thymus on x-rays. Diminished evidence of T-cell activity as assayed by the anergy panel or in vitro mitogen-induced lymphoblastic transformation.

► Treatment Steps

1. Supportive treatment; use aggressive antibiotic therapy, antifungal therapy.
2. Avoid whole blood transfusions, which may cause a fatal graft-versus-host reaction.
3. Avoid live virus vaccines (e.g., poliovirus; measles, mumps, rubella [MMR] vaccine).
4. Bone marrow transplantation.
5. Fetal thymus transplantation.
6. Lymphokines (e.g., aldesleukin—recombinant human interleukin-2).
7. Immunomodulators (e.g., filgrastim—recombinant human granulocyte colony-stimulating factor—as adjunctive treatment following immunosuppression).
8. Gene therapy, in selected cases, is being studied.

VI. HEREDITARY ANGIOEDEMA

► H&P Keys

This autosomal dominant inherited disorder is seen in childhood, although an acquired form is seen mostly in adults. Patients develop nonpitting localized subcutaneous or submucosol edema. The face, lips, tongue, and glottal structure are frequently involved. Upper airway obstruction may be fatal. Attacks may be precipitated by mild trauma (e.g., dental work). No pruritus is present. Patients do not respond to epinephrine. Gastrointestinal involvement may simulate an acute abdomen.

► Diagnosis

C_1-esterase inhibitor qualitative levels are depressed. Quantitative levels may be present, but not functional.

C_1 levels depressed in the acquired but not the hereditary form. Skin biopsy reveals no inflammatory changes and lacks eosinophilia.

► Disease Severity

Severity can vary from episode to episode in an individual patient. Each episode involving the upper airway is potentially life threatening. Severely affected patients have attacks of angioedema regularly every few weeks, and mildly affected patients may go many months between attacks.

► Concept and Application

Most commonly is a congenital absence or decrease of the C_1-esterase inhibitor levels. The complement cascade is activated without functional C_1-esterase inhibitor levels. C_4 levels are decreased during asymptomatic periods. C_1 and C_3 levels are normal. Adult with newly developed disease may have the acquired form, which may be associated with underlying malignant neoplasm.

► Treatment Steps

1. Supportive therapy during acute attacks (e.g., mild analgesics or narcotics, IV fluids, intubation or tracheostomy before critical obstruction occurs).
2. Infusion of C_1-esterase inhibitor concentrate has been effective, but not currently available in the United States.
3. Fresh frozen plasma is not recommended. Some patients may worsen due to the addition of complement components.
4. Attenuated androgens (e.g., stanozolol, 1–2 mg bid) contraindicated in children who are not fully grown and during pregnancy.
5. ε-Aminocaproic acid (a fibrinolysis inhibitor) may be used in children.
6. Prophylaxis before surgical procedures with fresh frozen plasma (two units 12–24 hours before the procedure).
7. Epinephrine should not be relied on.

VII. ATOPIC DERMATITIS

► H&P Keys

Atopic dermatitis is a very common chronic pruritic skin disorder seen mostly in infants and children, although it occasionally occurs in adults. The infantile form tends to affect the head but may also present with a symmetrical eczematoid rash involving the extensor surfaces. As the child grows, the rash becomes most prominent in the flexural areas (i.e., popliteal fossae, antecubital fossae) and dry skin becomes a prominent feature. Over time, the skin becomes lichenified and often hyperpigmented. Pruritus and scratching may lead to excoriation and infection of eczematoid lesions.

► **Diagnosis**

Total IgE is significantly elevated in 80% of patients, often beyond the levels seen in allergic rhinitis or allergic asthma. The total eosinophil count is frequently elevated during acute exacerbations of the rash. Allergy skin tests are usually positive to a wide variety of allergens, as is the RAST. However, it is often difficult to correlate these positive allergy tests with the clinical course of this disease.

► **Disease Severity**

Although most infants presenting with atopic dermatitis have mild to moderate skin involvement, which can be managed on an outpatient basis, occasionally, affected patients suffer from a generalized eczematoid rash involving much of the body surface. Severely affected patients may become acutely ill and develop generalized erythroderma and infection of their open skin lesions. This latter group require hospitalization, hydration, and intensive topical care as well as systemic antibiotics. On the other hand, mild to moderate cases of atopic dermatitis often respond to antihistamines and topical agents with gradual resolution of their skin rash over a period of years. Some adults diagnosed with atopic dermatitis during childhood continue to have dry skin and occasional hand eczema when they are exposed to irritants.

► **Concept and Application**

The mechanism for atopic dermatitis is not well understood. However, most patients are clearly atopic, having high levels of IgE, positive allergy skin tests, and high incidence of allergic rhinitis and conjunctivitis. Paradoxically, these patients may reveal minor defects in their cellular immunity with suppressed delayed hypersensitivity tests, decreased T-suppressor cells (CD8) and an increased ratio of helper (CD4) to suppressor cells. Patients also demonstrate abnormal cutaneous vascular responses. Defects in cellular immunity are demonstrated clinically by patients with atopic dermatitis who contract herpes, which may lead to life-threatening infection.

► **Treatment Steps**

1. Identify and eliminate exacerbating factors such as allergens, irritants, and psychosocial stressors.
2. Prevent dryness of the skin by decreasing exposure to hot water and patting the skin dry rather than rubbing vigorously.
3. Moisturize the skin with over-the-counter fragrance-free moisturizers or with prescription agents such as Lac-Hydrin 12% (ammonium lactate). Ointments are more effective than creams, which are more effective than lotions. Apply when skin is wet.
4. Prevent irritation of the skin by wearing loose-fitting noncoarse garments, avoiding excessive sweating, and by avoiding irritating soaps.
5. Antihistamines to treat pruritus (e.g., hydroxyzine, 25–50 mg qid).
6. Antipruritics (e.g., Sarna or Zonalon) applied topically.
7. Topical immunomodulator (TIM) agents (Elidel and Protopic) inhibit T-cell–derived cytokines.
8. Topical corticosteroids. Fluorinated agents usually are more effective but have more side effects than nonfluorinated agents.
9. Systemic corticosteroids. Use sparingly due to side effects (e.g., prednisone, 1 mg/kg/day in divided doses for 5–10 days).
10. Antibiotics to cover *Staphylococcus aureus* if signs of infection are present (e.g., dicloxacillin, 500 mg qid).

11. Coal tar acts as anti-inflammatory agent (e.g., Zetar).

12. Wet dressings can promote absorption of topical medications, hydrate the skin, and protect against persistent scratching.

13. Ultraviolet light therapy can be useful for severe atopic dermatitis.

14. Immunomodulatory therapy (thymopentin, interferons, and cyclosporin A) have been used in severe cases.

VIII. CONTACT DERMATITIS

▶ H&P Keys

Contact dermatitis is an inflammatory reaction of the skin caused by an external stimulis. Inflammation may be allergic or nonallergic (irritant). Nonallergic contact dermatitis is a common occupational skin disease. Most of the skin is simply inflamed as a result of exposure to a nonspecific irritating substance (e.g., detergents, solvents, water), which is referred to as irritant dermatitis. Allergic contact dermatitis is related to a delayed hypersensitivity reaction and may be due to a natural exposure to antigens, such as those in poison ivy plants, or may result from exposure to nickel in tools, watches, or jewelry; or allergens in hair dye, rubber products, makeup, or preservatives (parabens) in creams and lotions. Allergic contact dermatitis can occur at any age but is most often seen in adults. The lesions are initially pruritic but with time become lichenified. The location of the rash usually indicates the site of exposure. For example, allergy to a leather dye may cause shoe dermatitis.

▶ Diagnosis

Allergy patch testing to common contact allergens will usually be positive within 72 hours of application. A skin biopsy of the affected skin reveals an intense inflammatory infiltrate characterized by a marked infiltration of lymphocytes and macrophages, which typify a delayed hypersensitivity reaction.

▶ Disease Severity

Acute contact dermatitis such as widespread poison ivy may incapacitate the patient. The lesions are highly pruritic and often blisters, erythema, and edema are noted in acute reactor. Moderate reaction: often limited areas of eczema, which ultimately become lichenified. Dark-skinned patients develop hyperpigmentation at the site of the rash. Once the allergen is identified and eliminated, the rash will gradually resolve. Patients with unavoidable chronic exposure will continue to have a rash even if they receive medication.

▶ Concept and Application

Allergic contact dermatitis is a type IV delayed or cellular allergic reaction. The hapten of the allergen passes into the skin, combining with Langerhans' cells, lymphocytes, and other carrier molecules to form a complete allergen. With repeated allergen exposure, hypersensitivity increases. Lymphocytes release mediators (macrophage inhibiting factor) that recruit macrophages, which attack the allergen and surrounding tissues.

▶ Treatment Steps

1. Avoidance of the precipitating factors.

2. Wet dressings for acute vesiculating dermatitis (e.g., Burow's solution, aluminum acetate solution, or aluminum sulfate).

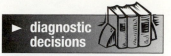

▶ **diagnostic decisions**

ALLERGIC DISEASES OF THE SKIN

Atopic Dermatitis
Pruritic, dry lesions may become lichenified and hyperpigmented. Elevated IgE, eosinophil count. Positive immediate allergy to prior skin tests. Skin biopsy is nonspecific.

Contact Dermatitis
Pruritic lesions may become lichenified or vesiculate. Positive patch tests within 72 hours. Skin biopsy shows marked infiltration of lymphocytes and macrophages.

Urticaria
Transient pruritic hives vary in size from 3 mm to 15 cm, usually with central clearing, often associated with angioedema.

Hereditary Angioedema
Nonpruritic nonpitting edema without hives. Skin biopsy reveals no inflammatory changes and lacks eosinophilia. Diminished functional C_1-esterase inhibitor level.

3. Antihistamines to treat pruritus (e.g., hydroxyzine, 25–50 mg qid). They do not affect the rash.
4. Antipruritics (e.g., calamine or Zonalon) applied topically.
5. Topical corticosteroids. Use ointments for thicker lesions; creams or lotions for exudative lesions or intertriginous regions; and lotions or gels for hairy regions such as the scalp.
6. Systemic corticosteroids (especially if lesions are on the face, hands, or other sensitive areas), e.g., prednisone, 1 mg/kg/day in divided doses for 5–10 days.
7. Antibiotics to cover *S. aureus* if signs of infection are present (e.g., dicloxacillin, 500 mg qid).
8. Ultraviolet light may be considered.

IX. ALLERGIC BRONCHOPULMONARY ASPERGILLOSIS

▶ H&P Keys

Allergic bronchopulmonary aspergillosis (ABPA) results from a manipulation reaction resulting from the presence of the fungus *Aspergillus fumigatus* present in the bronchial tree of asthmatic patients. Patients typically present with difficult-to-manage bronchial asthma associated with peripheral eosinophilia and high total IgE. Of asthmatic patients, 1–2% are affected by ABPA. Approximately 10% of corticosteroid-dependent asthmatics and 6% of patients with cystic fibrosis are also affected by ABPA. Affected patients often have a history of frequent use of or dependence on corticosteroids. At times, patients may complain of fever, general malaise, productive cough, and wheezing. Mucoid impaction may lead to atelectasis. Severely affected patients with pulmonary fibrosis may exhibit signs of chronic hypoxemia, including digital clubbing.

▶ Diagnosis

Total IgE is significantly elevated (> 1,000 IU/mL); elevated total eosinophil count (> 1,000/mm³); positive immediate-type hypersensitivity reaction to *A. fumigatus*. X-rays often reveal transient infiltrates. The presence of central or proximal bronchiectasis and absence of distal bronchiectasis is highly suggestive of ABPA. High-resolution CT (HRCT) is more sensitive and specific in detecting proximal bronchiectasis than plain films. Patients often have significant titers of precipitating IgG antibodies to *Aspergillus,* and *A. fumigatus* may be cultured from sputum of some patients, but a positive culture is not diagnostic. Examination of sputum may identify *A. fumigatus* hyphae and intense eosinophilia.

▶ Disease Severity

ABPA may vary from mild to moderate disease, with intermittent flares of asthmatic symptoms that quickly respond to corticosteroids, to severe progressive asthma associated with pulmonary fibrosis, progressive hypoxemia, digital clubbing, and end-stage pulmonary disease. ABPA can be staged as follows: acute, remission, exacerbation, corticosteroid-dependent asthma, and fibrotic.

▶ Concept and Application

The mechanism for ABPA is not entirely understood. However, it appears that certain asthmatic patients have a propensity to colonize *A. fumigatus* along their bronchial tree. The fungus does not infiltrate but remains in close proximity to the respiratory mucosa. *Aspergillus* antigens apparently diffuse to the mucosa and elicit a variety of reactions including a type I–IgE reaction as well as a type III or Arthus phenomenon. Specific IgE and IgG antibodies are produced against *Aspergillus.* Eventually, an acute inflammatory reaction ensues, leading to clinical symptoms.

► Treatment Steps

1. Inhaled short-acting β_2-adrenergic (e.g., albuterol) to treat the asthmatic component.
2. Oral corticosteroids (e.g., prednisone 0.5 mg/kg/day initially, then taper to a lower-dose maintenance program) can reduce clinical symptoms with attendant changes, including decreased total IgE and clearing of the CXR.
3. Immunotherapy is *not* effective.
4. Antifungal therapy (e.g., itraconazole, 200 mg bid) has shown promising results.

X. HYPERSENSITIVITY PNEUMONITIS

► H&P Keys

Hypersensitivity pneumonitis, or extrinsic allergic alveolitis, is caused by an immunopathologic reaction involving the alveoli, bronchioles, and surrounding pulmonary tissues resulting from exposure to organic dusts. Allergens causing hypersensitivity pneumonitis may be derived from bacterial (e.g., thermophilic actinomycetes in mushroom compost causing mushroom worker's lung), fungi (e.g., *Aspergillus* species in moldy tobacco causing tobacco worker's lung), insect proteins (e.g., *Sitophilus granarius* in infested flour causing wheat miller's lung), organic chemicals (e.g., isocyanates in various industries causing chemical worker's lung), or miscellaneous agents (e.g., avian proteins in pigeon droppings causing bird breeder's lung). An acute reaction or insidious chronic disease may occur depending on the concentration and duration of exposure of the allergen. Acute disease is associated with fever, chills, sweats, myalgia, dyspnea, and coughing; symptoms last for hours to days following exposure. Chronic disease usually lacks systemic symptoms, with patients complaining of dyspnea and perhaps cough. Physical examination may reveal bilateral fine rales and signs of hypoxemia. Patients with chronic disease may lack clinical symptoms initially but over time develop symptoms of dyspnea resulting from chronic pulmonary fibrosis and other signs of hypoxemia.

► Diagnosis

In part, the diagnosis is based on evidence of the immunologic reaction to the inhaled antigen. Affected patients reveal evidence of the presence of precipitating usually IgG, antibody directed against the offending antigen. Enzyme-linked immunosorbent assay (ELISA) may be used to detect circulating serum antibodies. Pulmonary function tests identify the presence of a restrictive lung disease, decreased diffusing capacity for carbon monoxide (DLCO), and arterial blood gases identify hypoxemia. CXR may be normal initially. However, eventually repeated or prolonged exposure to the antigen will be associated with roentgenologic evidence of interstitial fibrosis. HRCT is more sensitive and specific in chronic disease and reveals scattered, small, rounded opacities. Inhalation challenge is rarely used today because of the potential for serious damage. Bronchoalveolar lavage may reveal IgG and IgA antibodies.

▶ Disease Severity

Hypersensitivity pneumonitis may present as an acute disease associated with fever and elevated white count and sedimentation rates. Within a short time, signs, symptoms, and findings resolve. Repeated allergen exposure may lead to subacute episode in which pulmonary functions do not return to normal, and patients with chronic exposure to the allergen will develop irreversible restrictive lung disease and, eventually, end-stage lung disease.

▶ Concept and Application

Type III (immune-complex mediated) and type IV (cell-mediated delayed hypersensitivity) reactions occur to the inhaled organic antigenic matter.

▶ Treatment Steps

1. Avoid offending agent.
2. Inhaled short-acting β_2-adrenergic (e.g., albuterol).
3. Oral corticosteroids (e.g., prednisone 60 mg/day for 1 week, tapered slowly).
4. Immunotherapy with the offending antigens is not recommended.

XI. HYPEREOSINOPHILIC SYNDROME

▶ H&P Keys

Hypereosinophilic syndrome is characterized by high levels of peripheral eosinophilia and pulmonary infiltrates associated with eosinophilic infiltration into tissues and organs. Patients may initially be asymptomatic but over time show symptoms of organ pathology. Organ systems infiltrated with eosinophils are listed in descending order of frequency of involvement: hematologic, cardiovascular, cutaneous, neurologic, pulmonary, splenic, hepatic, ocular, and gastrointestinal. Symptoms may include coughing, dyspnea, symptoms of congestive heart failure, abdominal pain, and intravascular clotting abnormalities. Hypereosinophilic syndrome often affects young and middle-aged adult men. The ratio of male to female patients is 9:1.

▶ Diagnosis

Eosinophilia often exceeds 50% of the peripheral white count. The total IgE is not particularly elevated. Bone marrow biopsy reveals an intense myeloid hyperplasia of eosinophils. Biopsy of affected organs (e.g., lungs, heart, gastrointestinal tract) reveals an eosinophil infiltrate. The criteria for diagnosis include: eosinophilia of 1,500/mm³ for at least 6 months, tissue eosinophilia as exhibited on biopsy of specific organs, and no other known etiology for eosinophilia.

▶ Disease Severity

Hypereosinophilic syndrome can remain a limited disease with few clinical symptoms and marked primarily by very high eosinophil counts; or vital organs can sustain irreversible damage that ultimately results in the demise of the patient. Cardiac infiltration may lead to a restrictive carditis and congestive heart failure. High leukocyte counts (> 90,000/μL) are associated with a poor prognosis.

► Concept and Application

The mechanism for hypereosinophilic syndrome is unknown. It is thought to be related to overactive T-cell secretion of lymphokines, which stimulate the eosinophil line.

► Treatment Steps

1. General—treat the affected organ (e.g., inhaled bronchodilators if bronchospasm exists, diuretics if there is impaired left ventricular function). No therapy is required if there is no organ involvement.
2. Oral corticosteroids (e.g., prednisone 60 mg/day or 1 mg/kg/day).
3. Cytotoxic agents (e.g., hydroxyurea and etoposide) if there is significant organ involvement or unresponsiveness to steroids.
4. Interferon-α has shown promising results.

XII. DRUG ALLERGY

► H&P Keys

Drug allergy is an adverse immunologic reaction to an administered medication. The development of drug allergy is influenced by the type of medication, route of administration, frequency of administration, and underlying reactivity of the patient. Patients may suffer adverse drug reactions that are not immunologic in nature and are therefore nonallergic reactions. Examples of nonallergic drug reactions include overdosage, drug side effects, drug-to-drug interactions, and idiosyncratic reactions (e.g., primaquine-induced hemolytic anemia in a G6PD-deficient patient). Drug allergies can present as anaphylaxis, urticaria, or angioedema, serum sickness–like disease, vasculitis, ptomaine disease, drug fever, nephritis, or pathologic cutaneous conditions. Penicillin allergy is quite common and is often IgE mediated, presenting as urticaria or anaphylaxis. Nonimmunologic reactions simulating drug allergy may occur with mast cell degranulators, such as meperidine hydrochloride (Demerol) and codeine.

► Diagnosis

A good temporal correlation between the use of a medication and the onset of typical allergic symptoms (e.g., anaphylaxis, urticaria) sets the stage for a diagnosis of drug allergy. However, some supporting evidence of an immunologic reaction is needed to indicate that the origin of the reaction is immunologic. An elevated total or specific IgE, as well as eosinophilia, is supportive of the diagnosis of drug allergy. One of the most commonly diagnosed drug allergies is that of penicillin, confirmed by positive allergy skin test reactions to penicillin major or minor determinants.

► Disease Severity

Mild reversible or transient symptoms of drug allergy include cutaneous reactions, including urticaria, angioedema, and various exanthems. With cessation of the medications, symptoms subside without sequelae. On the other hand, drug reactions causing exfoliative dermatitis (e.g., sulfa drugs), severe anaphylaxis (e.g., penicillin), hepatitis (e.g., phenytoin [Dilantin]), pulmonary interstitial fibrosis (e.g., nitrofurantoin), interstitial nephritis (e.g., methicillin), Stevens–Johnson syndrome (e.g., sulfa) in some cases has led to permanent impairment and even death.

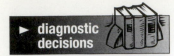

diagnostic decisions

ALLERGIC DRUG REACTIONS

Anaphylactic (Type I)
Immediate IgE-mediated anaphylaxis, angioedema, and urticaria. Penicillin is the most common cause of drug-induced anaphylaxis.

Cytotoxic (Type II)
IgG or IgM antibody against cell surface antigens cause hematologic reactions and nephritis. Drug-induced Coombs'-positive hemolytic anemia and methicillin-induced nephritis are good examples.

Serum Sickness (Type III)
Immune complex–mediated reaction involving fever, large-joint arthralgias, and multiorgan vasculitis. Drug-induced SLE from hydralazine and procainamide are examples.

Cell-Mediated (Type IV)
Delayed-type hypersensitivity reactions take days to occur. Reactions can range from contact dermatitis, if the drug is topical, to drug-induced interstitial nephritis.

► Concept and Application

The drug itself or its metabolite is often a low-molecular-weight hapten, which joins with body proteins to become an allergen. IgE-mediated drug reactions usually result in urticaria, angioedema, or anaphylaxis. Autoimmune disease or vasculitis may be a result of a reaction involving immune complexes containing antigen, antibody, and complement, whereas fixed drug eruptions and contact dermatitis appear to be caused by cellular or delayed-hypersensitivity reactions.

► Treatment Steps

1. Discontinue the offending medication.
2. Antihistamines to treat pruritus and urticaria.
3. Antipruritics applied topically for maculopapular rashes.
4. Oral corticosteroids are necessary if exfoliative dermatitis, vasculitis, or major organ involvement occurs.
5. Supportive treatment may include transfusions if a hemolytic drug reaction is present or IV fluids if hypotension is noted.
6. Epinephrine subcutaneously is often helpful in acute and severe IgE-mediated reactions.

BIBLIOGRAPHY

Adkinson NF Jr., *Middleton's Allergy: Principles and Practice,* 6th ed. Mosby, 2003.
Fireman P. *Atlas of Allergies and Clinical Immunology,* 3rd ed. Mosby, 2005.
Lichtenstein L. *Current Therapy in Allergy, Immunology, and Rheumatology,* 6th ed. Mosby, 2004.

Injuries, Wounds, Toxicology, and Burns | 7

I. EPISTAXIS

▶ H&P Keys

Control bleeding with direct pressure by squeezing nostrils or pack nasal passage with cotton soaked in lidocaine and Adrenalin. Remove blood, proceed with a careful exam to pinpoint the source of bleeding. Evaluate history for bleeding disorders and medication.

▶ Diagnosis

If indicated, rule out bleeding disorders (prothrombin time [PT], partial thromboplastin time [PTT], platelets), leukemia, and severe liver disease.

▶ Disease Severity

Severe bleeding without a visualized bleeding source is most often posterior. Monitor vital signs including pulse oximetry. Evaluate underlying conditions that exacerbate the bleeding (hypertension, liver disease).

▶ Concept and Application

Anterior bleeding arises from Kiesselbach's plexus; posterior, from external or internal carotids.

▶ Treatment Steps

Anterior—Pressure or packing, topical vasoconstrictors, cauterization (silver nitrate, using topical analgesia first).

Posterior—Posterior packing, antibiotics, volume resuscitation, if indicated: surgery.

II. CRANIAL INJURY

A. Facial Fracture (Frontal Bone, Mandible, Maxilla, Orbits, or Nose)

▶ H&P Keys

History and physical exam, roentgenographic studies, information from witness.

▶ Diagnosis

Primarily includes physical exam and x-ray studies. Pain, cerebrospinal fluid (CSF) rhinorrhea, diplopia, deformity, and tenderness suggest fracture.

Orbital Fracture—Swelling, difficulty with eye movement, vertical diplopia, and facial emphysema.

Frontal or Ethmoid—May have CSF rhinorrhea.

Nasal Bones—Deformity, epistaxis.

Mandible or Maxilla—Swelling, pain, airway compromise, jaw pain or deformity upon opening or closing the mouth (abnormal occlusion).

▶ Disease Severity

Neurologic deficits indicate poorer prognosis. Assess degree of trauma, neurologic status, and associated injuries via physical exam and x-rays.

► Concept and Application

Trauma. Evaluate neurologic status at intervals.

► Treatment Steps

1. Control of airway and hemorrhage, antibiotics, fracture reduction.

   Nasal—Closed reduction for simple fracture, open reduction in severe fracture cases. Always check for septal hematoma: requires immediate ear, nose, and throat (ENT) consult.

   Maxillary—Reduction, interdental wiring (simple fractures), orbital or zygoma wiring and traction (complex fractures).

   Mandibular—Internal fixation.

   Orbital—Surgery to resupport orbit.

B. Skull Trauma or Fracture

► H&P Keys

May be asymptomatic, or pain or swelling, central nervous system (CNS) signs, CSF leak (nose or ears). If CSF in nose or ears or blood in the middle ear, think basilar skull fracture. If ecchymosis behind ear (Battle's sign), think mastoid fracture. With raccoon eyes, think orbital roof or basilar fracture.

► Diagnosis

History and physical exam, computed tomographic (CT) scan or x-ray exam (remember, basilar fractures may not be evident on x-rays).

► Disease Severity

Frequent neurologic exams. Observe for epidural hematoma with linear fracture across middle meningeal artery.

► Concept and Application

Skull trauma may result in brain injury, hemorrhage, CSF leak, cranial nerve damage, or meningitis.

► Treatment Steps

Cardiopulmonary resuscitation (CPR) and ABCs (airway, breathing, circulation), then:

   Simple Linear (Closed)—Observation.

   Compound Linear (Open)—Antibiotics.

   Simple Depressed—Surgical treatment (fragment elevation).

   Compound Depressed—Urgent surgical treatment.

C. Concussion

► H&P Keys

Neurologic exam may be normal. History reveals a brief alteration of consciousness. May also have headache, amnesia, nausea, and vomiting.

► Diagnosis

History and physical exam (x-ray, CT scan, and magnetic resonance imaging [MRI] are all normal in concussions). Repeated neurologic assessments are important.

► Disease Severity

Determine neurologic status, degree of injury.

► **Concept and Application**

Head trauma, resulting in head injury and brief unconsciousness, without physical brain damage, secondary to disruption of the reticular activating system. Condition is the result of brain acceleration or deceleration.

► **Treatment Steps**

Careful observation (neurologic watch).

D. Subdural Hematoma

► **H&P Keys**

Symptoms may present after brief or prolonged time from injury: lethargy, headache, seizures, and coma. May have dilated ipsilateral pupil.

► **Diagnosis**

History and physical exam, CT or MRI.

► **Disease Severity**

Severity determined by neurologic exam and rate of deterioration.

► **Concept and Application**

Trauma resulting in vein or brain tear and hemorrhage under the dura.

► **Treatment Steps**

Surgical (especially in acute subdural), observation in some cases (small amount of bleeding, high-risk patient).

E. Epidural Hematoma

► **H&P Keys**

Symptoms usually present very shortly after injury: lethargy, headache, seizures, and hemiplegia. May have brief loss of consciousness, then return to normal prior to deterioration (lucid interval).

► **Diagnosis**

History and physical exam, CT or MRI.

► **Disease Severity**

Evaluate neurologic status.

► **Concept and Application**

Trauma-induced artery tear (middle meningeal artery common). Associated temporal bone fractures are common.

► **Treatment Steps**

Urgent surgery to avoid brain herniation.

F. Ocular Injury

► **H&P Keys**

May have pain, vision loss, subconjunctival hemorrhage. If light flashes noted, rule out retinal detachment.

► **Diagnosis**

History and physical exam, ophthalmoscopic and slit-lamp exam.

► **Disease Severity**

Evaluate vision. In chemical exposure, prognosis varies with type of agent, duration of exposure, and emergency care provided.

► Concept and Application

Chemicals—Chemical conjunctivitis, blindness.

Trauma—Hyphema, laceration, abrasion.

► Treatment Steps

Hyphema (Anterior Chamber Hemorrhage)—Ophthalmologist's evaluation needed as soon as possible.

Chemicals—Irrigation with normal saline.

Corneal Abrasion—Antibiotic ointment, pain control.

Corneal Laceration—Eye shield, immediate ophthalmologic consultation.

G. Auditory Injury

► H&P Keys

Swelling, pain, hearing loss, vertigo, and hemorrhage.

► Diagnosis

History, physical exam, and audiometric exam, x-ray of skull and temporal bone (rule out associated fracture).

► Disease Severity

Evaluate trauma to the pinna, external ear canal, and tympanic membrane.

► Concept and Application

Trauma.

► Treatment Steps

Tympanic Membrane Perforation
1. If small, supportive treatment (cotton earplug, systemic antibiotic for infection).
2. If large, surgical treatment.

Noise-Induced Hearing Loss—No treatment (except hearing aid).

Additional Information—Trauma to external ear may cause subperichondral hematoma. Calcified hematoma results in cauliflower ear. Prevent with early drainage.

H. Epidemiology and Prevention of Ocular and Auditory Injury

Epidemiology—Includes blunt ocular trauma (occupational, recreational, environmental), and ophthalmic foreign bodies and lacerations. Auditory injury may affect children (fireworks), teens (high-decibel music), and adults (occupational).

Prevention—Involves eye and ear protection along with education.

III. CHEST AND ABDOMINAL INJURY

A. Rib Fracture

► H&P Keys

Pain following trauma, increased with inspiration and palpation, ecchymosis. Rib x-rays may appear negative shortly after injury, yet show a "healing fracture" several weeks later.

► **Diagnosis**

History and physical exam, x-ray exam.

► **Disease Severity**

Assess cardiopulmonary status and consider possible trauma in adjacent areas. Rule out pneumothorax if patient remains dyspneic.

► **Concept and Application**

Fracture secondary to trauma. Without trauma, consider pathologic fracture causes.

► **Treatment Steps**

Simple rib fracture: Analgesics, ice initially, injection of local anesthetic (into intercostal nerve) as an option.

B. Pneumothorax

► **H&P Keys**

Dyspnea, chest pain, absent breath sounds, decreased tactile fremitus, hyperresonance. Tachycardia and hypotension may present in tension pneumothorax.

► **Diagnosis**

History and physical exam, chest x-ray (CXR).

► **Disease Severity**

Evaluate cardiovascular status, mentation, coexisting problems, oxygenation. Reduced venous return resulting from tension pneumothorax requires urgent treatment.

► **Concept and Application**

Air in pleural space, as a result of blunt or penetrating trauma (including iatrogenic trauma). May also be spontaneous, in patients with pulmonary disease, or menses-associated (catamenial).

► **Treatment Steps**

Tube Thoracostomy—Best treatment if > 50% or recurrent. Use fifth intercostal space, anterior axillary line.

Small (< 15%) or Stable Pneumothorax—Observe.

Urgent Tension Pneumothorax—Insert large-bore needle into second intercostal space, midclavicular line (MCL).

Catamenial—Medication to suppress ovulation.

C. Hemothorax

► **H&P Keys**

Dyspnea, chest pain.

► **Diagnosis**

History and physical exam (absent breath sounds), CXR.

► **Disease Severity**

Evaluate and monitor cardiac and pulmonary status. Prognosis worse in patients with significant preexisting condition.

► **Concept and Application**

Trauma or spontaneous. May be iatrogenic (central venous pressure [CVP] monitor insertion).

► **Treatment Steps**

Large chest tube (32–40 French) with 20-cm water suction.

Open Thoracotomy—For persisting hemorrhage or massive initial blood loss. Inadequate hemothorax drainage results in fibrothorax.

D. Flail Chest

► **H&P Keys**

Paradoxic chest wall motion, respiratory distress.

► **Diagnosis**

History and physical exam (chest palpation), x-ray exam.

► **Disease Severity**

Monitor for reduced vital capacity and respiratory distress secondary to multiple fractures.

► **Concept and Application**

Respiratory paradox with inspiration, secondary to multiple rib fractures.

► **Treatment Steps**

Intubation and positive pressure ventilation with positive end-expiratory pressure (PEEP).

► **Additional Information**

Pericardial Tamponade Symptoms—Diminished heart tones, narrow pulse pressure, electrocardiogram (ECG) with low voltage. Also Beck's triad (hypotension, reduced cardiac tones, high CVP).

E. Perforation of Viscus

► **H&P Keys**

Abdominal rigidity, pain, peritoneal irritation, reduced or absent bowel sounds, shoulder pain.

► **Diagnosis**

History and physical exam, x-rays, CT scan, diagnostic peritoneal lavage, exploratory laparotomy.

► **Disease Severity**

Determined by initial presentation, presence of coexisting medical problems, and baseline condition.

► **Concept and Application**

Trauma.

► **Management**

Laparotomy and surgical repair.

Spleen—Repair or splenectomy.

Colon—Repair (resection if severe injury).

Stomach—Repair.

► **Additional Information**

Blunt Abdominal Trauma—Spleen most often injured.

Penetrating Abdominal Trauma—Small bowel most often injured.

Positive Peritoneal Lavage Criteria—Red blood count (RBC) > 20,000 (in penetrating injury) or > 100,000 (in blunt injury).

F. Pelvic Fractures

► **H&P Keys**
Pain, with history of significant injury.

► **Diagnosis**
History and physical exam, x-ray studies, CT exam.

► **Disease Severity**
Review x-rays. Prognosis worse in elderly and with coexisting medical problems.

► **Concept and Application**
Trauma via falls, motor vehicle accidents, sports injuries, etc., resulting in fracture of innominate bone (ilium, ischium, or pubis), sacrum.

► **Treatment Steps**
1. Depends on multiple factors, with open reduction and internal fixation (ORIF), traction, and external fixation as choices.
2. Evaluation for coexisting injuries or trauma and treatment accordingly.

   Fracture of Ilium—Rest.

   Fracture of Anterior Superior Spine—Surgery.

   Fracture of Sacrum—Rest and support.

► **Additional Information**
Hemorrhage is the most important complication of pelvic fracture. Angiography with possible embolization may be required for severe, persisting hemorrhage.

G. Epidemiology and Prevention of Chest and Abdominal Injury

Epidemiology—Etiology most often cites motor vehicle accidents. Blunt injury due to occupational injury or falls play a role. Increased incidence of trauma-related abdominal and chest injury in low socioeconomic areas. Pneumothorax and hemothorax, perforation of viscera, and vascular tears are common.

Prevention—Involves driver education and vehicle safety modifications for automobiles. Community programs, education, job opportunity, and effective law enforcement reduce the incidence of street crime trauma.

IV. LACERATIONS

► **H&P Keys**
Observation; consider both history and source of injury; ascertain tetanus immunization status.

► **Diagnosis**
History and physical exam.

► **Disease Severity**
Evaluate neurovascular status and check for associated injuries, fractures, and hypotension.

► Concept and Application
Soft tissue injury secondary to trauma.

► Treatment Steps
1. Irrigation and debridement, antibiotics if indicated, tetanus toxoid, and primary closure (maintaining minimal wound tension and everting wound edges).
2. Use 1–2% lidocaine for anesthesia (with epinephrine, except for digits and end organs).
3. Remove sutures in 7–14 days. Utilize deep and subcuticular to relieve tension on skin edges. Try to remove facial sutures in 5 days.

► Additional Information
Increased infection is noted with primary closure of human bites.

V. FOREIGN BODIES

A. Eye, Ear, and Nose

► H&P Keys

Ear and Nose—Asymptomatic or odor, unilateral purulent drainage.

Eye—Pain, decreased visual acuity.

► Diagnosis
Physical exam.

► Disease Severity

Ear and Nose—Check tympanic membrane, test hearing.

Eye—Full ophthalmoscopic exam.

► Concept and Application

Ear and Nose—Commonly children.

Eye—Often work-related, trauma.

► Treatment Steps

Ear and Nose—Gentle removal (forceps, irrigation).

Eye—Removal of foreign body under local anesthesia. Avoid additional trauma during object removal. Ensure anesthesia is adequate and, in pediatric patient, control movement.

B. Aspiration

► H&P Keys
Wheezing and dyspnea may be present. History of child with object in mouth, reduced cough reflex secondary to anesthesia, disease, etc. Often an abrupt onset of cough or wheezing, dyspnea, and voice change. Most common in children under age 4.

► Diagnosis
CXR (opaque foreign body, atelectasis, or unilateral hyperinflation causing mediastinal shift).

► Disease Severity
Evaluate degree of respiratory distress.

► Concept and Application

Obstruction of trachea or bronchi by a foreign body.

► Treatment Steps

Removal via bronchoscopy.

► Additional Information

Epidemiology—Children are a high-risk group.

Prevention—Includes identification and management of high-risk patients (postop, sedated, or overdosed, with nasogastric [NG] tube, with neuromuscular disorders), reduction of gastric acidity (ranitidine [Zantac], etc.). In children: avoidance of grapes, hot dogs; checking toys and objects for small parts, and maintaining alertness. Peanuts are the most frequently aspirated object in children. Instruction in the Heimlich maneuver.

C. Swallowed

► H&P Keys

Sudden onset of gagging, pain, and choking.

► Diagnosis

Indirect laryngoscopy, x-rays, including barium swallow.

► Disease Severity

Observation and evaluation for esophageal perforation.

► Concept and Application

Increased frequency with motility disorders, stricture, and children results in lodged foreign body. Most common location is at the cricopharyngeus muscle.

► Treatment Steps

Endoscopic removal. Identify location (above or below gastro-esophageal sphincter). Observe. If perforation, antibiotics are given to avoid mediastinitis. Do not give meat tenderizer for obstruction by meat.

VI. BURNS

A. Eye Burns

See Ocular Injury section on page 185.

B. Thermal Burns

► H&P Keys

Assess degree of burn depth, determine etiology (thermal, chemical, etc.), duration of exposure, and emergency or home treatment rendered.

► Diagnosis

History and physical exam.

► Disease Severity

Erythema minor (first degree). Blisters (split thickness; second degree). Pain (first and second degree). No pain (third degree).

► Concept and Application

Burns result in thermal skin and tissue injury. Total epidermis destruction with partial dermis destruction is typical of second-degree burns. Total epidermis and dermis destruction is noted in third-degree burns.

▶ Treatment Steps

Removal of patient from source of burn, CPR, cooling burn, cleaning and debridement of burn, fluids (Ringer's initially), determination of area of burn, full history and physical exam, antibiotics, tetanus toxoid, grafting. For minor burn: loose gauze wrap on nonadhering dressing. For severe burns: CPR and airway control, fluid replacement (monitoring CVP and output), NG tube, pain and sepsis control (morphine), surgical treatment (grafting, etc.).

▶ Additional Information

Rule of nines to estimate burn extent: Each leg is 18%, each arm 9%, body front 18%, back 18%, head 9%, groin 1%.

C. Electrical Burns

▶ H&P Keys

Look for an entry or exit wound (high voltage, lightning). Massive tissue and bone destruction may be noted. Patients may be comatose and in cardiac arrest.

▶ Diagnosis

History and physical exam, serial arterial blood gases (ABGs), and hematocrit.

▶ Disease Severity

Prognostic factors include duration of electrical contact, amount of grounding present, path of the current, and amount of moisture present (moisture lowers skin resistance).

Massive tissue necrosis may precede infection, rhabdomyolysis. Assess and monitor cardiac and pulmonary status. Persisting myoglobinuria indicates significant muscle injury.

▶ Concept and Application

Direct electrical tissue trauma.

▶ Treatment Steps

1. Safe removal of patient from source, CPR, fluids and electrolyte treatment, cleaning and debridement of burns, surgical evaluation (fasciotomy, amputation), tetanus toxoid.
2. Significant fluid replacement may be required.
3. Monitor for arrhythmias.
4. Silver sulfadiazine cream may be employed topically.

VII. POISONING

A. Acetaminophen

▶ H&P Keys

Nausea and vomiting and diaphoresis.

▶ Diagnosis

Serum acetaminophen level.

► Disease Severity

Plot acetaminophen level on Rumack–Matthew nomogram to define risk. Monitor vital signs; may have hepatic failure or hepatic necrosis (jaundice, abnormal liver functions, right upper abdominal pain).

► Treatment Steps

1. Activated charcoal. Consider gastric lavage if < 1 hour from time of ingestion. Ipecac used in children only if < 1 hour from time of ingestion.
2. Antidote is acetylcysteine (Mucomyst).

B. Tricyclic Antidepressants

► H&P Keys

Transient hypertension, then hypotension, tachycardia, arrhythmias, conduction blocks, seizures, anticholinergic symptoms (dry mucosa or skin, urinary retention).

► Diagnosis

History and physical exam, ECG (wide QRS). Blood levels not routinely available as stat test.

► Disease Severity

Increasing serum levels correlated with increasing risk (seizures, arrhythmias). Monitor mentation, cardiac status, respiratory rate and exchange.

► Treatment Steps

1. Gastric lavage, activated charcoal, NG tube suction.
2. Sodium bicarbonate to correct acidosis.
3. Physostigmine, phenytoin (Dilantin) for seizures.

C. Sedatives

► H&P Keys

Lethargy, confusion, coma, hypotension, respiratory depression, disconjugate eye motion.

► Diagnosis

History and physical exam, urine drug screen, blood drug level available.

► Disease Severity

Coma scale, respiration depression. Length of time since ingestion and history of amount ingested may assist in severity determination.

► Treatment Steps

1. Control of airway, activated charcoal (if patient awake), cautious gastric lavage.
2. Supportive care.

D. Stimulants

► H&P Keys

Euphoria, dilated pupils, hypertension, tremors, tachycardia, hyperactivity, psychosis, hyperthermia, seizures, anxiety, nausea and vomiting.

► Diagnosis

History and physical exam (tremor, increased bowel sounds, etc.).

▶ Disease Severity

Determined by amount ingested (peak effects 1–2 hours after ingestion), coexisting medical problems, cardiac status.

▶ Treatment Steps

1. Supportive (treatment of hypertension, seizures, arrhythmias), charcoal.
2. Emesis may cause seizures.

E. Cocaine

▶ H&P Keys

Agitation, hyperthermia, hypertension, cardiac arrhythmia, tachycardia, seizures, pulmonary edema.

▶ Diagnosis

History and physical exam, urine drug screen.

▶ Disease Severity

Assess by history, cardiac status.

▶ Management

Supportive treatment, control of airway, monitor core temperature.

F. PCP (Phencyclidine)

▶ H&P Keys

Nystagmus, blank stare, psychosis, lethargy, incoordination, violent behavior, self-destructive behavior.

▶ Diagnosis

History and physical exam, urine drug screen. May have elevated creatine phosphokinase and myoglobinuria.

▶ Disease Severity

Physical exam.

▶ Treatment Steps

Control of airway, activated charcoal, supportive therapy.

G. Alcohol

▶ H&P Keys

Methanol—Blurred vision, headache, vomiting.

Ethanol—Incoordination, diplopia, drunkenness.

▶ Diagnosis

History and physical exam, blood alcohol level. May have elevated triglycerides, uric acid, and γ-glutamyl transferase (GGT).

▶ Disease Severity

Assess history, impact on the individual and the family, and clinical picture (withdrawal, abnormal lab tests, hepatic function).

▶ Treatment Steps

Methanol—Antidote (ethanol), sodium bicarbonate, detoxification, and rehabilitation.

Ethanol
1. Supportive care, airway protection/control.
2. Prevention includes continued support (Alcoholics Anonymous meetings) and medication (disulfiram).

H. Solvent Sniffing

▶ H&P Keys

Gastrointestinal (GI) irritation, CNS symptoms. Skin injury.

▶ Diagnosis

History and physical exam.

▶ Disease Severity

Assess duration and frequency of abuse; neurologic exam.

▶ Treatment Steps

Supportive treatment, control of airway, oxygen.

I. Heavy Metals and Arsenic

▶ H&P Keys

GI symptoms, arrhythmia, CNS symptoms, skin bronzing, cyanosis, delirium, Mees' lines, renal failure, vomiting, garlic odor.

▶ Diagnosis

History and physical exam, x-ray of abdomen (arsenic, lead, and iodides may be radiopaque), anemia, hematuria.

▶ Disease Severity

Assess by clinical exam (neurologic, cardiac, and pulmonary status).

▶ Treatment Steps

Emesis, gastric lavage, dimercaprol (BAL), 3–5 mg/kg IM q 4–6 h.

▶ Additional Information

Lead—Vomiting, lethargy, blue gum line; lavage, then use edetate calcium disodium (EDTA calcium).

Mercury—Give milk, gastric lavage, then dimercaprol. Chelators such as edetate calcium disodium (EDTA calcium), penicillamine, and BAL may be used for treatment of heavy metal toxicity.

J. Carbon Monoxide

▶ H&P Keys

Headache, confusion, nausea, dyspnea, clumsiness, cyanosis, or cherry-red skin.

▶ Diagnosis

History and physical exam (cyanosis), elevated blood carboxyhemoglobin.

▶ Disease Severity

Chronic exposure associated with parkinsonism.

▶ Treatment Steps

1. Removal from source, 100% oxygen.
2. Hyperbaric oxygen (if available) for comatose patients.

K. Diethyl-*m*-toluamide (DEET)

▶ H&P Keys

CNS symptoms, seizures, coma, hypotension, GI irritation.

▶ Diagnosis

History and physical exam.

► on rounds

POISONING SYMPTOMS AT A GLANCE

• Carbon monoxide	Headache, confusion, cyanosis, cherry-red skin
• DEET	CNS symptoms
• Iron	Diarrhea, abdominal pain, bloody stools
• Theophylline	Tremor, nausea, vomiting
• Aspirin	Respiratory alkalosis, metabolic acidosis, hyperventilation, tinnitus
• Stimulants	Dilated pupils, euphoria, hypertension, tremor
• Cocaine	Agitation, hyperthermia, hypertension, arrhythmia
• PCP	Nystagmus, blank stare, violent behavior, incoordination
• Acetaminophen	Nausea and vomiting
• Sedatives	Lethargy, confusion, coma, hypotension
• Heavy metal and arsenic	GI symptoms, CNS symptoms, skin bronzing

► Disease Severity

By clinical exam (neurologic status, time since exposure, degree of exposure).

► Treatment Steps

Emesis, gastric lavage.

L. Additional Information

1. Other Poisonings

Iron—Symptoms include diarrhea, abdominal pain, and bloody stools. Gastric lavage, parenteral deferoxamine.

Aspirin—Causes respiratory alkalosis and metabolic acidosis. Patient may be hyperventilating, diaphoretic, and report tinnitus.

Theophylline—Look for tremor, nausea and vomiting, and metabolic acidosis. Blood drug level can be checked.

Narcotics—Pinpoint pupils, hypotension; administration of naloxone hydrochloride (Narcan).

Barbiturates—Respiratory depression, hypotension; supportive care, charcoal, and alkalinization of urine.

2. Selected Antidotes

Folic acid for methyl alcohol poisoning. D-Penicillamine for copper poisoning. Protamine sulfate for heparin overdose. Latrodectus antivenin for black widow spider bites.

3. Drugs Visible on X-Ray

Heavy metals, phenothiazines, iodides, and chloral hydrate.

4. Poisoning Management Overview

1. Airway, breathing, circulation: history and physical exam; lab studies; gastric lavage and emesis; antidote after lavage; supportive care; laboratory workup.
2. Avoid ipecac with caustic ingestion and in somnolent patient.
3. If antidote available, cautious use of charcoal in addition. Used primarily in children.

VIII. FRACTURES

A. Vertebral Column

▶ H&P Keys

Pain, neurologic abnormalities.

▶ Diagnosis

History and physical exam, x-ray exam, CT exam.

▶ Disease Severity

Neurologic status, serial evaluations.

▶ Concept and Application

Vertebral body fracture (wedging, body fracture), articular process fracture, transverse process fracture.

▶ Treatment Steps

Simple Compression Fracture—Brace (some advocate surgical intervention, especially in young individual).

Initial Cervical Spine Treatment
1. Airway control with cervical spine protection, assess and support breathing, control shock and hemorrhage.
2. For unstable fracture or progressing neurologic deficit, cranial traction followed by surgical internal fixation.
3. Most other simple spinal fractures are treated with bracing or casting, with surgical intervention reserved for progressive neurologic symptoms.

B. Extremities

1. Tibia

▶ H&P Keys

Pain when pressure applied to the tibia.

▶ Diagnosis

History and physical exam, x-ray.

▶ Disease Severity

Determine severity via x-ray, coexisting medical problems.

▶ Concept and Application

Trauma.

▶ Treatment Steps

Tibial Shaft—Closed reduction and cast or internal fixation with intramedullary rodding.

Medial Tibial Condyle—ORIF.

Lateral Tibial Condyle—External reduction.

2. Fibula

▶ H&P Keys

Pain and swelling, with retained ability to walk.

▶ Diagnosis

History and physical exam, x-ray exam.

► **Disease Severity**

Rule out coexisting ankle injury.

► **Concept and Application**

Trauma.

► **Treatment Steps**

Walking cast or boot, followed by therapy.

3. Femur

► **H&P Keys**

Pain, swelling, deformity.

► **Diagnosis**

History and physical exam, x-ray studies.

► **Disease Severity**

Evaluate for coexisting medical problems, hypotension.

► **Concept and Application**

Usually significant trauma. With children, rule out child abuse.

► **Treatment Steps**

Femoral Neck
1. ORIF vs. long-term traction (usually in immobile patients).
2. Complications include avascular necrosis and nonunion of fracture.

4. Radius

► **H&P Keys**

Pain, reduced elbow-joint motion.

► **Diagnosis**

History and physical exam, roentgenographic studies.

► **Disease Severity**

Check neurovascular status.

► **Concept and Application**

Fall on hand common.

Colles' Fracture—Fall on extended wrist, fracture of distal radius and ulnar styloid (volar angulation and dorsal displacement).

Smith's Fracture—Fall on flexed wrist (dorsal angulation and volar displacement).

► **Treatment Steps**

Radial Head
1. Hemarthrosis aspiration and mobilization if simple.
2. Surgical (ORIF) if complete or displaced fracture.

Distal Radius Undisplaced—Cast 4–6 weeks, therapy.

5. Ulna

► **H&P Keys**

Pain, swelling, deformity.

► **Diagnosis**

History and physical exam, x-ray.

► **Disease Severity**
Check neurovascular status.

► **Concept and Application**
Trauma.

► **Treatment Steps**

Undisplaced—Closed or open reduction.

Displaced—ORIF.

Greenstick Radial or Ulnar Fractures in Children—Complete the break, then cast.

6. Humerus

► **H&P Keys**
Pain, swelling.

► **Diagnosis**
History and physical exam, x-ray studies.

► **Disease Severity**
Evaluate neurovascular status.

► **Concept and Application**
Trauma.

► **Treatment Steps**

Humeral Shaft or Distal Humerus—Reduction (traction), then splint and sling.

Surgical Neck of Humerus
1. Avoid immobilization, instead gentle range of motion.
2. ORIF for displaced tuberosity fracture.

► **Additional Information**

Childhood Medial or Lateral Epicondyle Fractures—If without displacement, splint elbow at 90°. With any displacement, ORIF.

IX. SPRAINS AND DISLOCATIONS

Sprains involve ligament injury; strains affect muscle; dislocations affect joints.

A. Hand

1. Distal Interphalangeal (DIP) Sprain

► **H&P Keys**
Pain, difficulty with joint flexion or extension.

► **Diagnosis**
History and physical exam, x-ray exam.

► **Disease Severity**
Evaluate strength and range of motion.

► **Concept and Application**
DIP joint injury or sprain, resulting in possible flexor–extensor tendon disruption.

► Treatment Steps

Symptomatic (if able to bend or extend joint).

► Additional Information

Mallet Finger—Tendon disruption, with loss of joint extension. Treat with splinting in hyperextension or surgery.

2. Proximal Interphalangeal (PIP) Dislocation

► H&P Keys

Pain. Displaced digit and motion loss.

► Diagnosis

History and physical exam. X-ray to rule out fracture.

► Disease Severity

Examine for neurovascular status.

► Concept and Application

Injury secondary to hyperextension, trauma.

► Treatment Steps

Flexion splint 2 weeks.

► Additional Information

PIP Sprain—Splint if a hyperextension injury or collateral ligament sprain (flexion splint). Extensor slip tear-splint in hyperextension.

3. Metacarpal Phalangeal (MCP) Sprain

► H&P Keys

Sprained finger or thumb MCP joint resulting in pain and motion loss.

► Diagnosis

History and physical exam, x-ray exam.

► Disease Severity

Evaluate for pinch, laxity of thumb ligaments. Use of hand contingent on adequate thumb strength.

► Concept and Application

Trauma, often hyperextension.

► Treatment Steps

Splint.

► Additional Information

Gamekeeper's Thumb—MCP joint of thumb sprained, affecting the ulnar collateral ligament. If suspected requires immobilization of thumb and urgent hand surgeon consultation.

B. Ankle

1. Lateral Ankle Pain

Injury to anterior talofibular ligament. May also include injury to fibulocalcaneal and posterior talofibular ligaments.

2. Medial Pain

Deltoid ligament injury.

► **Treatment Steps**

1. RICE (rest, ice, compression, elevation).
2. Nonsteroidal anti-inflammatory drugs (NSAIDs).
3. Ankle splint for second-degree sprain; cast for third-degree sprain.

C. Elbow Dislocation

Check vascular and neurologic status; if urgent reduction indicated, splint.

D. Shoulder Dislocation or Injury

Anterior inferior dislocation most common (in young patients).

► **Treatment Steps**

Dislocation—Urgent reduction (slow traction or reduction under anesthesia). Other dislocations include posterior and inferior.

Mild Sprain—Prevent external rotation for 6 weeks; sling.

X. DROWNING

► **H&P Keys**

Wheezing, tachypnea, vomiting, pulmonary edema, unconsciousness, shock, and cardiac arrest.

► **Diagnosis**

History and physical exam, CXR, ABGs, ECG.

► **Disease Severity**

Consider duration of immersion, patient's baseline medical status, water temperature, timing of rescue measures, cardiac and pulmonary status, electroencephalogram (EEG).

► **Concept and Application**

Dry (laryngospasm) or water-induced asphyxia results in hypoxia and brain damage.

► **Treatment Steps**

1. Urgent CPR and 100% oxygen.
2. Remember to continue CPR in hypothermic or prolonged cold-water submersion victims.

XI. INSECT AND SNAKE BITES

► **H&P Keys**

Insect Bite—Mild erythema to anaphylaxis and hypotension.

Snake Bite—Pain, swelling, hemorrhage, weakness, disseminated intravascular coagulation (DIC), possible systemic signs (lethargy, vomiting, shock).

▶ Diagnosis

History and physical exam. Leukocytosis and coagulation disorders.

▶ Disease Severity

Assess cardiac and pulmonary status. Consider patient's age and pre-existing medical problems, time since envenomation, location of bite (trunk has worse outcome than extremity), snake size (larger worse), and emergency treatment received.

▶ Concept and Application

Insects—Hymenoptera species commonly.

Snakes—In United States, pit vipers (copperhead, rattlesnake, water moccasin) are responsible for poisonous bites and are toxic to cardiac, vascular, and hematologic systems.

▶ Treatment Steps

Insect Bite—Remove stinger, ice, diphenhydramine hydrochloride (Benadryl).

Anaphylaxis—Epinephrine (1:1,000 0.3 mL SQ), antihistamines, prednisone.

Snake Bite—Tourniquet, antivenin.

▶ Additional Information

Black Widow Spider (**Latrodectus mactans**)—Red hourglass pattern on abdomen, bite results in muscle spasm and cramping. First, clean wound, give tetanus toxoid, muscle relaxant, antivenin.

Brown Recluse Spider (**Loxosceles reclusa**)—Violin design on back; possible skin necrosis; treat by cleaning wound and tetanus toxoid.

XII. ANAPHYLACTIC SHOCK

Systemic severe immunoglobulin E (IgE)-induced allergic reaction.

▶ H&P Keys

Hypotension, urticaria, dyspnea, tachycardia, vascular collapse, pruritus.

▶ Diagnosis

History (onset of symptoms in seconds to minutes) and physical exam.

▶ Disease Severity

Assess cardiac and pulmonary systems. Prognosis worse without early intervention.

▶ Concept and Application

Mast cell and basophils release histamine, platelet-activating factor (PAF), and arachidonic acid.

▶ Treatment Steps
1. CPR and control airway.
2. Epinephrine (1:1,000 0.3–0.5 mL SQ or 1:10,000 0.5–1 mg slow IV administration if in shock), Benadryl, fluids, dopamine, inhaled β-agonists, corticosteroids, oxygen.

XIII. ADDITIONAL MANAGEMENT INFORMATION

A. Traumatic Injury

Administer CPR, control airway, treat urgent problems (large pneumothorax, hemorrhage, etc.), administer oxygen, insert IV line, give fluids and medications, obtain history and physical exam, x-ray and lab studies.

B. Shock

Administer CPR, control airway, obtain history and physical exam, administer fluids (caution with cardiogenic shock, check CVP and output), administer vasopressors (dopamine), get lab studies, administer: corticosteroids, diuretic (protects kidneys), buffers, antibiotics (septic shock).

C. Child Abuse, Sexual Abuse, Sexual Assault

History and physical exam, medical treatment, documentation of evidence and appropriate reporting, psychological evaluation and support, separation from danger (child abuse), and long-term care plan.

D. Thermal Injuries

1. Frostbite

▶ H&P Keys

Tissue cold and hard without feeling.

▶ Diagnosis

History and physical exam; affected area may be white (superficial injury) or firm and frozen (deep injury).

▶ Disease Severity

Duration of exposure, prior presence of peripheral vascular disease or other medical problems.

▶ Concept and Application

Tissue damage as a direct result of thermal trauma. Skin and tissue damage from ice crystal formation. May be superficial or deep. Line of demarcation may develop.

▶ Treatment Steps

Rapid rewarming after body core temperature warming, tetanus toxoid, possibly antibiotics, surgical evaluation, amputation.

2. Hypothermia

▶ H&P Keys

Reduced core temperature (under 35°C), lethargy, coma, hypotension, confusion, miotic pupils.

▶ Diagnosis

History and physical exam, core temperature at or below 95°F (35°C), ECG (Osborne wave, elevated J-point; bradycardia; arrhythmias), flat EEG, metabolic acidosis.

▶ Disease Severity

Assess duration of exposure, age (mortality much worse in the elderly), emergency treatment rendered, and preexisting medical problems. Worse prognosis with lower temperatures.

► Concept and Application

Reduced core temperature from cold exposure resulting in decreased cardiac output, hypotension.

► Treatment Steps

1. CPR, core rewarming (heated oxygen), warming blankets, volume expansion.
2. Monitor ABGs, electrolytes, and rule out sepsis.

► Additional Information

Hypothermia Complications—DIC, pneumonia.

Hypothermic Death—Never declare dead unless patient rewarmed to 98.6°F.

3. Heatstroke

► H&P Keys

Confusion, elevated core temperature with or without diaphoresis, tachycardia, hypotension, hot skin, and headache.

► Diagnosis

History and physical exam, core temperature high, combined with CNS signs.

► Disease Severity

Assess cardiovascular status. Worse prognosis with significant preexisting disease.

► Concept and Application

Tissue injury from elevated temperature, with children and elderly at most risk.

► Treatment Steps

Urgent cooling (water spray, fans, ice packs).

► Additional Information

Heat Cramps—Cramps from salt depletion; skin cool; give fluids and salt, keep cool.

Heat Exhaustion—Salt and water loss; nausea, weakness, headache, thirst; give fluids and salt, keep cool.

Complications of Heatstroke—DIC, rhabdomyolysis, acidosis.

XIV. EPIDEMIOLOGY AND PREVENTION OF SELECTED ACCIDENTS

A. Home Accidents

Epidemiology—Involves all age groups and consists of a wide variety of hazards (electrical, thermal, poisoning, and trauma).

Prevention—Includes education, preventive planning (bicycle helmets, toy and playground equipment checks, removal of dangerous objects, obstacles, etc.).

B. Workplace Accidents

Epidemiology—Includes increased risk groups (meat cutters and packers, steelworkers, etc.), along with all employees.

Prevention—Includes both education and exercise of precautions (eye shield, hearing protection, hard hats, steel-tip shoes, etc.) and elimination of dangerous materials, practices, and procedures.

C. Athletic Accidents

Epidemiology—Includes home, school, recreational, and professional accidents. Impact and type of injuries are multiple, including falls, trauma, thermal injury, sprains and strains, fractures, concussions, contusions, and death.

Prevention—Includes education, correction of both training and performance errors (spearing in football), providing protective equipment of correct fit.

D. Automobile Accidents and Drunk Driving

Epidemiology—Includes all ages of society, with increased risk for both teenagers (drunk and reckless driving) and the elderly (visual impairment, cognitive functioning, and reaction time). Increased risk is associated with motorcycle and three-wheel all-terrain vehicle use.

Prevention—Includes education (driving, using seat belts, avoidance of drugs and alcohol), reduced speed limits, better roads, improved roadway markings and median barriers, and abutment protection. Numerous other factors play a role, such as larger-size vehicles, air bags, collapsible steering wheel, and padded dash regulations. Drunk driving prevention includes both education and modification of drinking age, along with effective legal deterrents (fines and jail terms).

E. Head and Spinal Cord Injury and Whiplash

Epidemiology—Includes motor vehicle accidents (the major cause of these injuries), falls, child abuse, occupational and trauma-induced accidents.

Prevention—Includes education, safety devices (automotive: air bags, seat and shoulder belts, padded dashboards, headrests; work: hard hats, etc.), and behavior modification (avoidance of high-risk activities or behavior). Appropriate emergency care may prevent permanent neurologic sequelae (sandbag, head stabilization).

F. Drowning

Epidemiology—Involves children most often.

Prevention—Centers on education (parents and children), swimming instruction, water and boating safety, dangers of hyperventilation, dangers of drug and alcohol use, and CPR training. Recognition of high-risk patients (epilepsy, syncope, divers, children, etc.).

G. Ingestion of Poisonous and Toxic Agents

Epidemiology—Includes accidental overdose in both children and adults and work and environmental toxicology and suicide in adolescents and adults.

Prevention—Includes education, awareness and labeling of dangerous substances, prevention of child access (keeping medication and toxins locked and in unaccessible locations, "childproof" containers), and easy access to emergency advice and treatment. Importance of home supply of ipecac.

H. Gunshot and Stab Wounds

Epidemiology—Demonstrates an increasing rate of violent crime and increasing use of handguns and automatic weapons. Elevated level of crime in poor socioeconomic areas. Impact includes an ever-increasing utilization of medical emergency facilities, financial burden on the medical insurance system, and morbidity and mortality, including innocent bystanders.

Prevention—Includes education, gun control, control of alcohol and drug use and abuse, law enforcement, and society efforts to diffuse inner-city neglect.

I. Thermal Injury

Prevention—Key points include education (increased heat disorders with alcohol; cystic fibrosis patients; dehydration; dark, non-breathable clothing; use of antipsychotics and diuretics; high-humidity days) and need for increased fluid intake and gradual heat acclimatization. Skin protection and early recognition of symptoms in frostbite and hypothermia patients is critical. Increased awareness for high-risk patients (elderly and children, alcohol and drug abusers, CNS disease, and sepsis) is important.

J. Child, Spouse, and Elderly Abuse

Epidemiology—Suggests that susceptible abuse victims include children, spouses, and the elderly. Impact is significant as a frequent society malady with great morbidity, mortality, and possible permanent psychological impact. Difficulty in obtaining accurate numbers of cases involved because of sensitivity of the subject and reluctance of many abused individuals to tell their stories.

Prevention—Physician and family education to obtain early diagnosis and screen for potentially abusive parents (observe and evaluate mother for postpartum depression). High index of suspicion may be required. Past medical history (abusers may have been abused themselves as children).

K. Sexual Abuse and Rape

Epidemiology—Suggests that adolescents and young children are at risk for sexual abuse (usually by family member).

Prevention—Includes education and early recognition by health care workers. Rape prevention includes patient education (how to avoid being a target) and self-defense.

L. Fire Prevention

Prevention—Includes education (not smoking in bed, proper storage of flammables, etc.), home precautions (smoke detectors and fire extinguisher, fireplace glass screen, fire safety plan, escape route, upkeep of electrical systems, etc.).

M. Falls

Epidemiology—Affect children, elderly, and adults (workplace injury, seizure-disorder patients, alcoholics) and are a frequent cause of accidental death. Significant morbidity and mortality associated with hip fractures.

Prevention—For children includes child-proofing the house, covering sharp corners, window locks, stair gates, and control of obstacles. For the elderly, medical and family assessment for need of cane, walker, or wheelchair; medical treatment or control of contributing illness (Parkinson's disease, visual impairment, anemia, stroke, etc.).

BIBLIOGRAPHY

Ballenger JJ. *Diseases of the Nose, Throat, Ear, Head, and Neck,* 14th ed. Philadelphia: Lea & Febiger, 1991.

Behrman RE. *Nelson Textbook of Pediatrics,* 17th ed. Philadelphia: W.B. Saunders, 2004.

Birnbaum JS. *The Musculoskeletal Manual,* 2nd ed. Orlando, FL: Academic Press, 1986.

Bryson PD. *Comprehensive Review in Toxicology,* 2nd ed. Rockville, MD: Aspen, 1989.

Cailliet R. *Neck and Arm Pain,* 3rd ed. Philadelphia: F.A. Davis, 1991.

D'Ambrosia RD. *Musculoskeletal Disorders, Regional Examination and Differential Diagnosis,* 2nd ed. Philadelphia: J.B. Lippincott, 1986.

Dreisbach RH. *Handbook of Poisoning: Prevention, Diagnosis and Treatment,* 13th ed. Norwalk, CT: Appleton & Lange, 2001.

Goldfrank LR, Flomenbaum NE, Lewin NA, et al (eds.). *Goldfrank's Toxicologic Emergencies,* 7th ed. Stamford, CT: Appleton & Lange, 2002.

Hardy JD. *Textbook of Surgery,* 2nd ed. Philadelphia: J.B. Lippincott, 1988.

Rockwood CA. *Fractures in Adults,* 3rd ed. Philadelphia: J.B. Lippincott, 1991; 1, 2.

Tierney LM, McPhee SJ, Papadakis MA (eds.). *Current Medical Diagnosis and Treatment.* Stamford, CT: Appleton & Lange, 2005.

Turek SL. *Orthopaedic Principles and Their Application,* 4th ed. Philadelphia: J.B. Lippincott, 1984; 1, 2.

Infectious Disease | 8

I. HUMAN IMMUNODEFICIENCY VIRUS (HIV) INFECTION AND THE ACQUIRED IMMUNE DEFICIENCY SYNDROME (AIDS)

A. HIV Infection

▶ H&P Keys

HIV infection is acquired by sexual transmission, direct blood contact, or from mother to child. About 4–6 weeks after exposure to HIV, a mononucleosis-like illness (fever, malaise, lymphadenopathy, rash, headache, arthralgias, or myalgias) occurs in most but not all people, lasting 1–2 weeks. Then there is an asymptomatic period with active viral replication and declining immune function. Ultimately, the patient may develop sweats, weight loss, diarrhea, and/or an opportunistic infection (see individual descriptions of common opportunistic infections [OIs] for clinical clues) or malignant disease associated with HIV-related immunosuppression.

▶ Diagnosis

HIV testing (enzyme-linked immunosorbent assay [ELISA], Western blot) is the first blood test. Further workup in the HIV-positive patient includes: (1) tracking immune function (CD4+-positive T-lymphocyte count [CD4+]); (2) following viral burden (quantitative viral RNA); (3) general tests such as complete blood count (CBC), chemistry (including liver tests), VDRL (Venereal Disease Research Laboratory) or rapid plasma reagin (RPR), purified protein derivative (PPD), hepatitis B serology, cytomegalovirus (CMV) serology, toxoplasmosis serology, Pap smear. Viral load measurements help to predict the initial rate of progression to AIDS and to select, maintain, and modify effective antiretroviral therapy.

▶ Disease Severity

Association between development of OIs and absolute (normal = 800–1,200) or percentage (normal = 55–70%) CD4+. As CD4+ declines, risk of OI increases substantially. With CD4+ > 800, risk of OI very small; CD4+ 200–500, increasing risk for *Mycobacterium tuberculosis, Histoplasma, Cryptococcus;* CD4+ < 200, risk for *Pneumocystis jiroveci* pneumonia (PCP; formerly known as *Pneumocystis carinii* pneumonia); CD4+ < 100, increasing risk for *Toxoplasma,* CMV, *Mycobacterium avium* complex (MAC). OIs are associated with the majority of AIDS deaths. High HIV viral load predicts rapid disease progression. Initiation or modification of antiretroviral therapy may be dictated based on these results. (See Tables 8–1 and 8–2.)

▶ Concept and Application

HIV attacks CD4+-positive T lymphocytes. Loss of CD4+ T cells results in progressive immune impairment with OI or cancer. Antiviral chemotherapy may be aimed at any point in the viral life cycle. Reverse transcriptase (nucleoside, nucleotide, and nonnucleoside reverse transcriptase inhibitors), viral fusion, and protease (protease inhibitors) are the viral targets thus far utilized in antiretroviral therapy. The HIV viral load is high during initial infection and then falls to a steady-state level that varies considerably (approximately 102–106 HIV RNA copies/mL). The CD4+ count also falls during acute HIV infection and then rebounds. The high mutational rate of HIV makes combination therapy necessary to escape or delay anti-

---

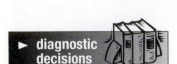

▶ diagnostic decisions

HIV DIAGNOSIS—FACTORS LEADING TO SUSPICION

Risk Factors
Sexual contact, sharing needles, unscreened blood or blood products, maternal/fetal.

Clinical Features Before Developing Opportunistic Infection
Weight loss/wasting, fatigue, adenopathy, diarrhea, oral lesions, cognitive deficits.

Opportunistic Infections
Pneumocystis jiroveci pneumonia, *Mycobacterium avium* complex infection, toxoplasmosis, cryptococcal meningitis, unexplained thrush or esophageal candidal infection.

Unexplained "Normal Infections"
Tuberculosis, syphilis, severe pneumococcal disease, histoplasmosis.

Malignancies
Kaposi's sarcoma, lymphoma, Hodgkin's disease.

8-1

1993 REVISED CLASSIFICATION SYSTEM FOR HIV INFECTION AND EXPANDED AIDS SURVEILLANCE CASE DEFINITION FOR ADOLESCENTS AND ADULTS[a]

	Clinical Categories		
CD4+ T-cell Categories	(A) Asymptomatic, Acute (Primary) HIV or PGL	(B) Symptomatic, not (A) or (C) Conditions	(C) AIDS- Indicator Conditions[b]
1. ≥ 500/µL	A1	B1	C1
2. 200–499/µL	A2	B2	C2
3. < 200/µL AIDS-indicator T-cell count	A3	B3	C3

[a]Persons with the AIDS-indicator conditions (category C) as well as those with CD4+ T-lymphocyte counts < 200/µL are reportable as AIDS cases.

[b]See text AIDS case definition.

PGL, persistent generalized lymphadenopathy.

retroviral resistance. The initial steady-state HIV load has predictive value for the rapidity of disease progression. The HIV viral load on treatment has important implications for adjusting antiretroviral therapy.

► Treatment Steps

1. There are five classes of antiretroviral agents approved for use in the United States. There are seven nucleoside reverse transcriptase inhibitors: zidovudine (AZT, ZDV, Retrovir), didanosine (ddI, Videx), zalcitabine (ddC, Hivid), stavudine (d4T, Zerit), lamivudine (3TC, Epivir), abacavir (Ziagen), and emtricitabine (Emtriva). There are seven approved HIV protease inhibitors: saquinavir (Invirase, Fortovase), ritonavir (Norvir), indinavir (Crixivan), lopinavir/ritonavir (Kaletra), atazanavir (Reyataz), amprenavir (Agenerase), and fos-amprenavir (Lexiva). There are three nonnucleoside reverse transcriptase inhibitors currently

8-2

CONDITIONS INCLUDED IN THE 1993 AIDS SURVEILLANCE CASE DEFINITION

- Candidasis of bronchi, trachea, or lungs
- Candidiasis, esophageal
- Cervical cancer, invasive
- Coccidioidomycosis, disseminated or extrapulmonary
- Cryptococcosis, extrapulmonary
- Cryptosporidiosis, chronic intestinal (> 1 mo duration)
- Cytomegalovirus disease (other than liver, spleen, or nodes)
- Cytomegalovirus retinitis (with loss of vision)
- Encephalopathy (HIV-related)
- Herpes simplex: chronic ulcer(s) (> 1 mo duration), or bronchitis, pneumonitis, or esophagitis
- Histoplasmosis, disseminated or extrapulmonary
- Isosporiasis, chronic intestinal (> 1 mo duration)
- Kaposi's sarcoma
- Lymphoma, Burkitt's (or equivalent term)
- Lymphoma, immunoblastic (or equivalent term)
- Lymphoma, primary, of brain
- *Mycobacterium avium-intracellulare* complex of *M. kansasii*, disseminated or extrapulmonary
- *M. tuberculosis,* any site (pulmonary or extrapulmonary)
- *Pneumocystis jiroveci* pneumonia
- Pneumonia, recurrent
- Progressive multifocal leukoencephalopathy
- *Salmonella,* septicemia, recurrent
- Toxoplasmosis of brain
- Wasting syndrome caused by HIV

available: nevirapine (Viramune), delaverdine (Rescriptor), and efavirenz (Sustiva). Tenofovir (Viread) is a nucleotide reverse transcriptase inhibitor. An injectable fusion inhibitor (T-20, Fuzeon) is available.

2. Therapy of HIV is based on CD4+ count, HIV RNA level, and clinical status. Antiretroviral therapy is given in symptomatic HIV disease, in asymptomatic individuals with a CD4+ of < 300, and in asymptomatic persons with a CD4+ of > 300 but with a high viral load and/or a rapidly declining CD4+ count.

3. Preferred initial antiretroviral regimens include combinations of three or more drugs. Drugs of different classes are combined, and care is taken to be sure that drugs with different potential resistance mechanisms are used together. Once-a-day regimens are also available and seem to have a high rate of compliance.

4. Changes in therapy are frequent. HIV RNA levels on effective therapy should have > 0.5 log decrease. The goal level of HIV RNA after initiation of treatment is undetectable or at least < 400 copies/mL. However, some patients who are clinically stable and are tolerating their medications may be able to meet a less rigorous goal. A return of the HIV RNA level to within 0.3–0.5 log of the pretreatment value suggests treatment failure. Modifications can be based on in vitro susceptibility testing (preferred) or on clinical judgment.

5. New drugs should not be added one at a time since this favors the gradual emergence of resistance.

6. HIV RNA measurements should be obtained at baseline, 3–4 weeks after initiating or changing therapy, and every 3–4 months along with CD4+ counts.

Health Maintenance—Pneumococcal vaccine, hepatitis B vaccine (if seronegative), and annual influenza vaccine should be given. (See comments in the specific OI section for prophylaxis recommendations for PCP, MAC, etc.) Those patients who are able to achieve more normal immune function (CD4+ counts above the level associated with a given infection) can stop their prophylaxis for that OI. During the restoration of immune function, some patients will experience exacerbations of symptoms related to OIs (immune reconstitution). Counseling and HIV testing should be offered to all pregnant women. Antiretroviral therapy administration and cesarean section delivery have been documented to significantly reduce perinatal transmission of HIV to < 5%. Postexposure prophylaxis for health care workers may reduce HIV transmission. The Centers for Disease Control and Prevention (CDC) has published recommendations for this indication. An example of a postexposure prophylaxis regimen would be efavirenz plus lamivudine plus tenofovir.

B. *Pneumocystis jiroveci* (formerly *carinii*) Pneumonia (PCP)

▶ H&P Keys

The most common AIDS-defining illness in the United States. Usually presents with subacute shortness of breath and dry cough (median symptom duration before presentation is 4 weeks).

▶ Diagnosis

Usually develops when CD4+ < 200. Arterial blood gas: hypoxemia, increased A-a gradient. Chest x-ray (CXR) usually shows bilateral infiltrates. Definitive diagnosis by demonstrating organism in pulmonary specimen (induced sputum, bronchoalveolar lavage [BAL], biopsy).

► Disease Severity

Mild disease (patient may be candidate for oral, outpatient therapy): $Po_2 > 70$ mm Hg, able to take oral medication, reliable follow-up. More severe hypoxemia and tachypnea are poor prognostic features.

► Concept and Application

P. jiroveci is a fungus. Infection can occur early in life but rarely causes disease in the normal host. HIV-related immunosuppression, severe malnutrition, lymphopoietic malignancy, and organ transplantation allow *P. jiroveci* to cause disease.

► Treatment Steps

1. Mild disease may be treated orally; severe disease is treated parenterally.
2. Drug of choice is considered to be trimethoprim–sulfamethoxazole (TMP-SMZ).
3. Alternative agents include pentamidine, dapsone and trimethoprim, clindamycin and primaquine, or atovaquone.
4. Duration of therapy is usually 21 days. For nonventilated patients with more severe disease (room air $Po_2 < 70$, A-a gradient > 35 mm Hg), a short course of corticosteroids is recommended.

Health Maintenance—Primary PCP prophylaxis is recommended for all HIV-infected individuals with a CD4+ < 200. Secondary prophylaxis is indicated for all with a previous episode of PCP. Drug of choice is TMP-SMZ with alternatives, including dapsone with or without trimethoprim or pyrimethamine, aerosolized or IV pentamidine, or clindamycin and primaquine. People receiving active treatment for toxoplasmosis need not take PCP prophylaxis. For people with stable increase in CD4+ cells above $250/mm^3$, prophylaxis can be discontinued.

C. Cytomegalovirus (CMV) Infection

► H&P Keys

CMV infection is the most common viral OI in advanced AIDS. The most common infections are retinitis, gastrointestinal (GI) tract (colitis, esophagitis), and systemic (viremia associated with wasting syndrome). Ocular complaints include "floaters," decreased vision, or blindness. Ophthalmoscopic exam is diagnostic. Colitis is associated with persistent diarrhea and crampy abdominal pain. Esophagitis presents with odynophagia. Wasting syndrome consists of significant weight loss with fever or diarrhea. CMV encephalitis is characterized by cognitive and focal neurological changes, periventricular lesions on brain scan, and sometimes a polyradiculopathy.

► Diagnosis

CMV retinitis diagnosed by ophthalmoscopic exam revealing exudates and inflammatory changes following a vascular distribution. Isolation of CMV from other body sites confirms the ophthalmoscopic impression. CMV colitis or esophagitis is diagnosed by endoscopy revealing edema, erythema, erosions, and hemorrhage. Cytomegalic inclusions seen on histopathologic exam are diagnostic. CMV may be recovered from buffy coat blood culture in some patients with the wasting syndrome.

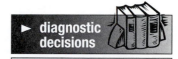

► **diagnostic decisions**

ELEMENTS TO FOLLOW IN HIV-INFECTED ADULT

Clinical
Weight loss, sense of well-being, cognitive function, functional status, new infection, new malignancy.

Laboratory—Immune
CD4+ absolute count, CD4+/CD8+ ratio, skin test reactivity.

Laboratory—Virologic
Level of HIV RNA (by PCR of b-DNA), genotypic.

► Disease Severity

The severity of CMV retinitis often is dictated by the anatomic location of lesions. Macular involvement severely affects vision; optic nerve involvement may cause blindness.

► Concept and Application

CMV infection is common in the general population, but significant disease is rare in the normal host. HIV-related immunosuppression allows for reactivation of latent viral infection or severe, progressive new infection. Finding CMV in urine, saliva, or blood documents viral presence but does not prove disease.

► Treatment Steps

1. For patients with symptomatic infection (e.g., GI disease or retinitis), a two-step approach to therapy is recommended.
2. Induction therapy is given with either ganciclovir or foscarnet for an average of 14–21 days.
3. Both drugs effectively suppress retinitis but cannot cure infection.
4. Maintenance therapy must be given lifelong to prevent recurrence, although patients with CD4+ counts exceeding 200 can stop therapy.
5. Neutropenia or thrombocytopenia with ganciclovir and renal insufficiency and electrolyte disturbance with foscarnet are frequently dose limiting.
6. Long-term maintenance therapy with ganciclovir is associated with a risk of emergence of ganciclovir resistance, dictating treatment with foscarnet.
7. Cidofovir is available for the treatment and maintenance therapy of CMV retinitis in patients with AIDS. Because of its long half-life, cidofovir is given once weekly for therapy and every other week for maintenance. Pharmacokinetics may allow for outpatient induction and maintenance without long-term IV access. Nephrotoxicity and neutropenia limit this therapy.
9. Oral valganciclovir is also approved for maintenance/preventive therapy of CMV retinitis. It is much better absorbed than oral ganciclovir.

Health Maintenance—Oral valganciclovir is available as prophylaxis for CMV disease in AIDS.

D. Tuberculosis (TB)

► H&P Keys

Symptoms of TB are usually pulmonary or may reflect extrapulmonary disease. The most common sites are peripheral lymph nodes and bone marrow. Other extrapulmonary sites include bone and joint, urine, liver, spleen, GI mucosa, and cerebrospinal fluid (CSF). TB may present as wasting syndrome. TB in early HIV infection tends to be similar to disease in non–HIV-infected patients. TB in later-stage HIV disease is more commonly atypical.

► Diagnosis

Pulmonary TB often occurs at a CD4+ of 250–500; extrapulmonary TB more commonly occurs at a lower CD4+, often < 200. Skin testing with PPD may be unreliable because of skin test anergy. CXR may show typical nodular infiltrates, with or without cavitation (apical lung fields most common), or more atypical lesions. Isolation of *M. tuberculosis* from pulmonary or other sites is diagnostic.

► Disease Severity

Response to therapy is usually good. Mortality rates are higher and median survival time shorter in the AIDS patient, although patients with restored immune function do well. Disseminated or extrapulmonary disease is more common with advanced immunodeficiency.

► Concept and Application

HIV-related immunosuppression increases the frequency and severity of TB disease. The HIV-infected person is at risk for developing active disease from a new exposure as well as from reactivation of previously acquired, inactive disease.

► Treatment Steps

1. A minimum treatment course of 9 months is recommended in AIDS patients.
2. In patients without previous treatment for TB and living in an area where drug resistance is low, a four-drug regimen (isoniazid [INH], rifampin, pyrazinamide, and ethambutol) is recommended for initial treatment.
3. In patients with a history of previous TB treatment, contact with multidrug-resistant TB, or living in an area with frequent drug resistance, five or more initial anti-TB drugs are indicated.
4. These regimens consist of the standard four drugs **plus** ofloxacin, ciprofloxacin, or streptomycin or other second-line anti-TB drugs.
5. Even with these regimens, the likelihood of response for documented multidrug-resistant TB is disappointing.
6. Direct observed therapy (DOT) should be used whenever possible.

Health Maintenance—Twelve months of INH is indicated for all HIV-infected people with a positive PPD. A 2-month course of rifampin and pyrazinamide is also effective but may be more toxic.

E. Disseminated *Mycobacterium avium-intracellulare* Complex (MAC)

► H&P Keys

Disseminated MAC is the most common systemic opportunistic bacterial infection in patients with AIDS. MAC most commonly causes lymphadenopathy and disseminated infection with persistent fever, significant weight loss, chronic diarrhea or malabsorption, and abdominal pain. Lymphadenopathy, organomegaly, or an abdominal mass may be present.

► Diagnosis

Abnormal liver tests, anemia, and leukopenia are common. Diagnosis is made by isolation of the organism from blood or tissue (bone marrow, lymph node, lung, or liver).

► Disease Severity

There are many organisms present in the blood and tissues of AIDS patients with disseminated MAC. Despite the number of organisms, most patients remain asymptomatic until late-stage disease. Survival without therapy is only about 4 months, although MAC is seldom the *cause* of death.

► Concept and Application

MAC is ubiquitous in the environment, and acquisition in AIDS is thought to result from ingestion or inhalation of organisms. MAC is minimally virulent and rarely cause disease in the immunocompetent host. The immune dysfunction in AIDS allows for disseminated infection. Disseminated MAC rarely occurs unless the CD4+ is < 100, usually when the CD4+ is < 50.

▶ Treatment Steps

1. MAC is resistant to most antituberculous agents.
2. Effective therapy can sterilize blood cultures and reduce the symptoms associated with infection. Not all patients enjoy a complete response.
3. Recommendations for therapy include either clarithromycin or azithromycin with ethambutol.
4. Sicker patients should receive one or more additional drugs from among rifabutin, ciprofloxacin, and amikacin.
5. Therapy is continued for life or until immune recovery (CD4+ > 150) has occurred.

Health Maintenance—Prophylaxis is indicated for HIV-positive patients with a CD4+ of < 100, as it appears to reduce disseminated MAC by approximately 55–85%. In order of decreasing efficacy, azithromycin **plus** rifabutin, clarithromycin, azithromycin, and rifabutin are all approved for MAC prophylaxis. The combination regimen is the least tolerated and most expensive. There is a risk of emergence of resistance with a macrolide regimen, potentially risking a loss of efficacy if a therapeutic regimen is needed.

F. *Toxoplasma* Encephalitis

▶ H&P Keys

Toxoplasma gondii is a common cause of latent central nervous system (CNS) infection in AIDS patients. *Toxoplasma* encephalitis often involves the cortex, brain stem, and/or basal ganglia, with associated neurologic abnormalities that may include focal deficit, change in reflexes or sensation, ataxia, or decreased cognition.

▶ Diagnosis

Blood tests for *Toxoplasma* are usually positive but can be unreliable. Brain imaging typically reveals multifocal disease. A presumptive diagnosis usually triggers empiric therapy. Definitive diagnosis requires visualization of the organism in brain tissue. Polymerase chain reaction (PCR) of CSF is promising.

▶ Disease Severity

Brain biopsy for definitive diagnosis usually is reserved for patients who are seronegative, have atypical radiologic imaging (single lesions), or do not improve on empiric therapy.

▶ Concept and Application

Reactivation of a latent infection generally occurs when the CD4+ is < 100. Up to one-third of seropositive AIDS patients may ultimately develop *Toxoplasma* encephalitis.

▶ Treatment Steps

1. The initial 6 weeks of therapy commonly consists of pyrimethamine, sulfadiazine, and folinic acid.
2. Response rates (at least partial improvement) are quite high, approximately 85%. Response is usually fast—failure to respond in a week casts significant doubt on the diagnosis.
3. Clindamycin may replace sulfadiazine in the sulfa-allergic patient.
4. Chronic maintenance, often at reduced dose, is required lifelong to prevent relapse.

Health Maintenance—Trimethoprim–sulfamethoxazole used for PCP prophylaxis is also effective prophylaxis for *Toxoplasma* encephalitis.

G. Cryptococcal Infection

► H&P Keys

Cryptococcal infections are the most common disseminated fungal infections in patients with AIDS. *Cryptococcus* may involve the lungs, skin, blood, bone marrow, prostate, and genitourinary tract, but usually presents as meningitis with subacute and nonspecific symptoms. The most common are fever and headache, with nausea, vomiting, and mental status changes occurring less frequently. Classic symptoms of meningismus, neck stiffness, and photophobia are uncommon.

► Diagnosis

CSF cryptococcal antigen allows for the most rapid diagnosis of cryptococcal meningitis, and culture is the standard confirmatory test. The India ink exam is no longer needed.

► Disease Severity

Mental status changes, very high serum or CSF cryptococcal antigen titers, and high opening pressure of CSF are associated with poor prognosis.

► Concept and Application

Cryptococcus neoformans is an encapsulated yeast commonly found in soil and associated with bird feces. Disease is acquired by inhalation, so the first site of infection is the lungs.

► Treatment Steps

1. Standard acute therapy includes an approximate 2-week course of amphotericin B with or without flucytosine. Ideally, the CSF should become culture negative.
2. Some patients with mild disease may be able to start with fluconazole.
3. All patients receive lifelong maintenance therapy to prevent relapse unless they achieve immune recovery.
4. Fluconazole is preferred for maintenance therapy.
5. Patients with very high CSF pressures may need frequent lumbar punctures to relieve headache and prevent serious sequelae such as blindness and herniation.

H. Herpes Simplex Virus (HSV)

► H&P Keys

HSV-1 and HSV-2 may cause ulcerative lesions at a variety of sites including orolabial, genital, anorectal, and esophageal ones. Lesions are characterized by pain and vesicle formation, followed by ulceration. Crusting and epithelialization may be delayed but resolves without scarring. Regional lymphadenopathy may be present. Esophagitis is associated with retrosternal pain and dysphagia. In the most severe cases ulcers can persist and expand without antiviral therapy.

► Diagnosis

The diagnosis of mucocutaneous HSV should be confirmed with HSV culture. Cultures are fairly inexpensive and rapid. Esophagitis requires endoscopy, with histopathologic and culture confirmation.

▶ Disease Severity

Severity depends on the site of infection and degree of immunosuppression.

▶ Concept and Application

Most AIDS patients have previously been infected with HSV and have latent infection in nerve root ganglia. Latent HSV often reactivates in the immunocompromised patient and can cause severe, prolonged disease.

▶ Treatment Steps

1. Usual therapy consists of oral or parenteral acyclovir until the lesions are healed.
2. Many patients will relapse after initial therapy and will require repeated therapy, followed by long-term maintenance.
3. Long-term maintenance therapy with acyclovir is associated with a risk of development of acyclovir resistance, dictating therapy with other agents such as foscarnet.

II. SEXUALLY TRANSMITTED DISEASES (STDs)

A. Gonorrhea

▶ H&P Keys

Uncomplicated gonococcal infections include urethritis, cervicitis, anoproctitis, and pharyngitis (pelvic inflammatory disease [PID] is discussed separately). Urethritis in men causes discharge and dysuria, whereas women report only dysuria. Cervicitis is generally asymptomatic. Pharyngitis generally causes no symptoms, but erythema and exudate may be present on exam. Anoproctitis may be associated with pain, and discharge may also be present. Disseminated gonococcal infection resulting from bacteremia may cause petechial or pustular skin lesions, tenosynovitis, septic arthritis, and occasionally, hepatitis, endocarditis, or meningitis.

▶ Diagnosis

Specific diagnosis is made by recovery of *Neisseria gonorrhoeae* from discharge, blood, or other body fluid. Therapy for uncomplicated disease is often empiric (without benefit of culture).

▶ Disease Severity

Of the uncomplicated gonococcal infections, pharyngitis is the most difficult to cure and dictates more specific therapy than does anal or genital infection (see Treatment Steps, below). Hospitalization may be advisable for initial therapy of disseminated infection.

▶ Concept and Application

Genital infections in women may produce minimal or no symptoms. PID as a sequela of gonorrhea or chlamydia may cause tubal scarring, resulting in infertility or ectopic pregnancy.

▶ Treatment Steps

1. Coinfection with chlamydia is common in people with gonococcal infections.
2. Treatment for gonorrhea should include therapy against *C. trachomatis* (see chlamydia Treatment Steps recommendations).
3. Resistance to penicillin and tetracycline is common. Recommended regimens for uncomplicated gonorrhea include ceftriax-

one, cefixime, ciprofloxacin, or ofloxacin, all as a single dose, plus a regimen effective against *Chlamydia.* Resistance to fluoro-quinolones has been increasing.

4. Ceftriaxone or ciprofloxacin should be used for pharyngeal disease.

5. Many additional antibiotics are effective for uncomplicated gonorrhea, including spectinomycin (intramuscular only) and a number of second- and third-generation cephalosporins (oral and parenteral).

6. The initial treatment of disseminated gonococcal infection consists of a parenteral cephalosporin (ceftriaxone, cefotaxime, ceftizoxime) or spectinomycin.

7. After clinical improvement, oral therapy with cefixime or ciprofloxacin is given to complete a week of treatment.

Health Maintenance—Persons treated for gonorrhea should be screened for syphilis by serologic testing. Sex partners should be referred for treatment. Safer sex is encouraged, and evaluation for HIV may be appropriate for many of these patients.

B. Chlamydia

▶ H&P Keys
C. trachomatis causes urethritis and cervicitis (PID is discussed separately). Urethritis is characterized by mucoid or purulent discharge and dysuria. Cervicitis is characterized by yellow endocervical exudate.

▶ Diagnosis
Nonculture tests for chlamydia are reliable and much more available and sensitive than cultures. Combined tests, e.g., ligase chain reaction, for gonorrhea and chlamydia.

▶ Disease Severity
As with gonococcal disease, chlamydial infection may go untreated in the female patient and result in tubal scarring, infertility, or ectopic pregnancy.

▶ Concept and Application
C. trachomatis is an obligate intracellular parasite of columnar or pseudostratified cells. The incidence of chlamydial infection is higher than that of gonorrhea.

▶ Treatment Steps
1. Coinfection with the gonococcus is common in patients treated for chlamydial infection.
2. Treatment for chlamydia should include therapy effective for gonococcal infection (see gonorrhea Treatment Steps recommendations).
3. Recommended regimens for chlamydial urethritis or cervicitis include doxycycline or azithromycin.
4. Alternatives include ofloxacin or erythromycin.

Health Maintenance—Sex partners should be referred for evaluation and treatment. Safer sex is encouraged.

C. Syphilis

▶ H&P Keys
Patients may seek treatment for signs or symptoms of primary infection (ulcer at the site of infection), secondary infection (rash, muco-

cutaneous lesions, adenopathy), or tertiary disease (cardiac, neurologic, ophthalmic, auditory, or gummatous lesions). Patients with latent infection may be identified by serologic testing.

► Diagnosis

Darkfield exam and direct fluorescent antibody tests of exudates or tissue allow the diagnosis of early syphilis but are seldom done except in STD clinics. Diagnosis may be made serologically with a nontreponemal test: e.g., RPR, confirmed with a treponemal test: e.g., fluorescent treponemal antibody absorption (FTA-ABS). Neurosyphilis can be diagnosed with CSF tests. At a minimum this would include a VDRL (which is diagnostic of neurosyphilis when positive), cell count, protein, and glucose. About one-half of the patients with neurosyphilis will have a positive CSF VDRL. Patients with primary, secondary, or latent syphilis need not undergo CSF exam unless there are: neurologic or ophthalmic signs or symptoms, other evidence of active disease (aortitis, gumma, iritis), treatment failure, HIV infection, or therapy not involving penicillin is planned. The CSF results can be difficult to interpret in the presence of HIV infection because even an asymptomatic person with HIV can have minor CSF cell count and protein abnormalities that mimic the changes of neurosyphilis. The VDRL test is still useful in this setting.

► Disease Severity

Patients are staged and treated according to clinical signs and symptoms (see above) or the duration of latency. Patients with latent disease for < 1 year are considered to have early latent disease, whereas others have late latent syphilis or syphilis of unknown duration. The duration or intensity of therapy is largely dictated by stage. The titer of the nontreponemal test correlates with disease activity.

► Concept and Application

Syphilis is a systemic disease caused by *Treponema pallidum.* Although CSF invasion in primary or secondary syphilis is common, few patients develop neurologic disease when treated appropriately.

► Treatment Steps

1. Patients with primary, secondary, and early latent syphilis are treated with one 2.4-million-units IM injection of benzathine penicillin.
2. Nonpregnant penicillin-allergic patients can be treated with a tetracycline for 2 weeks. This is less satisfactory than penicillin and needs closer follow-up.
3. Patients with late latent and tertiary syphilis are treated with three weekly 2.4-million-units IM injections of benzathine penicillin G.
4. Four weeks of a tetracycline offers alternative therapy.
5. Neurosyphilis is treated for 10–14 days with high-dose penicillin. Even patients with documented penicillin allergy should be considered for penicillin desensitization.
6. All patients require follow-up serologic testing (CSF if appropriate) to monitor response.
7. Although data are incomplete, HIV-infected patients are generally treated as above (although some recommend more intense treatment than is dictated by stage).

Health Maintenance—Sex partners should be referred for evaluation, although transmission occurs only when mucocutaneous lesions are present (uncommon after the first year). Patients should be considered for HIV testing.

► **diagnostic decisions**

GENITAL ULCER DISEASE

Syphilis
Clean, painless, usually single ulcer; large nodes.

Chancroid
Dirty, ragged, painful ulcer; large nodes.

Lymphogranuloma Venereum
Small ulcer, large nodes, "groove sign" between the inguinal and femoral nodes.

Herpes Simplex
Multiple painful, clustered vesicles or ulcers; variable nodes.

D. Chancroid

► H&P Keys

One or more painful genital ulcers, often in association with tender inguinal lymphadenopathy. Inguinal adenopathy may be suppurative.

► Diagnosis

Special cultures not readily available. Diagnosis probable with clinical signs and no evidence of syphilis or HSV.

► Disease Severity

In extensive cases, scarring may occur despite successful therapy.

► Concept and Application

Chancroid is caused by *Haemophilus ducreyi* and is endemic in many areas of the United States. It is a well-established cofactor for HIV transmission.

► Treatment Steps

1. Azithromycin or ceftriaxone single-dose therapy and 7 days of erythromycin are all successful.
2. Alternatives include 7 days of amoxicillin/clavulanate or 3 days of ciprofloxacin.

   Health Maintenance—Patients should be tested for HIV infection.

E. Pelvic Inflammatory Disease (PID)

► H&P Keys

PID represents a spectrum of upper genital tract inflammatory disorders, including endometritis, salpingitis, tubo-ovarian abscess, and pelvic peritonitis. Minimal clinical criteria for diagnosis of PID include lower abdominal tenderness, adnexal tenderness, and cervical motion tenderness. Fever and cervical discharge may be present.

► Diagnosis

Evidence of cervical infection with *N. gonorrhoeae* or *C. trachomatis* may be present. Endometritis on endometrial biopsy, tubo-ovarian abscess on ultrasound exam, or laparoscopic evidence is more definitive.

► Disease Severity

Patients with mild disease may be considered for outpatient therapy. Initial hospitalization is recommended if diagnosis is uncertain, abscess is suspected, pregnancy or HIV infection is present, patient is unable to tolerate oral medication, or compliance or follow-up is in question.

► Concept and Application

PID is caused by sexually transmitted organisms such as *N. gonorrhoeae* or *C. trachomatis,* as well as genital tract flora such as anaerobes Enterobacteriaceae and group B streptococcus.

► Treatment Steps

1. Outpatient regimens include cefoxitin plus probenecid or a third-generation cephalosporin plus 14 days of doxycycline or ofloxacin plus either clindamycin or metronidazole for 14 days.
2. Common parenteral regimens include cefoxitin or cefotetan plus doxycycline or clindamycin plus gentamicin.

   Health Maintenance—Sex partners should be referred for evaluation and treatment.

F. Epididymo-orchitis

► H&P Keys

Unilateral testicular pain and tenderness and palpable swelling of the epididymis are common.

► Diagnosis

Culture for *N. gonorrhoeae* and *C. trachomatis* and urine culture.

► Disease Severity

Failure to improve within 3 days requires reevaluation and consideration of hospitalization.

► Concept and Application

In men < 35 years of age, epididymo-orchitis is caused by gonococcal or chlamydial infection. Nonsexually transmitted disease associated with urinary tract infection caused by enteric bacilli is more common in men > 35 years of age.

► Treatment Steps

1. Treatment of sexually transmitted epididymo-orchitis includes therapy for both chlamydia and gonorrhea.
2. Single-dose ceftriaxone and 10 days of doxycycline or ofloxacin are recommended.

   Health Maintenance—Sex partners should be referred for evaluation and treatment.

G. Genital Herpes

► H&P Keys

Groups of painful vesicles that progress to shallow ulcerative lesions prior to crusting and healing. Commonly seen on external genitalia and on the cervix. Systemic symptoms such as fever, headache, and myalgias are not uncommon with initial episodes.

► Diagnosis

Viral culture for HSV.

► Disease Severity

Most infected persons never recognize signs of genital herpes; some have symptoms during the initial episode and then never again. A minority of infected persons have recurrent genital lesions.

► Concept and Application

Genital herpes, usually caused by herpes simplex virus type 2 (HSV-2), is a recurrent disease without cure. Serologic evidence suggests that 30 million people in the United States have been infected.

► Treatment Steps

1. Acyclovir and similar drugs such as valacyclovir and famciclovir speed recovery from initial episodes or recurrences and can be used to suppress recurrent disease.
2. Therapy cannot eradicate latent virus.

III. OTHER INFECTIOUS DISEASES

A. Infectious Mononucleosis

► H&P Keys

Fever, sore throat, lymphadenopathy, splenomegaly. Headache, myalgias, sweats, anorexia, and abdominal pain may also be present.

► Diagnosis

Atypical lymphocytosis, positive test for heterophile antibody (positive Monospot or Mono-Diff test), positive serology for Epstein–Barr virus (EBV) (especially immunglobulin M [IgM] antibody to viral capsid antigen [VCA-IgM]).

► Disease Severity

Complications of infectious mononucleosis include hemolytic anemia (positive Coombs' test), thrombocytopenia, granulocytopenia, splenic rupture rarely, neurologic problems (e.g., Guillain–Barré syndrome), myocarditis, or pericarditis.

► Concept and Application

Infectious mononucleosis is an acute, self-limited infection predominantly occurring in children and young adults and caused by EBV or CMV. Usual course of illness is 2–4 weeks.

► Treatment Steps

1. There is no specific therapy for EBV infection.
2. Corticosteroids are occasionally prescribed for severe tonsillitis with airway compromise, severe hemolytic anemia or thrombocytopenia, neurologic complications, myocarditis, or pericarditis.

B. Varicella (Chickenpox), Measles (Rubeola), Mumps, German Measles (Rubella)

► H&P Keys

These vaccine-preventable diseases occur rarely in the United States, although unvaccinated children and adults may still be susceptible.

► Diagnosis

Clinical clues supported by serologic tests are useful in diagnosing these illnesses. While an astute clinician can usually diagnose them easily, fewer and fewer doctors are seeing patients with these viral infections.

► Disease Severity

Varicella is occasionally complicated by pneumonia, encephalitis, or Reye's syndrome. Infection in the compromised host often includes severe skin disease and dissemination to visceral organs. Measles can be followed by pneumonia or encephalitis. Rubella is usually mild except for persistent arthralgia and arthritis. The greatest risk is to the fetus if a pregnant woman develops rubella. Mumps can lead to orchitis in men.

► Treatment Steps

1. The use of acyclovir in a usual episode of varicella, though approved, is controversial except in pregnancy.
2. Acyclovir therapy is routinely used for disseminated disease, CNS involvement, and pneumonia (zoster is discussed in Chapter 2).
3. Acyclovir is not likely to be effective if use is delayed beyond 3–4 days following onset of symptoms.
4. There is no standard treatment for measles or rubella.

Health Maintenance—Vaccine for varicella zoster virus is indicated for everyone older than 1 year without a history of clinical varicella. The duration of protection remains to be determined. Zoster immune globulin is given to seronegative immunosuppressed patients exposed to varicella.

C. Lyme Disease

▶ **H&P Keys**

Lyme disease has been divided into three stages:

Stage 1—erythema migrans.
Stage 2—neurologic or cardiac involvement.
Stage 3—arthritis or subtle neurologic complaints.

Lyme disease does not progress in an orderly manner from stage to stage, so there is greater clinical utility in determining whether the infection is localized or disseminated and whether it is acute or chronic. Current therapy is largely based on this determination. Erythema migrans (EM) is an expanding, annular, erythematous skin lesion at the site of tick attachment that clears centrally. Systemic symptoms often occur with EM and correlate with systemic dissemination. There may be secondary skin lesions. Nervous system manifestations early in Lyme disease include meningitis, cranial neuritis, and painful radiculopathy. Chronic nervous system manifestations may include subtle changes in cognitive function or significant focal abnormalities. The peripheral nervous system may also be involved. Cardiac involvement is manifested as varying degrees of heart block, myopericarditis, and cardiomyopathy. If untreated, nearly one-half of patients will develop arthritis, mainly affecting large joints such as the knee. Only a minority of patients progress to chronic arthritis. Some people with late-stage Lyme disease can have persistent neurologic complaints including forgetfulness, fatigue, and mild cognitive impairment.

▶ **Diagnosis**

The diagnosis is based on the clinical manifestations, with EM being most useful. Serologic evidence is supportive but not standardized. CSF (including serology) is examined with suspected CNS disease.

▶ **Disease Severity**

Disease severity varies considerably among patients.

▶ **Concept and Application**

Lyme disease is caused by the spirochete *Borrelia burgdorferi*. *Ixodes* ticks are the principal vector throughout the world. Though reported from most of the states, the majority of Lyme disease occurs in three regions: the Northeast, upper Midwest, and the far West, corresponding to the distribution of the tick vectors. Primary reservoirs for the tick include the white-footed mouse and other small rodents. The larval, nymphal, and adult ticks feed on progressively larger animals, with the adult tick favoring the white-tailed deer. Transmission to humans occurs during feeding and requires attachment for at least 24 hours.

▶ **Treatment Steps**

1. EM, Bell's palsy, mild cardiac disease, and early arthritis are treated with oral doxycycline or amoxicillin.
2. More serious CNS disease, more serious cardiac disease, and chronic arthritis are treated with parenteral ceftriaxone or penicillin G.
3. A single 200-mg dose of doxycycline can abort infection but only a small minority of tick bites transmit *B. burgdorferi*.

    Health Maintenance—One may attempt to limit tick exposure and the risk of Lyme disease by using repellents, reducing exposed skin, and promptly removing any attached ticks.

BIBLIOGRAPHY

Gorbach SL. *Infectious Diseases,* 3rd ed. Philadelphia: W.B. Saunders, 2003.

Forrest KV. *Manual of Clinical Microbiology,* 8th ed. Washington, DC: ASM Press, 2003.

Mandell GL. *Principles and Practice of Infectious Diseases,* 6th ed. New York: Churchill Livingstone, 2004.

Yu VL. *Antimicrobial Therapy and Vaccines.* Baltimore: Williams & Wilkins, 1999.

Musculoskeletal and Connective Tissue Disease

9

I. INFECTIONS

A. Osteomyelitis

▶ H&P Keys

More common in children, may be triggered by trauma, usual seeding is hematogenous. Presents with refusal to bear weight or move joint or extremity. Fever usually present.

▶ Diagnosis

White blood cell count (WBC), erythrocyte sedimentation rate (ESR), blood cultures. Radiographs may show soft tissue swelling early, followed by periosteal elevation and finally bone infarct and involucrum. Bone scan shows focal increased activity. Magnetic resonance imaging (MRI) shows marrow changes and soft tissue involvement early in course of disease.

▶ Disease Severity

Clinical evaluation following a change in ESR may be useful, and C-reactive protein.

▶ Concept and Application

In children, osteomyelitis is usually hematogenous. Seeding occurs in the small arterioles of the metaphysis where there is sluggish blood flow. Infection elevates pressure, creating pain. Pus lifts the periosteum and may cause cortical necrosis, resulting in a sequestrum (a fragment of dead bone). The most common organism is *Staphylococcus aureus,* except in neonates, where *Streptococcus* B is most common. From 6 months to 5 years *Haemophilus influenzae* is the most common.

▶ Management

Aspiration is useful to recover organisms for antibiotic selection. Blood cultures may substitute if positive. IV antibiotics, followed by oral medication after temperature is normalized for 6 weeks or until ESR is normal. Immobilization for symptomatic relief. Surgical debridement for refractory cases with involucrum and sequestra.

B. Septic Arthritis

▶ H&P Keys

Pain, erythema, joint effusion, and soft tissue swelling. Refusal to bend joint or bear weight in children.

▶ Diagnosis

Joint aspirate, high white count > 50,000 suspicious, > 100,000 presumptive of infection pending culture results of infection. Polymorphonuclear leukocytes predominate. High peripheral WBC, elevated ESR.

▶ Disease Severity

Coexisting morbidity predisposes to infection (chronic disease, cancer, drug abuse, immune deficiency).

▶ Concept and Application

H. influenzae most common in children < 5 years old, *S. aureus* in children > 5 years old, gonococci in adults and adolescents. In children, joint may be seeded from area of contiguous osteomyelitis.

► Treatment Steps
1. In children, hip joint requires early surgical drainage to prevent joint destruction.
2. Adults may be treated with serial aspiration, following the WBC in the fluid.
3. If no response (fall in WBC in synovial fluid), surgical debridement, often arthroscopically.
4. IV antibiotics, followed by oral antibiotics.

C. Lyme Disease

► H&P Keys
Variable presentation: joint effusions, arthralgia, myalgia, fatigue, occasional cardiac arrhythmia, central nervous system (CNS) involvement (Bell's palsy, headaches). May have characteristic rash, erythema chronicum migrans ("bull's-eye" rash).

► Diagnosis
Joint aspirates negative by culture, x-rays normal, serologic testing: enzyme-linked immunosorbent assay (ELISA) screen, confirmatory Western blot.

► Disease Severity
Cardiac and CNS symptoms.

► Concept and Application
Disease caused by *Borrelia burgdorferi,* a spirochete borne by the deer tick (*Ixodes dammini*). The disease occurs in three stages: rash, neurologic symptoms (neuritis, neuropathy, encephalopathy), arthritis. Immune complexes and cryoglobulin accumulate in the synovial fluid and tissues of the host.

► Treatment Steps
1. Treatment with oral doxycycline 100 mg bid or amoxicillin 2 g/day for 3–4 weeks.
2. Recalcitrant cases: IV ceftriaxone (Rocephin) 2 g/day for 6 weeks.

D. Gonococcal Tenosynovitis

► H&P Keys
Acute loss of joint motion with fusiform swelling of digit. Erythema, redness, fever, migratory polyarthritis, multiple arthralgia.

► Diagnosis
Diagnosis confirmed by aspiration and culture (Gram stain showing intracellular gram-negative diplococci). Radiographs normal.

► Disease Severity
Multiple-location presentation.

► Concept and Application
Presentation of systemic gonococcal infection.

► Treatment Steps
Penicillin G or ceftriaxone.

II. DEGENERATIVE DISORDERS

A. Degenerative Joint Disease; Arthralgia

▶ H&P Keys

Eighty percent of adults 65 years and older demonstrate radiographic signs of osteoarthritis (OA). Signs and symptoms are usually localized. If diffuse symptoms exist, collagen vascular disease should be considered. Pain occurs after use and is relieved with rest; in later stages, rest pain and night pain may be present. Crepitation occurs with passive motion and may be associated with pain. Joint enlargement from osteophyte and synovial hypertrophy is present late.

▶ Diagnosis

Characteristic radiographic findings are joint-space narrowing, subchondral bony sclerosis, marginal osteophyte formation, subchondral cyst formation. Laboratory findings are normal.

Differential Diagnosis—Roentgenographic findings of OA of the hands are also seen with seronegative inflammatory arthritis. OA of the hip may be avascular necrosis or pigmented villonodular synovitis. OA of the knee may be meniscus pathology, osteochondritis dessicans, or a sequela of septic arthritis, osteonecrosis.

▶ Disease Severity

Disease severity is a clinical diagnosis with severe restriction of activities of daily living. Radiographs may be normal early, weight-bearing films demonstrate joint-space narrowing. Osteophyte formation with sclerosis and cyst formation occur late.

▶ Concept and Application

Disease is characterized by progressive loss of articular cartilage, followed by formation of new bone and cartilage at the joint margins (osteophyte). Incidence increases with age, obesity, repetitive occupational activities (coal miners, jackhammer operators, etc.). The pathology of OA reflects the damage to the joint and reaction of the surrounding tissues. There is an increase in water content of the cartilage, with increased proteoglycan synthesis. As the disease progresses, the joint surface thins and becomes fibrillated. Appositional bone growth in the subchondral region leads to the sclerosis seen on x-rays. With progression, clefts and fractures of the subchondral plate occur, with the formation of subchondral cysts. Growth of bone and cartilage at the joint margins form osteophytes. Synovitis and joint effusions may be present.

▶ Treatment Steps

1. Protection of the joints from excessive force and chronic overuse. Supportive splints, unloading braces, shoe wedges, and the use of ambulatory aids (cane, crutches, walker) are protective.
2. Avoidance of repetitive impact loading (jumping, running) in lower extremity OA. Weight loss is beneficial. Physical therapy to increase joint motion and strength is beneficial.
3. Drug therapy consists of analgesics (acetaminophen), aspirin, and nonsteroidal anti-inflammatory drugs (NSAIDs). Narcotics should be used only as short-term measures. Intra-articular corticosteroid may be helpful in the management of acute flares. In-

tra-articular injections of high-molecular-weight hyaluronic acid preparations may be used in knee arthritis. Nutriceuticals (glucosamine, chondroitin sulfate) may slow the course of disease progression.

4. Surgery is reserved for cases in which conservative therapy fails. Options include arthroscopic lavage and debridement if mechanical signs are present, osteotomy to realign mechanical axis, arthroplasty, or fusion.

B. Low Back Pain

▶ H&P Keys

Predisposing factors include age 30–50, repetitive movements requiring lifting, pulling, bending, and twisting. Exposure to chronic vibration and prolonged sitting. Personal behavior (sedentary lifestyle, cigarette smoking, poor posture, emotional stress, obesity).

Etiologic Factors—Acute or chronic muscle, tendon, or ligamentous strain, lumbar disk herniation, degenerative changes of the spine, facet joint dysfunction, metabolic conditions that result in mechanical failure (osteoporosis).

▶ Diagnosis

Radiographs show disk space narrowing, marginal osteophytes, facet joint sclerosis, and hypertrophy resulting in foraminal narrowing. MRI, computed tomographic (CT) scan not necessary for initial evaluation; indicated when symptoms persist with radicular neurologic symptoms.

▶ Disease Severity

Physical evaluation, with loss of spine motion in all planes. Perivertebral muscle spasm. The presence of radicular pain below the knee suggests neurologic involvement (e.g., disk disease). Pain with hyperextension and activity is suggestive of spinal stenosis (neurogenic claudication).

▶ Concept and Application

Back pain is usually a self-limiting condition resulting from an acute strain or repetitive overload. The resulting inflammation and pain of ligaments, muscles, and tendons creates the short-term disability. Treatment addresses the cause of the overload and the underlying inflammation.

▶ Treatment Steps

1. Short period of rest (3–5 days).
2. Treatment of muscle spasm with ice massage and lumbar support.
3. Acetaminophen or NSAIDs for anti-inflammatory effect.
4. Major treatment is education in proper body mechanics to prevent recurrence.
5. Muscle strengthening for the back and abdomen combined with a flexibility program complete the treatment.
6. Aerobic fitness is beneficial in preventing recurrence.

C. Lumbar Disk Disease

▶ H&P Keys

Low back pain with radiation below the knee; leg pain is usually greater than back pain. Ten percent of backaches are related to some sort of nerve root irritation. Altered sensation, pins and needles, numbness may be present in the lower extremity. Pain increases with coughing, sneezing. Weakness may be present. Central disk may cause bilateral symptoms. Signs of limited spine motion, antalgic gait, sciatic list. Hip and knee flexed with standing, extended with sitting, absent or diminished reflexes, diminished sensation in a dermatome pattern. Positive tension signs with straight leg raising or sitting root tests.

► Diagnosis

Radiographic evaluation may demonstrate disk space narrowing or may be normal. CT scan and MRI allow visualization of the disk and neural elements. Electromyogram (EMG) will show changes only after several weeks of symptoms.

► Disease Severity

Dense paresthesias with complete motor loss are signs of severe nerve root impingement. Progressive loss of motor function and sensation is an indication for early surgical intervention. Loss of bowel and bladder function (cauda equina syndrome) requires emergency treatment with surgical decompression of the neural elements to prevent permanent dysfunction.

► Concept and Application

Nuclear material bulges, protrudes, or extrudes from the disk space to put pressure on the ligaments and nerve roots. Molecular changes in the disk with aging alter the structural properties of the disk and the annulus fibrosus that contains the disk. The disk loses water and becomes dry and friable, decreasing its ability to withstand axial loads. With sudden loading or repetitive loading in flexion and rotation, disk material is extruded beyond the confines of the annulus, resulting in the neurologic symptoms.

► Treatment Steps

1. Early intervention with a short period of bed rest 3–5 days, in conjunction with anti-inflammatory medication and ice.
2. This is followed by mobilization with back rehabilitation exercises.
3. Sixty percent of patients obtain relief in 4 weeks, 90% in 3 months, 96% in 6 months.
4. Surgical intervention is required for progression of symptoms and for those who are unresponsive to conservative management.

D. Disorders Secondary to Neurologic Disease

► H&P Keys

Stroke, diabetes, muscular dystrophy, cerebral palsy, and neuropathies all have musculoskeletal consequences.

► Diagnosis

Physical examination of joint motion and muscle balance. Examination for altered sensation. Painless swelling and joint deformity may be present with Charcot's joint arthropathy.

► Disease Severity

Clinical evaluation. Radiographs show progressive joint destruction and loss of position.

► Concept and Application

Neurologic conditions that alter muscle strength, balance, and protective sensation have musculoskeletal manifestations. Increased spasticity after stroke creates flexion deformities of the affected joints because of the increased strength of flexor over extensor musculature. This may result in functional problems, such as thumb-in-palm deformity, equinus deformity, gait abnormality. The loss of protective sensation and proprioceptive sensation as a result of neuropathy from diabetes leads to Charcot's arthropathy (painless destruction of a joint) as well as problems of skin ulceration from excess pressure (dropped metatarsal heads).

▶ Treatment Steps
1. Protective splinting to prevent contractures and physical therapy to preserve joint motion may prevent surgical intervention.
2. For severe muscle imbalance, corrective surgery with release and weakening of the flexors or augmentation of the extensors with muscle transfers may be required.
3. Protection of insensate joints with bracing and full-contact orthotics may delay or prevent joint destruction.
4. Patient education in skin care.

III. INHERITED, CONGENITAL, OR DEVELOPMENTAL DISORDERS

A. Congenital Hip Disorders

▶ H&P Keys

Congenital dislocation of the hip (CDH) is a serious condition if not diagnosed and treated in the first weeks of life. Girls are affected eight times more often than boys. Diagnosis is made by clinical exam at the time of birth. Backward and forward pressure on the femur in full flexion and abduction can demonstrate the femoral head moving in and out of the acetabulum.

▶ Diagnosis

Radiographs are not helpful because the femoral head is not calcified until at least 10 weeks of age. Ultrasonography of the hip is the diagnostic procedure of choice in the first weeks of life.

▶ Disease Severity

Delay in diagnosis gravely affects prognosis and treatment. If diagnosis delayed until 12–18 months as walking begins demonstrating a limp and rolling gait, surgery will only achieve a useful hip but one that will not be normal.

▶ Concept and Application

Risk factors include family history of dislocations, breech presentation at birth. Every birth should be screened for CDH.

▶ Management

Treatment at Birth—Treatment with splint or harness (Pavlik) to hold the hips in an abducted and forward-flexed position, worn for 12 weeks. Reduction is confirmed with x-rays and possibly arthrogram.

Treatment at 2 Months—Managed with traction and plaster immobilization.

Treatment at 12 Months—Surgery is indicated to achieve a stable joint. Hip is never normal, however.

B. Legg–Calvé–Perthes Disease

► H&P Keys

Painful hip in child ages 2–11. Child with limp.

► Diagnosis

X-ray may be normal in early disease. Later x-rays will demonstrate increased femoral head density or subarticular fracture line.

► Disease Severity

Age is key to prognosis: Presentation after age 8 represents a poor prognosis.

► Concept and Application

Noninflammatory self-limiting deformity of the weight-bearing surface of the femoral head secondary to avascular necrosis of the femoral head. Increased incidence with a positive family history, low birth weight, and abnormal birth presentation.

► Treatment Steps

1. Maintenance of the sphericity of the femoral head is most important factor for obtaining a good outcome.
2. Treatment is to first obtain normal range of motion with bed rest, traction.
3. This is followed with bracing or surgery to contain the femoral head in the acetabulum until revascularization and ossification occurs.

C. Slipped Capital Femoral Epiphysis

► H&P Keys

Presents as groin pain or as knee pain. Limp may be present with displacement. With complete displacement, leg may be shortened and externally rotated.

► Diagnosis

Radiographic images, especially lateral, are essential for showing displacement.

► Disease Severity

Degree of displacement determines residual problems. Significant displacement may result in the development of avascular necrosis. Chondrolysis may occur with the resultant osteoarthritis.

► Concept and Application

Adolescents with complaints of hip or knee pain should be considered to have a slipped capital femoral epiphysis. Occurs through the growth plate or epiphysis of the femoral neck during the adolescent growth spurt and is more common in boys than girls. The slip is probably caused by a weakening of the epiphyseal structures by hormonal changes of adolescence. Most often occurs in gynecoid boys.

► Treatment Steps

1. Slight to moderate displacement should be treated with percutaneous pinning to prevent further slip.
2. Manipulation may disturb the blood supply and create avascular necrosis.
3. For gross displacement, it is better to accept the deformity and correct it after growth has been completed with an osteotomy.

D. Intoeing

▶ **H&P Keys**

Patient presents with an intoed gait. May complain of falling and tripping over feet.

▶ **Diagnosis**

No diagnostic studies are necessary.

▶ **Disease Severity**

Clinical evaluation of degree of intoeing.

▶ **Concept and Application**

There are three causes of intoeing: (1) anteversion of the femoral neck, (2) metatarsus adductus, and (3) outward-curved tibiae (tibial torsion). Femoral anteversion allows for greater internal rotation of the hip than external rotation and is the major cause of intoeing. The condition corrects itself as growth continues. Most instances are corrected by age 10.

▶ **Treatment Steps**

No treatment other than reassurance is needed.

IV. METABOLIC AND NUTRITIONAL DISORDERS

A. Osteoporosis

▶ **H&P Keys**

Progressive loss of height. Spontaneous, multiple vertebral body compression fractures. Development of thoracic kyphosis. Fractures of the hip and wrist. May complain of bone pain in the axial skeletal or in the long bones of the lower extremity. History of multiple stress fractures. Family history of osteoporosis. Risk factors: alcohol, steroids, myeloma, postmenopausal, tobacco.

▶ **Diagnosis**

Plain x-rays may show osteopenia. Increase in medullary/cortex ratio of 2:1. Dual energy x-ray absorptiometry (DEXA) is the most sensitive of the monitoring techniques. Complete lab evaluation should include screens for thyroid, parathyroid, and renal disease; hematologic disorders; and malignant disease.

▶ **Disease Severity**

Loss of axial skeletal height, multiple compression fractures with thoracic kyphosis. Multiple fractures of hips, wrists, ribs, ankles. Recurrent stress risks.

▶ **Concept and Application**

Decrease in bone mineral content leading to spontaneous fractures of the spine, hip, and wrist. Commonly postmenopausal women; other risk factors include hereditary, drug use (steroids, heparin, thyroid), nutritional factors, activity (sedentary), cigarette smoking, alcohol. Disuse osteoporosis results when bones are not stressed normally, e.g., paralysis, prolonged bed rest or immobilization, space flight.

▶ **Treatment Steps**

Best treated with prevention, low-dose estrogen replacement in menopausal women. Calcitonin and bisphosphonates block bone resorption. Adequate intake of oral calcium and vitamin D are essential for prevention and treatment (400 IU/day of vitamin D and 1,500 g/day calcium. Fluoride causes increases in bone density, but the bone is more brittle. Weight-bearing exercise helps prevent development and progression of osteoporosis. Alendronate, 70 mg/week or 10 mg/day; residronate, 35 mg weekly; or ibandronate, 150 mg monthly is effective in the treatment of osteoporosis, but with a high rate of gastrointestinal (GI) side effects. Raloxifen (estrogen receptor antagonist) has been shown to decrease vertebral fractures, as has estrogen. Neither should be used with a history of stroke or thrombosis. Teriparatide used for 24 months seems to improve bone architecture and bone density.

B. Gout

▶ H&P Keys

Acute onset of painful, swollen, erythematous joints, deposition of crystals in soft tissue, tophi. Attacks may be preceded by trauma, alcohol, drugs, surgical stress, or acute medical illness. Great toe commonly involved; ankle, knee, tarsal bone may be affected.

▶ Diagnosis

Aspiration of joint fluid for birefringent crystals. Always send for culture and sensitivity.

▶ Disease Severity

Polyarticular attacks, soft tissue tophi formation, joint destruction, associated renal failure.

▶ Concept and Application

Tissue deposition of monosodium urate crystals from supersaturated extracellular fluids. Recurrent attacks of severe articular and periarticular inflammation: gouty arthritis. Accumulation of crystalline deposits in the soft tissue: gouty tophi. Renal impairment: gouty nephropathy. Causes: overproduction, 10%; underexcretion, 90%. Dehydration as a result of trauma, surgery, diuretics may precipitate attack.

▶ Treatment Steps

1. Treatment with anti-inflammatory medications; indomethacin (Indocin), 50 mg tid; or colchicine.
2. Aspiration and identification under polarized light microscopy diagnostic with birefringent crystals.
3. If attacks reoccur, treatment with allopurinol is helpful.
4. Intra-articular steroids effective if oral medication is not tolerated or contraindicated as in patients on anticoagulants or with chronic renal insufficiency.

C. Rickets

▶ H&P Keys

Brittle bones with ligamentous laxity, flattening of the skull, enlargement of the costal cartilages (rachitic rosary), dorsal kyphosis, bowing of long bones.

▶ Diagnosis

Radiographic evaluation: transverse radiolucent lines ("Looser's lines"), physeal cupping and widening. Laboratory evaluation: calcium levels are normal, with low phosphate and high alkaline phosphatase levels.

► Disease Severity

Clinical evaluation: long-bone bowing, rachitic rosary.

► Concept and Application

Decrease in calcium and/or phosphorus affecting the mineralization of the epiphyses of long bones. Histology: widened osteoid seams, distortion of the zone of maturation with poorly defined zone of provisional calcification. There are four causes of rickets:

1. Vitamin D deficiency resulting from inadequate diet or lack of exposure to sunlight.
2. Malabsorption of calcium secondary to steatorrhea.
3. Renal osteodystrophy caused by renal abnormality that affects the metabolism of vitamin D.
4. Hypophosphatemia resulting from defect in renal tubule (vitamin D–resistant rickets).

► Treatment Steps

1. Vitamin D produces rapid improvement.
2. Residual long-bone deformities may require surgical correction.
3. Vitamin D–resistant rickets requires treatment with phosphate replacement and vitamin D_3.

V. INFLAMMATORY OR IMMUNOLOGIC DISORDERS

A. Polymyalgia Rheumatica

► H&P Keys

Occurs in men and women > 60, and occurs twice as often in women. Patients complain of abrupt onset of pain affecting the shoulders, neck, upper arms, lower back, and thighs. Morning stiffness and gelling are predominant features. Physical examination reveals only tenderness and restriction of motion.

► Diagnosis

Radiographs are normal. Rheumatoid factor and antinuclear antibodies (ANAs) are normal, ESR is elevated. Diagnosis is by history and response to treatment with prednisone.

► Disease Severity

Elevated ESR, clinical impairment of activities.

► Concept and Application

Common syndrome of older patients, characterized by stiffness and pain in neck, shoulders, and hip lasting at least 1 month. Inflammation is present without joint destruction.

► Treatment Steps

1. Responds rapidly to low-dose prednisone.
2. If response is not seen in 1 week, diagnosis should be questioned.
3. Start prednisone, 10–20 mg/day, with taper to 5–7.5 mg/day.
4. Therapy may continue for > 1 year.

B. Lupus Arthritis

► H&P Keys

Disease of young females ages 14–40, with a 5:1 female-to-male ratio. The acute arthritis may involve any joint but usually involves the small joints of the hand, wrists, and the knee. It may be persistent and chronic or migratory. Soft tissue swelling and effusion are mild. Fatigue, rash, and fevers are common.

► Diagnosis

Clinical symptoms of morning stiffness, myalgia, arthralgia. Serologic testing: ANA positive in 95%.

► Disease Severity

Articular complaints are usually mild and reversible without erosions. Disease activity, however, can severely impair renal function and cause pulmonary and cardiac involvement. Neuropsychiatric manifestations may also be present. Increased tendency for thrombosis.

► Concept and Application

Autoimmune disease characterized by the production of autoantibodies to components of the cell nucleus. Pathologic findings are manifested by inflammation, vasculitis, and immune complex deposition disease (lupus kidney). Lupus arthritis is a polyarthritis characterized by low-grade synovitis without joint destruction. Joint distention may cause ligamentous laxity of the metacarpal phalangeal (MCP) and proximal interphalangeal (PIP) joints of the hand with resulting instability and deformity (swan-neck deformity, ulnar deviation of the fingers) without articular erosions.

► Treatment Steps

Treatment consists of periods of rest, avoidance of sun exposure, NSAIDs, hydroxychloroquine, and corticosteroids and other immunosuppressants such as cyclophosphamide, azathioprine, mycophenolate mofetil, and methotrexate. Splinting may preserve function in weakened joints. Methotrexate is used in recalcitrant disease. Fertility and carcinogenesis issues need to be discussed prior to immunosuppressant and immunomodulation therapy.

C. Polymyositis–Dermatomyositis

► H&P Keys

Complaints of proximal hip weakness, with difficulty on stairs and getting out of cars. Arm symptoms with difficulty lifting above the horizontal and lack of endurance strength. Physical examination may show diffuse symmetric muscle wasting and weakness. Affected muscles may be sore to palpation. Gait may be slow and wide based.

► Diagnosis

Clinical presentation of symmetric proximal muscle weakness. Elevated serum creatine kinase, aldolase, lactic dehydrogenase, and transaminase. Characteristic EMG abnormalities. Autoantibodies may be present. Muscle biopsy.

► Disease Severity

Involvement may extend to the heart, GI tract, lungs, peripheral joints.

► Concept and Application

This disease is an idiopathic inflammatory myopathy characterized by proximal limb weakness. Other disorders such as hypothyroidism, statin-induced myopathy need to be excluded.

▶ Treatment Steps

1. High-dose corticosteroid medication is the initial treatment.
2. Graded exercise after inflammation restores some strength and range of motion.
3. Methotrexate or azothioprine is used in patients not responding to corticosteroid.

D. Rheumatoid Arthritis (Juvenile, Adult)

▶ H&P Keys

Characteristically presents with morning stiffness with symmetric painful swelling in the small joints in young women ages 15–35. It may involve other joints not seen in OA such as elbows, shoulders, ankles, hips, and spine. Fatigue may be present.

▶ Diagnosis

Radiographs show juxta-articular erosions around the small joints of the hands and feet. Positive rheumatoid factor (RF), elevated ESR, and anemia are usually present.

▶ Disease Severity

Functional impairment in activities of daily living. Systemic involvement of other organ systems such as the lung, heart, skin, eye, GI and genitourinary systems is possible.

▶ Concept and Application

Etiology is unclear but is related to cell-mediated immune response (T cells) that incites an inflammatory response, initially against soft tissue and later cartilage, with subsequent bone loss secondary to periarticular bone resorption. Lymphokines and other inflammatory mediators initiate the cascade that leads to cartilaginous destruction.

▶ Treatment Steps

1. Aimed at controlling the inflammation with acetaminophen, NSAIDs, antimalarial immunosuppressives (such as methotrexate, azathioprine, leflunomide, mycophenolate mofetil, and anti–tumor necrosis factor [TNF] agents). Corticosteroids may be used to improve patient functional levels. Remicade (infliximab) is a monoclonal antibody used in conjunction with methotrexate. Opportunistic infections are reported. Evaluate for latent tuberculosis (purified protein derivative [PPD]) prior to using these agents.
2. Severely affected joints can be protected with splints and braces to prevent destruction. Synovectomy prior to joint destruction, total arthroplasty for severe disease.

E. Ankylosing Spondylitis

▶ H&P Keys

Common in young men aged 15–30. Presents with complaint of diffuse low backache without radicular symptoms. Profound morning stiffness. Usually a rapid response to anti-inflammatory medication. May have painless or painful effusions of large joints. May have uveitis and aortic valve disease, diminished spine motion in all three planes.

▶ Diagnosis

History and physical examination are most important. Restriction of chest expansion and spine flexion. Elevated ESR. May be human

► on rounds

MUSCULOSKELETAL DISORDERS, FOCUS ON INFLAMMATORY/IMMUNOLOGIC CONDITIONS

Polymyalgia Rheumatica
- Women over age 60, more common in women.
- Pain in the shoulders, neck, upper arms, low back, thighs; morning stiffness, gelling.
- X-rays are normal, RF and ANA are normal, ESR is elevated.
- Treat with prednisone

Ankylosing Spondylitis
- Common in men ages 15–30.
- Low back pain, profound morning stiffness.
- Elevated ESR, may be HLA-B27 positive, sacroiliitis on x-ray.
- Treat with anti-inflammatory medication.

Rheumatoid Arthritis
- Women ages 15–35.
- Symmetric painful swelling in the small joints, morning stiffness, fatigue; may affect elbows, ankles, hips, spine, and shoulders.
- X-rays positive for erosions, positive RF, elevated ESR, anemia.
- Treat with acetaminophen, NSAIDs, antimalarial, gold, penicillamine, and immunosuppressives.

Lupus Arthritis
- Females 14–40 (5:1 female/male ratio).
- Acute arthritis most often affecting the small joints of the hand, wrists, and knee.
- ANA positive in 95%.
- Treatment includes NSAIDs and corticosteroids.

Polymyositis–Dermatomyositis
- Symmetric proximal hip weakness, symmetric muscle wasting, weakness, slow gait, muscle tenderness to palpation.
- Elevated serum creatine kinase, aldolase, LDH, and transaminase; EMG abnormalities, may have autoantibodies.
- Treat with corticosteroids or methotrexate.

leukocyte antigen (HLA)-B27 positive. Radiographs of the sacroiliac joints show the earliest changes of sacroiliitis. Later, the spine films demonstrate progressive ankylosis.

► Disease Severity
Restriction of spine motion, chin-on-chest deformity, restriction of chest expansion with restrictive lung disease.

► Concept and Application
An inflammatory disease of the spinal joints and sacroiliac joints. Inflammatory changes and new bone formation occur at attachments of tendons and ligaments to bone (enthesopathy). If left untreated, there can be complete loss of spinal motion from the occiput to the coccyx. Treatment is to preserve motion through exercise and control inflammation with medication.

► Treatment Steps
1. Initial flair is treated with rest and anti-inflammatory medication.
2. Mobilization and flexibility exercises are started as the inflammation is controlled. Etanercept for spondylitis.

F. Bursitis

▶ H&P Keys

Soft tissue swelling that may be either painful or nonpainful, usually over a bony prominence. Swelling may occur spontaneously or as a result of trauma or an inflammatory disease (gout, rheumatoid arthritis).

▶ Diagnosis

Clinical evaluation. Additional evaluation for underlying inflammatory diseases. Radiographs to evaluate for bony prominences and soft tissue calcifications.

▶ Disease Severity

Clinical evaluation.

▶ Concept and Application

Bursae form wherever two tissue planes move in opposite direction or where tissues travel over a bony protuberance. Normal bursal locations are in the subacromial space of the shoulder, over the olecranon of the elbow, and over the tibial tubercle, and in the prepatellar space. This normal structure allows skin and tendon and muscle to slide over each other easily. If the bursa becomes infected, injured, or inflamed, fluid will accumulate in the bursa and produce visible swelling. Fibrinous loose bodies may also be formed in the bursa. After the inflammation subsides, adhesions and fibrosis may occur in the bursa, resulting in crepitation and, sometimes, pain.

▶ Treatment Steps

1. Avoidance of repetitive motions and trauma will prevent bursal inflammation.
2. Treatment of any underlying collagen vascular disease or crystalline arthritis will control the bursal swelling.
3. Acute treatment consists of rest, ice, anti-inflammatory medication. Aspiration to identify crystals or elevated WBC and bacteria may be required. Steroid injection may be used.
4. The use of protective padding, elbow and knee pads, can prevent recurrence. Steroid injection may be used.
5. Surgical excision is sometimes needed if the size or the location interferes with activities of daily living.

G. Tendinitis

▶ H&P Keys

Pain over tendon or at tendon insertion. May be acute in onset or as a result of repetitive overload, often seen after a sudden change in activity or sporting activity.

▶ Diagnosis

Physical signs of localized inflammation with point tenderness over the tendon. Weakness may be present secondary to pain.

▶ Disease Severity

Functional assessment of impairment.

▶ Concept and Application

Tendinitis is an inflammation of the tendon secondary to overload. This may be due to acute overload with partial tearing of the tendon or as a result of repetitive stress. A sudden change in activity or sporting activity that exceeds the body's reparative capabilities will result in an "overuse" tendinitis.

► Treatment Steps

1. Local treatment with ice massage and oral NSAIDs.
2. Splinting to restrict motion and rest injury zone.
3. Restoration of normal motion through a gentle stretching program followed by strength exercises and endurance training.
4. Return to sport and activity is gradual.
5. Assessment of work activity and sport intensity with adaptation of program will prevent recurrence. Training and equipment must also be adapted to prevent recurrence.

H. Fibromyalgia

► H&P Keys

Patients present with diffuse achiness, stiffness, fatigue, associated with multiple areas of clinical tenderness. Seventy-five percent are female, with an age distribution of 20–60 years. Pain tends to be localized to axial locations such as the neck and lower back. The upper trapezius is a common location of pain. On physical examination tenderness is present with moderate pressure. Common locations: occiput, trapezius, supraspinatus at ridge of scapula, lower back, lateral epicondyle.

► Diagnosis

Clinical examination makes the diagnosis. Laboratory evaluation (ESR, RF, ANA, complete blood count [CBC]) to exclude collagen vascular diseases and infectious causes (Lyme disease). Thyroid function tests are also valuable.

► Disease Severity

Clinical examination.

► Concept and Application

Etiology is unknown; fatigue is felt to be due to sleep disturbances, with loss of rapid eye movement (REM) sleep patterns. Highly correlated with abnormal sleep patterns and previous physical and sexual abuse.

► Treatment Steps

1. Patient education and reassurance.
2. Aerobic exercise is more beneficial than stretching alone.
3. NSAIDs are not effective as single agents but are effective in conjunction with bedtime dose of amitriptyline or cyclobenzaprine.

VI. NEOPLASMS

A. Osteosarcoma

► H&P Keys

Most common in second and third decade of life. Often presents as a painless mass. Found after rather minor trauma on routine x-ray.

► Diagnosis

Radiographs are diagnostic: demonstrate increased radiodensity with areas of radiolucency and permeative destruction and soft tissue extension. Elevated periosteum (Codman's triangle) may be present. Bone scans and MRI will show extent of lesion and skip lesions.

► Disease Severity

Extent of disease with involvement of multiple compartments.

► Concept and Application

A malignant tumor of bone characterized by the production of osteoid directly from a malignant spindle cell stroma. The knee and proximal humerus are the most commonly affected locations. Early diagnosis is difficult because of the disease's painless nature. Secondary osteosarcomas can arise from Paget's disease of bone and post–radiation therapy fields.

► Treatment Steps

1. Adjunctive chemotherapy pre- and postoperatively profoundly improves survival.
2. Limb salvage surgery may be offered to those patients who are good responders, with 95% tumor necrosis. Otherwise, amputation and prosthetic fitting is the treatment of choice, with the best survival and lowest recurrence rates.

B. Metastases to Bone

► H&P Keys

Presentation is usually with pain or with a pathologic fracture.

► Diagnosis

Radiographs demonstrate lytic and blastic lesions. Lesions involving > 50% of the cortex or that are > 2.5 cm in diameter are at risk for spontaneous fracture. Bone scanning sensitive for detection of early metastatic disease. MRI will accurately show extent of metastatic tumor involvement of bone. Alkaline phosphatase is usually elevated.

► Disease Severity

Lesions > 2.5 cm in diameter or > 50% of the cortex are at risk for spontaneous fracture and should be prophylactically stabilized.

► Concept and Application

Metastatic tumors are the most common malignancies of bone. Spread to bone can be either arterial or venous. Classically, lytic lesions are found in the axial skeleton and long-bone diaphyses and usually multiply. Most common lesions are breast, prostate, lung, kidney, and thyroid. Prostate and breast metastases are typically blastic. The most common metastases in children are Wilms' tumor and neuroblastoma.

► Treatment Steps

1. Radiation therapy is often helpful to control the pain and metastatic activity. Adenocarcinoma of lung does not respond to radiation therapy.
2. For impending fractures, stabilization with load-sharing devices (intramedullary rods) is preferred. For collapse of bony support of joint surfaces, replacement arthroplasties may be useful procedures if survival is expected beyond 6 months.

C. Pulmonary Osteoarthropathy

► H&P Keys

Clubbing of the fingers is the characteristic feature. In some patients, especially those with malignant lung tumors, severe bone pain may be present. Obtain family history of clubbing.

► Diagnosis

Physical feature of bulbous deformity of the digits (clubbing). Periostitis and thickening of the bones is present radiographically.

► Disease Severity

Clinical evaluation; evaluate for occult pulmonary tumor, especially if long-bone pain is present.

► Concept and Application

Disease characterized by excessive proliferation of skin and bones at the ends of the digits (clubbing).

► Treatment Steps

1. An NSAID is useful in controlling the pain of the periostitis.
2. Occult malignant tumor of the lung must be ruled out.

VII. OTHER DISORDERS

A. Shoulder–Hand (Frozen Shoulder) Syndrome

► H&P Keys

Decreased range of motion in the shoulder, often painful. May occur following minor trauma. Associated with diabetes, hypothyroidism, surgery; and higher in females.

► Diagnosis

Diagnosis is clinical; arthrogram will show decreased joint-space volume.

► Disease Severity

Clinical evaluation of functional loss of shoulder motion.

► Concept and Application

Adhesive capsulitis of the shoulder. Inflammatory condition with fibrosis and loss of normal joint space secondary to capsular contracture.

► Treatment Steps

1. Institution of early, aggressive range-of-motion exercises.
2. Adjunctive treatment with NSAIDs and ice.
3. May take 1 year to resolve. Surgical releases and manipulation are reserved for nonresponders to physical therapy.

B. Dupuytren's Contracture

► H&P Keys

Patients are usually males older than 40, of northern European ancestry, with a family history of the condition. Alcohol, smoking, diabetes, and seizures are contributory. Forty percent are bilateral. Ulnar digits are more commonly involved.

► Diagnosis

Clinical evaluation.

► Disease Severity

Interference with hand function, inability to get the fingers out of the palm of the hand.

► Concept and Application

Proliferative fibrodysplasia of the palmar subcutaneous tissue. Myofibroblast proliferation and increased type III collagen. Leads to progressive contracture from these nodules and cords of tissue.

► Treatment Steps

Surgical intervention for deformities of > 30–45° of the MCP or of any PIP involvement.

C. Carpal Tunnel Syndrome

► H&P Keys

Patients usually complain of night symptoms with paresthesias in the median distribution (the front of the thumb, index and long finger, and the radial half of the ring finger). May have weakness of pinch with thenar atrophy late in the disease process.

► Diagnosis

Other causes (thyroid disease, diabetes, pregnancy, amyloidosis) need to be excluded. Physical examination is usually diagnostic. Diminished sensation in the median nerve distribution. Positive Tinel's sign of the carpal canal. Positive Phalen's test. Nerve conduction velocity delays across the carpal ligament.

► Disease Severity

Progressive median nerve dysfunction with loss of two-point discrimination and weakness of thumb adduction. Thenar atrophy.

► Concept and Application

The median nerve and common flexors pass through a common tunnel in the wrist, bounded volarly by the transverse carpal ligament. Any process that decreases the volume of the canal will compress the median nerve and create symptoms.

► Treatment Steps

1. Primary treatment is rest with a cock-up resting splint.
2. Injection of hydrocortisone may be effective.
3. Surgical decompression for those not responding to conservative treatment.
4. Treatment of underlying disease process.

D. Paget's Disease of Bone

► H&P Keys

The most common sites are the spine, pelvis, skull, femur, and tibia. In most cases patients are asymptomatic. However, disease becomes clinically present with pain, progressive deformity, compression of neurologic structures, pathologic fractures.

► Diagnosis

Laboratory evaluation: increased alkaline phosphatase, increased urinary hydroxyproline excretion. Radiographic appearance: initial lesion is a focal area of radiolucency (osteoporosis circumscripta of the skull). In the long bones, resorption is characterized by an advancing wedge of radiolucency. Attempts at repair create sclerotic-appearing bone with thickening of the cortex.

► Disease Severity

The major complication of Paget's disease is sarcomatous transformation. This occurs in < 1% of cases. Presents with severe pain and extremely elevated serum alkaline phosphatase activity. Increased local circulation in hypervascular bone can create high-output congestive heart failure. Paget's fracture risk due to brittle bones. Increased bone density results in early osteoarthritis of surrounding joints. Spinal stenosis may occur with Paget's involvement of the spine.

▶ Concept and Application

Disorder of unknown etiology characterized by excessive bone resorption followed by excessive bone formation. Creates classic lamellar mosaic bone pattern.

▶ Treatment Steps

1. In most instances no treatment is necessary because of the paucity of clinical symptoms.
2. In symptomatic patients, NSAIDs may suppress the discomfort. Calcitonin administered subcutaneously may decrease pagetoid bone activity. Etidronate will decrease bone resorption.
3. With irreversible joint destruction, total joint arthroplasty offers relief of pain. Spinal decompression (laminectomy) for stenosis.

E. Eosinophil Granuloma

▶ H&P Keys

May present as progressive back pain, more often in the thoracic spine. Common locations: pelvis, femur, and spine. First and second decade of life. Lytic-appearing lesion characteristic. Periosteal thickening is common.

▶ Diagnosis

Classically, may cause vertebral flattening (vertebra plana), lytic lesions in long bones.

▶ Disease Severity

Lesions that compromise the structural integrity of long bones or cause neurologic compromise.

▶ Concept and Application

Bracing in children may be necessary to prevent progressive kyphosis.

▶ Treatment Steps

1. Treatment consists of observation (many lesions heal spontaneously), low-dose radiation for neurologic deficits.
2. Curettage or excision may be indicated for persistent lesions.

VIII. ACUTE OR EMERGENCY PROBLEMS

A. Effusion of Joint

▶ H&P Keys

Swelling of the joint, either spontaneous in onset or posttraumatic. Physical examination reveals loss of the normal joint contours and possibly a restriction in motion.

▶ Diagnosis

Aspiration of the joint classifies the fluid as noninflammatory (WBC < 2,000/mm³), inflammatory, or infectious (WBC > 100,000/mm³). Evaluation for crystals is essential to differentiate gout and pseudogout. Culture and Gram stain are needed to rule out infection. A bloody effusion with the history of trauma is suggestive of a severe injury, either a fracture or ligament injury; 85% of hemarthroses of the knee are anterior cruciate injuries.

► **Disease Severity**

High WBC indicates infectious etiology until proven otherwise. Prompt treatment is needed, or rapid joint destruction can occur as a result of proteolytic enzymes produced by the bacteria.

► **Concept and Application**

Any synovium-lined joint can have an effusion. The effusion is the production of excess synovial fluid in response to an inflammatory event. This event can be trauma, as in a hemorrhagic effusion; inflammatory, as in gout or rheumatoid arthritis; or an infection.

► **Treatment Steps**

1. Management depends on the etiology of the effusion.
2. Treatment of the inflammatory condition with oral anti-inflammatory medications or intra-articular steroids.
3. Infectious effusions are treated with serial aspirations or surgical drainage in combination with antibiotics.
4. Traumatic effusions resolve with rest, but treatment must address the injury pattern.

B. Spinal Stenosis

► **H&P Keys**

Elderly patients with complaints of back and buttock pain. Pain is made worse with walking and descending stairs and relieved only with prolonged rest. If activity continues, paresthesia and weakness may develop. Pain is increased with hyperextension of the spine and relieved with forward flexion of the spine. Sensory changes are described as water or candle wax dripping down the leg.

► **Diagnosis**

Radiographs often show degeneration of the facet joints. CT scan is the best noninvasive test for bony stenosis. MRI underestimates the degree of stenosis. Myelogram and postmyelogram CT are useful to fully define the disease, especially stenosis of the lateral recesses of the neural foramina.

► **Disease Severity**

Clinical impairment of activities with neurogenic claudication. Pain is increased with any activity that causes hyperextension of the spine. Acute trauma in the presence of stenosis may cause catastrophic neurologic symptoms with paraplegia and cauda equina symptoms and demands prompt surgical decompression.

► **Concept and Application**

The maturing of the skeleton results in degenerative changes involving the disk margins and facet joints. The bony overgrowth constricts the nerve roots. This may be exacerbated by ligamentous thickening and diskogenic protrusions.

► **Treatment Steps**

1. Adjustment to the limitations of the disease in conjunction with anti-inflammatory medications, ice or heat, and an exercise program.
2. If symptoms are severely disruptive to the patient, surgery (laminectomy) to decompress the nerve roots will give relief. Fu-

sion may be required if facetectomies are needed to decompress the neural elements.

C. Contusions

▶ **H&P Keys**

Contusions are a result of direct trauma. Localized erythema and swelling are present with palpable tenderness. There may be loss of adjacent joint motion if swelling is pronounced.

▶ **Diagnosis**

Diagnosis is by history and clinical examination. Radiographs rule out fracture or late myositis ossificans.

▶ **Disease Severity**

Clinical loss of function of the joint and affected extremity define severity. Large hematomas and contusions to a large area of the muscle mass will produce greater disability. Myositis ossificans, or calcification of the muscle, is a late sequela of a severe contusion or a result of repetitive contusions to the same muscle before primary healing has occurred or early application of heat.

▶ **Concept and Application**

Contusions are a result of direct trauma. Following the trauma there is local damage to blood vessels and muscle. As bleeding and swelling continue, there is increased muscle stiffness and loss of joint motion. Secondary agents of inflammation produced as response to the local tissue trauma produce the ache and stiffness that characterize the early period after a contusion.

▶ **Treatment Steps**

1. Treatment consists of ice and compression to control the swelling and bleeding.
2. Adjunctive use of NSAIDs is useful in controlling the secondary inflammation.
3. Early therapy is provided to restore painless range of motion, followed by flexibility and strengthening exercises.
4. Return to activity is allowed when there is full, painless range of motion and strength equal to the unaffected extremity.

D. Fractures and Dislocations

1. Cervical Spine

▶ **H&P Keys**

Fractures of the cervical spine are caused in four ways: (1) flexion, (2) extension, (3) vertical compression, and (4) rotation.

Flexion Injuries—The most common and usually involve the lower cervical spine. May be associated with compression of the vertebral body, rupture of the supraspinous ligament, dislocation of the posterior facets.

Extension Injuries—Generally less serious than flexion, with the most common being fractures of the odontoid; hyperextension injuries can result in damage to the anterior spinal artery, with the resultant anterior spinal artery syndrome. The hangman's fracture or fracture of the pedicles of C2 and spondylolisthesis of C2 on C3 results from hyperextension during falls.

Vertical Compression—Axial loading injuries cause vertical compression and result in fractures of the atlas or burst fractures.

► **Diagnosis**

Radiographs: anteroposterior (AP), lateral, oblique, and open-mouth odontoid are the standard views. Flexion and extension lateral x-rays evaluate instability. CT scan and MRI are useful in determining the geometry of fracture fragments and evaluating the degree of cord compression.

► **Disease Severity**

Disease severity is based on clinical findings of neurologic compromise.

► **Concept and Application**

The pattern of injury is dependent on the mechanism of injury. Treatment is based on decompression of the neurologic elements and stabilization of the spine, either surgically or with bracing.

► **Treatment Steps**

1. Treatment is stabilization of the unstable elements with surgery or bracing.
2. For neurologic compromise, prompt intervention to decompress the neural elements and stabilize the bony and ligamentous structures.

2. **Thoracic Spine**

► **H&P Keys**

Usually, high energy is necessary to produce these injuries unless significant osteoporosis is present. The pattern of injury depends on the position of the axis of flexion and direction of the force at the time of injury. These result in compression fractures, burst fractures, flexion–distraction injuries (seat belt), and fracture dislocations.

► **Diagnosis**

Radiographic evaluation with plain x-rays is usually adequate for thoracic fractures. CT scan is beneficial to define fracture geometry and neurologic compromise.

► **Disease Severity**

The degree of bony compression, displacement, and neurologic compromise defines the severity of the injury.

► **Concept and Application**

Compression fractures are common in falls from heights and falls onto the backsides by elderly osteoporotic patients. The injury occurs at the thoracic–lumbar junction where the thoracic kyphosis and lumbar lordosis meet. This results in loading forces on the anterior aspect of the vertebral body, with the resulting vertebral wedge fractures. Burst fractures are caused by pure axial loading and cause retropulsion of material, resulting in cord compromise with neurologic symptoms. The rapid deceleration injury of the seat-belted passenger results in the flexion–distraction fracture with a splitting of the vertebral body; displacement can be significant. Fracture dislocations are a result of a combination of flexion, compression, and rotation.

► **Treatment Steps**

1. Compression fractures of < 50% are usually treated with a short period of rest with supportive bracing and restorative exercise.
2. For those > 50%, surgical stabilization may be indicated.

3. Persistent back pain may occur after even minor compression in-juries.
4. Burst fractures associated with neurologic symptoms require op-erative stabilization and may require decompression.
5. Fracture dislocations often result in paraplegia; early operative stabilization will allow for early rehabilitation.

3. Lumbar Spine

► H&P Keys
Mechanism of injury is usually flexion or a combination of flexion and rotation. Pain is present in the posterior elements of the spine, and neurologic compromise may be present. Compression fractures are caused by pure axial loading. Differentiating between cord and root lesions is essential for prognosis.

► Diagnosis
Radiographs (AP, lateral, oblique), CT scan.

► Disease Severity
Based on level of neurologic compromise.

► Concept and Application
The cord ends at L1 and therefore only the lower motor and sensory nerves are involved in this injury. There is greater room in the lum-bar spine for displacement, and therefore greater displacement is necessary before neurologic compromise is present. The neurologic picture cannot be determined until spinal shock has passed, as ex-hibited by the return of the bulbocavernous reflex.

► Treatment Steps
Serial monitoring of the neurologic status and early stabilization and decompression of compressed neural elements provide for the best outcomes.

4. Closed Fracture of Hand Phalanges

► H&P Keys
Fractures are usually caused by twisting or angular forces. With frac-ture, there is loss of ability to use the hand fully, with associated pain and swelling. The location of the swelling and pain, as well as the pattern of altered motion, will suggest which of the phalanges has been injured. Loss of extension at the distal interphalangeal (DIP) joint is characteristic of a mallet finger or avulsion of the distal inser-tion of the extensor tendon onto the base of the distal phalanx and is the result of a sudden violent hyperflexion injury. Fractures of the phalanges may also present with acute angular deformities or rota-tion deformities, often seen with spiral fractures. Fractures of the distal phalanx are usually a result of a crushing blow.

► Diagnosis
Clinical examination correlated with biplanar x-rays is usually diag-nostic.

► Disease Severity
Intra-articular comminution is associated with poor function out-comes. Spiral fractures may result in rotation residuals if great care is not taken in the treatment of the fracture. Fractures of the distal phalanx often result in injuries to the nail bed, which can result in nail deformities if not anatomically repaired.

► Concept and Application

Fractures of the phalanges are caused by sudden, violent blows to the hand. They result in loss of joint function and angular deformities, accentuated by the pull of the tendons that act across the injured joints.

► Treatment Steps

1. Mallet fingers are treated with hyperextension splinting. Phalangeal fractures can be treated with splinting and buddy taping. Care must be taken to ensure flexion at the MCP and gentle flexion of the PIP to prevent loss of motion secondary to contraction of the collateral ligaments seen with prolonged splinting in full extension.
2. When there is loss of articular congruency, open reduction or percutaneous pinning is indicated. Unstable fracture geometries also require surgical stabilization.
3. Distal phalangeal fractures that involve the nail bed require repair of the nail bed with sutures.

5. Fracture of Neck of Femur

► H&P Keys

In the adolescent and young adult, femoral neck fractures occur as a result of high-energy accidents. In the elderly, they may occur with relatively minor trauma secondary to osteoporosis. Fractures may occur as a result of a direct fall on the greater trochanter or from a rotational force along the shaft of the femur. Symptoms include groin pain and inability to bear weight with the hip held in mild adduction and external rotation. The pain is exaggerated by motion, especially rotation of the hip. In an impacted fracture in the elderly, the symptoms may consist of groin pain only with ambulation; the pain may be referred to the knee or thigh.

► Diagnosis

AP and lateral x-rays usually confirm the diagnosis. In the elderly with groin pain and osteopenia, CT and a bone scan may be necessary to confirm the diagnosis.

► Disease Severity

Displaced fractures of the femoral neck have a high rate of complications, with delayed unions and the development of avascular necrosis of the femoral head from disruption of blood supply to the femoral head by the circumflex vessels. In young patients with axial loading fractures, posttraumatic chondrolysis may also be a complication. Even with minimal displacement, avascular necrosis and collapse of the femoral head may occur.

► Concept and Application

Femoral neck fractures should be considered in any elderly patient with groin pain. In younger patients, the diagnosis should be considered with high-energy trauma and associated groin pain. Displaced fractures of the femoral neck disrupt the blood supply to the femoral head and result in avascular necrosis.

► Treatment Steps

1. In young patients, the fracture of the femoral neck should be promptly reduced and internally fixed.
2. In the elderly, impacted and nondisplaced fractures may be pinned in situ. Because of the osteopenia, the fixation hardware may fail and require revision to a joint replacement. Displaced

fractures in the elderly should be treated with hemiarthroplasty or total hip arthroplasty if degenerative arthritis is present.

6. Fractures of the Foot and Leg

▶ H&P Keys

Fractures are a result of trauma but may also occur as a result of repetitive stress that results in a stress fracture. Fractures usually present with acute pain and swelling. Ecchymosis develops secondary to the fracture hematoma. Inability to bear weight, or pain exacerbated with weight bearing is usually present. Obvious angular deformity may be present with severely displaced fractures.

▶ Diagnosis

Radiographs are usually diagnostic. AP and lateral films are standard. Special views are necessary to evaluate the ankle (mortise view) and the foot (oblique views) to fully assess the injury pattern. The mortise view evaluates whether there has been injury to the syndesmosis with widening of the ankle mortise. The oblique foot views evaluate Lisfranc's joint. Injury to this region is often missed with plain x-rays. When pain is present only with activity and there is no history of trauma, bone scan may be necessary to evaluate for a stress injury. The most common locations for stress fractures in the foot and leg are the metatarsal, tibia, and fibula.

▶ Disease Severity

The location and the degree of comminution and displacement are predictive for rates of healing and complications of stiffness and lost joint motion. The distal third of the tibia is notorious for slow bony union, with a high percentage of delayed unions or nonunions. The fifth metatarsal in the diaphyseal region is also prone to nonunion, especially if weight bearing is allowed. Lisfranc's joint at the base of the second metatarsal is another region for complications following injury, with late arthritis and stiffness often present.

▶ Concept and Application

Fractures of the lower extremity require definition of their location and fracture geometry to ensure proper treatment.

▶ Treatment Steps

Fractures of the lower extremity require immobilization for adequate healing. This may be provided with casting, fracture bracing, or internal fixation with plates and screws or intramedullary devices. Principles of treatment are restoration of joint congruity and bony length with correction of angular and rotation deformities.

7. Dislocations and Separations

▶ H&P Keys

Any joint may suffer a dislocation. A dislocation occurs when a violent force applied to the joint results in the disruption of the supporting ligamentous structures. Pain is usually present, with ecchymosis over the injured ligamentous structures. Joint deformity and loss of motion may be present if the joint does not reduce spontaneously. There is joint instability with stress testing and a sense of insecurity with weight bearing.

▶ Diagnosis

Radiographs are used to show displacement or associated fractures. Stress testing of ligamentous supports confirms damage to and instability of the joint.

► Disease Severity

The residuals of joint dislocation depend on the joint injured. Hip dislocations have a high rate of complication with avascular necrosis. Dislocations of the knee may result in arterial injury to the popliteal vessels and loss of perfusion to the lower leg. Shoulder dislocations may result in injuries to the axillary or musculocutaneous nerves and persistent instability of the shoulder. Dislocations of Lisfranc's joint may result in persistent pain, stiffness, and ambulatory dysfunction.

► Concept and Application

Joint dislocations are serious injuries. They result when the forces that are applied to the joint exceed the ligaments' ability to withstand the stress. Instability occurs as a result of the loss of the passive restraints provided by the ligaments. The displacement of the normal joint structures may result in secondary injury to adjacent structures. Chronic instability may be a result of the injury.

► Treatment Steps

1. Rapid reduction of the dislocation and assessment of secondary injury patterns are the mainstays of treatment.
2. Fracture bracing and early protected motion programs may be useful in decreasing the morbidity associated with prolonged immobilization with rigid casting.
3. Operative repair is indicated for irreducible dislocations and for stabilization of grossly unstable joints.

8. Rotator Cuff Syndrome

► H&P Keys

Rotator cuff insufficiency may occur as an acute event after a fall into the shoulder. The injury usually occurs when the extremity is extended to break the fall and the weight of the body is suddenly applied to the tendon while it is under tension. The injury may result in sudden loss of shoulder function with inability to abduct the shoulder. The tear may occur by attrition in the older patient, with gradual deterioration of shoulder strength. Immediate symptoms are pain and swelling in the shoulder region. Pain may be increased with passive motion. There is weakness in shoulder abduction. Pain may be increased in activity above the horizontal and with resistance to abduction. There may be a positive drop arm test, with inability to hold the arm at the horizontal against any resistance.

► Diagnosis

X-rays may be normal or may show superior migration of the humeral head, impinging on the inferior surface of the acromion. In an acute injury, the humeral head may be low in the glenoid fossa secondary to intra-articular hematoma. Arthrography and MRI will define the magnitude and location of the tear.

► Disease Severity

The degree of symptoms depends on the magnitude of the tear. Partial or small tears may result in only minimal dysfunction and present with the predominant feature of pain. Larger tears will result in loss of shoulder strength. Long-standing cuff tears will result in cuff arthropathy, arthritis characterized by a high-riding humeral head impinging on the acromion, with glenohumeral arthritis.

► Concept and Application

Rotator cuff tears may occur as a sudden failure or as a result of slow attrition. Loss of balance in the musculature of the shoulder results in altered mechanics of the shoulder. The humeral head migrates superiorly and may herniate through the hole in the cuff to impinge on the acromion. The altered mechanics result in the late development of glenohumeral arthritis.

► Treatment Steps

1. Initial treatment is with ice, rest, and anti-inflammatory medications.
2. As the pain of the acute injury subsides, rehabilitation is started to increase strength in the cuff and restore muscle balance. If the shoulder does not improve with rehabilitation, surgery is indicated for repair of the cuff.
3. In young patients and those who require overhead strength in the shoulder, early surgical repair is advised. Decompression of the subacromial space by partial acromionectomy is indicated to decrease the compressive forces on the shoulder.
4. In older patients with irreparable tears, symptomatic relief may be obtained with debridement of the cuff and rehabilitation.

E. Other Orthopedic Emergencies

Other orthopaedic emergencies include compartmental syndrome, cauda equina syndrome, joint infections, open fractures, and fractures and dislocations with vascular involvement.

1. Compartment Syndrome

A rise in the interstitial compartment pressures as a result of bleeding or soft tissue swelling that prevents the perfusion of the compartment. Presents first with severe pain, which increases with passive stretch of the compartment. Diagnosis with intracompartmental pressure assessment; > 30 mm Hg warrants surgical decompression.

2. Cauda Equina Syndrome

Progressive loss of lower extremity function, with loss of bowel and bladder control. Secondary to pressure on the cauda equina. Requires immediate surgical decompression.

3. Joint Infections

Painful inflammation with pain on passive motion of the joint. Serial aspiration or surgical lavage is needed promptly to prevent the destruction of the joint by chondrolytic enzymes.

4. Open Fractures

Fractures in which the bone is exposed through the skin surface either from within or without. Grading is dependent on the size of the wound and zone of injury and the degree of soft tissue contamination. The greater the zone of injury and the greater the degree of contamination, the greater the increase in risk of infection and limb loss.

5. Vascular Compromise Following Fracture and Dislocation

Fractures and dislocations that cause loss of perfusion require prompt attention, with reduction usually restoring blood flow. Angiography is necessary if pulses are not restored. Knee dislocations mandate an angiogram because of the high rate of intimal injury to the popliteal artery and late thrombosis and subsequent limb loss.

BIBLIOGRAPHY

Ball GV. *Clinical Rheumatology.* Philadelphia: W.B. Saunders, 1993.

Cailliet R. *Neck and Arm Pain,* 3rd ed. Philadelphia: F.A. Davis, 1991.

Callen JP. Cutaneous manifestations of collagen vascular disease and related conditions. *Med Clin North Am,* September 1989.

Connolly JF. *The Management of Fractures and Dislocations: An Atlas,* 3rd ed. Philadelphia: W.B. Saunders, 1997.

D'Ambrosia RD. *Musculoskeletal Disorders,* 2nd ed. Philadelphia: J.B. Lippincott, 1986.

Dieppe PA. *Atlas of Clinical Rheumatology.* Philadelphia: Lea & Febiger, 1986.

Enneking WF. *Musculoskeletal Tumor Surgery.* New York: Churchill Livingstone, 1983.

Morrissy RT. *Pediatric Orthopedics,* 5th ed. Philadelphia: J.B. Lippincott, 2001; 1, 2.

Niwayama G, Resnick D. *Diagnosis of Bone and Joint Disorders,* 2nd ed. Philadelphia: W.B. Saunders, 1988.

O'Donoghue DH. *Treatment of Injuries to Athletes,* 4th ed. Philadelphia: W.B. Saunders, 1984.

Pettid, FJ. *Practical Orthopedics,* 5th ed. Mosby, 2000.

Stone J. *Current Rheumatology Diagnosis & Treatment.* New York: McGraw-Hill, 2004.

Turek SL. *Orthopedics: Principles and Their Application,* 4th ed. Philadelphia: J.B. Lippincott, 1984; 1, 2.

Neurology | 10

I. INFECTIOUS DISEASES OF THE CENTRAL NERVOUS SYSTEM (CNS) / 259

II. NEUROMUSCULAR DISORDERS / 264

III. NUTRITIONAL AND METABOLIC DISORDERS / 267

IV. PAROXYSMAL DISORDERS / 268

V. CEREBROVASCULAR DISORDERS / 271

VI. TOXIC DISORDERS / 275

I. INFECTIOUS DISEASES OF THE CENTRAL NERVOUS SYSTEM (CNS)

A. Viruses

1. Human Immunodeficiency Virus (HIV)

▶ H&P Keys

Risk factors include blood transfusion, needle sharing, unsafe sex; presentations include: headache and fever (meningitis) 1%, progressive dementia with impaired saccadic eye movements (15–20%), paraparesis (myelopathy) 20%, pain and numbness (neuropathy) 30%; focal deficits in CNS, lymphoma, toxoplasmosis, or progressive multifocal leukoencephalitis (PML).

▶ Diagnosis

HIV antibodies by enzyme-linked immunosorbent assay (ELISA) (if positive, confirm with Western blot); magnetic resonance imaging (MRI) of affected area to exclude mass lesion in myelopathy, dementia, or focal deficits; cerebrospinal fluid (CSF) for pleocytosis; cultures in meningitis; CSF protein and electromyography (EMG) and nerve conduction velocities (NCV) in neuropathy; vitamin B_{12} level.

▶ Disease Severity

CD4+ count < 200 associated with severe immunosuppression and opportunistic infections; viral load > 100,000 copies/mL correlate with CD4+ decline and clinical progression; dementia, myelopathy, lymphoma, and PML carry poor prognosis.

▶ Concept and Application

Etiology of dementia and myelopathy unknown; direct invasion in meningitis; reduced immunocompetence in toxoplasmosis, lymphoma, neuropathy, or PML.

▶ Treatment Steps

1. For parenchymal mass lesion, pyrimethamine and sulfadiazine for 2 weeks; biopsy if not better.
2. Radiation for CNS lymphoma.
3. Amphotericin for fungal meningitis.
4. IV immunoglobulin G (IgG) if neuropathy is demyelinating; otherwise, biopsy to rule out specific infectious or vasculitic etiologies.
5. Pain treatment with tricyclic antidepressants, gabapentin, lamotrigine, carbamazepine.
6. For dementia, treatment protocols include reverse transcriptase and protease inhibitors.
7. Vacuolar myelopathy has no specific therapy.

2. Herpes Simplex Virus (HSV)

▶ H&P Keys

In the CNS, usually presents with encephalitic symptoms including clouding of consciousness, aphasia, fever, headache, seizures; exam denotes aphasia, hemiparesis, nuchal rigidity, confusion, and variable somnolence.

▶ Diagnosis

Brain computed tomography (CT) shows edema and hemorrhage in the temporal lobe and orbitofrontal cortex; MRI demonstrates areas of high signal intensity on T2-weighted images (Fig. 10–1); electroencephalogram (EEG) shows periodic lateralized epileptiform discharges (PLEDs) (Fig. 10–2); CSF has increased protein and mild lymphocytic pleocytosis and, at times, xanthochromia; polymerase chain reaction (PCR) of CSF is helpful for the diagnosis; biopsy makes definitive diagnosis.

► Disease Severity

Sequelae directly related to duration of disease prior to therapy; often fatal if not treated; age > 30 associated with poor prognosis.

► Concept and Application

Virus accesses brain by reactivation from fifth cranial nerve; direct invasion causes necrosis, hemorrhage, edema; sporadic occurrence.

► Treatment Steps

1. IV acyclovir when diagnosis suspected.
2. Biopsy of lesion, but therapy should not be delayed while waiting for biopsy.
3. Anticonvulsants for seizures.
4. Supportive care.

B. Meningitis

1. Aseptic

► H&P Keys

Preceding upper respiratory infection, exanthem, exposure to rat excreta; headache, fever, photophobia, nuchal rigidity.

► Diagnosis

CT scan to rule out abscess; CSF examination shows pleocytosis, predominantly lymphocytic, mild protein elevation, normal glucose;

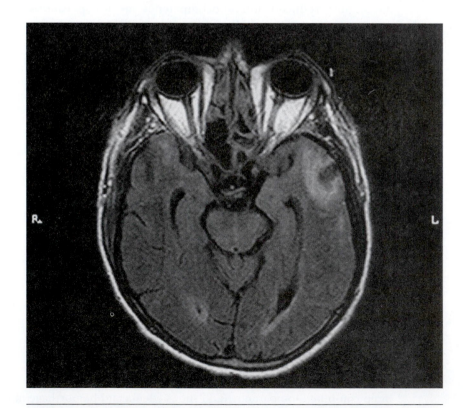

Figure 10–1. MRI of HSV encephalitis with increased T2 signal in both temporal lobes. R, mesial; L, lateral with T1 hypodensity secondary to hemorrhage.

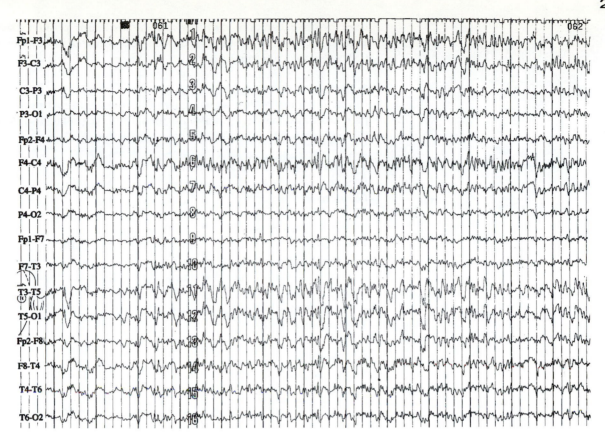

Figure 10–2. Electroencephalogram with periodic lateralizing epileptiform discharges escalating to electrographic seizure in a patient with herpes encephalitis.

negative bacterial cultures and Gram's stain; acute and convalescent viral titers helpful.

► Disease Severity

Usually benign course, without sequelae; decreased mentation; focal neurologic signs, seizures suggest concurrent encephalitis and worse outcome.

► Concept and Application

Meningeal infection with virus, most often enterovirus or mumps virus; initial infection with Lyme disease, HIV, leptospirosis, and syphilis may present similarly.

► Treatment Steps

Supportive management.

2. Bacterial (Septic)

► H&P Keys

History of sinusitis, ear infection, epidemic meningitis, pneumonia; presents with headache, fever, photophobia, seizures, nuchal rigidity, and obtundation; suspect meningococcus with petechial rash, pneumococcus with pneumonia or sinus infection in adults, *Haemophilus influenzae* with similar symptoms in children.

► Diagnosis

Negative CT of head (if timely); CSF pleocytosis up to 10,000, mainly neutrophils; low (< 40% of serum) glucose; protein elevation; positive bacterial cultures and Gram stain; positive bacterial antigens if partially treated; positive blood cultures in 60%; elevated CSF pressure (200 mm/H_2O).

▶ **Disease Severity**

Coma, focal neurologic signs, signs of herniation, seizures bear poor prognosis and may suggest abscess formation; sequelae and outcome directly related to time of institution of therapy.

▶ **Concept and Application**

Pyogenic infection of meninges with prominent vascular changes (small to medium arteritis).

▶ **Treatment Steps**

1. Blood culture; CT of head, lumbar puncture (LP).
2. Do not delay antibiotics for LP or LP for CT; cefotaxime in adults and children > 3 months; ampicillin and cefotaxime in neonates and infants.
3. Steroids may lessen hearing loss in children.
4. Supportive care.

3. Fungal

▶ **H&P Keys**

Progressive dementia, headaches, nuchal rigidity, lack of fever, cranial nerve involvement, often immunosuppression or history of lymphoma or other malignant disease; exposure to birds; suspect *Cryptococcus* in the immunosuppressed, mucormycosis in diabetics.

▶ **Diagnosis**

CSF with predominantly lymphocytic and monocytic pleocytosis; positive cryptococcal antigen and positive India ink in cryptococcal meningitis; positive fungal cultures in weeks.

▶ **Disease Severity**

Hydrocephalus; arteritis, thrombosis, and infarction of the brain.

▶ **Concept and Application**

Granulomatous meningitis composed of fibroblasts, giant cells, and necrosis.

▶ **Treatment Steps**

1. Amphotericin B along with antifungal agents (fluconazole, itraconazole).
2. Supportive care.

4. Tuberculous (TB)

▶ **H&P Keys**

Positive purified protein derivative (tuberculin) (PPD) in 75%; fever, malaise, headache; development of nuchal rigidity, decreased mental status, confusion, dementia, lower cranial nerve involvement.

▶ **Diagnosis**

Chest x-ray (CXR); PPD; CSF shows lymphocytic pleocytosis, elevated protein (often to several hundred), low glucose (normal in 30%), positive acid-fast bacillus (AFB) stain or immunofluorescence; cultures take several weeks and often require multiple LPs.

► Disease Severity

Residual deficits depend on onset of therapy in relation to stage of disease; obtundation, seizures, hydrocephalus, or focal signs indicate poor prognosis.

► Concept and Application

Caseating granulomas surrounded by epithelioid cells, lymphocytes, and connective tissue; exudate results from fibrin, lymphocytes, and areas of caseation necrosis; exudate spreads along pial vessels and invades underlying brain.

► Treatment Steps

1. Isoniazid can cause peripheral neuropathy and seizures.
2. Daily addition of pyridoxine; addition of rifampin and pyrazinamide; use of streptomycin when resistance is suspected.
3. Careful observance for liver toxicity.
4. Use of steroids for treatment of all cases of TB meningitis.
5. Treatment of increased intracranial pressure; hydrocephalus treated with ventriculoperitoneal shunt.

C. Abscesses

► H&P Keys

History of sinus, ear, periodontal, pulmonary, or head wound infection, endocarditis; suspect congenital heart disease in children; presents with focal severe headache, nausea and vomiting, seizures; focal signs dependent on location.

► Diagnosis

MRI or CT with contrast of affected area shows ring-enhancing lesion with edema, mass effect, "daughter lesion"; LP shows "aseptic" pleocytosis but is usually not necessary and may be contraindicated because of possible herniation.

► Disease Severity

Untreated cases produce major disability or death; mortality rate in treated cases is 30%; 50% suffer neurologic sequelae.

► Concept and Application

Focal infection of brain parenchyma, usually without meningitis; encapsulated with central necrotic material and pus; solitary 75% of the time; usually caused by anaerobes or microaerophilic organisms, most commonly anaerobic streptococci or bacteroides.

► Treatment Steps

1. Biopsy using stereotaxic CT guidance.
2. Steroids for management of intracranial pressure.
3. Mechanical hyperventilation and P_{CO_2} of < 30 may be needed if severe.
4. Anticonvulsants for seizures.
5. IV antibiotics include penicillin and metronidazole if pathogen is unknown; vancomycin for methicillin-resistant staphylococci and third-generation cephalosporin for gram-negative bacteria.

D. Spirochetes

1. Lyme Disease

► H&P Keys

History of tick bite in about 50% of patients; history of erythema chronicum migrans in about 60% of patients; influenza-like symptoms; can present as an aseptic meningitis; weeks to months later neurologic involvement will happen in 15% of the cases; most common neurologic presentation is one of meningoencephalitis with cranial or peripheral neuritis; chronic symptoms include encephalopathy and axonal neuropathy; peripheral nervous system presentations include Bell's palsy, mononeuritis multiplex, myositis, and peripheral neuropathy.

▶ Diagnosis

Lyme titers by ELISA, confirmed by Western blot; perform CSF examination in all neurologic cases; typical CSF abnormalities include mononuclear cell pleocytosis as high as 3,000 and increased protein level up to 400; check for intrathecal production of Lyme-specific antibodies, cultures and PCR testing in equivocal cases.

▶ Disease Severity

Myelitis-causing quadriparesis, seizures, and dementia have infrequently been described but are likely to leave sequelae. Radiculoneuritis is commonly reported in Europe but rare in the United States.

▶ Concept and Application

Arthropod-borne infection. *Borrelia burgdorferi* is a spirochete inoculated into humans by the *Ixodes* or deer tick; endemic in northeastern United States.

▶ Treatment Steps

1. Treat erythema migrans or Bell's palsy with oral doxycycline or amoxicillin for 30 days; for any other neurologic symptoms or conditions, treat with IV ceftriaxone 2 g daily for 14 days.
2. Corticosteroids are used in failure to respond to antibiotics.

II. NEUROMUSCULAR DISORDERS

A. Carpal Tunnel Syndrome

▶ H&P Keys

Nocturnal pain or numbness in first three digits of the hand, weakness on thumb opposition, wrist pain with rare shoulder pain; exacerbation with repetitive motion of wrist; positive Tinel's sign at median nerve at the wrist.

▶ Diagnosis

Wrist x-rays show bony deformities; MRI of wrist demonstrates focal compression of median nerve; EMG and NCV will show focal median nerve conduction velocity slowing at the wrist, axonal loss; depending on history, check for diabetes, rheumatoid arthritis, Lyme disease.

▶ Disease Severity

Severe atrophy of thenar muscles, marked thumb opposition weakness, permanent pain or numbness of first three digits, absent sensory early and, later, motor potentials on nerve conduction of the median nerve.

▶ Concept and Application

Compression of median nerve or traumatic injury of nerve by repetitive motion; diabetes, amyloidosis, acromegaly, hypothyroidism, sarcoidosis, rheumatoid arthritis, and pregnancy increase risk of syndrome.

▶ **Treatment Steps**
1. Mild cases will respond to wrist splint.
2. Recurrence of pain or numbness will respond to steroid injection.
3. Surgery offers excellent results in > 90% of cases of well-demonstrated carpal tunnel syndrome.
4. Reduction of repetitive activity.
5. Modification of work environment.

B. Guillain–Barré Syndrome (Acute Inflammatory Demyelinating Polyneuropathy)

▶ **H&P Keys**
Progressive ascending weakness a few weeks after an upper respiratory or gastrointestinal (GI) illness or surgery; back discomfort in 60%; no sensory level; areflexia; distal, but may be proximal, progressive weakness mainly in the legs; no fever on presentation; very symmetrical; maximum evolution of disease in 2 weeks in 50% of patients, in 4 weeks in 90% of patients.

▶ **Diagnosis**
CSF with high protein but < 10 white blood cells (WBCs) (50 in HIV patients); slowing of conduction velocities to conduction block on EMG and NCV studies; check for Lyme, HIV, urine porphyrins, hepatitis; culture stools for *Campylobacter jejuni*. GM1, Gd1a, and GD1b myelin glycolipid antibodies in CSF support the diagnosis.

▶ **Disease Severity**
Poor prognostic indicators include severe tetraparesis, hyperacute onset, assisted ventilation, low nerve amplitudes on EMG and NCV (suggesting axonal involvement and likely to result in prolonged sequelae), and abnormal phrenic nerve studies; autonomic instability may increase morbidity.

▶ **Concept and Application**
Proximal and later distal segmental demyelination with inflammatory cell infiltration in nerve.

▶ **Treatment Steps**
1. Plasmapheresis in first week for quickly progressing cases (inability to stand) or ventilator dependence.
2. Supportive care.
3. Recent evidence favors intravenous immune globulin (IVIG) as treatment.
4. Corticosteroids are not helpful.

C. Myasthenia Gravis

▶ **H&P Keys**
Diplopia, ptosis; symptoms worsen at end of day; young females; elderly males; demonstrable fatigue on examination, such as worsening of ptosis on prolonged upward gaze.

▶ **Diagnosis**
Dramatic improvement with IV edrophonium chloride (Tensilon) (test double blind); positive antibodies to acetylcholine receptors

(80% in generalized, only 50% in ocular myasthenia); decrement of motor nerve potential with repetitive stimulation; may need single-fiber analysis; thoracic MRI for thymic abnormalities (hyperplasia in 85%, thymomas in 10–15%).

▶ Disease Severity

Bulbar weakness increases risk of aspiration; low pulmonary vital capacity indicates respiratory compromise; thymoma requires surgery.

▶ Concept and Application

Antibodies that block or permanently bind to the acetylcholine receptors, presumably resulting from autoimmune reaction possibly triggered by or cross-reactive with thymic acetylcholine receptors; this leads to disturbance in the neuromuscular synaptic transmission and decreased muscle excitation.

▶ Treatment Steps

1. Acetylcholinesterase inhibitor increases available acetylcholine.
2. Corticosteroids reduce the immunologic process; other immuno-suppressants are used in severe cases.
3. Thymectomy, although controversial, can eliminate the need for medications in some cases or reduce the doses in others.
4. Acute worsening is best treated by discontinuation of medications and ventilatory support.
5. Plasmapheresis is useful for short periods to hasten improvement.

D. Myopathies and Dystrophies

▶ H&P Keys

History of progressive proximal weakness in most cases; myalgias and cramps are more the exception than the rule; weakness is noted raising arms overhead and in related activities, or getting up from a chair; myotonic dystrophy will show myotonia on percussion of small muscles (e.g., tongue); Duchenne's dystrophy shows calf muscle enlargement.

▶ Diagnosis

Creatine kinase (CK) is elevated in most cases of myopathy and muscular dystrophy; EMG and NCV demonstrate small, brief (myopathic) motor unit potentials and normal nerve conduction velocities; muscle biopsy is diagnostic in most cases; metabolic myopathies may require biochemical studies; ischemic exercise test is abnormal in some glycogen metabolic myopathies because of the inability to utilize energy substrate; electrocardiogram (ECG) is needed for high incidence of cardiac abnormalities.

▶ Disease Severity

Severe weakness could be associated with respiratory compromise; high CK might cause myoglobinuria and renal failure in metabolic myopathies; many myopathies associated with life-threatening cardiac abnormalities; swallowing and respiratory difficulties could result in death.

▶ Concept and Application

Duchenne's dystrophy is the result of lack of dystrophin (muscle fiber surface membrane protein resulting in disturbance of structural integrity of sarcolemma); a severe inflammatory process of the muscle results in polymyositis; other myopathies are the result of metabolic derangements (McArdle's), protein serine-threonine kinase enzyme defect (result of triple nucleotide repeats expansion) in myotonic dystrophy, or intrinsic sarcomere dysfunction (congenital myopathies).

► Treatment Studies
1. Appropriate genetic studies facilitate diagnosis and genetic counseling along with prenatal diagnosis.
2. Corticosteroids in polymyositis and Duchenne's dystrophy; anticonvulsants in myotonic dystrophy to reduce cramps.
3. Orthoses and ambulatory aides might be helpful in activities of daily living.

III. NUTRITIONAL AND METABOLIC DISORDERS

A. Vitamin B$_{12}$ Deficiency

► H&P Keys
Painful dysesthesias in feet and hands followed by difficulty ambulating; ataxia, leg weakness, spasticity, changes in mentation, visual loss.

► Diagnosis
Vitamin B$_{12}$ levels can be obtained in most laboratories; because neurologic presentation does not necessarily parallel the hematologic picture, a high level of suspicion is needed; a few cases may have "normal" levels, and these may require measurement of methylmalonic acid and homocysteine, both of which are elevated in B$_{12}$ tissue deficiency. Measure parietal cell antibodies. Gastroscopy to evaluate atrophic gastritis with risk of gastric carcinoma.

► Disease Severity
Progressive leg weakness and spasticity leading to the need for ambulatory aids; in general, symptoms lasting > 3 months are unlikely to revert; the etiology for the deficiency should be established.

► Concept and Application
White matter degeneration of the spinal cord and occasionally of the brain; changes begin in the posterior column of the lower cervical segment and spread downward, forward, and laterally.

► Treatment Steps
1. Initial management is emergent.
2. Daily B$_{12}$ (1,000 mg) is needed in the first 7 days to replete stores. Subsequently, needs are supplied by 1,000 mg of B$_{12}$ monthly.

B. Thiamine Deficiency

► H&P Keys
Usually undernourished alcoholics, but sometimes patients with gastric carcinoma or hyperemesis gravidarum, who present with ataxia of gait, gaze palsies or nystagmus, and mental confusion and amnesia (Wernicke's encephalopathy); ocular abnormalities might include nystagmus that could be either horizontal or vertical, weakness or paralysis of conjugate gaze, or weakness of the external rectus muscle, which is always bilateral; the ataxia is one of stance and gait with no evidence of tremor, and the confusion could present as a global confusional state, stupor, and coma or as a hallucinatory state with overactivity; Wernicke's encephalopathy might progress to an amnesic syndrome with severe short-term memory impairment and confabulation (Korsakoff's psychosis).

▶ Diagnosis

CSF is almost always normal; blood pyruvate may be elevated; red blood cell (RBC) transketolase or plasma thiamine activity is markedly reduced, but the diagnosis remains a clinical one.

▶ Disease Severity

Transition to the Korsakoff state heralds poor outcome, even with therapy; other symptoms are likely to improve with treatment; concurrent septicemia, pneumonia, and liver disease result in about 15% mortality rate.

▶ Concept and Application

Thiamine deficiency results in necrotic lesions of the mamillary bodies, periaqueductal region, thalamus, hypothalamus, and floor of the fourth ventricle.

▶ Treatment Steps

1. Administer IV thiamine, 50 mg and IM 50 mg initially; and IM 50 mg daily subsequently until normal diet is resumed.
2. Avoid glucose infusion prior to thiamine administration.
3. Provide supportive care.
4. Evaluate for infections and other conditions.

C. Metabolic Encephalopathy

▶ H&P Keys

Progressive clouding of consciousness in general without any focal symptomatology; history of medication overdose, infections, anoxia, hypo- or hyperglycemia, renal insufficiency, liver disease, alcohol intoxication; examination demonstrates normal pupillary reactions with small pupils, normal oculovestibular responses, normal corneal responses, and no focal deficits in a mentally obtunded patient.

▶ Diagnosis

CT of the head is used to rule out mass lesions in patients with focal neurologic deficits (hypoglycemia, hypoxia, azotemia, and hepatic encephalopathies might cause focal neurologic signs); EEG to rule out nonconvulsive status epilepticus or postictal state; drug screen and metabolic parameters including sodium, glucose, oxygen, P_{CO_2}; CXR and urinalysis (UA) to rule out infections.

▶ Disease Severity

Prolonged hypoxia or hypoglycemia may result in permanent neurologic injury; ventilatory support might be needed in many instances of coma; fever should raise suspicion of meningitis or abscess.

▶ Concept and Application

Usually reversible; nonstructural injuries resulting in generalized cerebral dysfunction.

▶ Treatment Steps

Correction of metabolic derangement.

IV. PAROXYSMAL DISORDERS

A. Seizures

▶ H&P Keys

History of abrupt stereotypic transitory loss or alteration of consciousness with or without involuntary movements; short or no warning (aura); confusional state after recovery of consciousness; bowel and bladder incontinence and tongue biting may happen, usually accompanied by bodily injuries; physical examination usually normal after the event; may have upgoing toes and abnormalities of tone immediately at the end of the episode; if witnessed, the event can start focally in one limb, with automatism or behavioral manifestations or generalized increase or decrease in tone; brief alteration of consciousness without postictal confusion happens in absence seizures in children.

► Diagnosis
CT or MRI of brain to rule out irritative lesion (stroke, tumor, abscess); routine EEG might be diagnostic in ≤ 20% of patients; prolonged EEG monitoring might be necessary in difficult cases; single photon emission computed tomography (SPECT) and positron-emission tomography (PET) studies helpful in epileptogenic focus localization; diagnosis remains a clinical one; cardiac evaluation might be needed to rule out convulsive syncope in selected cases.

► Disease Severity
Seizures, although most often idiopathic, can be the presentation of otherwise treatable conditions such as brain tumors, abscesses, arteriovenous malformations; repeated seizures during the day might result in severe functional and social disability along with bodily injuries; the disease carries a number of social limitations with it; status epilepticus markedly increases morbidity and mortality.

► Concept and Application
Usually caused by an irritative lesion capable of causing abnormal neuronal discharges that can spread and perpetuate themselves.

► Treatment Steps
1. Treatment depends on seizure type.
2. When no seizures, patients respond best to valproic acid.
3. Generalized and partial seizures respond to phenytoin, valproate, zonisamide, lamotrigine, topiramate, tiagabine, carbamazepine, and levetiracetam.
4. Febrile seizures do not require chronic anticonvulsant therapy.
5. Refractory cases may require surgery or vagal nerve stimulator placement.
6. Status epilepticus (continuous seizure activity lasting < 20 minutes or multiple seizures without interictal recovery) are medical emergencies requiring immediate use of IV benzodiazepines followed by IV phenytoin or valproic acid and, if necessary, barbiturate coma with mechanical ventilation.

B. Trigeminal Neuralgia

► H&P Keys
Brief, sharp, lancinating pain mainly in the third or second division of the fifth cranial nerve. Precipitated by touch, cold, or chewing.

► Diagnosis
Normal neurologic exam; if abnormal, consider other conditions such as posterior fossa mass lesion; beware of young multiple sclerosis (MS) patients with similar symptoms; any neurologic abnormality should cause a prompt investigation of the posterior fossa with CT or MRI for cerebellar pontine angle tumors, tumors of the fifth nerve, and MS.

► Disease Severity

The condition is a painful disease that results in no permanent sequelae to the patient if untreated; however, the pain is severe
enough to have caused some patients to commit suicide.

► Concept and Application

The specific etiology is unknown, but may involve arterial ectasia
with nerve compression in some cases.

► Treatment Steps

1. Medical management is highly satisfactory; oral carbamazepine is
   usually started at the beginning (75% response rate); refractori-
   ness may require the addition of baclofen, gabapentin, lamotrigine, or amitriptyline.
2. Monitoring for dizziness, unsteadiness, bone marrow suppression
   with carbamazepine.
3. Acute confusional state and seizures may occur with abrupt discontinuation of baclofen.
4. Microvascular decompression of the nerve might result in long-
   standing relief.

C. Headaches

► H&P Keys

History of intermittent or persistent head pain with or without associated vegetative symptoms; migraines are usually unilateral, pulsating
headaches and if classic are associated with visual scotomata;
hemisensory disturbances; nausea and vomiting; and photo-, phono-,
and osmophobia; cluster headaches are retro-orbital, occurring in
the adult smoker associated with lacrimation; ipsilateral Horner's syndrome usually lasts 90 minutes, may occur at the same time of day;
tension headaches are chronic, bandlike headaches with no other
symptomatology; examination should be normal.

► Diagnosis

CT or MRI of the head to rule out intracranial mass lesion; early
generalized, pulsating headaches might mean nocturnal hypoxemia
and may require oximetry; LP should be done on patients with
nuchal rigidity or fever; sinus x-rays should be done on patients with
percussion tenderness.

► Disease Severity

Headaches might be the initial and sole presentation of intracranial
lesions such as brain tumors, abscesses, hydrocephalus, and other
space-occupying lesions (Fig. 10–3); otherwise, these are benign conditions.

► Concept and Application

Migraine is a familial disorder characterized with abnormal cerebral
and intra- and extracranial vascular reactivity; chronic tension
headaches are secondary to self-perpetuating muscle tension; cluster
headaches could be paroxysmal parasympathetic discharges through
the superficial petrosal nerve.

► Treatment Steps

1. Abortive therapy can be provided by means of nonsteroidal anti-
   inflammatory drugs (NSAIDs).
2. 5HT1B and 5HT1D agonists (sumatriptan, zolmitriptan, rizatrip-
   tan, frovatriptan, eletriptan, and naratriptan) are highly effective

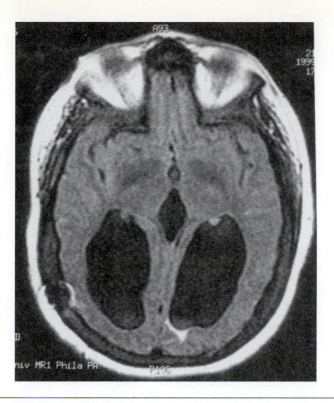

Figure 10–3. T1-weighted MRI image of acute obstructive hydrocephalus revealing dilated third and lateral ventricles.

migrainous attack abortive agents except in patients with known vascular disease or hypertension.

3. Migraine prophylaxis can be achieved by using β-blockers, valproic acid, topiramate, tricyclic antidepressants, riboflavin, magnesium supplementation.

4. Cluster headaches respond well acutely (> 70% of cases) to oxygen inhalation.

5. Ergotamine orally and intranasal lidocaine can provide abortive therapy as well.

6. Prophylaxis is achieved by oral corticosteroids or verapamil.

V. CEREBROVASCULAR DISORDERS

A. Ischemic Thrombotic Strokes

▶ **H&P Keys**

Predisposing risk factors include diabetes, hypertension, hypercholesterolemia, smoking, elevated homocysteine and C-reactive protein; acute onset of fixed neurologic deficit, usually while sleeping; possible prior history of short-lived deficits or unilateral visual loss (transient ischemic attacks); contralateral hemiparesis and aphasia in middle cerebral or carotid distribution; contralateral leg and shoulder weakness in anterior cerebral territory; dense visual field cut in posterior cerebral territory.

▶ **Diagnosis**

CT or MRI of head to further localize lesion and exclude bleeding (Figs. 10–4 and 10–5); carotid noninvasive or magnetic resonance angiogram (MRA) study to assess for stenosis; blood count and chem-

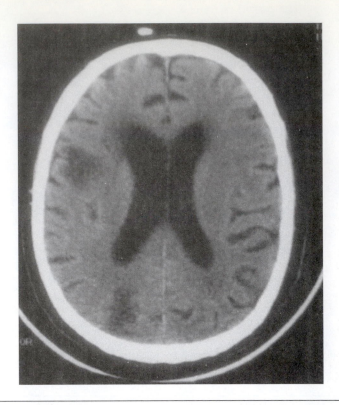

Figure 10–4. CT scan demonstrating right frontal and occipital infarcts in a patient with carotid artery thromboembolism.

istry for risk factors; antinuclear antibodies (ANAs), sedimentation rate, rapid plasma reagin (RPR), coagulation factor deficiency studies, homocysteine, C-reactive protein; arteriography and hypercoagulable and collagen vascular disease workup in young individuals.

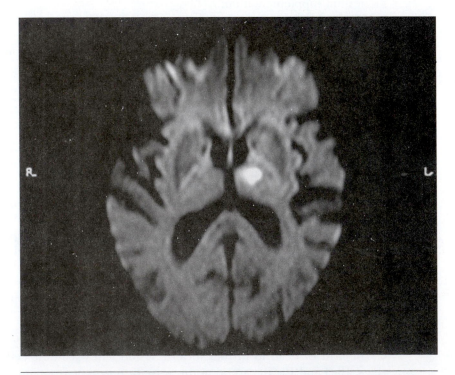

Figure 10–5. Diffusion-weighted MRI demonstrating hyperintense lesion in the L thalamus due to acute infarction.

► Disease Severity

Large clinical or radiologic deficits correlate with large areas of infarction and have increased risk of edema and herniation or hemorrhagic conversion; rehabilitation is also limited.

► Concept and Application

Predisposing factors reduce resilience of large arteries; atherosclerosis at branching and curves of cerebral arteries cause stenosis with subsequent embolization or narrowing of lumen (Fig. 10–6). Migraines and oral contraceptives increase risk of infarction.

► Treatment Steps

1. Includes reduction of risk factors, management of stroke complications, secondary prevention with antiplatelet or anticoagulant agents.
2. Surgery in carotid arteries if stenosis > 70%.
3. Discontinuation of oral contraceptives.
4. Physical therapy.
5. Periodic follow-up for recurrences.

B. Cardioembolic Strokes

► H&P Keys

History of rheumatic fever, cardiac dysrhythmias; abrupt onset; hemorrhagic strokes or multifocal distribution. Evidence of cortical signs including aphasia, seizures, more than one arterial distribution in addition to findings similar to thrombotic strokes.

► Diagnosis

CT or MRI of head, ECG, transthoracic and transesophageal echocardiogram if ECG is normal and suspicion for cardiac source still high, Holter monitor, blood cultures if endocarditis suspected.

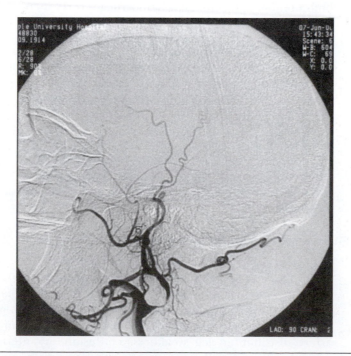

Figure 10–6. Digital subtraction carotid angiogram revealing large atherosclerotic plaque in the common carotid artery extending to internal and external carotid branches.

► Disease Severity

Embolic strokes tend to be larger and more commonly hemor-rhagic, higher incidence of edema with mass effect and seizures in-crease morbidity and mortality.

► Concept and Application

Sources of embolization include atrial fibrillation (with or without valvular disease), prosthetic valves, endocarditis, left ventricular hy-pokinesis or thrombus, cardiac tumors (myxomas).

► Treatment Steps

1. With the exception of myxoma and recent heart attack, long-term anticoagulation is needed.
2. Anticoagulation with heparin can be started within a few hours if stroke is not too large or there is no hemorrhage.
3. Switch to warfarin (Coumadin) when therapeutic and follow in-ternational normalized ratio (INR) recommendations depending on cause of stroke.

C. Intracerebral Hemorrhage

► H&P Keys

Usually, history of uncontrolled hypertension or coagulation deficits, sudden apoplectic onset, severe headache, nausea, vomiting, and fo-cal neurologic deficits; exam shows hemiparesis, obtundation, sen-sory deficits, conjugate eye deviation contralateral to hemiparesis (toward hemiparesis if brain stem), rapidly developing coma in pon-tine or cerebellar hemorrhage, elevated blood pressure.

► Diagnosis

CT or MRI of head to assess extent of bleeding; LP may be bloody but nonspecific and may induce herniation.

► Disease Severity

Both pontine and cerebellar hemorrhages carry increased risk; cere-bellar hemorrhage is usually treated surgically if large.

► Concept and Application

Hypertensive hemorrhages are due to aneurysmal dilatation (Char-cot–Bouchard aneurysms) of small-caliber arteries as a result of lipo-hyalinosis. Amyloid deposition in older patients (amyloid angiopa-thy).

► Treatment Steps

1. Supportive therapy, management of intracranial hypertension, careful control of systemic hypertension.
2. Lobar and cerebellar hemorrhages may be amenable to surgical resection.

D. Subarachnoid Hemorrhage

► H&P Keys

Acute onset of worst headache of patient's life, nausea, vomiting, variable loss of consciousness, may have had previous "warning" headaches; nuchal rigidity, obtundation; hemiparesis in middle cere-bral territory; third cranial nerve palsy in posterior communicating artery distribution; leg weakness, confusion in anterior cerebral artery territory. Two-thirds of ruptured aneurysms occur in anterior circulation.

► Diagnosis

CT of head positive in about 90% of cases; MRI may miss initial picture; LP shows elevated pressure, markedly bloody and xanthochromic, protein elevated, leukocytosis in 48 hours. Cerebral angiography is mandatory for definitive diagnosis; if initially negative (vasospasm), repeat in 6–12 weeks. Delay study if severe vasospasm present.

► Disease Severity

Outcome depends on mental status at time of ictus. Lethargic or obtunded patients have poorer outcome. Vasospasm and seizures add to morbidity. Disease associated with polycystic kidneys. Multiple aneurysms in many cases.

► Concept and Application

Hypertension, arteriosclerosis cause weakness of large-artery walls at bifurcations, leading to saccular dilatation. Rupture of this dilatation with associated arterial pressure results in symptoms. Reflex vasospasm causes oligemia and in severe cases, infarcts. Arteriovenous malformation can also rupture.

► Treatment Steps

1. Control of hypertension.
2. Reduction of Valsalva with stool softeners, quiet room.
3. Reduction of vasospasm with nimodipine.
4. Reduction of increased intracranial pressure with osmotic agents.
5. Hyperventilation and ventriculostomy if necessary.
6. Treatment of seizures with anticonvulsants.
7. Surgery when stable.

VI. TOXIC DISORDERS

A. Medications

1. Opioids

► H&P Keys

High incidence of addiction; inadvertent poisoning or suicidal attempts, results in varying degrees of obtundation followed by decreased ventilation, miosis, bradycardia, and hypothermia.

2. Barbiturates

► H&P Keys

High incidence of addiction; suicide attempts or accidental poisoning result in progressive unarousal, respiratory depression; pupillary response present and pulmonary edema.

3. Benzodiazepines

► H&P Keys
Similar to barbiturates.

4. Antipsychotic Drugs

► H&P Keys

Use of phenothiazines and butyrophenones, treatment of schizophrenia; side effects are parkinsonian syndrome, buccolingual involuntary movements (tardive dyskinesias), inability to sit still (akathisia), and a syndrome of severe rigidity, fever, and confusion (neuroleptic malignant syndrome), which can prove fatal in 20% of cases even when treated.

5. Cocaine

▶ **H&P Keys**

History of dependency; can be administered nasally, intravenously, or smoked; symptoms of intoxication include tremor, myoclonus, seizures, and psychosis. Stroke, seizures, and subarachnoid hemorrhages have been described.

VII. NEOPLASMS

A. Glioblastoma

▶ **H&P Keys**

Most common type of primary CNS tumor in adults (Fig. 10–7); history of hemiparesis or other focal neurologic signs, also seizures, confusion, obtundation, and late headache. No clear predisposing factors; most common cause of new-onset seizures in middle age. Exam correlates with complaints.

▶ **Diagnosis**

Contrast CT or MRI will show characteristic ring-enhancing lesion; rarely may be multicentric or across corpus callosum. Other studies are negative, including search for a metastatic origin. MR spectroscopy, PET, functional MRI, and cerebral blood flow techniques add to the current diagnostic arsenal. Biopsy shows typical

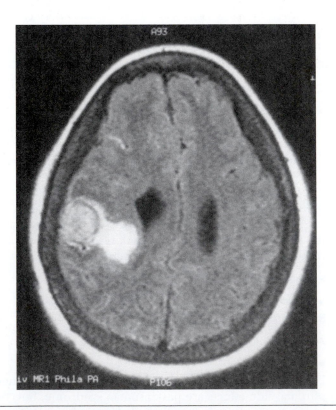

Figure 10–7. Fluid-attenuated inversion recovery MRI of right frontal glial tumor demonstrating vasogenic edema and midline shift.

pseudopallisading, hemorrhage, pleomorphism, and hypercellularity, and necrosis and endothelial hyperplasia.

▶ Disease Severity
Younger patients have better prognosis than older ones. Less than one-fifth of all patients survive more than a year.

▶ Concept and Application
Likely arises from anaplasia of astrocytes. Secondary characteristics of the tumor lead to further tissue invasion and mass effect.

▶ Treatment Steps
1. Surgery to debulk tumor.
2. Radiation accompanied by use of corticosteroids (vasogenic edema) and anticonvulsants is routine because of patient's symptoms.
3. Chemotherapy with timazolamide or bis chloroethyl nitrosourea (BCNU).
4. New radiothearapy techniques include radioactive implants, stereotactic radiosurgery, radiation with radiosensitizers, hyperthermia.
5. Monoclonal antibodies did not prove useful.
6. Genetic modification is the most promising future approach.

B. Meningioma

▶ H&P Keys
Benign tumor, causes symptoms by compression or irritation. Convexity tumors present with hemiparesis, seizures, and headaches; parasagittal with bicrural asymmetric weakness and spasticity, with sphincter disorder. Can happen in spinal canal (mainly females) or on optic nerve. Exam relates to complaints and presentation.

▶ Diagnosis
CT of head will show a usually rounded dural lesion with mass effect; MRI may only show lesion clearly with contrast enhancement (Fig. 10–8). It may calcify and show on plain x-rays.

▶ Disease Severity
Location of the tumor and potential for surgical resection determine outcome. Usually, tumor recurs if not completely resected.

▶ Concept and Application
Arise from arachnoid cells and may attain great size prior to development of symptoms. Usually cause exostosis rather than bone erosion. Some have progesterone, somatostatin, epidermal growth factor, and estrogen receptors and enlarge because of this. Psammoma bodies can be seen microscopically.

▶ Treatment Steps
1. Surgical resection when accessible; otherwise, radiation if symptomatic.
2. Incidental tumors can be observed because of slow growth.
3. Corticosteroids for edema; anticonvulsants for seizures.

C. Metastases

▶ H&P Keys
History of smoking, breast cancer, or other predisposing factors. Usually presents with focal neurologic signs, behavioral changes, headaches, or seizures. May be apoplectic if it bleeds.

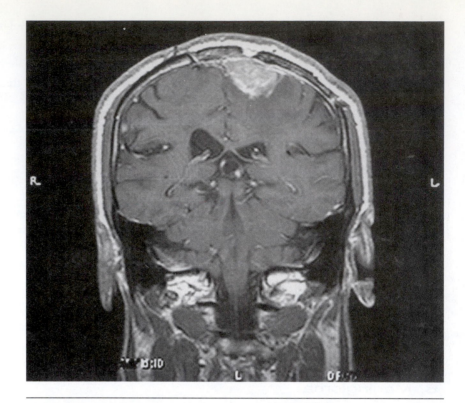

Figure 10–8. Gadolinium-enhancing meningeal mass (meningioma) with compression of underlying brain and surrounding T1 hypointensity due to edema.

▶ Diagnosis

MRI or CT scan shows single or multiple lesions with surrounding edema and enhancement. Physical examination including breast, gynecologic, and rectal exam; CXR; blood count may lead to diagnosis of primary. Biopsy of lesion if primary unknown will lead to separation from other etiologies.

▶ Disease Severity

Choriocarcinoma, melanoma, thyroid carcinoma, and hypernephroma may present with high incidence of bleeding. Solitary lesions have better prognosis and can be resected in some cases. Final outcome is relative to the primary disease itself.

▶ Concept and Application

Most commonly arises from lung, breast, or melanoma.

▶ Treatment Steps

Radiation, steroids, and anticonvulsants. Chemotherapy in appropriate cases.

VIII. DEGENERATIVE DISEASES

A. Alzheimer's Disease

▶ H&P Keys

Onset in late fifties or sixties; presents initially with deficit in retentive memory followed by dysnomia, spatial disorientation, personality changes, and gait disorder. The mental status examination shows findings related to these complaints. Seizures, paraparesis, and abulia can be seen in advanced cases.

► Diagnosis

CSF is normal, EEG is diffusely slow late in the disease, and the CT or MRI show atrophy; SPECT scan shows biparietal perfusion defects. PET scans and T2-weighted MRI proven useful in diagnosis. Efforts are being made to develop a biologic marker.

► Disease Severity

Progressive dementia leads to both physical and mental dissolution and eventually death.

► Concept and Application

The etiology is unknown, but a relationship exists with chromosome 21 in familial cases, the same chromosome involved in Down syndrome. The latter condition has pathologic similarities to Alzheimer's disease. In familial autosomal dominant cases, mutations in presenilin 1 and 2 and amyloid precursor protein genes are found. E4 alelle inheritance of apolipoprotein E gene carries genetic risk.

► Treatment Steps

1. Treatment includes memantine and acetylcholine esterase inhibitors (tacrine, donepezil, rivastigmine, galantamine) with effect on cognition and global measures.
2. Psychotic symptoms are controlled with newer atypical antipsychotics.
3. Depression is treated with selective serotonin reuptake inhibitors (SSRIs).

B. Amyotrophic Lateral Sclerosis (ALS)

► H&P Keys

Progressive weakness, usually asymmetrically, involving all voluntary muscles except extraocular ones. Prominent cramps, fasciculations, accompanied by "stiffness," dysarthria, and dysphagia. Exam shows mainly distal weakness with atrophy and fasciculation. Reflexes are exaggerated, tone is increased (spastic), toes are extensor. Combination of weak limb with atrophy and hyperreflexia is very suggestive.

► Diagnosis

Do MRI of cervical spine if exam shows atrophy and weakness of arms with hyperreflexia of legs to rule out cervical lesion. EMG shows denervation and reinnervation, as does the muscle biopsy. CK is minimally elevated in some cases. Do lead blood levels, hexosaminidase A, serum protein electrophoresis to exclude conditions that will mimic it, particularly when upper motor neuron signs are absent or mild. Familial cases secondary to SOD1 gene mutations are diagnosed with genetic testing.

► Disease Severity

The disease is fatal; bulbar forms have a shorter course. Respiratory failure and malnutrition are causes of death.

► Concept and Application

Neuronal loss in the anterior horn and motor cortex. Etiology is unknown, but glutamate excitotoxicity and free radical injury are implicated. Familial cases are associated with mutation of calcium or zinc superoxide dismutase gene.

► Treatment Steps

Riluzole is the first U.S. Food and Drug Administration (FDA)-approved drug for ALS treatment.

C. Parkinson's Disease

▶ H&P Keys

Progressive tremor, slowness, festinating gait, stooped posture. Early on, symptoms may be nonspecific ("arm discomfort"). Exam shows a resting tremor of 4–6 Hz, difficulty with passive motion (rigidity) evenly through the full range, decreased expression, paucity of movements (bradykinesia), and difficulty with posture. When tremor is added to the rigidity, "cogwheeling" results. Dementia occurs in 30% of cases.

▶ Diagnosis

No routine diagnostic studies exist; have decreased basal ganglia dopamine activity on PET scan. Exclude medications, progressive supranuclear palsy, olivopontocerebellar degeneration.

▶ Disease Severity

The disease eventually leads to disability in spite of therapy. Swallowing can be markedly affected.

▶ Concept and Application

Neuronal loss of the substantia nigra and other pigmented nuclei. Reduced dopamine levels. Similarity to a syndrome caused by the designer drug methylphenyltetrahydropyridine (MPTP) has raised question of environmental factor.

▶ Treatment Steps

1. Replace dopamine with L-dopa; added carbidopa (Sinemet) reduces peripheral effects. This medication can cause variations in clinical state not associated with dosing (on–off phenomenon).
2. Dopamine receptor agonists are also helpful (bromocriptine, pergolide, pramipexole, ropinirole).
3. Anticholinergics improve tremor but can worsen dementia.
4. Rasagaline, a selective monoamine oxidase (MAO)-B inhibitor, is used to slow down the disease progression.
5. Catechol-*O*-methyltransferase (COMT) inhibitors prolong L-dopa availability.

D. Huntington's Disease

▶ H&P Keys

Progressive mental deterioration; becoming irritable, impulsive, exhibiting poor self-control. Hand and face chorea develops and eventually all muscles follow. The exam shows chorea, dementia, oculomotor disturbances.

▶ Diagnosis

The CT or MRI shows caudate head atrophy; genetic studies can define the patient at risk and the subject with overt disease.

▶ Disease Severity

The disease is transmitted as autosomal dominant with complete penetrance; it is fatal. Childhood cases present with rigidity and seizures also. Mode of transmission leads to anticipation (subsequent generations show earlier and more severe signs).

▶ Concept and Application

Autosomal dominant inheritance; gene located on the short arm of chromosome 4; multiple erroneous repeats of nucleic acid triplets (CGA) results in defective Huntington's gene.

► Treatment Steps
1. No known treatment. Genetic counseling available for receptive individuals.
2. Because there is no cure, patients or individuals at risk may commit suicide.

IX. TRAUMA

A. Subdural Hematoma

► **H&P Keys**
History of head trauma with progressive change in mentation, focal neurologic signs, often loss of consciousness but not always, hemiparesis, large unreactive pupil with ophthalmoplegia if acute; seizures, headache, progressive change in mentation if chronic.

► **Diagnosis**
CT of head (Fig. 10–9), if performed without contrast, may miss an isodense (chronic) subdural hematoma. MRI of head with contrast (gadolinium) is the study of choice. Both will show crescentic lesion with signal compatible with blood.

► **Disease Severity**
Progressive focal neurologic deficit, progressive obtundation, requires quick intervention. Mass effect and shift of intracranial contents in radiologic studies also are usually suggestive of increased severity.

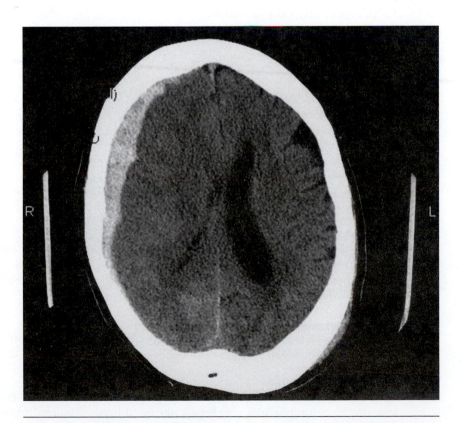

Figure 10–9. Hyperintense acute subdural hematoma with compression of underlying brain.

▶ Concept and Application

Ruptured bridging superficial cortical veins are responsible for blood accumulation. Chronic subdural may have recent rebleeding. Mass effect and cortical irritation are responsible for symptoms.

▶ Treatment Steps

1. Subdural hematomas with rapidly or incapacitating symptoms are best treated with surgical evacuation of the clot.
2. Prudent observation or corticosteroids can be used for small, incidental, or symptom-free subdural hematomas.

B. Epidural Hematoma

▶ H&P Keys

Severe head trauma accompanied by loss of consciousness, transient recovery of consciousness followed by progressive obtundation, posturing, shallow respirations, seizures, focal neurologic signs, coma.

▶ Diagnosis

CT of head or MRI will show concave blood clot, white on CT, bright on T1- and T2-weighted images on MRI. Skull x-rays will show fracture through area of middle meningeal artery or, less commonly, across venous sinus.

▶ Disease Severity

If untreated, the condition is lethal; timing is of the essence.

▶ Concept and Application

Tear of middle meningeal artery or venous sinus results in accumulation of blood at great pressure in a potential space.

▶ Treatment Steps

1. Emergent surgical evacuation.
2. Supportive.

C. Contusion

▶ H&P Keys

History of moderate to severe head trauma (unconscious for > 5 minutes); returns to alertness with confusion and mild mutism. Exam shows extensor plantar reflexes, mild hemiparesis, elevated blood pressure and heart rate.

▶ Diagnosis

CT or MRI may show focal parenchymal swelling (most commonly frontal or temporal tip) or delayed hemorrhage.

▶ Disease Severity

Degree of alertness at the time of evaluation, time unconscious, degree of retrograde amnesia determine severity of injury if otherwise uncomplicated. Temporal lobe herniation is main cause of morbidity and mortality.

▶ Concept and Application

Sustained head trauma results in neuronal swelling and axonal shearing, often maximal 24–48 hours after event.

▶ Treatment Steps

Control of intracranial pressure with hyperventilation, ventriculostomy; barbiturate coma may lessen neuronal injury. Delayed physical and cognitive deficits may occur and will require therapy.

X. DEMYELINATION

A. Multiple Sclerosis

▶ H&P Keys

History of arm, leg, hand, or foot numbness (50% of patients); visual loss (25%); diplopia; incoordination; weakness; bladder dysfunction. Exam shows sensory loss in spinal distribution, afferent pupillary deficit, ataxia, dysarthria, hyperreflexia, internuclear ophthalmoplegia.

▶ Diagnosis

MRI will show periventricular white matter demyelination or lesion in the spinal cord or optic nerve (Fig. 10–10). LP shows lymphocytic pleocytosis (< 100 cells/mL), increased protein (< 100 mg/mL), normal glucose, increased IgG intrathecal production, and oligoclonal bands. Large myelinated pathways can be assessed with evoked potentials (visual, auditory, somatosensory). The disease can be mimicked by syphilis, Sjögren's syndrome, systemic lupus erythematosus, sarcoidosis, and Lyme disease. The diagnosis remains clinical and depends on finding different lesions on separate occasions.

▶ Disease Severity

Pure spinal forms, chronic progressive, and early presentation are correlated with worst outcome. Elevation of body temperature (Uhthoff's phenomenon), stress, and infection can cause exacerbation.

▶ Concept and Application

The etiology of the disease is multifactorial, with environmental factors, increased incidence in temperate regions, immunogenetic factors such as certain human leukocyte antigen (HLA)-Dw or DR, followed by an aberrant immunologic response against CNS myelin.

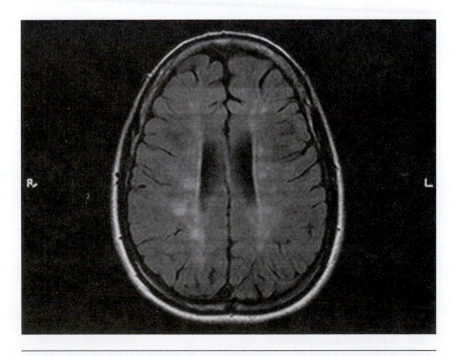

Figure 10–10. MRI of patient with multiple sclerosis demonstrating multiple white matter lesions with characteristic periventricular localization and perpendicular to ventricle orientation.

► Treatment Steps

1. Acute attacks respond to IV corticosteroids.
2. Chronic prophylaxis can be obtained with interferon-β or glatiramer acetate.
3. The tremor responds to isoniazid, propranolol, clonazepam, or primidone; baclofen orally or intrathecally or tizanidine reduces spasticity.
4. Fatigue responds to amantadine, pemoline, or modafinil.
5. Gait disability, bladder disorders require appropriate care.

XI. SLEEP DISORDERS

A. Sleep Apnea

► H&P Keys

Obesity, short neck, large tongue, large tonsils in children, myxedema, acromegaly, myotonic dystrophy in obstructive type; poliomyelitis, syringobulbia, and brain stem infarct in central type; history of heavy snoring, daytime sleepiness, fatigue, early morning headache, impotence.

► Diagnosis

Thyroid studies to rule out hypothyroidism; polysomnogram to exclude other etiologies of daytime sleepiness and to assess apneas and differentiate between central or obstructive type; multiple sleep latencies to assess the degree of nocturnal disturbance.

► Disease Severity

Six or more apneas per hour; oxygen desaturation; nocturnal cardiac arrhythmias. Sleep apnea is associated with cerebrovascular accidents, heart attacks.

► Concept and Application

Upper airway laxity and collapse on inspiration; reduced nocturnal respiratory drive in central type.

► Treatment Steps

1. Weight reduction of as few as 5 pounds may reduce symptoms.
2. Continuous positive airway pressure (CPAP) for obstructive type, repeat studies and adjust settings.
3. Protriptyline for central apnea.

B. Narcolepsy

► H&P Keys

Present with excessive daytime sleepiness; multiple daytime naps; paralysis with strong emotions in 70% (cataplexy); sleep paralysis; hypnagogic hallucinations; normal examination.

► Diagnosis

Sleep study (polysomnogram) is normal and will exclude other pathologies; multiple sleep latencies show rapid eye movement (REM) sleep onset in at least 2 out of 4–5 recordings; same abnormality can be seen with use of drugs, drug withdrawal, or sleep deprivation; therefore, needs good clinical correlation.

► Disease Severity

Most patients have narcolepsy and cataplexy by history; there could be milder cases; few have all symptoms.

► Concept and Application

The disease may be due to abnormalities in the orexin neurotransmitter system.

► Treatment Steps

1. Nondrug therapy consists of short naps, avoidance of heavy meals.
2. Drug therapy (often needed) consists of pemoline, and if unsuccessful, methylphenidate (Ritalin). Imipramine may be useful in controlling cataplexy. Modafinil, a newer drug, is effective and has fewer side effects in the treatment of narcolepsy and excessive daytime sleepiness.

BIBLIOGRAPHY

Bradley WG, Daroff RB, Fenichel GM, Marsden CD. *Neurology in Clinical Practice,* 4th ed. Boston: Butterworth Heinemann, 2004.

Brazis PW, Marsden JC, Biller J, Brazis P. *Localization in Clinical Neurology.* Philadelphia: Lippincott Williams & Wilkins, 2001.

Campbell WW, DeJong RN. *DeJong's The Neurologic Examination,* 6th ed. Philadelphia: Lippincott Williams & Wilkins, 2005.

Goetz CG, Pappert EG. *Textbook of Clinical Neurology.* Philadelphia: W.B. Saunders, 2003.

Joynt RJ, Griggs RC (eds.). *Baker's Clinical Neurology.* Philadelphia: Lippincott Williams & Wilkins, 2002.

Mayo Clinic Department of Neurology. *Mayo Clinic Examinations in Neurology,* 7th ed. St. Louis: Mosby, 1998.

Ropper AH, Brown RJ. *Adams & Victor's Principles of Neurology.* New York: McGraw-Hill, 2005.

Rowland LP (ed.). *Merritt's Neurology,* 11th ed. Lippincott Williams & Wilkins, 2005.

Samuels MA (ed.). *Hospitalist Neurology.* Boston: Butterworth–Heinemann, 1999.

Male and Female Reproduction

11

I. UTERUS

A. Malignant Neoplasm

1. Endometrial Cancer

▶ H&P Keys

Obesity, nulliparity, chronic anovulation, diabetes, hypertension, postmenopausal bleeding, history of tamoxifen therapy, unopposed estrogen therapy.

▶ Diagnosis

Endometrial biopsy, transvaginal ultrasonography (thickened endometrial "stripe"), hysteroscopy, fractional dilatation and curettage.

Advanced Disease—Chest x-ray (CXR), intravenous pyelogram (IVP), computed tomographic (CT) scan, barium enema, cystoscopy.

▶ Disease Severity

International Federation of Gynecology and Obstetrics (FIGO).

FIGO Staging (1988)

Stage I—Endometrium, myometrium.

Stage II—Cervix.

Stage III—Serosal, adnexal involvement:
- Positive peritoneal cytology.
- Vaginal mets.
- Pelvic/periaortic nodes.

Stage IV—Bladder, bowel mucosa.
- Distant mets.

▶ Concept and Application

Relationship between estrogen production and endometrial proliferation; overgrowth of the endometrium in response to unopposed estrogen.

▶ Treatment Steps

Early Disease—Total abdominal hysterectomy and bilateral salpingo-oophorectomy (with or without lymph node sampling).

Adjunctive Therapy
1. External beam radiation.
2. Preoperative radiation.

Recurrent Endometrial Carcinoma
1. High-dose progestins, e.g., medroxyprogesterone.
2. Chemotherapy, e.g., adriamycin, platinum.

B. Leiomyomata Uteri

▶ H&P Keys

Most common solid pelvic tumor in women; pain, abnormal uterine bleeding, pressure, uterine enlargement, urinary frequency, rectal pressure (Fig. 11–1).

▶ Diagnosis

Complete blood count (CBC), physical exam, pelvic ultrasound.

▶ Disease Severity

Severity of pain, anemia, urinary symptoms, hydronephrosis, uterine size beyond 12 weeks.

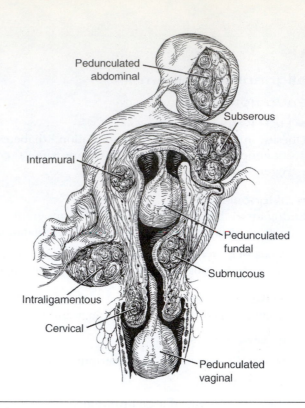

Figure 11–1. Common types of uterine fibroids. (Reproduced, with permission, from Pernoll ML, Benson RC [eds.]. *Current Obstetric & Gynecologic Diagnosis & Treatment,* 9th ed. Appleton & Lange, 2002.)

► **Concept and Application**

Localized proliferation of smooth muscle cells, estrogen-dependent, shrinkage after menopause. Arises from a single smooth muscle cell.

► **Treatment Steps**

1. *Observation:* bimanual exams, ultrasonograms, monitoring for growth.
2. *Medical:* Gonadotropin-releasing hormone (GnRH) agonists to induce a hypoestrogenic state, thus resulting in shrinkage.
3. *Surgical:* Myomectomy, uterine artery embolization, myolysis, total abdominal hysterectomy.

C. Other Disorders

1. Endometriosis

► **H&P Keys**

Premenstrual dysmenorrhea, premenstrual spotting or staining, dyspareunia, infertility, chronic pelvic pain, retroverted uterus, uterosacral nodularity, nonmobile uterus.

► **Diagnosis**

History and physical examination, bimanual examination, pelvic ultrasonography (for presence of endometrioma), laparoscopy (gold standard of diagnosis; Fig. 11–2), biopsy if possible (histology shows endometrial glands and stroma). (CA 125 of questionable help and very nonspecific.)

► **Disease Severity**

American Fertility Society stages I to IV (minimal through severe), extent of pelvic pain.

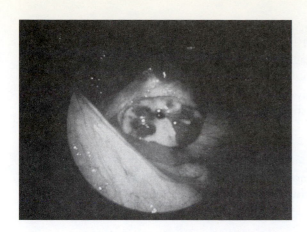

Figure 11–2. Implants of endometriosis are seen on the ovarian surface at the time of laparoscopy. These are "powder burn" in appearance and characteristic of classical endometriosis.

► Concept and Application

Retrograde menstruation (most commonly accepted theory), hematogenous spread, lymphogenous spread, genetic and family predisposition, coelomic metaplasia, estrogen-dependent growth of endometriosis, resolves after menopause.

► Treatment Steps

Depends on age of patient, duration of infertility, severity of symptoms, extent of disease.

1. Expectant therapy.
2. Medical therapy consists of GnRH agonist (medical treatment of choice), progestogens, oral contraceptives, nonsteroidal anti-inflammatory drugs (NSAIDs).
3. Conservative surgery.
4. Radical surgery via laparoscopy, laparotomy.
5. Danazol not currently used because of androgenic side effects.

II. OVARY

A. Malignant Neoplasm

1. Ovarian Cancer

► H&P Keys

Fifth most common of all cancers in women, higest mortality rate; two-thirds present with advanced disease. Affects 1 in 70 women in the United States.

► Diagnosis

Symptoms of ascites, abdominal distention in advanced stages. History and physical exam, pelvic ultrasonography, CA 125, CXR, surgical staging.

► Disease Severity

Surgical Staging—Stage I limited to the ovaries; stage II, pelvic extension; stage III, intraperitoneal metastases outside the pelvis; stage IV, distant metastases.

Main Histologic Types—Epithelial tumors (80%), sex-cord stromal tumors (3%), germ cell tumors (5%).

► Concept and Application

Spread to adjacent peritoneal surfaces; lymphatic and hematogenous spread. Familial or hereditary association in 5–10% of cases.

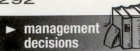

► management decisions

BENIGN ADNEXAL MASSES

Ovarian Corpus Luteum Cyst
Observation; serial ultrasonography; cyst usually resolves within 9 weeks, with or without oral contraceptive suppression. Rarely, surgical intervention is needed.

Ovarian Hemorrhagic Corpus Luteum Cyst
As above.

Ovarian Follicular Cyst
Observation; usually associated with anovulatory cycle; ultrasound for size; progestin to bring on menses; occasionally, oral contraceptives will help shrink cyst. Rarely, surgery is needed.

Endometrioma
Observation; analgesics, GnRH agonists to suppress growth of endometriosis, serial ultrasonography to check response to GnRH agonist. Surgery may be needed to drain cyst, remove cyst wall, or even perform oophorectomy.

Pedunculated Fibroid
Observation, serial ultrasonography; rarely need surgery if rapid growth in size, or pain from torsion or pressure.

Ovarian Cyst with Torsion
Stat admission to OR, to detorse ovary if no ischemia present; otherwise, emergency oophorectomy performed.

► **Treatment Steps**
1. Total abdominal hysterectomy, bilateral salpingo-oophorectomy, omentectomy, staging.
2. Adjunctive chemotherapy.

Overall 5-year survival depends on age, stage, grade, and residual disease after initial surgery.

B. Ovarian Cysts

► **H&P Keys**
Abdominal pain; anovulation, irregular bleeding, irregular periods, reproductive age group; usually unilateral, bimanual exam.

► **Diagnosis**
CBC and differential, pelvic ultrasonography (size, loculations, unilaterality versus bilaterality, calcifications), β-human chorionic gonadotropin (β-hCG) to rule out ectopic pregnancy.

► **Disease Severity**
Amount of pain, cyst size, presence of loculations, fluid in the peritoneal cavity (rare).

► **Concept and Application**
Most common is functional cyst related to anovulation. Follicular cyst continues to develop and enlarge without ovulation, thereby causing pain, possibly intraperitoneal rupture, and irregular menses. Eighty-five percent will resolve by 9 weeks.

► **Treatment Steps**
1. Observation, recheck at 3-week intervals.
2. Serial ultrasonograms.
3. Serial CBC with differential if suspicion of intraperitoneal bleeding.
4. Surgery if danger of torsion.
5. Possible laparotomy, ovarian cystectomy, or oophorectomy.

III. CERVIX

A. Malignant Neoplasm

► **H&P Keys**
Human papillomavirus (HPV) infection plays a main role in the pathogenesis of cervical cancer, cigarette smoking, high-risk sexual behaviors. Postcoital bleeding, abnormal discharge, abnormal Pap smears.

► **Diagnosis**
Pap smear, colposcopy, cervical biopsy, cone biopsy, endocervical curettage (ECC), CXR, IVP, barium enema, cystoscopy, proctosigmoidoscopy, magnetic resonance imaging (MRI) (optional).

► **Disease Severity (FIGO Staging, 1985)**
Staging is clinical.

Stage I—Confined to cervix.

Stage II—Upper vagina, not pelvic sidewall.

Stage III—Extending to pelvic sidewall.

Stage IV—Beyond pelvis: distant organs.

► Concept and Application

Slow progression from preinvasive to invasive disease. Screening is key.

► Treatment Steps

1. Total abdominal hysterectomy (cure rate 95%).
2. Stage IB–IIA: Radical hysterectomy or radiotherapy.
3. Recurrence of advanced stage: chemotherapy, radiotherapy.
4. Possible pelvic exenteration.

B. Cervicitis and Sexually Transmitted Diseases (STDs)

► H&P Keys

Herpes —Herpes simplex virus (HSV); multiple tender vesicles.

Gonorrhea—Neisseria gonorrhoeae; discharge, asymptomatic.

Syphilis—Treponema pallidum; chancre, fever, secondary skin rash, condyloma latum.

Chlamydia—Chlamydia trachomatis; mucopurulent discharge. Asymptomatic.

Chancroid—Haemophilus ducreyi; ulcerative disease: soft, painful ulcers.

HPV—Multifocal fleshy warts.

Lymphogranuloma Venereum (LGV)—C. trachomatis; "groove sign" (line between lymph nodes), buboes.

► Diagnosis

HSV—Clinical examination; viral culture.

Gonorrhea—Gram-negative intracellular diplococci seen on Gram stain. Culture on Thayer–Martin medium.

Syphilis—Venereal Disease Research Laboratory (VDRL), fluorescent treponemal antibody (FTA), rapid plasma reagin (RPR).

Chlamydia—Culture.

Chancroid—Biopsy, LGV, complement fixation.

► Disease Severity

HSV—Primary lesions 2–3 weeks, recurrent lesions.

Gonorrhea—Severity of symptoms may progress to overt pelvic inflammatory disease (PID) with tubo-ovarian abscess formation; advanced stages: arthritis.

Syphilis—Primary, secondary, tertiary syphilis; neurosyphilis.

Chlamydia—Cervicitis may progress to overt PID with tubo-ovarian abscess formation.

Chancroid—Severity of symptoms.

HPV—HPV serotyping: high-risk types versus low-risk types for progression to dysplasia.

LGV—Severity of symptoms.

► Concept and Application

Transmitted sexually via oral, vaginal, and anal contact; also associated with specific microorganism; also with body fluid contact.

► Treatment Steps

HSV—Acyclovir, famciclovir, valacyclovir.

Gonorrhea—Ofloxacin or ceftriaxone or cefoxitin. Also treat for chlamydia.

Syphilis—Benzathine penicillin.

Chlamydia—Azithromycin, doxycycline.

Chancroid—Oral sulfonamides, tetracycline.

HPV—Chemical destructive techniques (podophyllin), cryotherapy, electrocautery, laser vaporization, 5-fluorouracil, interferon, bichloroacetic acid.

C. Cervical Dysplasia and Management of Abnormal Pap Smear

► H&P Keys

Early age of coitus, sexual promiscuity, multiple sexual partners, cigarette smoking, high-risk male partner, abnormal Pap, HPV infection.

► Diagnosis

Pap smear, colposcopy, biopsy, ECC, cone biopsy.

► Disease Severity

Based on Bethesda 2001 classification:

- Negative for squamous intraepithelial lesion (SIL).
- Atypical squamous cells of undetermined significance (ASCUS).
- ASCUS, cannot exclude high-grade SIL (HGSIL).
- Low-grade SIL (LGSIL).
- HGSIL.
- Squamous cell carcinoma.

► Concept and Application

Identify preinvasive disease to prevent invasive disease.

► Treatment Steps

1. Cervical intraepithelial neoplasia (CIN) 1:
   - Observation with follow-up cytology.
   - Local ablation.
2. HGSIL, CIN 2–3; carcinoma in situ (CIS): ablation or excision, e.g., cryosurgery, electrocautery, loop electrosurgical excision procedure (LEEP), cone biopsy.
3. All patients with noninvasive lesions should have Pap smears every 4–6 months for about 2 years.

IV. VAGINA AND VULVA

A. Malignant Neoplasms

1. Vulvar Carcinoma

► H&P Keys

Chronic vulvar irritation or itching, labial lesion that does not heal, history of condyloma; age range 60–80 years.

► Diagnosis and Evaluation

Biopsy.

► Disease Severity

Staging based on T-N-M system (FIGO, 1988). Clinical assessment of tumor size (T), node assessment (N), metastases (M). Some associated with HPV.

► Treatment Steps

1. Depends on size of lesion, location, and patient factors.
2. Wide local incision to radical vulvectomy. Groin node evaluation is important.
3. Adjunct radiation therapy or exenteration for advanced stages III and IV.

2. Vaginal Cancer

► H&P Keys

Vaginal discharge, urinary symptoms.

► Diagnosis

Pap smear, colposcopy, biopsy.

► Disease Severity

Staging: stage I limited to the vaginal mucosa; stage II, subvaginal tissue involvement; stage III, extension to pelvic sidewall; stage IV, beyond true pelvis.

► Concept and Application

Ninety-five percent are squamous cell carcinoma: most commonly in upper vagina, possibly of STD origin. Most frequently a nonprimary cancer.

► Treatment Steps

1. Depends on stage.
2. Radiation therapy, surgery, chemotherapy.

B. Candidiasis of the Vulva and Vagina

► H&P Keys

Thick whitish discharge, cottage cheesy, itching, nonmalodorous, burning, swelling, dysuria. Obesity, frequent douching, diabetes, human immunodeficiency virus (HIV) disease, antibiotic usage, immunosuppressed patients.

► Diagnosis

Microscopic specimen examination including potassium hydroxide (KOH) and saline wet mount; hyphae on wet-mount exam; culture.

► Disease Severity

Severity of symptoms.

► Concept and Application

Candida albicans.

► Treatment Steps

Topical and oral antifungals.

C. Vaginitis and Vulvovaginitis

► H&P Keys

Trichomoniasis—May be asymptomatic, greenish-gray, frothy, malodorous discharge, strawberry spots on cervix and vagina, vaginal pH between 5 and 6.

Bacterial Vaginosis—Watery malodorous discharge, pH 5.0–5.5.

► Diagnosis

Trichomoniasis—Saline wet mount and KOH prep show trichomonad organisms intermixed with clumps of white blood cells (WBCs).

Bacterial Vaginosis—"Clue" cells (squamous cells with coccobacilli bacteria obscuring the sharp borders and cytoplasm), fishy odor, positive "whiff" test when mixed with KOH.

► Disease Severity
Severity of symptoms.

► Concept and Application

Trichomoniasis—*Trichomonas vaginalis.*

Bacterial Vaginosis—*Gardnerella vaginalis.*

► Treatment Steps

Trichomoniasis—Metronidazole (PO).

Bacterial Vaginosis—Metronidazole (PO or intravaginal).

D. Pelvic Relaxation/Urinary Incontinence

► H&P Keys
Varies, based on structure or structures involved and the degree of prolapse, pressure, heaviness, urinary (stress) incontinence, frequency, hesitancy, incomplete voiding, recurrent infections, painful or incomplete defecation. Ten to fifteen percent of women suffer significant recurrent urinary loss.

► Diagnosis
History and exam, Q-tip test; evaluation of urinary function, urodynamic testing, anoscopy, sigmoidoscopy.

► Disease Severity
First degree, second degree, third degree, procidentia (uterus completely outside vagina).

► Concept and Application
Loss of uterine support, paravaginal tissue support, bladder wall and urethrovesicle angle support, and support overlying the distal rectum, associated with aging and multiple childbirth.

► Treatment Steps
1. Order of treatment depends on severity and etiology of prolapse and/or urinary incontinence.
2. Bladder training, biofeedback, anticholinergic drugs, β-sympathomimetic agonists, antidepressants, estrogen replacement therapy, Kegel exercises, pessaries, surgery: colporrhaphy, obliteration of the rectovaginal space (Moschowitz procedure), vaginal hysterectomy.

V. MENSTRUAL DISORDERS

A. Dysmenorrhea

► H&P Keys
Pelvic pain with menses with variable onset of pain compared to day 1 of flow; nausea, diarrhea, headache, ovulatory menstrual cycles.

► **Diagnosis**

Ovulatory menses, menstrual pain history.

► **Disease Severity**

Severity of symptoms, from mild to incapacitating.

► **Concept and Application**

Result of uterine contractions, caused by prostaglandins.

> *Primary Dysmenorrhea*—No associated pelvic pathology.

> *Secondary Dysmenorrhea*—Associated with pelvic pathology: endometriosis, fibroids, etc.

► **Treatment Steps**

Primary Dysmenorrhea
1. NSAIDs to inhibit prostaglandin synthetase and thereby decrease smooth-muscle contractility.
2. Combination oral contraceptives to inhibit ovulation.
3. GnRH agonists in severe cases if suspicion of endemetriosis is present.
4. If no relief, laparoscopy may be needed to rule out pelvic pathology (e.g., secondary dysmenorrhea).

B. Premenstrual Syndrome (PMS)

► **H&P Keys**

Anxiety, breast tenderness, crying spells, depression, fatigue, irritability, weight gain around the luteal phase of the cycle; prior to the onset of menses, usually relieved with the onset of bleeding.

► **Diagnosis**

Basal body temperature charts; symptom-recording diaries; daily weight recordings.

► **Disease Severity**

Severity of symptoms and impact of symptoms on daily life. Premenstrual dysphoric disorder (PMDD).

► **Concept and Application**

Unknown, but progesterone deficiency is one of the more popular theories.

► **Treatment Steps**

There are no studies in evidence-based medicine with respect to any specific treatment to be effective. Treatments include exercise, vitamin B_6, progesterone, diuretics, oral contraceptives. Treatment of PMDD with antidepressants in the luteal phase.

C. Disorders of Menstruation

1. Amenorrhea

► **H&P Keys**

Primary amenorrhea is defined as no menses by age 16. *Secondary* is 3 months or longer of amenorrhea in a normally cycling individual. Possible sexual ambiguity or virilization; possible absence of secondary sex characteristics.

► **Diagnosis**

History and physical examination, β-hCG, prolactin, follicle-stimulating hormone (FSH), luteinizing hormone (LH), progesterone with-

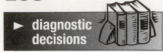

► diagnostic
decisions

SECONDARY AMENORRHEA

Pregnancy
Most common etiology of secondary amenorrhea in reproductive age women. Look for sexual activity with partner—unprotected intercourse. Usually 1–2 weeks beyond expected date of menses. Check pregnancy test.

Menopause
Most common etiology of secondary amenorrhea in older women. Average age of menopause is 51.4 years in the United States. Look for a history of hot flashes; vaginal dryness; abnormal menstrual bleeding patterns, followed by amenorrhea. If this occurs before age 40, it is called premature ovarian failure. Check FSH levels and estradiol levels.

Hypothalamic Amenorrhea
History of exercise; eating disorder (usually anorexia); decreased body fat; high-stress lifestyle; heroin or opiate usage. Measure patient's height, weight, and body mass index (BMI); check bone density for osteoporosis. Obtain good dietary history.

Polycystic Ovarian Disease (PCOD)
History of obesity, hirsutism, and infertility. Usually familial as well; look for height, weight; ↑ BMI; hirsutism on face, chest, abdomen, male escutcheon; bilateral ovarian cystic enlargement; obtain LH, FSH, and check if positive withdrawal bleed to progestins.

---

drawal test. If virilization, testosterone, dehydroepiandrosterone sulfate (DHEAS). *Primary:* karyotype, FSH, estradiol.

► **Disease Severity**

Presence or absence of secondary sex characteristics; no breast development by age 14.

► **Concept and Application**

Primary—Müllerian agenesis, testicular feminization (androgen insensitivity), Turner's syndrome.

Secondary—Pregnancy, Asherman's syndrome (intrauterine synechiae), polycystic ovarian disease, congenital adrenal hyperplasia, hyperandrogenism, hypothyroidism, hyperprolactinemia.

Hypothalamic—Associated with weight loss, chronic anxiety, excessive exercise, eating disorder (anorexia nervosa), marijuana, tranquilizers, head injury, chronic medical illness, central nervous system (CNS) tumor, IV drug use (opium derivatives).

Note—In the absence of all the above, diagnosis is dysfunctional uterine bleeding.

► **Treatment Steps**

1. *Primary:* Obtain karyotype if < 30 years old. If abnormal karyotype, phenotypic female: estrogen replacement therapy for completion of secondary sex characteristics. Müllerian agenesis requires surgery.
2. *Secondary:* Requires cyclic menstrual function to prevent endometrial hyperplasia: cyclic combination oral contraceptive therapy or monthly progestin therapy.
3. *Hypothalamic:* Hormone replacement therapy to prevent osteoporosis and maintain normal physiologic status.
4. *Asherman's syndrome:* Amenorrhea not responsive to estrogen–progesterone cycle; hysteroscopic surgical intervention.

VI. MENOPAUSE

► **H&P Keys**

Changes in menstrual cycle regularity, decreased cycle interval, finally cessation of menses; mean age 51.4 years; atrophy of estrogen-dependent tissue (uterus, breasts, vagina), vasomotor symptoms (hot flashes), osteoporosis, urethral changes, increased frequency of cystitis, insomnia.

► **Diagnosis**

FSH; estradiol. Menopause prior to age 40 means premature ovarian failure; if menopause prior to age 30, check karyotype.

► **Disease Severity**

1. Skin collagen content decreases.
2. Worsening serum lipid profile.
3. Vaginal dryness with atrophy.
4. Breast atrophy.
5. Osteopenia leading to osteoporosis and possibly stress fractures.
6. Atherosclerotic coronary vessel disease.
7. Senility, Alzheimer's disease.

► Concept and Application

Sequelae of decreased estrogen result of loss of all remaining follicles. Estrone is principle estrogen in menopause, produced from androgen precursor androstenedione.

► Treatment Steps

1. Diet, exercise, lifestyle changes.
2. Herbal and natural treatments.
3. Hormone therapy if symptoms interfering with life.
4. For bone protection, increase calcium intake to 1,500 mg/day. Bisphosphonates may be helpful as well as selective estrogen receptor modulators (SERMs).
5. Increase exercise.
6. Decrease fat intake.
7. Treatment of individual symptoms associated with menopause.

VII. BREAST

A. Malignant Neoplasm

► H&P Keys

Family history (5–10% of breast cancers show genetic component), long history of estrogen exposure, nulliparity, high fat intake; discrete lump, retracted nipple, puckering of breast skin (peau d'orange), axillary lymphadenopathy, nipple bleeding or discharge (Table 11–1).

► Diagnosis

Mammography, physical examination, biopsy.

11-1

RISK FACTORS FOR BREAST CANCER

Factor	Relative Risk
Family history of breast cancer	
First-degree relative (sister or mother)	1.2–3.0
Menstrual history	
Menarche < 12 years of age	1.3
< 40 menstrual years	1.5–2.0
Oral contraceptive use	No effect
Estrogen replacement < 10 years	No effect
Pregnancy	
First delivery > 35 years of age	2.0–3.0
Nulliparous	3.0
Other neoplasms	
Contralateral breast cancer	5.0
Carcinoma of uterus or ovary	2.0
Carcinoma of major salivary gland	4.0
Other conditions	
Atypical hyperplasia	4.0–6.0
Previous biopsy	1.9–2.1
North American (white or black)	5.0
Age 60 vs. age 40 years	2.0
Moderate alcohol use	1.5–2.0
Radiation exposure (> 90 rads)	4.0
Obesity	Suggested but unknown
Large-bowel cancer	Suggested but unknown
Increased dietary fat	Suggested but unknown

Reproduced, with permission, from Gant NF, Cunningham FG. *Basic Gynecology and Obstetrics.* Norwalk, CT: Appleton & Lange, 1993.

► **Disease Severity**

Stated by T (tumor size), N (regional lymph nodes), and M (distant metastases). Evaluations done for hormone receptors reflect tumor responsiveness to chemotherapy.

► **Concept and Application**

Unknown, possibly related to hormones or high-fat diet; surgical menopause appears to be protective; complex combination of environmental and genetic influences.

Tumor is analyzed for the presence of estrogen receptors and/or progesterone receptors.

► **Treatment Steps**

Surgery
1. Mammography.
2. Biopsy.
3. Lumpectomy.
4. Simple mastectomy (if necessary).
5. Radical mastectomy (if necessary).

Hormonal Therapy—If positive hormone receptors, progestins.

B. Fibroadenoma

Benign breast neoplasm.

► **H&P Keys**

Younger women, ages 20–35; single breast mass, smooth, well-circumscribed, firm, mobile, and rubbery nodule.

► **Diagnosis**

Mammography, sonography.

► **Disease Severity**

Severity of symptoms.

► **Concept and Application**

Unknown.

► **Treatment Steps**
1. Fine-needle aspiration to make diagnosis.
2. Subsequent observation.
3. Possible lumpectomy needed.

C. Intraductal Papilloma

Benign breast lesion.

► **H&P Keys**

Unilateral bloody or serous nipple discharge, no palpable mass.

► **Diagnosis**

History, exam, mammogram, and duct evaluation.

► **Disease Severity**

Amount of nipple discharge.

► **Concept and Application**

Unknown.

► **Treatment Steps**

Local excision of lesion and duct.

D. Fibrocystic Disease

► H&P Keys

Cyclic bilateral pain (mastalgia) and breast engorgement, may radiate to shoulders or upper arms, diffuse bilateral nodularity, "lumpy-bumpy" pattern.

► Diagnosis

History, examination, mammography, ultrasound.

► Disease Severity

According to symptoms.

► Concept and Application

May be hormone related as symptoms are frequently cyclic.

► Treatment Steps

Regular breast exams.

1. Diet therapy.
2. Avoidance of caffeine and tobacco.
3. Occasionally, medical therapy is helpful, e.g., progestins.
4. Medication treatments.

VIII. OTHER PROBLEMS

A. Infertility, Male and Female

► H&P Keys

Primary Infertility—Never having conceived, despite 12 months of unprotected intercourse.

Secondary Infertility—Previous history of conception but currently unable to establish a subsequent pregnancy despite 12 months of unprotected intercourse.

► Diagnosis

Complete history and physical on both partners, semen analysis, postcoital test, hysterosalpingogram, progesterone level (midluteal phase), endometrial biopsy (Fig. 11–3).

► Disease Severity

Directly proportional to the duration of the infertility; worse prognosis with longer duration of infertility.

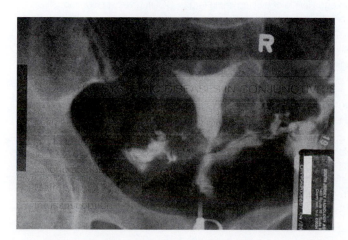

Figure 11–3. A normal hysterosalpingogram is shown in this photograph. The uterus takes on a classic "goblet" shape, and both tubes are patent. There is free dye throughout the peritoneal cavity.

► **Concept and Application**

Forty-five percent male factor, 45% female factor; 10% unexplained. One-sixth of all U.S. couples are infertile.

Male Factor—Most commonly associated with varicocele (etiology of infertility uncertain). Other factors include infection, trauma, impotence, antisperm antibodies, etc.

Female Factor—Blocked tubes, ovulatory dysfunction, peritoneal factor (pelvic adhesive disease, endometriosis, etc.).

► **Treatment Steps**

Ovulatory Dysfunction—Ovulation-induction agents.

Tubal Factor
1. Surgery.
2. Assisted reproductive technology (ART):
   • In vitro fertilization (IVF).
   • Gamete intrafallopian transfer (GIFT).

Cervical Mucus Factor—Intrauterine insemination, bicarbonate douching.

Peritoneal Factor
1. Laparoscopy confirms diagnosis.
2. If endometriosis, ablation of peritoneal implants, lysis of adhesions, restoration of normal pelvic anatomy with or without GnRH agonist.
3. If pelvic adhesions, as above with or without antibiotic postop therapy.

► **management decisions**

INFERTILITY

Ovulatory Dysfunction
One-third of all infertility etiologies. Determine cause of oligo/anovulation. If abnormal thyroid function, replace thyroid hormone, then await resumption of menses. If elevated prolactin levels, determine etiology—use bromocriptine (dopamine agonist) to decrease prolactin, then await resumption of menses. If elevated androgen levels of adrenal origin, give glucocorticoid to inhibit adrenals, then add ovulation induction agent (e.g., clomiphene, human menopausal gonadotropins). If elevated androgen levels of ovarian origin (e.g., PCOD), give ovulation induction agents. If hypothalamic amenorrhea, remove etiologic agent if possible (e.g., dietary correction, ceasing drug usage, decreasing severe exercise, etc.).

Tubal Obstruction
One-third of all infertility etiologies. Associated with poor prognosis if long-standing. Also risk of ectopic pregnancies. Surgery is first-line treatment; attempt to open tube(s) via laparoscopy/hysteroscopy or laparotomy. Overall success rate is 10%. ART if surgery not possible. IVF provides up to 20–25% success rate/cycle. Involves ovulation induction with potent injectable gonadotropins, oocyte retrieval, and embryo transfer.

Male Factor
Third main cause of overall infertility. Semen analysis shows most abnormalities, although sperm antibody testing and postcoital testing very important. If low count, or antisperm antibody positive, then intrauterine insemination is suggested (with/without ovulatory induction drugs). If unsuccessful, ART with intracytoplasmic sperm injection. Finally, donor semen is used in the most severe cases.

Male Factor—Intrauterine insemination, ART, intracytoplasmic sperm injection, donor sperm.

B. Pelvic Inflammatory Disease (PID)

▶ H&P Keys

Pain, abdominal/adnexal tenderness, fever, dysuria, vaginal discharge, adnexal masses, peritoneal signs, cervical motion tenderness.

▶ Diagnosis

Physical exam, ultrasound, elevated WBC count, elevated sedimentation rate, cervical cultures, laparoscopy.

▶ Disease Severity

Depends on extent of signs and symptoms, multiple episodes of PID may result in infertility, chronic pelvic pain, increased ectopic pregnancy rate. Tubo-ovarian abscess (TOA).

▶ Concept and Application

Infection of the upper genital tract, usually polymicrobial consisting of *C. trachomatis*, *N. gonorrhoeae*, endogenous aerobes (*Escherichia coli*, *Proteus*, etc.), and endogenous anaerobes (*Bacteroides*, *Peptostreptococcus*), *Mycoplasma hominis*. *Chlamydia* is most common pathogen associated with PID.

▶ Treatment Steps

Outpatient

1. Ofloxacin (levofloxacin) for 14 days with or without metronidazole.
2. One dose of ceftriaxone, 250 mg, and doxycycline for 14 days with or without metronidazole.
3. Recheck patient in 2–3 days for possible need to admit.

Inpatient

1. IV antibiotics. Doxycycline plus intravenous cefoxitin, or clindamycin plus gentamicin.
2. Pelvic ultrasound. If TOA present and unresponsive, then drainage.
5. In severe cases, patient may require surgery with total abdominal hysterectomy and bilateral salpingo-oophorectomy.

IX. HEALTH MAINTENANCE

A. Gynecologic Examination and Screening

▶ H&P Keys

History—Age at menarche, cycle length, duration of flow; vaginal discharge; pelvic pain; sexual history; history of abnormal cervical cytology; obstetrical history (gravidity and parity), contraception usage.

Review of Systems—Gastrointestinal, urinary, endocrine, metabolic, cardiovascular, hematologic.

Physical Examination—Vital signs, breast exam (sitting and supine), thyroid exam, axillary lymph nodes, abdomen, hair distribution.

Pelvic Examination—External genitalia, speculum examination.

Bimanual Examination—Cervix, uterus, adnexa.

Rectal Examination—Rectovaginal exam, guaiac test.

▶ **diagnostic decisions**

CHRONIC PELVIC PAIN

Endometriosis
Chronic pelvic pain of more than 6 months' duration; family history positive (mother, sister, daughter, etc.); dysmenorrhea several days to a week *before* onset of menses; premenstrual spotting or staining; dyspareunia (deep thrusting); afebrile, pain usually diffuse, bilateral; uterine retroversion, decreased mobility; abnormal vaginal discharge usually absent; rectovaginal nodularity; uterosacral implants; bilateral adnexal tenderness, normal WBC; check ultrasound for ovarian cysts.

Chronic PID
Chronic pelvic pain of more than 6 months' duration; STD etiology; history of more than one chlamydial infection; fever, chills; mucopurulent cervical thick copious discharge; cervical motion tenderness; bilateral adnexal tenderness; peritoneal signs; elevated WBCs, elevated sed rate; check ultrasound for tubo-ovarian abscesses.

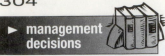

► **management decisions**

FAMILY PLANNING

Teenage Girl
The most important two issues here are to prevent pregnancy *and* to prevent transmission of STDs, especially in light of multiple partners. Condoms plus hormonal contraception would provide this coverage. Hormonal contraception consists of either oral contraceptives or long-acting injectable progestins (e.g., Depo-Provera), contraceptive patch, or vaginal ring.

Woman in Long-Term Monogamous Relationship
Completed childbearing: Laparoscopic tubal sterilization or vasectomy is most highly recommended if permanent contraception desired. Otherwise, long-acting progestins, or IUD.
Not completed childbearing: Long-acting progestins, or oral contraceptives, or IUD.

Woman over 35, Smoker, in Monogamous Relationship
Condoms or long-acting injectable progestins, or IUD.

Perimenopausal Woman
Ultra-low-dose oral contraception assuming no contraindications to estrogen; long-acting progestins; tubal sterilization if permanent contraception desired.

► **Diagnosis**
Pap smear, lipid profile, STD screening, mammogram, colonoscopy, bone density at appropriate ages.

Note—General gynecologic exam should be done annually along with counseling about tobacco, alcohol, caffeine, exercise, and diet.

B. General Counseling for Contraception

Types—Natural family planning; spermicides and barrier contraceptives (spermicide, condoms, diaphragms, sponges, cervical caps); intrauterine devices (IUDs) (Progesta-Sert, Paraguard); steroid contraceptives: contraceptive patch, vaginal ring, combination oral contraceptive, progestin-only contraceptives; injectable and implantable contraceptives (medroxyprogesterone acetate); postcoital contraception (emergency contraception), oral abortifacients (RU-486, methotrexate and misoprostol).

Effectiveness (Given as Failure Rate)—Oral contraceptives, < 1–2%; IUD, 2–4%; diaphragm with spermicide, 10–20%; condom, 5–15%.

Surveillance of Prescribed Contraceptives—Oral contraceptives: regular breast, thyroid, liver, and pelvic examinations, initial blood pressure check; IUD: string check 6 weeks after insertion.

C. Sterilization
Most frequent method of controlling fertility in the United States.

Male Sterilization—Vasectomy failure rate 1%.

Female Sterilization—Postpartum failure rate 1 in 250; interval (between pregnancies) failure rate 1 in 500.

Counseling must include permanent nature of procedure, operative risk, failure rate. Despite careful counseling, approximately 1% of patients undergoing sterilization subsequently request reversal. Most common reason: new sexual partner.

BIBLIOGRAPHY

Beckman CRB, Ling FW, et al. *Obstetrics and Gynecology,* 4th ed. Baltimore: Lippincott Williams & Wilkins, 2002.

DeCherney AH, Pernoll ML. *Current Obstetric and Gynecologic Diagnosis and Treatment.* Norwalk, CT: Appleton & Lange, 2002.

Gant NF, Cunningham FG. *Basic Gynecology and Obstetrics.* Norwalk, CT: Appleton & Lange, 1993.

Obstetrics | 12

I. UNCOMPLICATED PREGNANCY

A. Health and Health Maintenance

1. Prenatal Care

▶ **H&P Keys**

Accurate dating! Presumptive signs of pregnancy: amenorrhea with nausea and breast tenderness and bluish vaginal mucosa. Probable: positive pregnancy test (β-human chorionic gonadotropin [β-hCG]), uterine change, and outlining of fetus. Diagnostic: fetal imaging (ultrasonography, etc.), auscultation of the fetal heart.

▶ **Diagnosis**

Prenatal evaluation. Complete blood count (CBC), urinalysis (UA), urine culture and sensitivity (C&S), blood type and Rh factor, antibody screen, hepatitis B surface antigen, rubella titer, syphilis serology, Pap smear, gonorrhea and chlamydia cultures at first visit. Maternal serum α-fetoprotein (MSAFP) at 15–18 weeks and 50-g glucose screening at 24–28 weeks. All Rh-negative women need Rh immune globulin (Rh Ig) at 26–28 weeks (as well as at time of invasive procedures, trauma, or vaginal bleeding). Dose of 300 μg of Rh Ig neutralizes 15 cc Rh-positive red blood cells (RBCs). Must give within 72 hours of exposure. Also consider human immunodeficiency virus (HIV), hemoglobin electrophoresis screening for group B strep at approximately 36 weeks.

▶ **Disease Severity**

Surveillance for complications: preeclampsia, low birth weight, malnutrition, pre- and postterm delivery, anemia, common infections, gestational diabetes, abnormal lab tests.

▶ **Concept and Application**

Prevention and early treatment of pregnancy complications.

▶ **Treatment Steps**

Initial Care—Accurate dating and diagnosis, education.

Emergency Care—Refer to specific problems.

Continued Care—Routine education, surveillance, and maintenance.

B. Prenatal Diagnosis

▶ **H&P Keys**

Exposure to medications or teratogens (i.e., alcohol, radiation, tetracycline, antiepileptics, folic acid antagonists, warfarin, mercury, syphilis, rubella, toxoplasmosis), pedigree, accurate pregnancy dating, exam looking for expression of genotype.

▶ **Diagnosis**

Specific for condition evaluated: biochemical screening tests: MSAFP, unconjugated estriol, and β-hCG and inhibin A. Abnormal patterns are associated with neural tube defects and aneuploidy (trisomies 18 and 21). Ultrasound screening: major structural anomalies, thickened nuchal fold, growth lag, and abnormal amniotic fluid volume.

▶ **Disease Severity**

Specific for condition evaluated.

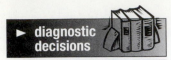
▶ diagnostic decisions

PRENATAL DIAGNOSIS

Chorionic Villus Sampling
Provides direct DNA analysis of fetus by sampling chorionic tissue. Evaluation can be done between 10 and 14 weeks.

Amniocentesis
Provides direct DNA analysis of fetus by sampling the somatic cells of the fetus. Evaluation is done after 15–16 weeks.

Biochemical Screen
Provides indirect biochemical analysis of AFP, estriol, and β-hCG as markers for fetal abnormalities, specifically open neural tube defects and chromosomal abnormalities. Evaluation is done between 15 and 18 weeks.

Ultrasound
Provides a visual image of the fetus at any gestational age.

▶ **Concept and Application**

Hundreds of biochemical, chromosomal, and genetic disorders can be diagnosed by condition-specific tests including ultrasonography, identified structural change, karotyping, DNA analysis technologies, fetal tissue enzyme activity, and metabolic product accumulation in fetal cells obtained by chorionic villus sampling (CVS), amniocentesis, percutaneous umbilical blood sampling, or fetal biopsy. Major congenital anomalies occur in 3% of all pregnancies.

▶ **Treatment Steps**
1. Specific for the condition evaluated.
2. Nondirective counseling is used.

C. Postpartum Care of the Mother

▶ **H&P Keys**

Childbirth in the preceding 6 weeks. Lochia changes from red to brown to serous over first 2 weeks. Episiotomy heals rapidly. Uterus is in pelvis at 2 weeks and normal size at 6 weeks. If mother is Rh negative, baby needs to be tested; if baby is Rh positive, Rh Ig must be given.

▶ **Diagnosis**

Pap smear at postpartum visit if no recent Pap smear.

▶ **Disease Severity**

Infection: endomyometritis (mixed aerobic and anaerobic flora), mastitis (*Staphylococcus aureus*), breast abscess. Depression: > 50% will have a week of "the blues," 10% will be depressed, and 0.05% suicidal.

▶ **Concept and Application**

Fifty percent of nonlactating women ovulate between 28 and 90 days postpartum. Cardiac output normalizes in several hours. Glomerular filtration rate (GFR) is down to normal in a few weeks.

▶ **Treatment Steps**

Initial Care
1. Evaluation, support, and problem-specific therapy.
2. Rh Ig if indicated.

Emergency Care—Problem specific.

D. Lactation

▶ **H&P Keys**

Absence of pain, erythema, localized induration, abscess, nipple fissures or cracks. Prefeeding engorgement and discomfort is common in the first few weeks. Limit medications to those necessary and not contraindicated.

▶ **Diagnosis**

None.

▶ **Disease Severity**

Same as history and physical examination.

▶ **Concept and Application**

Human breast milk is the best nutrition and immunologic stimulation for the baby. Prolactin is essential. Suckling stimulates the neurohypophysis to release oxytocin, which contracts the breast's myoepithelial cells, allowing milk "letdown." Less than 1% of most medications is found in breast milk. Nipple fissures and cracks allow ingress of bacteria, causing cellulitis to abscess.

► **Treatment Steps**

Initial Care—Encourage relaxation and hydration to facilitate breast-feeding.

Emergency Care
1. Treat mastitis with antibiotics effective against *S. aureus*, and continue breast-feeding.
2. Abscess may require surgical drainage.

E. Normal Labor and Delivery

► **H&P Keys**

Progressive uterine contractions associated with cervical change; progressively intense, about every 3 minutes and lasting 60 seconds.

► **Diagnosis**

Normal latent phase lasts a maximum of 20 hours in the nulligravida and 14 hours in the multipara. Normal active phase dilatation is at least 1.2 cm/hr in the nulligravida and 1.5 cm/hr in the multipara (Fig. 12–1).

Reassuring fetal heart tracing, normal rate between 120 and 160 beats per minute with adaquate variability and tolerance of the stress of the contractions. Reactive tracing with two accelerations in fetal heart rate in 20 minutes suggests fetal well-being in absence of stress of contractions.

► **Disease Severity**

Failure of acceptable progress.

► **Concept and Application**

Increased prostaglandins cause an increased number of myometrial gap junctions that allow cells to communicate and rhythmically depolarize in labor.

COMPLICATIONS OF LACTATION

Breast Engorgement
Diffuse distention, firmness and nodularity of the breast secondary to normal edema, and lymphatic engorgement as a result of the milk coming in. It is sometimes associated with tenderness and a transient fever. Treatment depends on whether the mother is breast- or bottle-feeding.

Galactocele
Blocked milk duct with collection of milk behind it. It is an isolated lump which may be mildly tender. Treatment includes warm compresses, massage, and breast-feeding.

Mastitis
Infection in the breast that presents with pain, erythema, fever, malaise. It usually presents in one segment of the breast. *S. aureus* is the most common organism. Treatment includes antibiotics along with hot compresses and continuation of breast-feeding.

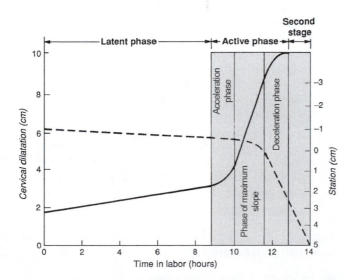

Figure 12–1. Stages of labor. (Reproduced, with permission, from Cohen W, Friedman EA, eds. *Management of Labor,* 2nd ed. University Park Press, 1988.)

► Treatment Steps

Initial Care—Make diagnosis by serial examinations and initiate management.

Continued Care
1. When cephalopelvic disproportion is diagnosed, cesarean section is used for delivery.
2. Hypotonic dysfunction is treated with oxytocin augmentation.

II. COMPLICATED PREGNANCY

A. Adolescent Pregnancy

► H&P Keys

Nineteen years old and younger, sexually transmitted disease (STD) surveillance, nutritional deficiency, substance abuse, sexual abuse.

► Diagnosis

Same for pregnancy; assist with social support network.

► Disease Severity

Disease specific.

► Concept and Application

Seventeen percent have *Chlamydia trachomatis,* and 3% *Neisseria gonorrhoeae* per year; increased need for calcium (1,600 mg/day) and calories (2,700 cal/day); 89% of 10th graders have alcohol exposure, and 8% have cocaine; up to 38% have had nonvoluntary sexual activity.

► Management

Routine prenatal care with a special emphasis in support services and screening and intervention for problems.

B. Ectopic Pregnancy

► H&P Keys

Early pregnancy symptoms and signs; amenorrhea; abnormal vaginal bleeding; and abdominal pain, colicky and lateralizing to the affected side. Shoulder pain, rectal pain, syncope, and peritoneal signs are associated with intraperitoneal bleeding. Passage of the decidual cast is confused with spontaneous abortion (SAB).

► Diagnosis

Quantitative β-hCG rising < 66% every 48 hours, serum progesterone < 5 ng/mL, and inability to identify an intrauterine pregnancy by transabdominal ultrasonography when the β-hCG is > 5,000 mIU/mL or by transvaginal ultrasonography if the β-hCG is > 2,000. Culdocentesis to identify hemoperitoneum if ultrasonography is not available. Blood type and Rh.

► Disease Severity

Transvaginal sonography and serial measurement of the β-hCG diagnose many unruptured ectopics.

► Concept and Application

Ectopic pregnancy is implantation outside of the uterine cavity; 78% are ampullary. Incidence of ectopic pregnancy has increased to 1 in

66 pregnancies. Risk factors include salpingitis, tubal surgery (including prior ectopic pregnancy), infertility treatments, and advanced age. Rh Ig if Rh negative.

► Treatment Steps

Initial Care
1. **Early diagnosis is key.**
2. Protocols are available for the nonsurgical management (methotrexate) of the small, unruptured ectopic pregnancy.
3. More commonly, conservative laparoscopic surgery, removing only the products of conception through a slit in the tube (slit salpingostomy), or removal of a limited portion of the tube is performed—partial salpingectomy (segmental resection).

Emergency Care—Salpingectomy for hemoperitoneum with a large ruptured ectopic pregnancy.

C. Spontaneous Abortion (SAB)

► H&P Keys

Spontaneous fetus loss at or before 20 weeks from first day of last menstrual period or 500 g. Vaginal bleeding, rupture of membranes, cervical dilatation, passage of tissue.

► Diagnosis

β-hCG, transabdominal and transvaginal ultrasonography, progesterone, blood type, and Rh factor.

► Disease Severity

Threatened Abortion—Bleeding in the first 20 weeks of an intrauterine pregnancy. This occurs in 20–25% of women, and approximately half of these go on to abort the pregnancy.

Inevitable Abortion—Cervix is dilated or membranes are ruptured.

Incomplete Abortion—Some tissue is retained.

Complete Abortion—All tissue is passed.

Missed Abortion—Retention of nonviable pregnancy in the uterus for 4–8 weeks after the demise.

► Concept and Application

Fifty to seventy-five percent of conceptions end in spontaneous abortion. Most of these are unrecognized. Fifteen to twenty percent of recognized pregnancies are lost in the first and early second trimester. At least 50% of SABs are caused by genetic factors, including nondisjunction and translocation. Endocrine problems, principally luteal-phase deficiency, are present in 25%. Second-trimester losses are more often related to maternal diseases and uterine structural anomalies.

► Treatment Steps

Initial Care
1. Threatened abortion is usually managed by observation and prevention of the introduction of infection. There is no evidence to support that bed rest will prevent early SAB.
2. Incomplete abortion is treated by uterine evacuation.
3. Rh Ig for the Rh-negative woman.

Emergency Care—Same as initial care.

► **management decisions**

TREATMENTS FOR ECTOPIC PREGNANCY

Methotrexate
Medical treatment for ectopic pregnancy that meets specific criteria. The treatment is given intramuscularly and under strict supervision.

Salpingectomy
Surgical treatment in which the fallopian tube is removed.

Salpingostomy
Removal of the ectopic pregnancy from the tube by making an incision in the antimesenteric side of the fallopian tube. After the tissue is removed, the incision in the tube is left open.

Salpingotomy
Removal of the ectopic pregnancy as above except the incision in the fallopian tube is then sutured closed.

Continued Care
1. Emotional support for the patient and family.
2. Prepregnancy evaluation if recurrent (three or more).

D. Induced Abortion

▶ H&P Keys

Termination of an otherwise viable pregnancy for medical or personal reasons. A legal termination is consistent with statutory authority. An illegal or criminal one is not.

▶ Diagnosis

Same as initial pregnancy evaluation.

▶ Disease Severity

Advanced gestational age.

▶ Concept and Application

Compliance with the patient's wishes. Procedures are safest when performed in the first trimester. They can be done either surgically or medically using a combination of methotrexate followed by prostaglandins.

▶ Treatment Steps

Initial—Same as routine early pregnancy care, Rh Ig.

Emergency Care
1. Patients having a criminal abortion are at increased risk for serious complications including sepsis, abscess, and structural damage.
2. Intravenous hydration, broad-spectrum antibiotics, expeditious uterine evacuation, and evaluation for associated injury are indicated.

E. Septic Abortion

▶ H&P Keys

Same as SAB, except for symptoms of infection, fever, foul-smelling discharge, and pain. Possible history of illegal abortion.

▶ Diagnosis

Same as SAB except for associated infection, septic shock, renal failure.

▶ Disease Severity

Same as SAB except for associated infection, septic shock, renal failure. Can be lethal.

▶ Concept and Application

Same as SAB except for increased risk of perforation and associated organ injury at dilatation and evacuation.

▶ Treatment Steps

Same as SAB, plus inspection of injury and administration of broad-spectrum antibiotics prior to or during procedure pending culture results.

F. Placenta Previa

▶ H&P Keys

Frequent incidental ultrasonographic finding in early pregnancy. Patients present with painless vaginal bleeding in the third trimester.

Most first bleedings are limited as long as digital examination does not occur.

► Diagnosis

Transabdominal and transvaginal ultrasonography is used in most cases (Fig. 12–2).

► Disease Severity

Degree of placenta previa present and the amount of bleeding.

► Concept and Application

Implantation of the placenta in the lower uterine segment covering the entire cervix (complete or central), partially covering the internal os (partial), or encroaching on the internal os (marginal). It is related to poor uterine vascularization (high multiparity, cesarean section) or large placental mass (multiple gestation or hydrops). Poor mechanical hemostasis causes heavy intra- and postpartum bleeding. Five percent of second-trimester pregnancies are found to have a placenta previa; 90% of these resolve by term. A patient with a previous cesarean section and placenta previa has a 25% risk of placenta accreta.

► Treatment Steps

Initial Care

1. Asymptomatic patient education, and coital restriction in the third trimester.
2. Serial ultrasonograms for fetal growth and placental location.

Emergency Care—A patient who has bleeding is hospitalized for hemodynamic stabilization and fetal assessment.

Continued Care

1. Delivery is usually by cesarean section after 36 weeks with documented fetal maturity or uncorrectable fetal compromise.
2. Patients with marginal placenta previa may attempt a vaginal delivery.

G. Abruptio Placentae

► H&P Keys

Painful contractions, tender uterus, fundus remains firm between contractions, and vaginal bleeding. Fetal monitoring may be nonreassuring.

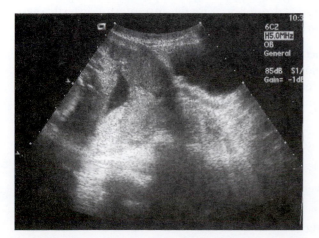

Figure 12–2. Placenta previa.

▶ Diagnosis

Clinical diagnosis, CBC, platelet count, fibrin split products, fibrinogen and prothrombin time (PT) and partial thromboplastin time (PTT) for disseminated intravascular coagulation (DIC). Ultrasonography is of limited value.

▶ Disease Severity

Shock out of proportion to the observed blood loss, especially if concealed hemorrhage. Fetal demise possible if > 50% abruption.

▶ Concept and Application

Bleeding into the decidua basalis. Couvelaire uterus is caused by blood extravasating into the myometrium (ecchymosis). Abruptio may be caused by hypertension, cocaine, smoking, uterine decompression, and trauma.

▶ Treatment Steps

Initial and Emergency Care
1. Hemodynamic stabilization, observation for complications, and delivery of the mature fetus.
2. Vaginal delivery is attempted if the patient is stable hemodynamically and the fetal monitoring is reassuring.
3. Immature fetus may be expectantly managed in mild abruptions.

H. Preeclampsia

▶ H&P Keys

Hypertension (140/90 mm Hg) and proteinuria (> 300 mg/24 hours) and edema after 20 weeks. Signs and symptoms of HELLP syndrome (**H**emolysis, **E**levated **L**iver functions, **L**ow **P**latelets).

▶ Diagnosis

Careful blood pressure (BP) measurement, 24-hour urine for protein and creatinine clearance, CBC with platelets, and uric acid. Aspartate aminotransferase (AST, formerly SGOT), bilirubin, and lactic dehydrogenase (LDH) may be elevated. Fetal growth and well-being assessment.

▶ Disease Severity

Mild preeclampsia is without symptoms and signs of severe preeclampsia. Severe preeclampsia if BP > 160/110 mm Hg, > 5 g of proteinuria in 24 hours, visual disturbances, headache, pulmonary edema, cyanosis, epigastric pain, right upper quadrant pain, liver dysfunction, oliguria, thrombocytopenia, intrauterine growth retardation (IUGR), or oligohydramnios.

▶ Concept and Application

Diffuse multiorgan vasospastic disease starting months before diagnosis, characterized by decreased sensitivity to angiotensin II and increased thromboxane-to-prostacyclin ratio. Delivery is the only specific therapy.

▶ Treatment Steps

Initial Care—Gestational age, fetal and maternal assessment.

Term—Delivery.

Preterm
1. Weighing the risks and benefits of expectant management for the baby and the mother.

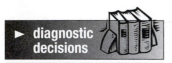

▶ **diagnostic decisions**

THIRD TRIMESTER BLEEDING

Placenta Previa
Look for painless bleeding with the placenta located low in the uterus in the area of the cervix.

Placental Abruption
Look for bleeding associated with pain and contractions. Look carefully for fetal compromise.

Bloody Show
Painless bleeding often mixed with mucus. Bleeding is usually minimal and is often accompanied by early labor.

2. Bed rest is the mainstay of expectant care.
3. Steroids should be given if preterm delivery is deemed likely.

Emergency Care
1. Magnesium sulfate (4- to 6-g load and 2 g/hr) is used for seizure prophylaxis.
2. Monitoring BP, respiration, reflexes, and urinary output.
3. Diastolic BPs over 110 mm Hg are treated with antihypertensive medications such as hydralazine (5-mg boluses).

I. Eclampsia

▶ H&P Keys

Preeclampsia with tonic–clonic seizures of no other etiology.

▶ Diagnosis

Same as preeclampsia.

▶ Disease Severity

Same as preeclampsia.

▶ Concept and Application

Same as preeclampsia.

▶ Treatment Steps

Initial and Emergency Care
1. Same as preeclampsia.
2. Treatment of seizures with magnesium sulfate.
3. Delivery when mother is stable.

J. Premature Labor

▶ H&P Keys

Uterine contractions with cervical change prior to 37 weeks. Symptoms: cramps, backache, pressure, and uterine contractions.

▶ Diagnosis

Monitor for contractions, rule out rupture of membranes, check for cervical change, culture vagina for group B streptococcus, evaluate for urinary tract infection or other processes that might be causing the contractions, confirm dating if indicated.

▶ Disease Severity

No tocolysis if rupture of membranes, advanced cervical dilatation (5+ cm), fetal distress, fetal anomalies, mature fetus, in utero infection, and conditions made worse by tocolysis.

▶ Concept and Application

Preterm labor associated with premature rupture of membranes (PROM), incompetent cervix, infection, uterine overdistention, abnormal placentation, dehydration, and idiopathic causes. Prostaglandin activation is a common final pathway. β-Sympathomimetics (ritodrine and terbutaline), magnesium sulfate, prostaglandin synthetase inhibitors (indomethacin), and calcium channel blockers (nifedipine) have been used to treat preterm labor (PTL). All tocolytics can be associated with serious complications. Steroid treatment to help with fetal lung maturity is also recommended.

► Treatment Steps

Emergency Care

1. Monitoring, hydration, and evaluation of the patient; administration of tocolytic (SQ terbutaline, 0.25 mg, 3–6 doses every 20–30 minutes or incremental increases from IV 0.050 mg/min or IV $MgSO_4$ 6-g load and 2–3 g/hr) and monitoring for complications (pulmonary edema, etc.).
2. Penicillin for group B streptococcus prophylaxis.
3. Betamethasone IM, 12 mg every 12 hours for two doses, to hasten pulmonary maturity and decrease hemorrhagic disorders and necrotizing enterocolitis.

Continued Care—Outpatient on oral β-sympathomimetics.

K. Infections of the Genitourinary Tract

► H&P Keys

Infection in the urinary tract is the most common type of infection in the pregnant female. Asymptomatic bacteriuria (> 100,000 colony-forming units [CFU] per milliliter) progresses to cystitis about 25% of the time and to pyelonephritis in 1–3% of gravidas. Increased nocturia, urgency, frequency, dysuria are common symptoms. Pyelonephritis is associated with a significantly elevated temperature, flank pain, costovertebral angle (CVA) tenderness.

► Diagnosis

UA positive for leukocyte esterase, nitrate, white blood cells (WBCs), RBCs; 10,000 CFU/mL is significant in the symptomatic patient.

► Disease Severity

Pyelonephritis: evaluate for intrauterine infection, sepsis in 2% of patients, rarely associated with septic shock and adult respiratory distress syndrome (ARDS).

► Concept and Application

Urinary stasis (decreased tone, mechanical ureteral or bladder compression) and glucosuria facilitate bacterial (*Escherichia coli*) overgrowth; 8% have asymptomatic bacteriuria.

► Treatment Steps

Initial Care

Lower Tract—Antibiotic therapy by local sensitivities (usually 7–10 days of ampicillin or nitrofurantoin).

Pyelonephritis—IV, then oral therapy. Monitoring for preterm labor.

Continued Care—Reculturing monthly. If recurrent infection, prophylactic antibiotics.

L. Incompetent Cervix

► H&P Keys

Painless preterm (second trimester) effacement and dilatation of the cervix. Patient complains of several days of vaginal or pelvic pressure, watery-to-pink vaginal discharge, or backache prior to rupture of the membranes. There is no history consistent with uterine contractions. The process usually recurs in multiple pregnancies if there is no intervention. Although there is no specific known cause, risk factors include trauma to the cervix including surgery and diethylstilbestrol (DES) exposure.

▶ Diagnosis

Internal os dilated > 1 cm or painless passage of a #8 Hegar dilator. The appearance of cervical funneling on ultrasound. No documentation of uterine contractions. History of similar occurrences in previous pregnancies.

▶ Disease Severity

Associated with deep lacerations or conizations and cervical amputations.

▶ Concept and Application

Cervix is not able to maintain closure pressure against the expanding gestation.

▶ Treatment Steps

Initial Care—Prophylactic transvaginal cerclage at 12–16 weeks.

Emergency Care—An emergency cerclage may be placed after PTL is ruled out.

Continued Care—Physical and coital activities may be restricted.

M. Central Nervous System (CNS) Malformation in the Fetus and Neural Tube Defect (NTD)

▶ H&P Keys

Ninety percent of NTDs occur in pregnancies in which there is no identifiable increased risk and are due to multifactorial inheritance. There is a 10-fold increased risk in a subsequent pregnancy. Preconceptional poor glycemic control increases risk in diabetics. Presents in the United States as an incidental ultrasonographic finding and during the evaluation of an elevated MSAFP.

▶ Diagnosis

Elevated MSAFP, amniotic fluid (AF) AFP, elevated AF acetylcholinesterase. Directed scan (Fig. 12–3).

▶ Disease Severity

Anencephaly (failure of development of the forebrain) occurs in 50% of NTDs. Spina bifida may occur at any level.

▶ Concept and Application

Failure of closure of at least a portion of the neural tube prior to the 28th day postconception. Prepregnancy folic acid decreases the risk.

▶ Treatment Steps

Initial Care—Diagnosis, nondirective genetic counseling and option counseling.

Emergency Care—Delivery by cesarean section is recommended for fetuses with isolated NTDs.

Continued Care—If pregnancy is maintained, monitoring for hydrocephalus.

N. Trisomy

▶ H&P Keys

Advanced maternal age, previous history, balanced translocation, low MSAFP. Trisomy 21 is most common, accounting for 1 in 800 live births.

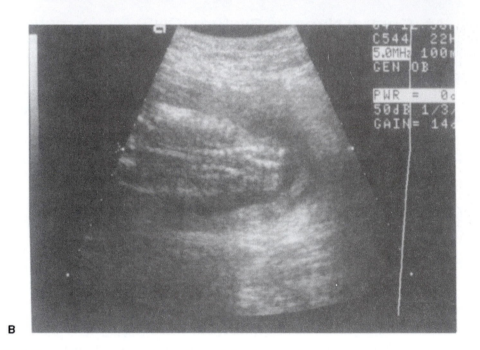

Figure 12–3. CNS malformation.

► Diagnosis
Fetal sampling via CVS, amniocentesis, or percutaneous umbilical blood sample (PUBS) is definitive.

► Disease Severity
Babies with a mosaicism may not fully express the typical phenotype.

► Concept and Application
Aneuploidy results from nondisjunction in the first meiotic division or from an unbalanced translocation. Trisomy 21 is most common, followed by trisomy 18 and trisomy 13.

► Treatment Steps

Initial Care—Nondirective counseling, support of the patient's decision within the legal and ethical framework.

O. Rh Incompatibility or Isoimmunization

► H&P Keys

Inadequate or no Rh Ig after Rh-positive RBC exposure in Rh-negative woman; Kell-negative recipient of Kell-positive transfusion.

► Diagnosis

Serial maternal antibody titering; amniocentesis or PUBS once greater than the critical titer. Middle cerebral artery (MCA) Dopplers can be used as a noninvasive measure for anemia in isoimmunization.

► Disease Severity

Delta OD450 (a measure of bilirubin in amniotic fluid) in zone III is associated with imminent fetal death from erythroblastosis fetalis. PUBS is used for both diagnosis (hemoglobin and hematocrit and antigen determination) and treatment (transfusion).

► Concept and Application

Maternal hemolytic immunoglobulin G (IgG) antibody formation to fetal red cell antigens (Rh, Kell, Duffy, Kidd, etc.), extramedullary hematopoiesis in the fetal liver, decreased oncotic protein production and edema, anasarca (erythroblastosis fetalis). Rh-negative woman has a 15% risk of sensitization in the first exposed Rh-positive, ABO-compatible pregnancy if not treated with RhoGAM.

► Treatment Steps

Initial Care

1. Serial measurement of the indirect Coombs' and antibody titering.
2. MCA Dopplers.
3. Amniocentesis or PUBS (diagnostic and therapeutic) is performed once critical titer is reached or MCA Doppler indicates severe anemia.

Emergency Care—PUBS or delivery.

Continued Care—Serial studies and therapy are determined by previous results.

P. Multiple Gestation

► H&P Keys

High index of suspicion when size greater than dates, multiple heartbeats, positive family history, ovulation induction; 1 of 80 black women, 1 of 100 white women.

► Diagnosis

Ultrasonogram, elevated MS-AFP. See Figure 12–4.

► Disease Severity

Serial ultrasonographic evaluation for growth and polyhydramnios.

► Concept and Application

Seventy percent of twins are dizygotic, wherein two eggs are fertilized by two sperm. This type of twinning is affected by race, heredity, age, and parity as well as infertility treatments.

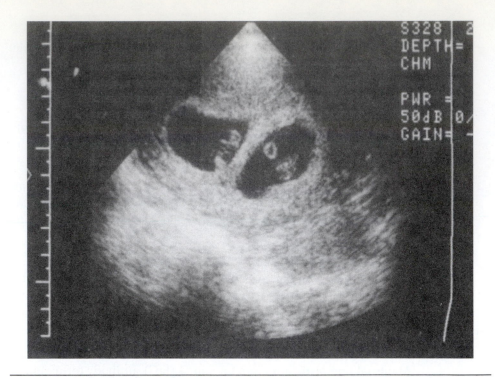

Figure 12–4. Multiple gestation.

Thirty percent are monozygotic—one egg fertilized by one sperm; 70% of monozygotic are monochorionic diamniotic (division days 3–8).

Risks: 15% perinatal mortality, preterm labor, discordant growth or IUGR, malformations, preeclampsia, anemia, abruption, polyhydramnios, malpresentation, twin–twin transfusion syndrome, diabetes.

► **Treatment Steps**

Initial Care—Increased calories and iron, preterm labor education, a management program of maternal and fetal surveillance.

Emergency Care—Treatment of specific complications.

Continued Care—Following through on the management plan.

Q. Maternal Mortality

► **H&P Keys**
Maternal mortality is defined as the death of a woman from any pregnancy-related problem during pregnancy or within 42 days of termination of pregnancy.

► **Diagnosis**
Self-evident.

► **Disease Severity**
Self-evident.

► **Concept and Application**
Causes: embolism (24%), hypertensive disease (20%), hemorrhage (16%), and infection (10%) are the most common. Rates have been declining since the mid-1970s.

► Management
Initial care: prevention.

R. Depression

► H&P Keys
Mean age 40 years; disturbance of mood, intense anguish, and loss of a sense of control; predisposing factors include victim of abuse, childhood loss of a parent, genetic predisposition, deprivation, and lifestyle stress.

► Diagnosis
High index of suspicion: a high score on the Beck Depression Inventory.

► Disease Severity
Suicide threats and attempts.

► Concept and Application
Most common psychiatric disorder in women.

► Treatment Steps

Initial Care
1. Mild to moderate depression is treated with psychotherapy.
2. Severe, chronic, recurrent depression is treated with antidepressants and psychotherapy.

Emergency—Hospitalization and psychotherapy for suicidal ideation.

S. Premature Rupture of Membranes

► H&P Keys
Leakage of AF from vagina prior to term.

► Diagnosis
Demonstration of ferning and nitrazine-positive fluid. Culture the cervix for gonorrhea, group B streptococcus, and *Chlamydia trachomatis*. Quantitative AF volume. Vaginal pool specimen for maturity studies.

► Disease Severity
Chorioamnionitis or fetal distress.

► Concept and Application
Rupture allows bacteria access to the fetus. If < 24 weeks, risks of pulmonary hypoplasia, contractures, and limb anomalies increase.

► Treatment Steps

Initial Care—Observation for symptoms and signs of infection (uterine tenderness or irritability, fever, maternal or fetal tachycardia, leukocytosis, purulent fluid), labor, and fetal well-being.

Emergency Care—Delivery if mature lungs or fetal or maternal indications.

Continued Care—Initial care plus periodic fetal assessment.

T. Hyperemesis Gravidarum

► H&P Keys
Intractable nausea and vomiting associated with significant weight loss, dehydration, electrolyte imbalance, or ketonemia. This occurs predominantly prior to 16 weeks of gestation.

► **management decisions**

EVALUATION OF RUPTURE OF MEMBRANES

Pooling
Speculum exam reveals large amount of fluid in the vagina. False-positive results can come from recent intercourse.

Nitrazine
Amniotic fluid turns nitrazine paper blue. False-positive results can result from urine, semen, cervical mucus, blood contamination, antiseptic solution, or vaginitis. False-negative results can be from minimal leakage or exam remote from the time of rupture of membranes.

Ferning
The deposition of salt crystals on a glass slide when the amniotic fluid dries. False-positive can result from cervical mucus. False-negative can result from contamination with blood or urine or antiseptic solution or very early gestational age.

► **Diagnosis**
Rule out other causes: gastroesophageal reflux, pancreatitis, hepato-biliary disease, and other gastrointestinal disorders.

► **Disease Severity**
Protracted negative protein balance and ketonemia adversely affect fetal growth.

► **Concept and Application**
Etiology unknown.

► **Treatment Steps**
Frequent small, bland meals with liquids at separate intervals, antiemetics.

Emergency Care
1. Intravenous hydration.
2. Antiemetics.
3. Psychosocial support.
4. Hyperalimentation is used rarely.

U. Abnormalities of Labor, Dystocia

► **H&P Keys**
Patient in labor with abnormal progress based on graphic analysis (see Table 12–1).

► **Diagnosis**
Graphic analysis of labor, assessment of pelvis and fetal attitude, position, and presentation.

► **Disease Severity**
Prolonged latent phase: no progress from latent to active phase (nulligravidas > 20 hours, multiparas > 40 hours). Protracted active phase dilatation: nulligravidas 1.2 cm/hr, multiparas 1.5 cm/hr. Arrest of dilatation: no change in 2 hours. Arrest of descent: no descent in 1 hour.

12-1

ABNORMAL LABOR PATTERNS, DIAGNOSTIC CRITERIA, AND METHODS OF TREATMENT

Labor Pattern	Diagnostic Criterion		Preferred Treatment	Exceptional Treatment
	Nulliparas	Multiparas		
Prolongation disorder				
Prolonged latent phase	> 20 hr	> 14 hr	Therapeutic rest	Oxytocin or cesarean deliveries for urgent problems
			Expectant and supportive	Cesarean delivery for CPD
Protraction disorders				
Protracted active phase dilatation	< 1.2 cm/hr	< 1.5 cm/hr		
Protracted descent	< 1.0 cm/hr	< 2 cm/hr		
Arrest disorders				
Prolonged deceleration rate	> 3 hr	> 1 hr	Without CPD: oxytocin	Rest if exhausted
Secondary arrest of dilatation	> 2 hr	> 2 hr	With CPD: cesarean delivery	Cesarean delivery
Arrest of descent	> 1 hr	> 1 hr		
Failure of descent	No descent in deceleration phase or second stage of labor			

CPD, cephalopelvic disproportion.

Source: Cohen W, Friedman EA (eds.). *Management of Labor.* University Park Press, 1983.

► Concept and Application

Reason for over one-quarter of all cesarean sections. Uterine contractions may be ineffective when associated with mechanical factors.

► Treatment Steps

Initial and Continuing Care
1. Prolonged latent phase, therapeutic rest or augmentation.
2. Protracted dilatation, augmentation if no disproportion.
3. Arrest of dilatation, same.
4. Arrest of descent, same or obstetric forceps if indicated.
5. Labor is augmented by IV pitocin. The pitocin is titrated to achieve three contractions in 10 minutes of adequate intensity.

V. Postpartum Hemorrhage

► H&P Keys

Uterine Atony—Predisposing factors: prolonged labor, precipitous labor, infection, uterine overdistention, multiparity, fibroids, oxytocin augmentation, and magnesium sulfate.

Genital Tract Laceration—Predisposing factors: instrumented vaginal delivery, precipitous delivery, macrosomic infant, previous genital tract laceration, and in utero manipulation.

Retained Placental Fragments—From incomplete removal of normal placenta, retained accessory lobe, or partial placenta accreta.

► Diagnosis

Vital signs, CBC, blood product availability, and search for the source of the bleeding.

► Disease Severity

Normal blood loss: singleton, vaginal, 500 mL; twin, vaginal, 1,000 mL; cesarean section, 1,000 mL. Normal parturient can lose 900 mL without any symptoms; 1,500 mL is associated with tachycardia, narrowed pulse pressure, positive blanch test; 2,000 mL is associated with hypotension; 2,400 mL is associated with profound hypotension and vasoconstriction.

► Concept and Application

Uterine blood flow is 500–600 mL/min. Interference with the normal mechanisms of hemostasis may result in significant blood loss.

► Treatment Steps

Emergency Care
1. Uterine massage, oxytocin, methylergonovine maleate (Methergine) or 15-methylprostaglandin $f_2\alpha$.
2. Transfusion if hemodynamically unstable.
3. Determination of etiology of the hemorrhage; definitive treatment.
4. Hysterectomy is last resort.

W. Postpartum Sepsis

► H&P Keys

Predisposing factors: cesarean section, prolonged rupture of membranes, chorioamnionitis, prolonged labor, multiple pelvic exams, internal monitors, obesity, and anemia. Febrile morbidity: temperature of > 100.4°F on two occasions at least 6 hours apart 24 hours postpartum.

▶ Diagnosis

Endomyometritis presents with uterine tenderness and fever; cultures are not reliable. Wound infection presents with fever, pain, tenderness, erythema, and swelling; wound cultures are helpful. Pyelonephritis, pneumonia, and atelectasis should be ruled out.

▶ Disease Severity

Evaluate for septic pelvic thrombophlebitis, which presents as persistent fever and tachycardia after presumed effective antibiotic treatment; responds to the addition of heparin.

▶ Concept and Application

Uncontrolled sepsis results in physiologic instability, organ failure, and death.

▶ Treatment Steps

Initial Care—Endomyometritis: broad-spectrum antibiotics until afebrile for 24–48 hours and patient is asymptomatic.

Wound Infection
1. Probe for fascial integrity.
2. Drainage, wound care, and broad-spectrum antibiotics until resolved.

Emergency Care—Same.

X. Obstetric Forceps and Vacuum Extractor

▶ H&P Keys

Adequate anesthesia, empty bladder (if not outlet), full cervical dilatation, known fetal attitude, position, and station.

▶ Diagnosis

Clinical assessment of fetal size and pelvis.

▶ Disease Severity

Mid: Station engaged but > +2. Low: Station is at least at +2 but not on the pelvic floor, and rotations of < 45 degrees. Outlet: Fetal head is at or on the perineum and the rotation is < 45 degrees.

▶ Concept and Application

Shortening of the second stage for a variety of fetal and maternal reasons.

▶ Treatment Steps

After prerequisites are met, apply instruments, check application, and apply traction with contractions. Inspect genital tract for injury after delivery. If unsuccessful, proceed to cesaerean section.

Y. Diabetes

1. Gestational

▶ H&P Keys

Universal screening or screen if risk factors are present (prior history, obesity, macrosomia, hydramnios, family history, excessive weight gain).

▶ Diagnosis

If 50-g glucola screen > 140 mg/dL, then proceed to 3-hour oral glucose tolerance test (GTT); abnormal if any two values exceed fasting blood sugar (FBS) > 105, > 190 at 1 hour, > 165 at 2 hours, or > 145 at 3 hours.

► **Disease Severity**

Start on diet of 30–35 kcal/kg of ideal body weight (IBW). If FBS is > 105 or 2-hour postprandial levels are > 120, evaluate for insulin. Fifteen percent of patients progress to insulin. Monitor for preeclampsia, bacterial infection, macrosomia, and hydramnios. See Table 12–2.

► **Concept and Application**

Pregnancy is diabetogenic. Prevalence 2%. Human placental lactogen (hPL) induces peripheral insulin resistance.

► **Treatment Steps**

Initial—Initiate diet, monitor blood sugar, culture urine monthly, fetal well-being assessment in third trimester.

Continued Care
1. As in initial management, normalize blood sugar in labor.
2. Test for diabetes at 6 weeks postpartum.

2. Overt

► **Diagnosis**

Hemoglobin A_{1c}, home glucose monitoring, ultrasound, 24-hour urine for protein and creatinine clearance, BP, MSAFP.

► **Disease Severity**

Elevated hemoglobin A_{1c} increases risk of congenital anomalies (neural tube and heart), maternal and fetal risks increase with duration of disease, presence of small-vessel disease (retinopathy, nephropathy, and IUGR). Increased incidence of preeclampsia.

► **Concept and Application**

Impaired insulin secretion and insulin resistance. Prone to ketoacidosis at lower blood sugar levels.

► **Treatment Steps**

1. Education, diet, exercise, normalization of blood sugar (FBS between 70 and 105, 2-hour postprandial < 120).
2. Monitor for complications.
3. Tight control of blood sugar in labor.

Z. Asthma

► **H&P Keys**

Acute dyspnea, wheezing, cough. One-third become better, one-third stay the same, one-third experience a worsening of the condition in pregnancy. Patients usually tolerate labor well.

12-2

PRISCILLA WHITE CLASSIFICATION				
Class	Age at Onset		Duration	Vascular Disease	Therapy
A	Any		Any	None	Diet
B	Over 20	OR	Under 10	None	Insulin
C	10–19	OR	10–19	None	Insulin
D	Before 10	OR	Over 20 Retinopathy	Benign	Insulin
F	Any		Any	Nephropathy	Insulin
R	Any		Any Retinopathy	Proliferative	Insulin
H	Any		Any	Heart disease	Insulin

► **on rounds**

PROBLEMS IN OBSTETRICS

Preeclampsia
- Hypertension and proteinuria or edema after 20 weeks.
- Diagnosis by blood pressure measurement, 24-hour urine for protein.
- Treatment includes bed rest (if preterm) and delivery (if term). Magnesium sulfate to prevent seizures.

Eclampsia
- Preeclampsia with tonic–clonic seizures.
- Diagnosis as in preeclampsia.
- Treatment includes stabilization of the mother and then delivery of the fetus.

Abruptio Placenta
- Vaginal bleeding, tender uterus, shock.
- Clinical diagnosis, ultrasound no help.
- Treatment includes hemodynamic stabilization and delivery (with mature fetus).

Placenta Previa
- Painless third-trimester vaginal bleeding, often at night.
- Diagnosis by ultrasound.
- Treatment for asymptomatic cases:
  Education
  Hematinics
  Serial ultrasounds
  Coital restriction in third trimester
- Urgent cases: hemodynamic stabilization.

► **Diagnosis**

Peak flow monitoring.

► **Disease Severity**

Accessory muscle usage, respiratory rate, pulse oximetry, arterial blood gases (ABGs).

► **Concept and Application**

Bronchospasm in response to allergens, antigens, or irritants; infection.

► **Treatment Steps**

Acute
1. β-Agonist inhalers, parenteral glucocorticoids.
2. Evaluation of fetal well-being.

Continued Care
1. β-Agonist, inhaled glucocorticoids, cromolyn.
2. Peak flow monitoring.

BIBLIOGRAPHY

ACOG. *Compendium of Selected Publications.* Washington, DC: American College of Obstetricians and Gynecologists, 2005.

Cunningham FG. *Williams Obstetrics,* 22nd ed. Stamford, CT: Appleton & Lange, 2005.

DeCherney AH, Pernoll ML (eds.). *Current Obstetric and Gynecologic Diagnosis and Treatment,* 9th ed. Norwalk, CT: Appleton & Lange, 2002.

Gabbe SG. *Obstetrics: Normal and Problem Pregnancies,* 4th ed. New York: Churchill Livingstone, 2002.

Martin DH. Sexually transmitted diseases. *Med Clin North Am.* Philadelphia: W.B. Saunders, 1990.

Niswander KR. *Manual of Obstetrics, Diagnosis and Therapy,* 5th ed. Boston: Little, Brown & Co., 1996.

Sweet RL. *Infectious Disease of the Female Genital Tract,* 4th ed. Baltimore: Williams & Wilkins, 2002.

Ophthalmology | 13

I. CONJUNCTIVITIS

Hyperemia of conjunctival blood vessels. Types: allergic, bacterial, viral; common, often not serious.

► H&P Keys

Red eye, usually without blurred vision, pain, or colored halos. Exudation is more severe in bacterial, moderate in viral, and least in allergic (watery). Itching is pronounced in allergic. Ciliary flush is absent. Conjunctival injection is prominent in bacterial, moderate in viral, and least in allergic. Corneal disturbance may be present in viral, absent in bacterial and allergic. Pupil, anterior chamber depth, and intraocular pressure are normal. Preauricular lymph node may be present in viral but absent in bacterial and allergic (Tables 13–1, 13–2).

► Diagnosis

Correct diagnosis for cause of red eye determines effectiveness of treatment and reduces complications. Aside from conjunctivitis, other causes of red eye must be ruled out. Differentiate from acute glaucoma, acute iridocyclitis, and keratitis corneal lesions (Tables 13–3, 13–4, 13–5).

Most cases are managed without laboratory studies. Smear of exudates. Conjunctival scrapings for culture and sensitivity studies.
1. Allergic conjunctivitis: eosinophils.
2. Bacterial conjunctivitis: polymorphonuclear cells and bacteria.
3. Viral conjunctivitis: lymphocytes.

► Disease Severity

Assess vision, pupils, amount of pain, and sensitivity to light. Rule out red eye caused by acute glaucoma, corneal lesions, or iridocyclitis.

Allergic Conjunctivitis—Itching, watery discharge, chemosis, history of allergies, edematous lids, and no preauricular nodes.

Bacterial Conjunctivitis—Severe purulent discharge; may have subconjunctival hemorrhage. Red eye subconjunctival hemorrhage. Gram stain for causative bacteria.

Viral Conjunctivitis—History of recent upper respiratory tract infection or contact with someone 7–10 days prior with a red eye. Usually gets worse the first few days after onset and may last for 2–3 weeks. Watery or mucous discharge, red and edematous eyelids. Eyelid sticking, worse in the morning. May have subconjunctival

---

► cram facts

RED EYE

Uveitis
Eye pain, blurred vision, injected conjunctiva, photophobia, diagnosis on slit lamp showing "cells and flare" (protein and white blood cells [WBCs] in aqueous humor).

Keratitis
Severe pain, photophobia, diagnosis with fluorescein stain showing multiple punctate lesions.

Glaucoma
Eye pain, nausea, vomiting, headache, hazy cornea diagnosis, pupil not reacting, increased ocular pressure.

Viral Conjunctivitis
Profuse water discharge.

Allergic Conjunctivitis
Itchy, bilateral.

Bacterial Conjunctivitis
Purulent discharge.

13-1

SYMPTOMS OF CONJUNCTIVITIS

Symptoms	Bacterial	Viral	Allergic
Exudation	+++	++	+
Itching	0	0	++
Blurred vision	0	0	0
Colored halos	0	0	0
Pain	0	0	0
Photophobia	0	0	0

+++, severe; ++, moderate; +, present; 0, absent.

13-2

SIGNS OF CONJUNCTIVITIS

Symptoms	Bacterial	Viral	Allergic
Conjunctival injection	+++	++	+
Discharge	+++	++	+
Preauricular lymph node	0	+	0
Corneal opacification	0	0/+	0
Corneal epithelial disruption	0	0/+	0
Ciliary flush	0	0	0
Pupil	N	N	N
Anterior chamber depth	N	N	N
Intraocular pressure	N	N	N

N, normal; +, present; 0, absent.

► **management decisions**

RED, INFLAMED EYE

Acute Conjunctivitis
Extremely common, minimal change in vision, minimal discomfort, diffuse conjunctival injection/hyperemia, tearing (purulent—bacterial, watery—viral), itchy—allergic.

Corneal Ulcer
Pain, photophobia, decreased vision, watery tearing, ciliary injection, contact lens use (especially soft lenses worn while sleeping).

Acute Iridocyclitis
Pain, photophobia, decreased vision, watery discharge, small pupil sometimes, ciliary injection, history of recent trauma (blunt or corneal abrasion) or autoimmune diseases.

Acute Angle-Closure Glaucoma
Severe pain, nausea/vomiting, elderly, markedly decreased vision (halo around light), mid-size dilated nonreacting pupil, diffuse conjunctival hyperemia, cloudy/opaque cornea.

hemorrhages and corneal irritations. Palpable preauricular lymph nodes suggests viral cause.

► **Concept and Application**
Viral conjunctivitis is associated with systemic problems, upper respiratory infection and fever, pharyngoconjunctival fever, adenovirus type 3 or type 7. Allergic conjunctivitis is associated with seasonal rhinitis of hay fever, erythema multiforme, serious systemic disorders with ocular involvement, Stevens–Johnson syndrome, allergic reaction to medication (see Table 13–5).

► **Treatment Steps**
(See Table 13–6.)

Allergic Conjunctivitis
1. Detection and removal of source of irritants.
2. Cold compress for comfort during waking hours.
3. Vasoconstrictor/antihistamine or mild topical steroids to the affected eyes. Improvement should be noted immediately or within 2–3 days.
4. Persistent irritation requires consultation and further investigation.

Bacterial Conjunctivitis
1. Appropriate topical antibiotic drops during the waking hours of the day and ointment at night.
2. Washing away exudates and warm soaks of eyes for comfort.
3. Avoidance of topical steroids.

13-3

SYMPTOMS OF RED EYE

Symptoms	Acute Conjunctivitis	Acute Iritis	Acute Glaucoma	Corneal Lesions
Exudation	+/+++	0	0	0/+++
Itching	0/++	0	0	0
Blurred vision	0	+/++	+++	+++
Colored halos	0	0	++	0
Pain	0	++	++/+++	++
Photophobia	0	+++	+	+++

+++, severe; ++, moderate; +, present; 0, absent.

13-4

SIGNS OF RED EYE

Signs	Acute Conjunctivitis	Acute Iritis	Acute Glaucoma	Corneal Lesions
Conjunctival injection	+/+++	++	++	++
Discharge	+/+++	0	0	0/+
Preauricular lymph node	0/+	0	0	0
Corneal opacification	0/+	0	+++	0/+++
Corneal epithelial disruption	0/+	0	0	+/+++
Ciliary flush	0	++	+	+++
Pupil	N	Mid-dilated Irregular	Small/irregular	N/small
Anterior chamber depth	N	N	Shallow	N
Intraocular pressure	N	Low	High	N

+, present; ++, moderate; +++, severe; N, normal; 0, absent.

Viral Conjunctivitis

1. Usually subsides after its natural course. It is very contagious about 5 days after onset. Patients with red and weeping eyes should avoid spreading to other people.
2. Isolation from group gatherings.
3. Artificial tears and cold compresses as often as needed for comfort.
4. Frequent hand washing.

II. DISORDERS OF THE EYELIDS

A. Blepharitis

Chronic bilateral inflammation of the lid margins.

► H&P Keys

Itching, irritation, burning of lid margins, red rims, scales of lashes, ulcerated areas along lid margins.

► Diagnosis

Lid margin ulceration or no ulceration, scales oily or dry.

► Disease Severity

Check scalp, brows, ears for seborrhea. Smear and stain of scraping from lid margins. Stain cornea. Evaluate for ulceration.

13-5

ASSOCIATED SYSTEMIC DISEASES IN CONJUNCTIVITIS

Systemic Diseases	Bacterial Conjunctivitis	Viral Conjunctivitis	Allergic Conjunctivitis
Pharyngoconjunctival fever (adenovirus type 3, type 7)	0	+	0
Seasonal rhinitis of hay fever	0	0	+
Erythema multiforme (Stevens–Johnson syndrome)	0	0	+

+, present; 0, absent.

13-6

MANAGEMENT OF CONJUNCTIVITIS			
	Bacterial Conjunctivitis	Viral Conjunctivitis	Allergic Conjuctivitis
Topical antibiotics	Sulfa, tobramycin polymixin B, erythromycin	0	0
Topical mast cell stabilizers, NSAIDs	0	0	+++
Antihistamines (oral)	0	0	±
Isolation precaution	0	++	0
Remove irritants	+	++	+++

+, of some benefit; ++, moderate benefit; +++, treatment of choice; ±, may or may not help; 0, no benefit; NSAIDs, nonsteroidal anti-inflammatory drugs.

▶ Concept and Application

Seborrheic Blepharitis—Associated with seborrhea of scalp, brows, ears. Nonulcerative lid margin, scales oily, *Pityrosporum ovale* present.

Staphylococcal Blepharitis—*Staphylococcus aureus* or *Staphylococcus epidermidis,* coagulase-negative, ulcerative lid margin, hordeola, chalazia, epithelial keratitis lower one-third of cornea, marginal infiltrates, recurrent conjunctivitis.

▶ Treatment Steps

Seborrheic Blepharitis—Soap-and-water shampoo of scalp. Removal of scales from lid margins with baby shampoo.

Staphylococcal Blepharitis
1. Daily antibiotic ointment against *Staphylococcus.*
2. Long-term low-dose systemic antibiotic therapy.

B. Stye

External hordeolum (glands of Zeis or Moll, hair follicles).

▶ H&P Keys

Recent onset; localized red, swollen, tender area of the lid, frequently preceded by diffuse edema of the lid.

▶ Diagnosis

Red, swollen gland with pore opening can be seen at the lid margin. Tender area can be identified with a cotton tip.

▶ Disease Severity

Pain is related to the amount of swelling. Pus tends to point to the skin surface of the lid margin.

▶ Concept and Application

Common staphylococcal infection of Zeis's or Moll's glands of the lids. A small abscess sometimes is formed.

▶ Treatment Steps
1. Warm compresses over affected lids 10 minutes three times a day after application of antibiotic ointment.
2. Incision and drainage of pus when needed.

C. Chalazion

Internal hordeolum (meibomian gland).

▶ H&P Keys

Persistent nontender lump palpable or visible along the margin of upper or lower eyelid. Inflammation and swelling develop over a period of days and can remain for months.

▶ Diagnosis

When the lid is everted, the nodules usually point toward the conjunctival side and can be detected as reddened, elevated areas. Absence of acute inflammation is seen in fully developed chalazion.

▶ Disease Severity

1. Evaluate for malignancy if recurrent at same site.
2. Assess visual disturbance caused by the lump on the lids.
3. Perform biopsy if recurrent.

▶ Concept and Application

A granulomatous inflammation of the meibomian gland. Seldom subsides spontaneously. Langhans' giant cells, yellowish, fatty content. Large chalazion pressing on the eyeball, can cause astigmatism. Recurrence at same site after excision suggests malignant disease.

▶ Treatment Steps

1. Warm compresses.
2. Topical antibiotics.
3. Local steroid injection.
4. Excision if large and disturbs vision.
5. Biopsy if recurrent.

D. Entropion

Turning inward of the lid margin, usually affects the lower lid.

▶ H&P Keys

Tearing, irritation of the cornea. Eyelashes turn inward, touching cornea.

▶ Diagnosis

Check the lid margin, position of the eyelashes, and the integrity of the cornea. Early detection of corneal ulcer.

▶ Disease Severity

Entropion can cause trichiasis, the turning inward of the lashes so that they rub on the cornea. Irritation of the cornea can predispose to corneal ulcer.

▶ Concept and Application

Senile type caused by degeneration of fascial attachments in the lower lid. *Cicatricial* type caused by scarring of the palpebral conjunctiva and the tarsus. Common in trachoma, Stevens–Johnson syndrome, chemical burns, and trauma.

▶ Treatment Steps

1. Temporary taping to evert lid.
2. Corrective surgery.

E. Ectropion

Turning outward of lower lid.

▶ H&P Keys

Tearing, irritation. Sagging and eversion of lid margin.

► **Diagnosis**

Test closure of lids and integrity of cornea.

► **Disease Severity**

Exposure keratitis. Fluorescein stain for corneal integrity.

► **Concept and Application**

Bilateral. Older persons. Relaxation of orbicularis oculi. Present in aging and seventh cranial nerve palsy.

► **Treatment Steps**

1. Protection of cornea.
2. Lubrication with artificial tears or ointment.
3. Surgical correction of deformed lid.

F. Epicanthus

Wide nasal folds.

► **H&P Keys**

Vertical folds of skin over medial canthi; in Asians and most children of all races.

► **Diagnosis**

Corneal light reflex test is normal. So-called esotropia, or turning in of the eye, appears present on side gaze.

► **Disease Severity**

Prominent epicanthal folds in children becomes less obvious as child grows older.

► **Concept and Application**

The large skin fold covers the nasal sclera and causes pseudo-esotropia. Frequent concern as strabismus. A common cause for referral.

► **Treatment Steps**

Explanation and understanding. No treatment needed.

G. Blepharoptosis

Droopy eyelids.

► **H&P Keys**

May be noted at birth; congenital or acquired. Drooping of upper lids when both eyes are open. Unilateral or bilateral. Constant or intermittent.

► **Diagnosis**

Determine amount of movement of upper lid and severity in blocking of vision. Assess cosmesis and skin position.

► **Disease Severity**

Degree of upper lid movement and occlusion of pupillary axis for vision. Concern with visual development in children. May cause amblyopia.

► **Concept and Application**

Congenital—Developmental failure of levator muscle of the lid, anomalies of superior rectus muscle, complete external ophthalmoplegia. Dominant transmission.

Acquired

Mechanical Factors—Edema of lids, swelling, tumor, fat.

Myogenic Causes—Muscular dystrophy, myasthenia gravis.

Neurogenic (Paralytic)—Weakness of cranial nerve III.

► Treatment Steps
1. Conservative: no cosmetic or visual acuity disturbance.
2. Myasthenia gravis: neostigmine.
3. Special spectacle frames.
4. Surgery for improvement of vision or cosmesis: frontalis sling for no action of levator, to lift upper lid; levator strengthening for partial weakness of levator.

III. DISORDERS OF THE LACRIMAL SYSTEM

A. Undersecretion

Dry-eye syndrome, Sjögren's syndrome.

1. Dry-Eye Syndrome (Keratoconjunctivitis Sicca)

► H&P Keys

Dry, irritative conjunctiva. Dry, sore mouth. Foreign-body sensation, scratchy and sandy feeling of the eyes. Itchy, burning, photosensitivity, excessive mucus, redness, pain, dry lids. Grossly, normal-looking eyes.

► Diagnosis

Dry undersecretion is confirmed by Schirmer's test with strip of blotting paper (4 mm × 30 mm). The strip is inserted onto the lower lid margin so that the strip protrudes forward from the eye. The rate of lacrimation is measured. By the end of 5 minutes the strip should be moistened for at least 15 mm in a normal response. In Sjögren's syndrome, the moistening rarely extends beyond 5 mm along the strip, suggesting inadequate tear production.

► Disease Severity

Undersecretion of tears. Evaluation studies for corneal epithelium and conjunctival defects with vital stain such as rose bengal (1%). The affected areas will be colored bright red. Collagen-vascular diseases, conjunctival scarring, drugs, and vitamin A deficiency should be investigated, if not yet diagnosed.

► Concept and Application

Dryness of eye may have many causes. Hyposecretion, excessive evaporation, mucin deficiency are predisposing factors.

Sjögren's syndrome is a general glandular atrophy. It affects the lacrimal and salivary glands and is associated with rheumatic diathesis. Postmenopausal women. Dryness affects conjunctiva, cornea, mouth, trachea.

► Treatment Steps
1. Search for cause.
2. Artificial tears, methylcellulose are used frequently.

B. Acute Dacryocystitis

▶ **H&P Keys**

Infection of lacrimal sac. Common acute or chronic in infants or in patients over 40. Tearing and discharge. Swelling lump, redness, pain, tenderness over tear sac area. May have fever.

▶ **Diagnosis**

Persistent tearing. Purulent material can be expressed from tear sac. Nasolacrimal duct is blocked. Staining of conjunctival smear to identify infectious organisms.

▶ **Disease Severity**

Tearing in mild cases. Purulent discharge in moderate to severe blockage of nasolacrimal ducts.

▶ **Concept and Application**

Blockage of nasolacrimal duct is the cause of infection. May be developmental.

▶ **Treatment Steps**

In children, forceful massage of the tear sac is tried initially. Irrigation and probings of nasolacrimal duct are usually effective in adults.

Acute
1. Warm compresses.
2. Appropriate antibiotics.
3. Incision and drainage if necessary.

Chronic—Surgical removal of obstruction of nasolacrimal duct (dacrocystorhinostomy).

IV. DISORDERS OF THE OPTIC NERVE

A. Elevation of the Disc

1. Congenital Anomalous Disc Elevation

Blurred optic disc since birth, caused by developmental anomaly.

▶ **H&P Keys**

No symptoms, blurred disc margin, elevated disc substance, obliterated cup, no edema, no hemorrhage.

▶ **Diagnosis**

Dilated ophthalmoscopy; document with optic disc photography, pseudopapilledema; visual field, intravenous fluorescein angiography (Tables 13–7, 13–8).

▶ **Disease Severity**

Benign, nonprogressive; rule out true papilledema.

▶ **Concept and Application**

Hyperopia, glial tissue, persistent hyaloid remnants, drusen of the disc.

▶ **Treatment Steps**

Detection and follow-up through serial examinations to monitor possible progression.

13-7

SYMPTOMS OF BLURRED OPTIC NERVE HEAD

Symptoms	Papilledema	Papillitis	Pseudopapilledema
Etiology	Acute swelling of optic disc • Increased intracranial pressure • Brain tumor • Hypertension • Pseudotumor cerebri	Acute blurred disc margin • Ischemia • Inflammation • Multiple sclerosis	Blurred disc • Congenital, developmental anomalies • Hyperopia
Acute loss of vision	+	+++ (Severe)	0
Headaches	+++	0/+	0
Retrobulbar pain on eye movement	0	+/+++	0

+, present; ++, moderate; +++, severe; 0, absent.

2. Papilledema

Swelling of optic disc caused by increased intracranial pressure (Fig. 13–1).

► H&P Keys

Symptoms of brain tumor, hyperemia of optic disc, tortuosity of veins and capillaries, blurring and elevation of disc margin, hemorrhages on and surrounding nerve head.

► Diagnosis

Studies for brain lesions, computed tomographic (CT) scan, magnetic resonance imaging (MRI), magnetic resonance angiography (MRA), intravenous fluorescein angiography.

► Disease Severity

Brain tumor, pseudotumor cerebri, severe systemic hypertension.

► Concept and Application

Swelling of optic disc secondary to increased intracranial pressure, brain tumor 50%.

► Treatment Steps

Detection and referral for evaluation by neurologists or neurosurgeons.

3. Papillitis

Anterior optic neuritis. Inflammatory edema of the optic nerve head visible by ophthalmoscope.

13-8

SIGNS OF BLURRED OPTIC NERVE HEAD

Signs	Papilledema	Papillitis	Pseudopapilledema
Hyperemia of disc	+++	+++	0
Hemorrhages	+++	+	0
Tortuosity of veins, capillaries	+++	++	+
Disc margin blurred,	+++	+++	+++
elevated	+++	0/+	++
One eye affected	Rare	+++	++
Both eyes affected	+++	Rare	Rare
Afferent pupillary defect	0	+++	0/+
Visual field defect	0/+	+++	0/+

+, present; ++, moderate; +++, severe; 0, absent.

Figure 13–1. (A) Mild papilledema with blurred disc margins superiorly and inferiorly. (B) Acute papilledema with cotton-wool spots and hemorrhages. (Reproduced, with permission, from Vaughan DG [ed.]. *General Ophthalmology,* 15th ed. Stamford, CT: Appleton & Lange, 1999).

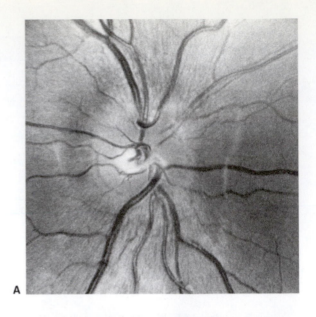

A

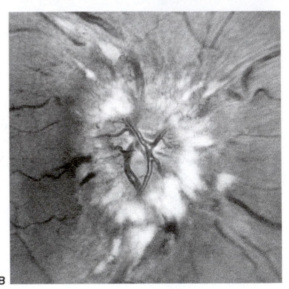

B

► H&P Keys

Sudden loss of central vision, usually in one eye. Pain behind the eyeball on movement of the affected eye. Reduced vision. Swinging light test for relative afferent pupillary defect.

► Diagnosis

Ophthalmoscopy, visual field test for central scotoma, CT of orbits and chiasm, MRI and MRA of the brain.

► Disease Severity

Search for multiple sclerosis, Lyme disease, and neurosyphilis. Rule out compressive lesions of optic nerve and chiasm.

► Concept and Application

Inflammation of optic nerve. Idiopathic. Associated with multiple sclerosis, Lyme disease, and neurosyphilis. Prognosis for return vision after single attack is good. Spontaneous resolution can follow in weeks to months.

▶ Treatment Steps
1. IV corticosteroid versus no treatment for acute phase.
2. Oral prednisone treatment is contraindicated in the treatment of idiopathic optic neuritis.

B. Pallor of the Disc, Optic Atrophy
Optic nerve degeneration.

▶ H&P Keys
Decreased vision, visual field loss, relative afferent pupillary defect, fixed dilated pupil, pale optic disc.

▶ Diagnosis
Vision, pupillary reaction to light, swinging light test, ophthalmoscopy; compare both discs for asymmetry of color, cupping, fine-vessels pattern.

▶ Disease Severity
Intraocular pressure for glaucoma, orbital mass compression of nerve. Intravenous fluorescein angiography of disc.

▶ Concept and Application
History of diseases that damage nerve fiber layer of retina, optic nerve, optic chiasm, optic tracts. Common causes: optic neuritis, long-standing papilledema, compression of the nerve by a mass, meningioma, ischemic optic neuropathy, glaucoma.

▶ Treatment Steps
Detection and referral for investigation and treatment.

V. DISORDERS OF THE VISUAL PATHWAYS

A. Monocular Defects (Central Scotomas)
Anterior to chiasm.

▶ H&P Keys
Loss of central vision in one eye. Reduction of visual acuity (Fig. 13–2).

▶ Diagnosis
Visual acuity testing, pupillary reaction to light, swinging light test for relative afferent pupillary defect, ophthalmoscopy, visual field testing, red-color appreciation, Amsler grid.

▶ Disease Severity
Ophthalmoscopy for macular and optic nerve diseases. Rule out retinal detachments, vascular occlusions, such as central retinal artery occlusion, branch retinal artery occlusion, central retinal vein occlusion. Intravenous fluorescein angiography.

▶ Concept and Application
Prechiasmal lesions mean monocular loss of vision. Optic nerve lesions. Scotoma is a blind or partially defective area in the visual field.

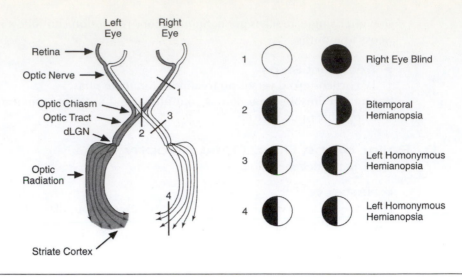

Figure 13–2. Visual pathways with associated field defects. (Reproduced, with permission, from Schwartz SH. *Visual Perception,* 2nd ed. New York: McGraw-Hill, 1999).

Central scotoma means central vision is affected. Optic neuritis. Ischemic optic neuropathy. Multiple sclerosis.

► **Treatment Steps**
Detection and referral.

B. Bitemporal Defects

At the chiasm.

► **H&P Keys**
Visual field defect affects both eyes, bitemporal hemianopsia, side vision defect of both eyes (see Fig. 13–2). Confrontation testing with red object.

► **Diagnosis**
Vision, visual fields testing, CT scan, MRI/MRA.

► **Disease Severity**
CT scan. Check out enlarged sella turcica for pituitary tumor.

► **Concept and Application**
Bitemporal visual field defects means chiasmal lesions; suspect pituitary tumor.

► **Treatment Steps**
Detection and referral.

C. Homonymous Defects

Posterior to chiasm.

► **H&P Keys**
Loss of visual fields of both eyes on the same side (see Fig. 13–2). Visual field defects on the right or left side. Confrontation testing with red object.

► **Diagnosis**
Visual field testing, intracranial studies, CT scan, MRI.

► **Disease Severity**

Check out neurologic symptoms and signs for brain tumor and cerebral vascular lesions, stroke.

► **Concept and Application**

Defects indicate lesions behind the chiasm. Lesions affect optic tract opposite the defects, extending to occipital cortex. The more posterior the lesion, the more similar in shape, size, and severity the damage in the two eyes. Check out tumor, cerebral vascular diseases.

► **Treatment Steps**

Detection and referral.

VI. AMBLYOPIA

Defective vision, uncorrectable by glasses, in an otherwise normal eye.

► **H&P Keys**

Eye fixation pattern, vision test, ophthalmoscopy.

► **Diagnosis**

Refraction, check out anisometropia.

► **Disease Severity**

Check out visual loss caused by organic diseases, congenital cataracts, retinoblastoma.

► **Concept and Application**

Preventable blindness. Strabismus in 50% of patients with amblyopia. Amblyopia secondary to strabismus. Organic visual loss causes strabismus. Predisposing factors: strabismic amblyopia, refractive amblyopia, form-deprivation and occlusion amblyopia.

► **Treatment Steps**

Early detection. Early treatment before age 5 (Table 13–9).

► **diagnostic decisions**

THREE COMMON CAUSES OF VISION LOSS

Amblyopia
Child, positive family history, decreased vision in one eye uncorrectable with glasses, no organic disease, strabismus in 50% (exotropia—eye turns out, esotropia—eye turns in).

Diabetic Retinopathy
Frequency increases with duration of disease, vision may be normal, decreased vision is often a late sign, hypertension, exacerbated with puberty and pregnancy.

Glaucoma (Open-Angle)
Positive family history, advanced age (especially 80+ years), diabetes, hypertension, normal vision, constricted peripheral vision, thinning of optic disc rim/asymmetrical optic nerve rims, increased intraocular pressure (> 21 mm Hg).

► **management decisions**

Amblyopia	Glasses
	Occlusion therapy
	Surgery for strabismus
Diabetic retinopathy	Retinal laser treatment for clinically significant macular edema and/or proliferative retinopathy
	Vitrectomy

13-9

PROGRESSION OF DIABETIC RETINOPATHY

Nonproliferative retinopathy
  Microaneurysms
  Hemorrhages (dot and blot, flame)
  Hard exudates
  Retinal edema
Preproliferative retinopathy
  Retinal nerve fiber layer infarcts (cotton-wool patches)
  Venous dilation, loops, and beading (irregularities of the vein caliber)
  Telangiectasias (intraretinal microvascular abnormalities)
Proliferative diabetic retinopathy
  Neovascularization of the retina, optic disc, or vitreous
  Preretinal and vitreous hemorrhages
  Fibrous proliferation
  Tractional retinal detachment

VII. STRABISMUS

Misalignment of two eyes so that both eyes cannot be directed toward the object of fixation (Fig. 13–3).

▶ H&P Keys

Family history, head trauma, systemic disease, neurologic disorder.

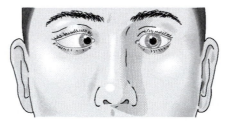

Primary position: right esotropia

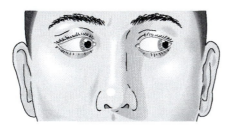

(A)   Left gaze: no deviation

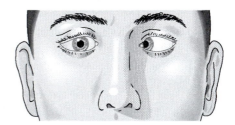

Right gaze: left esotropia

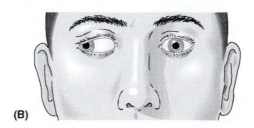

(B)

Figure 13–3. (A) Right esotropia. (B) Right exotropia. (Reproduced, with permission, from Vaughan DG [ed.]. *General Ophthalmology,* 15th ed. Stamford, CT: Appleton & Lange, 1999).

13-10

CLASSIFICATION OF STRABISMUS

	Comitant (Nonparalytic) Strabismus	Noncomitant (Paralytic) Strabismus
Onset	Childhood (under 6 yr)	Later in life
Angle of misalignment *varies* with direction of gaze	0	+
Extraocular muscles palsy	0	+
Associated neurologic disease*	0	+

*Blowout fracture; palsy of cranial nerve III; orbital diseases; thyroid.

+, present; 0, absent.

► **Diagnosis**

General inspection, corneal light reflex, cover test, dilated ophthalmoscopy.

► **Disease Severity**

Check for intraocular lesions, cataract, retinoblastoma, other retinal abnormalities. Examine for neurologic disorder.

► **Concept and Application**

Early detection (Tables 13–10, 13–11). Delayed diagnosis affects vision, eye, and systemic problems.

► **Treatment Steps**

1. Detection early to allow diagnosis and treatment.
2. Search for serious organic conditions that cause strabismus.

VIII. DIABETES WITH OPHTHALMOLOGIC MANIFESTATIONS

► **H&P Keys**

Decreased vision often a late symptom that may not be evident until ocular damage is severe. The longer a patient is diabetic, the more likely the retinopathy and visual loss. Age of onset, type of diabetes, history of hypertension, and presence of obesity are relevant to disease severity and management. Changes in refraction of lens, decreased or abnormal pupillary responses, extraocular muscle palsy, cataract, iris neovascularization, optic neuropathy, or retinopathy. Diabetic retinopathy progresses in severity from nonproliferative or background retinopathy to preproliferative and proliferative changes (see Table 13–11).

13-11

TYPES OF IMBALANCE OF THE TWO EYES

	Tropia (Visible Turning)	Phoria (Tendency to Turn)
Horizontal		
Inward turning	Eso*tropia*	Eso*phoria*
Outward turning	Exo*tropia*	Exo*phoria*
Vertical		
Upward turning	Hyper*tropia*	Hyper*phoria*
Downward turning	Hypo*tropia*	Hypo*phoria*

► Diagnosis

Direct ophthalmoscopy detects most ophthalmic clinical manifestations of diabetes, including retinopathy, optic neuropathy, blockage of the red reflex by cataract (Fig. 13–4). Indirect ophthalmoscopy: wider, stereoscopic view of retina. Biomicroscopy with a slit lamp: useful in evaluating for diabetic changes in anterior segment including cataracts and iris neovascularization. Pupillary dilation for easier, more thorough examination of retina and lens. Ultrasonography for internal structure (e.g., tractional retinal detachment), when blood, debris, or membranes impede direct visualization of retina.

► Disease Severity

Biomicroscopy with a contact lens system provides stereoscopic, detailed view of structures of retina; especially valuable in diagnosis of macular edema. Fluorescein angiography to assess extent of disease, such as leakage from abnormal vessels in suspected neovascularization, and in guiding laser photocoagulation treatment of clinically evident macular edema by revealing characteristic lesions and pathologic processes of retinopathy, e.g., microaneurysms, capillary leakage, and nonperfusion areas. Images of retina.

► Concept and Application

Cellular edema, pericyte destruction, endothelial damage and dysfunction from increased intracellular sorbitol and hypoxia lead to capillary hyperpermeability. Abnormal retinal vascular permeability leads to macular edema, which threatens vision and may be an indication for laser therapy. Increased hemoglobin A_{1c} oxygen affinity impairs oxygen release, resulting in retinal hypoxia. Basement membrane thickening and increased platelet and red blood cell aggregability predispose to regions of microvascular occlusions, retinal hypoxia, and release of vasogenic factors with subsequent neovascularization of the retina, optic nerve, or iris. Widespread panretinal laser photocoagulation reduces release of vasogenic stimuli and therefore neovascularization.

► Treatment Steps

1. Tight medical control with long-term near-normalization of blood sugar level slows the progression of diabetic retinopathy. Aggressive control of blood pressure to 130/80 or better.

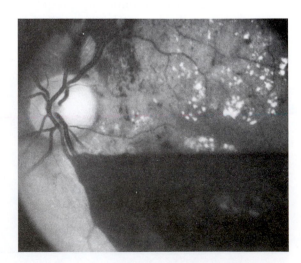

Figure 13–4. Proliferative diabetic retinopathy with preretinal hemorrhage obscuring the inferior macula. Macular exudate, microaneurysms, and intraretinal hemorrhages are also present. (Reproduced, with permission, from Vaughan DG [ed.]. *General Ophthalmology,* 15th ed. Stamford, CT: Appleton & Lange, 1999).

2. Laser photocoagulation for diabetic retinopathy with clinically significant macular edema and high-risk proliferative retinopathy.

3. Vitrectomy may be indicated for severe vitreous or preretinal hemorrhages, or tractional retinal detachment.

IX. DISORDERS OF THE CORNEA

See Table 13–12.

A. Corneal Ulcers

▶ H&P Keys

Pain, photophobia, blepharospasm, lacrimation, discharge, and decreased vision often present. The lesion begins as a dull, grayish, circumscribed, superficial infiltration of the cornea that subsequently ulcerates. Conjunctival and limbal injection is usual and blood vessels may grow in from the limbus in long-standing cases (pannus). Pus may appear in the anterior chamber (hypopyon). Corneal perforation with iris prolapse may occur.

▶ Diagnosis

The ulcer stains green with fluorescein. Bacterial and fungal cultures from corneal scrapings should be obtained prior to starting antibiotic treatment.

▶ Disease Severity

Slit-lamp biomicroscopy may be used to determine the extent of corneal thinning and infiltration and the presence of hypopyon.

▶ Concept and Application

Bacterial or fungal infection following trauma, corneal foreign body, contact lens wear, or previous corneal disease. Assume bacterial until proven otherwise.

▶ Treatment Steps

1. Cycloplegia (scopalamine), broad-spectrum or fortified topical antibiotics, subconjunctival antibiotics.

13-12

DISEASES OF THE GLOBE

A. Cornea
  1. Ulcers
  2. Herpes simplex keratitis
  3. Ophthalmic herpes zoster
  4. Dry eye (keratoconjunctivitis sicca)
  5. Interstitial keratitis
B. Sclera
  1. Scleritis
C. Uvea
  1. Uveitis
    a. Anterior
    b. Posterior
D. Retina
  1. Retinal detachment
  2. Vascular occlusions
    a. Arteriolar
    b. Venous
  3. Hypertensive retinopathy
  4. Retinitis pigmentosa
  5. Age-related macular degeneration
E. Penetrating injuries

2. Eye shield if corneal thinning.
3. Pain medication (acetaminophen).
4. Avoid steroids.

B. Herpes Simplex Keratitis

► H&P Keys
Red eye, foreign-body sensation, photophobia, tearing, decreased vision, skin vesicles. Decreased corneal sensation. Dendritic corneal branching lesion. Possible recent topical steroids, systemic steroids, or immune deficiency state.

► Diagnosis
Edge of herpetic lesions are heaped up with swollen epithelial cells, which stain with rose bengal, whereas the central ulceration stains with fluorescein. Corneal or skin lesion scraping for multinucleated giant cells and intranuclear inclusion bodies. Viral culture.

► Disease Severity
Slit-lamp examination with intraocular pressure measurement. Concomitant corneal infiltrates, iritis, hypopyon, or glaucoma may occur. Bacterial superinfection must be ruled out.

► Concept and Application
Self-limited primary ocular herpes keratoconjunctivitis, regional lymphadenitis, vesicular blepharitis, or skin involvement. Herpesvirus establishes presence in trigeminal ganglion, allowing chronic recurrent disease.

► Treatment Steps
1. Skin vesicles (antibiotic ointment); eyelid margin involvement, conjunctivitis, corneal epithelial disease (topical trifluorothymidine or vidarabine).
2. Consider mechanical debridement of infected corneal epithelium.
3. Topical steroids contraindicated for corneal epithelial involvement.

C. Ophthalmic Herpes Zoster

► H&P Keys
Acute vesicular skin rash of fifth cranial nerve dermatome. Fever, malaise, blurred vision, eye pain, red eye. Conjunctivitis, corneal involvement (e.g., pseudodendrites), uveitis, optic neuritis, retinitis, glaucoma. Postherpetic neuralgia may occur late. Involvement of tip of nose by vesicles (Hutchinson's sign) associated with corneal involvement. Immunocompromised or risk factors for acquired immune deficiency syndrome (AIDS).

► Diagnosis
Clinical diagnosis based on pattern of skin rash. Pseudodendrites stain poorly with fluorescein. Regional lymphadenopathy with associated pain occurs in primary disease.

► Disease Severity
Slit-lamp examination with intraocular pressure measurement. Dilated optic nerve and retinal examination. Immunodeficiency workup if < 40 years old or immunodeficiency suspected.

► Concept and Application
Primary herpes zoster: acute infection of dorsal root ganglion by chickenpox virus. Secondary eruption following ganglion involve-

ment may be associated with immune compromise from neoplastic, inflammatory, or infectious processes.

► Treatment Steps
1. Systemic acyclovir if started in first 5–7 days of skin rash.
2. Antibiotic ointment to skin lesions.
3. Consider systemic steroids and cimetidine in nonimmunocompromised, nondiabetic patients over age 60 to reduce postherpetic neuralgia.

D. Interstitial Keratitis

► H&P Keys
Acute: pain, tearing, photophobia, red eye. Corneal stromal blood vessels, corneal edema, anterior uveitis. Old disease: deep corneal scarring and haze, corneal stromal thinning, and ghost vessels. Associated with maternal venereal disease, saddle nose, frontal bossing, Hutchinson's teeth, chorioretinitis, optic atrophy (congenital syphilis); hearing deficit, tinnitus, vertigo, polyarteritis nodosa (Cogan's syndrome); hypopigmented or anesthetic skin lesions, loss of temporal eyebrow or eyelashes, thickened corneal nerves, iris nodules (leprosy); tuberculosis.

► Diagnosis
Slit-lamp and dilated fundus examination. Rapid plasma reagin (RPR), fluorescent treponemal antibody absorption (FTA-ABS), purified protein derivative (PPD) (tuberculin) tests with anergy panel, chest x-ray, sedimentation rate.

► Disease Severity
Slit-lamp examination for corneal edema, scarring or thinning, or uveitis.

► Concept and Application
Chronic nonulcerative infiltration of the deep layers of the cornea with uveal inflammation.

► Treatment Steps
1. Acute corneal involvement: topical cycloplegia, topical steroids, treatment of underlying disease.
2. Corneal transplant surgery for central corneal scarring with impaired vision.

X. DISORDERS OF THE LENS

A. Glaucoma

► H&P Keys

Primary Open-Angle Glaucoma—Usually asymptomatic in the early stages. Risk factors include advanced age, African ancestry, immediate family members with glaucoma, myopia (nearsightedness), diabetes mellitus, hypertension. The optic nerve may show an increased ratio of the physiologic cupping diameter to disc diameter, pallor, displacement of retinal vessels to the rim, and asymmetry compared to the contralateral eye.

Acute Angle-Closure Glaucoma—Presents with severe ocular pain, blurred vision, halos around lights, headache, nausea, and vomiting. Examination shows red eye, mid-dilated sometimes oval pupil, cloudy cornea, marked elevation of intraocular pressure, shallow anterior chamber, and closed angle by gonioscopy. Highly farsighted patients are at greater risk. An attack may be precipitated by dim light, emotional stress, or dilating drops.

Congenital Glaucoma—Presents with light sensitivity, corneal cloudiness, and excessive tearing. Chronically, there may be slow development and learning disabilities.

Secondary Glaucomas—May occur with chronic exposure to steroids (topical generally), ocular trauma, retinal vein occlusion, intraocular inflammation, intraocular tumor, diabetes mellitus, and carotid vascular disease.

► Diagnosis

Intraocular pressure measurement may be performed with Schiøtz's (indentation) or applanation tonometry. Individuals may present with normal intraocular pressures and have glaucoma. A patient who has elevated intraocular pressure but shows no sign of optic nerve damage or visual field loss is generally considered to be a glaucoma suspect. Visual field defects start insidiously. They are characterized by arcuate-shaped scotomas or a silent contraction of the peripheral field, sparing the central vision until late in the disease process.

► Disease Severity

The severity of disease is based on the clinical appearance of the optic nerve and on the visual field. Response to treatment is evaluated with regard to relationship of lowering of intraocular pressure to stability of changes in the optic nerve appearance and visual field (Fig. 13–5).

► Concept and Application

Glaucoma is in general a condition in which the intraocular pressure is too elevated for the health of the optic nerve, resulting in damage and visual field loss. This is generally due to increased resistance to aqueous outflow. In primary open-angle glaucoma, there appears to be an increased resistance to aqueous outflow through the trabecular meshwork. In primary angle-closure glaucoma, the peripheral iris closes off the angle structures, preventing aqueous outflow. Neovascularization, pigmentary or inflammatory debris, traumatic damage, or cellular changes from chronic steroid exposure all increase resistance to aqueous outflow. Both the medical and surgical treatment of glaucoma is based on the reduction of in-

► management decisions

GLAUCOMA	
Open-angle	β-Adrenergic antagonists, α-adrenergic agonists, prostaglandin analogs, topical carbonic anhydrase inhibitors, miotics, adrenergic agonists. Laser trabecular burns. Surgical filtration procedures.
Closed-angle	Topical β-blockers, pilocarpine, carbonic anhydrase inhibitors. Oral carbonic anhydrase inhibitors, osmotics (glycerin), IV mannitol. Laser peripheral iridotomy—for definitive treatment.

traocular pressure by promoting aqueous outflow or reducing aqueous production.

► **Treatment Steps**

Open-Angle Glaucoma

1. β-Adrenergic antagonists (e.g., timolol), topical carbonic anhydrase inhibitors (e.g., dorzolamide, brinzolamide), and adrenergic agonists (e.g., epinephrine) decrease aqueous production.

   α-Adrenergic agonists (e.g., brimonidine, clonidine, apraclonidine), prostaglandin analogs (e.g., latanoprost, travaprost), and miotics (e.g., pilocarpine) reduce outflow resistance.
2. Laser trabecular burns promote aqueous outflow.
3. Surgical filtration procedures promote aqueous outflow.

Angle-Closure Glaucoma

1. Acutely treat with topical β-blockers, topical pilocarpine, oral carbonic anhydrase inhibitors, and osmotic agents such as oral glycerin or intravenous mannitol.
2. A laser or surgical peripheral iridectomy must be performed for definitive treatment of the anatomic problem.

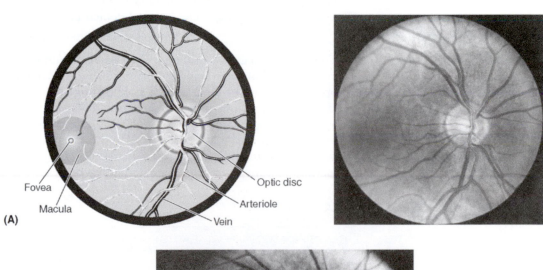

(A)

Fovea

Macula

Optic disc

Arteriole

Vein

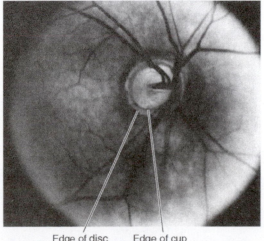

(B)   Edge of disc   Edge of cup

Figure 13–5. (A) Normal optic disc. (Photo by Diane Beeston.) (B) Glaucomatous optic disc. (Reproduced, with permission, from Vaughan DG [ed.]. *General Ophthalmology,* 15th ed. Stamford, CT: Appleton & Lange, 1999).

B. Cataract

► H&P Keys

A cataract is a lens opacity. Complaints of painless blurred vision, glare, increasing nearsightedness, or monocular double vision. History of previous eye conditions, injury, surgery, or concurrent diseases may suggest cause of cataract. Assessment of visual acuity with optical correction by means of Snellen letter chart or a number chart, or picture charts or ability to fixate on and follow or reach for a moving object for young children or adults with severe mental disability. Preferential viewing techniques may estimate visual acuity in infants. The lens is best examined for cataracts with a dilated pupil. The simplest way is with a handheld direct ophthalmoscope showing dark lenticular opacities blocking the normal red reflex of the retina. The slit-lamp biomicroscope is routinely used to detect the location and density of any opacity within the lens.

► Diagnosis

Potential visual acuity that might be expected with removal of the cataract may be estimated by the use of a potential acuity meter (PAM) or a laser interferometer. Both instruments are based on the ability of a patient to resolve letters or lines projected onto the retina.

When significant lens opacification prevents direct retinal examination, B-scan ultrasonography may be used to detect severe abnormalities of the retina, such as retinal detachment or tumors.

► Disease Severity

The clinical degree of cataract formation, assuming that no other eye disease is present, is judged primarily by visual acuity. With direct ophthalmoscopy of the posterior pole through the cataract, the ocular fundus becomes increasingly more difficult to visualize as the lens opacity becomes denser. Slit-lamp biomicroscopy allows judgment of lens clarity and location of the cataract. Glare testing and contrast sensitivity testing are new methods for quantitatively estimating the functional impact a cataract has on vision.

13-13

CLASSIFICATION OF CATARACTS

A. Age related
   1. Nuclear sclerotic
   2. Posterior subcapsular
   3. Cortical
   4. Mature
   5. Morgagnian and hypermature
B. Congenital
C. Juvenile
   1. Inborn errors of metabolism
   2. Chromosomal abnormalities
D. Secondary
   1. Traumatic or physical damage
   2. Associated with intraocular disease
      a. Chronic or recurrent uveitis
      b. Retinitis pigmentosa
      c. Retinal detachment or tumors
   3. Associated with systemic disease (e.g., hypoparathyroidism, Down syndrome, diabetes mellitus)
   4. Toxic
      a. Steriods
      b. Miotic agents
      c. Intraocular metals: copper or iron

► Concept and Application

A cataract is an opacity or loss of transparency within the lens. Cataracts may be classified by their age of onset, location, and etiology (Table 13–13). The most common indication for cataract surgery is the patient's desire for improved visual function. Medical indications for cataract surgery include phacolytic glaucoma, phacomorphic glaucoma, phacotoxic uveitis, and dense cataracts that obscure the view of the fundus and interfere with the diagnosis and management of other ocular diseases such as diabetic retinopathy or glaucoma. In children, cataract extraction is performed early to prevent otherwise irreversible visual impairment from amblyopia, the loss of visual maturation from visual sensory deprivation.

► Treatment Steps

No current medical treatment conclusively delays, prevents, or reverses the development of cataracts in adults.

1. Pupillary dilation, increased ambient illumination, or improved spectacle correction may be temporarily helpful until cataract progression causes additional symptoms.
2. Surgical removal of the cataract with or without artificial lens implantation is the definitive treatment.

BIBLIOGRAPHY

Foundation of the American Academy of Ophthalmology. *Ophthalmology Monographs.* Italy: 1999.

Kanski JS. *Clinical Ophthalmology: A Systematic Approach,* 5th ed. Boston: Butterworth–Heinemann Medical, 2003.

Spalton DJ, Hitchings RA, Hunter PA. *Atlas of Clinical Ophthalmology,* 2nd ed. London: Wolfe Publishing, 1994.

Vaughan D. *General Ophthalmology,* 16th ed. Stamford, CT: Appleton & Lange, 2003.

I. NEUROLOGY

A. Febrile Seizures

► H&P Keys

Occurs in children 6 months to 6 years of age. Signs and symptoms include generalized, tonic, atonic, tonic–clonic, or focal seizures and fever. Risk factors include positive family history, developmental delay, day care, prematurity, perinatal maternal smoking.

► Diagnosis

Diagnosis of exclusion based on history and physical exam. Evaluate for source of infection or metabolic imbalance. May include lumbar puncture (LP), blood and urine cultures, electrolytes, glucose, calcium, and complete blood count (CBC) based on clinical presentation.

► Disease Severity

Simple Febrile Seizure—Generalized seizure lasting < 15 minutes, occurring once in a 24-hour period.

Complex Febrile Seizure—A focal seizure or a generalized seizure lasting > 15 minutes, or more than one seizure in a 24-hour period.

► Concept and Application

Increased incidence in a first-degree relative. Thirty percent recurrence after first seizure. Unclear etiology.

► Treatment Steps

1. ABCs (airway, breathing, circulation).
2. Lorazepam (Ativan) or diazepam (Valium) for prolonged seizures.
3. Prophylactic anticonvulsants are controversial.

B. Infantile Botulism

► H&P Keys

Caused by the toxin of *Clostridium botulinum*. *C. botulinum* spores can be found in soil, dust, lakes, and contaminated food products, including honey. Signs and symptoms include weakness, poor feeding, weak cry, constipation, respiratory failure, symmetric descending flaccid paralysis, loss of a gag reflex, and ptosis.

► Diagnosis

Stool culture for *C. botulinum* and toxin, electrophysiologic studies.

► Disease Severity

Neurologic changes, pulmonary function tests, arterial blood gases (ABGs).

► Concept and Application

Botulinum toxin irreversibly binds to the neuromuscular junctions and inhibits exocytosis of acetylcholine, which results in flaccid paralysis.

► Treatment Steps

1. Supportive care.
2. Antitoxin (neutralizes circulating toxin before it binds to nerve endings). Must be given expediently.
3. No antibiotics. Aminoglycosides contraindicated.

C. Neural Tube Defects (NTDs)

► H&P Keys

Failure of neural tube to close in utero (normally closes by day 26). Signs and symptoms depend on the region of spinal cord involved and the extent of the lesion. Clues to diagnosis are a tuft of hair, dimple, or birthmark over the spine.

► Diagnosis

Prenatal ultrasonography, maternal α-fetoprotein (AFP), clinical exam, magnetic resonance imaging (MRI), and computed tomographic (CT) scanning.

► Disease Severity

Asymptomatic or disturbances of bowel, bladder, motor function. Degrees of severity include: spina bifida occulta (incomplete closure of the posterior lumbosacral spinal cord) (see Fig. 14–1), meningocele (herniation of the meninges through the spinal canal defect without neural tissue), encephalocele (herniation of the meninges and brain substance through a skull defect), myelomeningocele (severe spinal dysraphism with herniation of the meninges and spinal cord), anencephaly (congenital absence of the cerebral hemisphere and cranial vault). More than 75% of myelomeningoceles are associated with hydrocephalus (usually related to an Arnold–Chiari malformation). Majority have normal intelligence.

► Concept and Application

Multifactorial. Maternal folate supplementation during pregnancy has decreased its frequency.

► Treatment Steps

Multidisciplinary approach.

Figure 14–1. Spina bifida. Radiographic study of an 11-month-old with a lumbothoracic myelomeningocele who had undergone a surgical repair as a neonate. A right ventriculoperitoneal shunt was placed for the associated hydrocephalus.

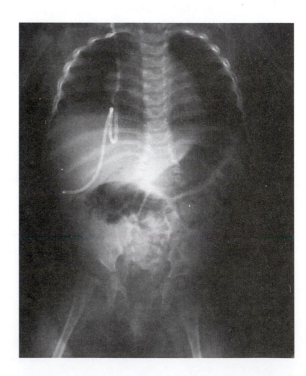

D. Malformations

1. Hydrocephalus

► **H&P Keys**

A congenital or acquired condition resulting from impaired circulation, absorption, or overproduction of cerebrospinal fluid (CSF). Can cause increased intracranial pressure. Signs and symptoms include headaches, vomiting, nausea, irritability, lethargy, third and sixth cranial nerve palsies, papilledema, bulging anterior fontanelle, rapid increase in head circumference, setting-sun sign, long-tract signs, vital sign changes.

► **Diagnosis**

Clinical exam, CT scan. Avoid LPs (risk of herniation).

► **Disease Severity**

Evidence of herniation: Cushing's triad (bradycardia, hypertension, and irregular breathing), vomiting, change of mental status.

► **Concept and Application**

Communicating—Results from either an obstruction of CSF flow from outside the ventricular system or an overproduction of CSF. Etiologies include intraventricular hemorrhages (premature infants), postinfectious state, tumors, hemorrhagic trauma.

Noncommunicating—Results from obstruction of CSF flow within the ventricular system. Etiologies include aqueductal stenosis, Chiari malformation (low cerebellar tonsils), and Dandy–Walker malformation of the fourth ventricle.

► **Treatment Steps**

Placement of a ventriculoperitoneal (VP) shunt if needed.

2. Congenital Glaucoma

► **H&P Keys**

Incidence of about 1 in 100,000 births; 30% are unilateral. Signs and symptoms include photophobia, tearing, blepharospasm, and clouding or enlargement of the cornea.

► **Diagnosis**

Intraocular pressure measurements. Clinical exam.

► **Disease Severity**

Blindness if not treated promptly.

► **Concept and Application**

Maldevelopment of the trabecular meshwork of the eye resulting in increased intraocular pressure as a result of decreased aqueous humor outflow. Autosomal recessive. Associated with conditions such as congenital rubella, neurofibromatosis, Sturge–Weber syndrome (facial port-wine stain, seizures, central nervous system [CNS] calcifications), chromosomal abnormalities, and retinopathy of prematurity.

► **Treatment Steps**

Surgery.

3. Congenital Cataracts

▶ **H&P Keys**

Unilateral or bilateral opacification of the lens. Signs and symptoms include decreased visual attentiveness, light sensitivity, decreased vision, and opacification of the lens.

▶ **Diagnosis**

Ophthalmologic exam, ocular ultrasonography. Rule out associated systemic conditions.

▶ **Disease Severity**

Varies by the degree of opacification. Blindness, amblyopia.

▶ **Concept and Application**

Often idiopathic but may have an autosomal dominant inheritance pattern. May occur as part of a systemic disease including intrauterine infections (rubella, cytomegalovirus [CMV]), metabolic diseases (galactosemia), syndromes (Marfan, Alport's), or be associated with chromosomal disorders (trisomies).

▶ **Treatment Steps**

1. Surgical removal of lens.
2. Evaluate for associated underlying problems.

II. RHEUMATOLOGY

A. Henoch-Schönlein Purpura

▶ **H&P Keys**

Small-vessel vasculitis occurring in children ages 1–7 years. Male-to-female ratio 2:1. Signs and symptoms include abdominal pain, rash, vomiting, hematemesis, and joint pain. Purpura, most commonly found on the buttocks and lower extremities, is the first sign in > 50% of cases. Patients may also have fever, gastrointestinal (GI) bleeding, intussusception (3%), and hematuria.

▶ **Diagnosis**

No pathognomonic laboratory tests. Normal platelet count and coagulation studies. Mild increase in white blood cell count (WBC) and erythrocyte sedimentation rate (ESR). Elevation of serum immunoglobulins A (IgA) and M (IgM) in 50% of cases. Skin lesions show leukocytoclastic vasculitis.

▶ **Disease Severity**

Morbidity and mortality related to the extent of GI or kidney involvement. May lead to GI hemorrhage, intussusception, or end-stage renal disease.

▶ **Concept and Application**

Leukocytoclastic vasculitis often involving the synovium, GI tract, or renal glomerulus. An immune complex disease (IgA involved).

▶ **Treatment Steps**

1. Supportive care.
2. Corticosteroids (if GI hemorrhage).
3. Anti-inflammatory agents if needed for arthritis.
4. Urinalysis (UA) to evaluate for hematuria.

B. Kawasaki Disease

► H&P Keys

Fever of ≥ 5 days associated with at least four of the following: bilateral conjunctival injection, cervical lymphadenopathy, rash, mucous membrane changes (strawberry tongue, erythema of the lips or oropharynx), extremity changes (edema, erythema).

► Diagnosis

Clinical presentation. Findings may include an elevated WBC with an elevated ESR and C-reactive protein, pyuria, uveitis, hydrops of the gallbladder, thrombocytosis (second week of illness), desquamation of the hands and feet.

► Concept and Application

Etiology unknown.

► Disease Severity

Aneurysms of the coronary arteries and other large arteries. Electrocardiographic (ECG) changes.

► Treatment Steps

1. Intravenous γ globulin.
2. Aspirin.
3. Cardiac evaluation (ECG, echocardiogram).

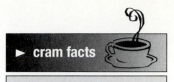

► **cram facts**

DIAGNOSTIC FEATURES
OF KAWASAKI DISEASE

- Fever (≥ 5 days)
- Bilateral nonsuppurative conjunctival injection
- Cervical lymphadenopathy
- Rash
- Mucous membrane changes (strawberry tongue, erythema of lips or oropharynx)
- Extremity changes (edema, erythema)

III. GENITOURINARY SYSTEM

A. Hypospadias

► H&P Keys

Urethral meatus located proximal to its normal position at the tip of the glans (any point along the course of the anterior urethra from the perineum to the tip of the glans). Abnormal urinary stream.

► Diagnosis

Clinical presentation.

► Disease Severity

Dependent on the location.

► Concept and Application

Failure of the urethral folds to fuse completely over the urethral groove.

► Treatment Steps

Surgical correction. Avoid circumcision (foreskin used in repair).

B. Posterior Urethral Valves

► H&P Keys

Most common cause of anatomic bladder outlet obstruction in male children. Signs and symptoms include a poor urinary stream, dribbling, absence of voiding, abdominal distention, vomiting, and failure to thrive.

► Diagnosis

Voiding cystourethrogram.

► Disease Severity

Chronic renal failure, hydronephrosis.

► Concept and Application

Mucosal folds obstruct the posterior urethra.

► Treatment Steps

Early surgical repair.

C. Vesicoureteral Reflux

► H&P Keys

Often asymptomatic. May develop features of urinary tract infection (fever, vomiting, flank pain, dysuria, frequency, urgency, irritability).

► Diagnosis

Voiding cystourethrogram.

► Disease Severity

Renal scarring, pyelonephritis.

► Concept and Application

Abnormal backflow of urine from the bladder into the ureters or kidneys. Increased incidence of reflux in siblings.

► Treatment Steps

Management depends on grade of reflux and the amount of renal scarring.

1. Medical management includes treatment of the urinary tract infection and prophylactic antibiotics.
2. Surgical correction of the anatomic defect if severe reflux or scarring.

D. Infantile Polycystic Disease

► H&P Keys

Signs and symptoms include enlarged palpable kidneys, oliguria, and respiratory insufficiency in the neonate. Older infants may present with hepatosplenomegaly, flank masses, renal tubular acidosis, and hypertension.

► Diagnosis

Renal ultrasonography.

► Disease Severity

Renal insufficiency, hypertension, portal hypertension, hepatic fibrosis, variable cortical atrophy.

► Concept and Application

Bilateral renal cystic disease, autosomal recessive inheritance.

► Treatment Steps

1. Treatment of hypertension.
2. Management of chronic renal failure.
3. Management of portal hypertension.

E. Multicystic Kidney Disease

► H&P Keys

A unilateral, dysplastic, nonfunctioning kidney. Usually an asymptomatic abdominal mass.

► Diagnosis

Renal ultrasonography.

► **cram facts**

CONGENITAL KIDNEY DISEASE

	Involvement	Inherited
Multicystic kidney disease	Unilateral	No
Polycystic kidney disease	Bilateral	Yes

► Treatment Steps
1. Evaluation of renal function.
2. Monitoring.
3. Kidney not routinely removed.

F. Undescended Testis

► H&P Keys
Nonpalpable testis.

► Diagnosis
Clinical exam, ultrasonography (location of testis).

► Disease Severity
More prone to testicular torsion, malignant degeneration, and impaired fertility.

► Concept and Application
Result of mechanical hindrance, abnormal epididymal development, or endocrine dysfunction during fetal development.

► Treatment Steps
1. Surgical orchiopexy before 2 years of age.
2. Consider hormonal therapy.

IV. NEONATOLOGY

A. Transient Tachypnea of the Newborn (TTN)

► H&P Keys
Mild self-limited respiratory disorder seen more frequently in infants born by cesarean section. Signs and symptoms include increased respiratory rate, mild cyanosis, and retractions.

► Diagnosis
Chest x-ray (CXR) shows prominent vascular markings with fluid in the fissures. Diagnosis of exclusion.

► Disease Severity
Respiratory rate, cyanosis, ABGs, pulse oximetry.

► Concept and Application
Delayed resorption of fetal lung fluid.

► Treatment Steps
1. ABCs.
2. Supportive care.

B. Respiratory Distress Syndrome

► H&P Keys

Incidence inversely proportional to the newborn's gestational age and birth weight. Signs and symptoms include respiratory distress (tachypnea, grunting, nasal flaring, retractions) soon after delivery.

► Diagnosis

CXR shows a fine reticular granularity of the lung fields and air bronchograms (Fig. 14–2). Must differentiate from other causes of respiratory distress in newborns (sepsis, heart disease, CNS disorders, lung anomalies).

► Disease Severity

ABGs, pulse oximetry, hemoglobin, metabolic disturbances, cardiovascular compromise. Long-term complications include bronchopulmonary dysplasia (BPD), cor pulmonale, retinopathy of prematurity, poor growth, and persistent patent ductus arteriosus.

► Concept and Application

Secondary to lung immaturity (surfactant deficiency), incomplete structural lung development, and highly compliant chest wall. Results in atelectasis, hyaline membrane formation, and pulmonary edema.

► Treatment Steps

1. Prevention of prematurity.
2. Maternal steroid administration 48–72 hours prior to delivery to stimulate fetal surfactant production.
3. Neonatal surfactant via endotracheal tube at delivery for premature infants (surfactant serves to reduce surface tension of the alveoli).

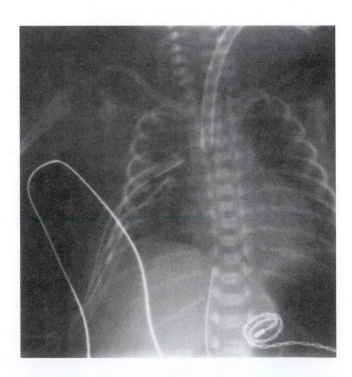

Figure 14–2. Respiratory distress syndrome. Radiographic study of a 2-week-old infant who was prematurely born at 23 weeks' gestation. This neonate requires ventilator support for his persistent respiratory distress. The lung fields show a fine reticular granularity and air bronchograms. Two chest tubes noted in right lung field.

4. Supportive care (correction of hypoxia, acidosis, and hypercapnia).

C. Meconium Aspiration

▶ **H&P Keys**

Presence of meconium in the amniotic fluid and the newborn's trachea. Signs and symptoms include retractions, increased respiratory rate, cyanosis, and hypoxia.

▶ **Diagnosis**

Clinical presentation, CXR.

▶ **Disease Severity**

Severe respiratory distress with increased respiratory rate, retractions, and hypoxia requiring ventilatory support; pneumothorax; pulmonary hypertension.

▶ **Concept and Application**

Aspiration of meconium-contaminated amniotic fluid leading to airway obstruction and poor gas exchange.

▶ **Treatment Steps**

1. Suctioning the infant on the perineum.
2. Direct visualization and suctioning of the trachea in distressed infants.
3. ABCs.
4. Chest physiotherapy.
5. Supplemental oxygen.
6. Mechanical ventilation if needed.

D. Rh Incompatibility

▶ **H&P Keys**

Infant of a gravida 2 Rh-negative mother. Signs and symptoms include pallor, respiratory distress, cardiomegaly, edema.

▶ **Diagnosis**

Rh type, ABO group, Coombs' test (positive), hemoglobin, blood smear (hemolysis), reticulocyte count (increased), and bilirubin (increased).

▶ **Disease Severity**

Hydrops fetalis; severe anemia leading to heart failure, ascites, pleural and pericardial effusions; thrombocytopenia; organomegaly; elevated bilirubin leading to kernicterus (staining of the basal ganglia).

▶ **cram facts**

EMESIS IN CHILDREN

	Bilious	Abdominal Mass	Serum pH
Pyloric stenosis	No	Yes	Elevated
Malrotation	Yes	No	Decreased
Intussusception	Yes	Yes	Decreased

► **Concept and Application**

Sensitization and antibody formation in an Rh-negative mother exposed to Rh-positive fetal blood (contains D antigen). This antibody crosses the placenta, causing hemolytic disease in the fetus. Rarely occurs during the first pregnancy.

► **Treatment Steps**

1. Supportive therapy, including volume expansion, red blood cell (RBC) transfusion, and ventilatory support if needed.
2. Exchange transfusion in extreme cases.
3. Prevention in Rh-negative mothers with the administration of Rh_o(D) immune globulin (RhoGAM).

E. Neonatal Hyperbilirubinemia

► **H&P Keys**

Signs and symptoms depend on the etiology. Ascertain a maternal history (blood type, race, illnesses during pregnancy, drug usage, family history of anemia), and an infant history (birth weight, onset of jaundice, stooling pattern, trauma, feeding pattern [breast-feeding], emesis).

► **Diagnosis**

Total and direct bilirubin (normal total levels rise to a mean of 6.5 ± 2.5 mg/dL in a full-term formula-fed infant). Hemoglobin, smear, reticulocyte count, maternal and infant blood type, direct Coombs' (evidence of hemolysis), albumin level; urine Clinitest; culture if sepsis is suspected.

► **Disease Severity**

Elevated bilirubin in the first 24 hours of life is pathologic. Kernicterus (bilirubin staining and necrosis of neurons in the basal ganglion) especially with hemolytic disease.

► **Concept and Application**

Physiologic jaundice is found in 60% of newborns with maximum values reached in the second to fourth day (6–8 mg/dL) as a result of inefficient bilirubin conjugation and excretion. Jaundice due to breast-feeding reaches a maximum level of 7.3 ± 3.9 mg/dL. The etiology is unknown. Elevated levels of bilirubin also occur with increased turnover of RBCs from hemolysis (ABO or Rh incompatibility), significant bruising, cephalhematomas, structural or metabolic abnormalities of RBCs, or hereditary defects of bilirubin conjugation (Crigler–Najjar syndrome, Gilbert disease).

► **Treatment Steps**

1. Evaluation and treatment for underlying pathologic etiologies.
2. Encouragement of fluid intake.
3. Phototherapy with pathologically elevated bilirubin levels.
4. Exchange transfusion in severe cases.

F. Developmental Dysplasia of the Hip

► **H&P Keys**

A higher incidence with breech deliveries, first-born children, females, and oligohydramnios. Left hip more commonly involved. Twenty percent have a positive family history. Signs and symptoms include Barlow sign (posterosuperior movement of the femur over the limbus with adduction and posteriorly directed pressure), Or-

► **management decisions**

Febrile Seizures
ABCs (airway, breathing, circulation); lorazepam (Ativan) or diazepam (Valium) for prolonged seizures; prophylactic anticonvulsants are controversial.

Kawasaki Disease
Intravenous γ globulin; aspirin; cardiac evaluation (ECG, echocardiogram).

Neonatal Hyperbilirubinemia
Evaluation and treatment for underlying etiology; encouragement of fluid intake; phototherapy with pathologically elevated bilirubin levels; exchange transfusion in severe cases.

tolani sign (relocation of the hip with abduction, causing a dull clunk) (see Fig. 14–3), asymmetric leg lengths, and asymmetric thigh creases. A limitation of abduction is seen in older infants.

► Diagnosis
Clinical exam, hip ultrasonogram, radiography.

► Disease Severity
Three degrees of hip dysplasia in order of increasing severity: subluxable, dislocatable, dislocated. Can lead to avascular necrosis and decreased range of motion.

► Concept and Application
Multifactorial (mechanical, hormonal, and hereditary).

► Treatment Steps
1. Goal is to restore contact between the femoral head and the acetabulum.
2. Management depends on the degree of hip dysplasia and the age at diagnosis. Harness, closed reduction (traction), open reduction.

V. INFECTIOUS DISEASES

A. Bronchiolitis

► H&P Keys
Common (60% of infants). Winter-to-spring months. Peak age < 24 months. Signs and symptoms include cough, rhinorrhea, with or without low-grade fever, scattered wheezing with or without rales, labored breathing.

► Diagnosis
Clinical features (age, season, physical). Evaluation of nasopharyngeal secretions (viral culture, enzyme-linked immunosorbent assay [ELISA], or immunofluorescence). CXR has nonspecific changes (hyperinflation, atelectasis, with or without interstitial infiltrates).

► Disease Severity
General appearance, mental status changes, labored breathing (tachypnea, nasal flaring, retractions, accessory muscle use), cyanosis, pulse oximetry, ABG if severe distress. Higher morbidity and mortality if infant has underlying pulmonary or cardiac disease, immunodeficiency disease, underlying chronic disease, history of prematurity, or is < 6 weeks old.

► Concept and Application
Viral infection (primary cause is respiratory syncytial virus) of lower respiratory tract. Transmission by direct contact. Respiratory mucosal injury, inflammation or edema, mucus production.

► Treatment Steps
1. Prevention by hand washing and monoclonal antibody injections (for children at risk).
2. Supportive care including oxygen if hypoxic.
3. Aerosolized β_2-adrenergic agent trial.
4. Use of ribavirin and steroids controversial.

► **on rounds**

PEDIATRIC INFECTIONS

Croup
- Ages 6–36 months, also termed *laryngotracheitis.*
- Barklike cough, hoarseness, inspiratory stridor, CXR positive steeple sign (subglottic swelling).
- Worse at night.
- Supportive treatment, mist, O_2.

Epiglottitis
- Ages 2–7.
- Fever, drooling, dysphagia, stridor, may have abnormal lateral neck x-ray, possible toxic appearance, anxious.
- Winter most often.
- Support airway, visualization in OR followed by intubation.

Bronchiolitis
- Peak age < 2 years.
- Cough, wheezing, labored breathing, nonspecific CXR.
- Winter to spring occurrence.
- Supportive treatment.

B. Otitis Media

► H&P Keys
Peak age < 24 months. Winter season. Signs and symptoms include pain, fever, hearing loss, cough, and congestion as well as hyperemia, dullness, decreased mobility, retraction or bulging (loss of landmarks) of tympanic membrane. Asymptomatic in 50% of cases.

► Diagnosis
Pneumatic otoscopy, tympanometry, audiometry.

► Disease Severity
Overall appearance, degree of discomfort or hearing loss, response to therapy. Higher morbidity if young age (< 6 months), environmental setting (passive smoking, day care), genetic factors (familial, trisomy 21, Native American), immunodeficiency, congenital anomalies (cleft palate, choanal atresia).

► Concept and Application
Bacterial infection (usually *Streptococcus pneumoniae,* nontypable *Haemophilus influenzae, Moraxella catarrhalis*) of middle ear. Viral co-pathogens (40%). Often results from a dysfunctional eustachian tube.

► Treatment Steps
1. First-line antibiotics include aminopenicillins.
2. Consider coverage for pneumococcal resistent organisms in high-risk groups (e.g., day care, age < 2 years, recent antibiotic use).
3. Consider myringotomy tubes if persistent effusion with hearing loss, failure of prophylaxis, or high-risk groups (e.g., trisomy 21, cleft palate, known sensorineural hearing loss).
4. Prevention with pneumococcal vaccine.

C. Epiglottitis (Supraglottitis)

► **H&P Keys**

Ages 2–7 years if unvaccinated. Winter months. Signs and symptoms include acute hyperpyrexia (39°C), hoarseness, drooling, dysphagia, anxious or toxic appearance, stridor, and respiratory distress. Rare in vaccinated children.

► **Diagnosis**

Clinical presentation (high index of suspicion!). Lateral neck x-ray (thumb-shaped epiglottis, ballooning of hypopharynx) only if presentation not classical. Cultures of epiglottis and blood after airway secured.

► **Disease Severity**

Overall appearance. Mental status changes. Respiratory distress (tachypnea, inspiratory stridor, retractions, cyanosis). Hypoxia and hypercapnia.

► **Concept and Application**

Edema or cellulitis of epiglottis resulting in glottic narrowing. Primarily *H. influenzae* type b (> 90%).

► **Treatment Steps**

1. Prevention is key (Hib vaccine).
2. Early suspicion.
3. ABCs.
4. Minimal disturbance to child.
5. Direct visualization and culture of epiglottis in operating room followed by intubation.
6. Emergent cricothyrotomy if complete airway obstruction.

D. Laryngotracheitis (Croup)

► **H&P Keys**

Ages 6–36 months. Nocturnal. Severity of disease peaks at 3–5 days. Signs and symptoms include barklike cough, hoarseness, upper respiratory symptoms, inspiratory stridor.

► **Diagnosis**

Clinical presentation, steeple sign (subglottic swelling) on CXR.

► **Disease Severity**

Overall appearance, mental status changes, respiratory distress, hypoxia and hypercapnia.

► **Concept and Application**

Mucosal edema and swelling of subglottis and trachea leading to hypoxia and atelectasis. Primarily caused by parainfluenza virus.

► **Treatment Steps**

1. Supportive (especially airway).
2. Minimal disturbance.
3. Mist.
4. Oxygen if hypoxemia.
5. Racemic epinephrine or dexamethasone if severe respiratory distress.

E. Varicella (Chickenpox)

► **H&P Keys**

Incubation period of 14–15 days. Winter or spring months. Contagious period is 4–5 days prior to exanthem and until rash scabs.

Signs and symptoms include fever, malaise, vesicles with erythematous base ("teardrop on rose petal") beginning on hairline or trunk and spreading to extremities.

▶ **Diagnosis**

Characteristic rash. Fluorescein monoclonal antibody.

▶ **Disease Severity**

Worse course if < 1 year of age, teenager or adult, or visceral involvement (lungs, CNS, liver, joints, heart, kidneys).

▶ **Concept and Application**

Human herpes varicella-zoster virus. Respiratory (direct contact) transmission. Cutaneous tissue involvement after primary or secondary viremia. Lifelong immunity after infection.

▶ **Treatment Steps**

1. Prevention is key (varicella vaccine).
2. Antipruritic drug.
3. Antimicrobial therapy if secondary infection (usually group A streptococcus).
4. Acyclovir if child is immunocompromised, older, or severely involved.

F. Pharyngitis

▶ **H&P Keys**

Signs and symptoms include fever, sore throat, hoarseness, cough, abdominal pain, tonsillar erythema or enlargement or exudate, petechiae of palate, anterior cervical adenopathy, "sandpaper" rash. Concomitant nasal symptoms suggest viral etiology.

▶ **Diagnosis**

Throat culture, rapid *Streptococcus* antigen test.

▶ **Disease Severity**

Clinical discomfort. Suppurative complications (cervical adenitis, otitis media, septicemia). Nonsuppurative complications (rheumatic fever, nephritis).

▶ **Concept and Application**

Cellulitis of pharynx and tonsils. Organisms include group A β-hemolytic streptococci, adenovirus, influenza virus, Epstein–Barr virus.

▶ **Treatment Steps**

1. Self-limiting if viral etiology.
2. Penicillin (erythromycin if penicillin allergy) for 10 days if group A β-hemolytic streptococci.

G. Bacterial Meningitis

▶ **H&P Keys**

Signs and symptoms include fever, lethargy, irritability, neck stiffness or pain, headache, altered consciousness, nuchal rigidity, Kernig's sign, Brudzinski's sign.

▶ **Diagnosis**

Bacterial culture of CSF is gold standard. CSF cytology and biochemical parameters. Bacterial antigen test if child currently on antibiotics.

► **Disease Severity**

Mental status change, focal or persistent neurologic deficit, syndrome of inappropriate secretion of antidiuretic hormone (SIADH), neonatal infection, focal or late-onset seizures. Long-term sequelae include learning disability, hearing impairment, seizure disorders.

► **Concept and Application**

Primarily hematogenous spread to CSF. *S. pneumoniae* and *Neisseria meningitidis* are usual pathogens in childhood (group B streptococcus, *Escherichia coli,* or other gram-negative enteric bacilli, *Listeria monocytogenes* in neonates).

► **Treatment Steps**

1. Age-specific antibiotics pending cultures. Respiratory isolation.
2. Identification and treatment of associated complications if necessary.
3. Prevention (vaccine, treatment of carrier state).
4. Consider dexamethasone in infants > 6 weeks with Hib meningitis.

H. Congenital Infections (STORCH)

1. Congenital Syphilis

► **H&P Keys**

Characteristic features include skin rash (palms and soles), hepatosplenomegaly, snuffles (blood-tinged nasal discharge), Parrot's pseudoparalysis (periostitis), saber shins, Hutchinson (peg) teeth, thrombocytopenia, anemia, jaundice, saddle nose, hepatitis.

► **Diagnosis**

Serology (rapid plasma reagin [RPR], fluorescent treponemal antibody absorption [FTA-ABS]), darkfield examination (organism).

► **Concept and Application**

Spirochete (*Treponema pallidum*).

► **Treatment Steps**

1. Prevention.
2. Prenatal screening.
3. Penicillin for all infected mothers and infants with positive serology without documented adequate treatment.

2. Congenital Toxoplasmosis

► **H&P Keys**

Characteristic features include chorioretinitis, scattered CNS calcifications, hydrocephalus, developmental delay.

► **Diagnosis**

Serology (organism isolation).

► **Concept and Application**

Intracellular protozoan parasite (*Toxoplasma gondii*).

► **Treatment Steps**

1. Prevention (avoid cat litter and undercooked meat).
2. Multidisciplinary approach.
3. Pyrimethamine and/or sulfadiazine have variable effectiveness.

3. Human Immunodeficiency Virus (HIV)

► **H&P Keys**

One-third of infants of HIV-positive mothers will develop acquired immune deficiency syndrome (AIDS). Presentation variable (e.g.,

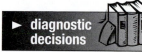

► **diagnostic decisions**

CONGENITAL INFECTIONS (STORCH)

Syphilis
T. pallidum; snuffles, palm and sole rash, anemia, hepatosplenomegaly, periostitis, peg teeth, saddle nose; prescription penicillin.

Toxoplasmosis
T. gondii; oocysts from cat litter and meat; hydrocephalus, chorioretinitis, scattered CNS calcifications; prescription pyrimethamine.

Other
HIV, hepatitis B, varicella.

Rubella
Blueberry muffin lesions, hepatosplenomegaly, anemia, cardiac lesions, deafness, cataracts.

Cytomegalovirus
Most common congenital infection; usually asymptomatic; hepatosplenomegaly, jaundice, deafness, microcephaly, periventricular CNS calcifications.

Herpes Simplex
Usually acquired at birth; seizures (temporal lobe); encephalitis, vesicles, overwhelming sepsis, hepatitis; prescription acyclovir.

frequent infections, developmental or growth delay, lymphadenopathy, persistent thrush).

► Diagnosis
1. Polymerase chain reaction (PCR) useful in diagnosis and viral load detection.
2. Serology.

► Concept and Application
Human retrovirus that infects tissue cells (including helper T cells).

► Treatment Steps
Azidothymidine (AZT). Antimicrobial therapy for infections. Poor prognosis.

1. Prevention is key.
2. Treatment of infected pregnant women has decreased the incidence of vertical transmission.
3. Antiretroviral drugs and immunomodulators.
4. Vaccines are under investigation.

4. Congenital Rubella Infection (German Measles)

► H&P Keys
Characteristic features include intrauterine growth retardation (IUGR), congenital cardiac defects, cataracts, deafness, thrombocytopenia, "blueberry muffin" skin lesions, hepatosplenomegaly.

► Diagnosis
Serology (organism isolation).

► Concept and Application
Multiorgan damage by the virus.

► Treatment Steps
1. Prevention is key (rubella vaccine).
2. Prenatal screening.
3. Multidisciplinary approach.

5. Congenital Cytomegalovirus Infection (CMV)

► H&P Keys
Majority of cases are asymptomatic. Characteristic features include jaundice, hepatosplenomegaly, microcephaly, chorioretinitis, deafness, periventricular CNS calcification, IUGR.

► Diagnosis
Organism isolation (serology).

► Concept and Application
Herpesvirus. Multiorgan involvement. Transmission with primary or recurrent maternal infection.

► Treatment Steps
1. Prevention by hand washing.
2. Multidisciplinary approach.
3. Antiviral treatment controversial.

6. Herpes Simplex Virus (HSV)

► H&P Keys
Incidence of HSV: 1 in 5,000 deliveries. Characteristic features include vesicular skin rash, chorioretinitis, meningoencephalitis, seizures, microcephaly.

► Diagnosis

Organism isolation (Tzanck test, immunofluorescent studies).

► Concept and Application

HSV-2 (70%). Transmission more likely during primary maternal infection.

► Treatment Steps

1. Antiviral (acyclovir) therapy.
2. Supportive care.

I. Hemolytic–Uremic Syndrome

► H&P Keys

Children usually between 2 months and 8 years of age. Triad of uremia, thrombocytopenia, and microangiopathic hemolytic anemia. Signs and symptoms include preceding illness (diarrhea or upper respiratory infection [URI]), irritability, bloody diarrhea, poor urinary output, pallor, petechiae, edema, hypertension.

► Diagnosis

CBC with platelets and smear (red blood cell [RBC] morphology), Coombs' test (negative), electrolytes with blood urea nitrogen (BUN) and creatinine (Cr).

► Disease Severity

Seizures, stroke, coma, cardiac failure, metabolic imbalance (metabolic acidosis).

► Concept and Application

No one causative factor (viral, bacterial, drugs). Peripheral destruction of platelets, RBC hemolysis secondary to mechanical destruction by fibrin strands in small renal vessels.

► Treatment Steps

1. Supportive care.
2. Correction of fluid and electrolyte imbalance.
3. Correction of hypertension.
4. Dialysis and RBC transfusion if needed.

VI. GASTROENTEROLOGY

A. Cleft Lip or Palate

► H&P Keys

Common (1/1,000 live births). Family history.

► Diagnosis

Clinical.

► Disease Severity

Feeding problems, frequent ear infections, speech problems. Associated with many anomalies.

► Concept and Application

Failure of primary (lip) and secondary (cleft) palate closure. Multifactorial inheritance (3–5% recurrence with an affected parent or sibling; 10% if two affected parents or siblings).

► Treatment Steps

1. Multidisciplinary approach.
2. Surgical repair.

B. Tracheoesophageal Fistula (TEF)

▶ **H&P Keys**

Signs and symptoms of TEF include excessive oral secretions, coughing or choking on foods, tachypnea, wheezing, rales.

▶ **Diagnosis**

Inability to pass nasal catheter to stomach. Surgical exploration. Barium studies rarely needed.

▶ **Disease Severity**

Respiratory distress, signs and symptoms of aspiration pneumonia.

▶ **Concept and Application**

Failure of trachea and esophagus to separate during embryogenesis. Proximal esophageal atresia with a tracheal-to-distal esophageal fistula is most common type (85%).

▶ **Treatment Steps**

Surgery.

C. Pyloric Stenosis

▶ **H&P Keys**

Average age 3–4 weeks of life. First-born males. Signs and symptoms include progressive nonbilious projectile emesis, peristaltic abdominal waves in epigastrium, palpable right upper quadrant mass ("olive").

▶ **Diagnosis**

Clinical. Sonogram or upper GI (UGI) series ("tram-track" sign) if necessary. Hypochloremic hypokalemic metabolic alkalosis.

▶ **Disease Severity**

Cachexia, profound dehydration, severe metabolic imbalance.

▶ **Concept and Application**

Mechanical gastric outlet obstruction results from congenitally hypertrophied pyloric muscle.

▶ **Treatment Steps**

1. Correction of fluid and electrolyte abnormality.
2. Surgical repair (pyloromyotomy).

D. Malrotation of the Small Intestine

▶ **H&P Keys**

Bilious projectile emesis, abdominal distention.

▶ **Diagnosis**

Clinical. Barium study.

▶ **Disease Severity**

Melena (secondary to intestinal ischemia), sepsis, signs and symptoms of peritonitis or perforation.

▶ **Concept and Application**

Mechanical obstruction from either poor fixation of cecum to abdominal wall (midgut volvulus or twisting) or extrinsic bands.

▶ **Treatment Steps**

Surgery (15–20% mortality rate).

E. Intussusception

► H&P Keys

Most common cause of intestinal obstruction ages 3–12 months. Signs and symptoms include intermittent colicky pain, bilious emesis, mental status changes, palpable "sausage-shaped" abdominal mass, "currant jelly" stools (Fig. 14–3).

► Diagnosis

Clinical. Barium enema.

► Disease Severity

Severe metabolic acidosis, evidence of intestinal ischemia or infarction, severe dehydration.

► Concept and Application

Invagination or telescoping of proximal bowel into more distal bowel. Lymphatic and venous compromise. Primarily ileocolic region. Leadpoint lesion (e.g., polyp, lymphoma) in older children.

► Treatment Steps

1. Barium enema reduction.
2. Antibiotics if peritoneal signs.
3. Occasionally, surgical reduction.

F. Necrotizing Enterocolitis (NEC)

► H&P Keys

Characteristic features of NEC include prematurity (75%), poor feeding or regurgitation, emesis, hematochezia, temperature instability, gastric retention, abdominal distention with decreased bowel sounds.

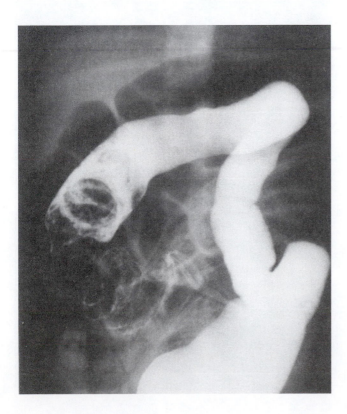

Figure 14–3. Intussusception.
Barium enema of a 4-month-old infant with intermittent colicky pain, pallor, poor tone, and a palpable "sausage-shaped" abdominal mass. The contrast material did not descend into the ileocecal region. The diagnosis was confirmed during an explorative laparoscopy.

► Diagnosis

Clinical. Blood or reducing substances in stool, thrombocytopenia, prolonged prothrombin time (PT) and partial thromboplastin time (PTT). Pneumatosis intestinalis, bowel wall edema, biliary air, or free air in peritoneum on abdominal x-ray.

► Disease Severity

Evidence of sepsis, hemorrhage, disseminated intravascular coagulation (DIC), shock, severe metabolic acidosis, mental status changes.

► Concept and Application

Unknown. Presentation consistent with bowel ischemia or infarction.

► Treatment Steps

1. Bowel rest.
2. Fluid resuscitation.
3. Parenteral nutrition.
4. Broad-spectrum antibiotics.
5. Surgery if failure of medical management or if complications.

G. Colonic Aganglionosis (Hirschsprung's Disease)

► H&P Keys

Absence of meconium stools in first week of life. Signs and symptoms include emesis, abdominal distention, minimal stool in rectal vault.

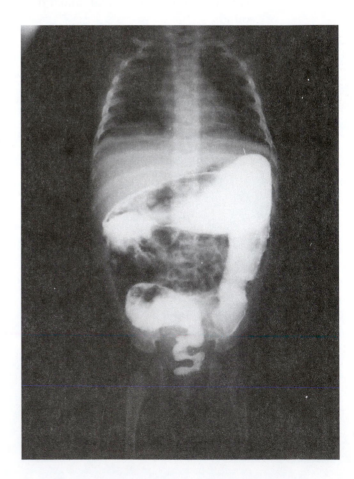

Figure 14–4. Hirschsprung's disease. Barium enema of a 4-day-old infant with abdominal distention, green emesis, a tight rectum, and an explosive liquid stool following the rectal examination. The lumen of the rectum is contracted with proximal colonic dilatation, suggesting congenital aganglionosis. The diagnosis was confirmed with a rectal biopsy.

► **Diagnosis**

Clinical. Rectal biopsy. Barium study in older children (Fig. 14–4).

► **Disease Severity**

Presentation can simulate sepsis or NEC.

► **Concept and Application**

Absence of colonic ganglia resulting in persistent colonic contraction.

► **Treatment Steps**

Surgery.

VII. GENETICS

A. Down Syndrome (Trisomy 21)

► **H&P Keys**

Characteristic features include epicanthal folds, upslanting palpebral fissures, transverse palmar (simian) creases, cardiac anomalies (40%) including septal defects, atlantoaxial instability (12%), duodenal atresia (4–7%), short stature, leukemia (1%), thyroid disease, sterility in males, early Alzheimer's disease, shortened life span (Fig. 14–5).

► **Diagnosis**

Clinical. Chromosome analysis (classical trisomy [95%], translocation [4%], mosaic [1%]). Prenatal screening (amniocentesis, chorionic villus sampling) in high-risk groups (advanced maternal age).

► **Treatment Steps**

1. Supportive care.
2. Cardiac evaluation.
3. Correction of anomalies.
4. Genetic counseling.
5. Special education.

B. Trisomy 18

► **H&P Keys**

Characteristic features include IUGR, micrognathia, clenched hands with overlapping fingers, congenital heart disease (ventricular septal defect [VSD], patent ductus arteriosus [PDA]), mental retardation.

► **Diagnosis**

Clinical. Chromosome analysis.

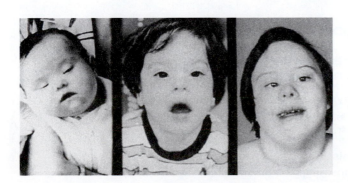

Figure 14–5. Typical phenotype in Down syndrome.

► **diagnostic decisions**

CHROMOSOMAL ABNORMALITIES

Trisomy 21
Down syndrome; 1/700 births; mental retardation, cardiac (atrioventricular canal), duodenal atresia, simian creases, epicanthal folds.

Trisomy 13
Poor prognosis; 1/10,000 births; cleft lip/palate, CNS malformations (holoprosencephaly), renal and ocular malformations.

Trisomy 18
Poor prognosis; 1/5,000 births; IUGR, clenched hands, rocker-bottom feet, cardiac (VSD, PDA).

5P
Cri du chat; catlike cry, mental retardation, microcephaly.

45,XO
Turner syndrome; 1/2,000 newborn girls; short webbed neck, horseshoe kidney, coarctation of aorta, primary amenorrhea.

47,XXY
Klinefelter's syndrome; 1/1,000 boys, seminiferous tubule dysgenesis, hypogonadism, tall stature, gynecomastia, infertility.

► Treatment Steps
Same as for trisomy 21.

C. Trisomy 13

► **H&P Keys**
Characteristic features include cleft lip or palate (60–80%), microcephaly, urinary tract malformations, CNS and ocular malformations, aplasia cutis congenita, polydactyly.

► **Diagnosis**
Clinical. Chromosome analysis.

► **Treatment Steps**
Same as for trisomy 21.

D. Gonadal Dysgenesis 45,XO (Turner's Syndrome)

► **H&P Keys**
Characteristic features include transient lymphedema of feet and hands at birth (80–90%), short stature, short webbed neck, short fourth metacarpal bone, cardiac defects (coarctation of aorta), renal anomalies (horseshoe kidney), lack of secondary sex characteristics with primary amenorrhea. Normal intelligence. Most spontaneously abort in early pregnancy.

► **Diagnosis**
Clinical. Chromosome analysis.

► **Treatment Steps**
1. Evaluation for and correction of anomalies.
2. Psychosocial counseling.
3. Estrogen replacement at puberty.
4. Consider growth hormone therapy.

E. Fragile X Syndrome

► **H&P Keys**
Characteristic features include mental retardation, hyperactivity, seizures, prominent ears, long face, macro-orchidism. Common cause of mental retardation in males (1/1,000).

► **Diagnosis**
Chromosome analysis with fragile X studies.

► **Treatment Steps**
1. Genetic counseling.
2. Supportive.

VIII. PULMONOLOGY

A. Congenital Laryngeal Stridor (Laryngomalacia)

► **H&P Keys**
Signs and symptoms include noisy "crowing" respirations (positional) and stridor.

► **Diagnosis**
Clinical. Fluoroscopy or direct visualization.

► Disease Severity

Respiratory distress (tachypnea, retractions, poor air movement).

► Concept and Application

Delayed maturation of newborn larynx, resulting in increased flexibility.

► Treatment Steps

Positioning (self-limited).

B. Congenital Lobar Emphysema

► H&P Keys

Most common congenital lung lesion. Respiratory distress in early infancy.

► Diagnosis

CXR (radiolucent lobe, mediastinal shift). Mimics pneumothorax.

► Disease Severity

Severe respiratory distress or cyanosis.

► Concept and Application

In utero bronchial obstruction with normal alveolar histology. Usually unilateral.

► Treatment Steps

Surgical resection.

C. Cystic Adenomatoid Malformation

► H&P Keys

Respiratory distress in infancy.

► Diagnosis

CXR (mediastinal shift, multiple cystic areas). Mimics diaphragmatic hernia.

► Concept and Application

Early embryonic insult with cysts and little normal lung tissue.

► Treatment Steps

Surgical resection. Significant mortality and morbidity.

D. Pulmonary Sequestration

► H&P Keys

Fever, hemoptysis, and respiratory symptoms if intralobar. Respiratory symptoms, heart failure, or no symptoms if extralobar. Dullness to percussion, heart murmur.

► Diagnosis

CXR (mass). Further investigation includes bronchoscopy, sonogram, and aortogram.

► Concept and Application

Segments of nonfunctioning embryonic lung tissue that are nourished by anomalous systemic circulation. Intralobar type occurs within normal visceral pleura. Extralobar type has separate visceral pleural covering.

► Treatment Steps

Surgical resection.

IX. DISORDERS OF THE MUSCULOSKELETAL SYSTEM

A. Scoliosis

▶ Description

A lateral curvature of the spine involving the thoracic and/or lumbar vertebrae.

▶ Diagnosis

Clinical evaluation of patient's back in an erect and a bent-at-the-hips position. X-rays can quantitate any curvature > 10 degrees.

▶ Treatment

Depends on severity of curvature. Follow curves < 15–20 degrees closely at interval health maintenance visits. If curvature is > 20 degrees, the patient should be referred to an orthopedic surgeon for additional therapy, which may include bracing or surgical intervention.

B. Kyphosis

▶ Description

An excessive roundback of the thoracic spine.

▶ Diagnosis

Physical examination. X-rays may be used to differentiate a postural and structural defect.

▶ Treatment

Improvement of posture, back exercises, braces.

C. Slipped Capital Femoral Epiphysis

▶ Description

Posterior-medial displacement of femoral head. Occurs most frequently in males and is associated with obesity.

▶ Diagnosis

History significant for pain in hip or knee region. X-ray of the hip shows femoral head displacement.

▶ Treatment

Surgical intervention required.

D. Osgood–Schlatter Disease

▶ Description

Stress changes at the tibial tuberosity. Most commonly seen in adolescent males during growth spurt.

▶ Diagnosis

Clinical. Point tenderness at tibial tuberosity with occasional associated swelling.

▶ Treatment

Supportive.

BIBLIOGRAPHY

Avery GB, Fletcher MA, MacDonald MG. *Neonatology: Pathophysiology and Management of the Newborn,* 5th ed. Philadelphia: Lippincott Williams & Wilkins, 1999.

Behrman RE, Kliegman RM, Jenson HB. *Nelson Textbook of Pediatrics,* 17th ed. Philadelphia: W.B. Saunders, 2004.

Burg FD, Ingelfinger JR, Polin RA, Gershon AA. *Gellis & Kagan's Current Pediatric Therapy,* 17th ed. Philadelphia: W.B. Saunders, 2002.

McMillan JA, DeAngelis CD, Feigin RD, Warshaw JB. *Oski's Pediatrics: Principles & Practice,* 3rd ed. Philadelphia: Lippincott Williams & Wilkins, 1999.

Psychiatry | 15

I. PSYCHOSES

A. Schizophrenia

▶ H&P Keys

History—Family history; onset late teens through twenties, often triggered by stress; may have premorbid schizotypal features; symptoms for at least 6 months.

Physical and Mental Status Exam—Hallucinations, delusions, disorganized speech, bizarre behavior (positive symptoms); agitated, constricted, inappropriate affect; social withdrawal, poor self-care, anhedonia, poverty of speech, lack of motivation, attentional impairment (negative symptoms); may have soft neurologic signs.

▶ Diagnosis

No pathognomonic signs or lab studies; rule out general medical etiology (e.g., substance abuse, temporal lobe epilepsy, delirium, medications, central nervous system [CNS] infections, trauma, tumors, endocrine and metabolic disorders); psychotic affective, schizophreniform, schizoaffective, delusional, personality disorders; obtain complete history, physical, neurologic exam, routine labs (including complete blood count [CBC], electrolytes, renal and liver function tests [LFTs]), thyroid function tests (TFTs), serology, urine toxicology, erythrocyte sedimentation rate (ESR), human immunodeficiency virus (HIV), toxicology, B_{12}, folate; electroencephalogram (EEG), brain imaging indicated with first episode, unusual presentation (e.g., older age, rapid onset of new symptoms, visual or olfactory hallucinations, clouded sensorium, catatonia, focal neurologic signs).

▶ Disease Severity

Worse prognosis with poor premorbid social history, early onset, insidious onset, lack of insight, nonparanoid subtype, absence of mood symptoms, neurologic abnormalities, male gender, negative symptoms, brain imaging abnormalities. Increased risk for medical illness, incarceration, violence, substance use, victimization, poverty, suicide (10–15%).

▶ Concept and Application

Associated with altered dopaminergic activity in the mesolimbic and mesocortical tracts. Negative symptoms associated with enlargement of cerebral ventricles and cortical atrophy. Functional neuroimaging demonstrates hypofrontality. Both (polygenic) genetic and environmental contributions.

▶ Treatment Steps

Acute

1. Hospitalization for stabilization, protection of self and others (may require involuntary commitment).
2. Benzodiazepines and antipsychotics for acute agitation.
3. Rule out general medical, substance-induced etiologies.
4. Antipsychotic medication: "atypicals" (olanzapine, risperidone, quetiapine) may treat negative symptoms better than older antipsychotics. Clozapine indicated for refractory symptoms (weekly CBC to rule out agranulocylosis).

▶ diagnostic decisions

PSYCHOSIS

Mood Disorders
Bipolar, unipolar, schizoaffective—40%.

Drug-Induced States
Withdrawal delirium, intoxication—25%.

Schizophrenia
Spectrum disorders—5–10%.

Neurologic Disease
Epilepsy, head trauma, CVA, dementia (especially subcortical), basal ganglia disease, delirium, masses, infection, others—20–25%.

Modified from Taylor, MA, *The Fundamentals of Clinical Neuropsychiatry.* New York: Oxford University Press, 1999, p. 264.

▶ cram facts

SYMPTOMS SUGGESTING MEDICAL OR SUBSTANCE-INDUCED PSYCHOSIS

- Abrupt onset
- Older age
- Physical or laboratory abnormalities
- Disorientation, clouded sensorium, memory impairment
- Visual, olfactory, tactile hallucinations *without* auditory hallucinations

► **management decisions**

ACUTE PSYCHOSIS

Maintain Safety, Manage Agitation/Arousal
Calming environment and staff behavior. "Show of force" if necessary. Benzodiazepine, e.g., lorazepam, 2 mg PO or IM, and/or neuroleptic, e.g., haloperidol, 5 mg PO or IM, given q 30–60 min until patient is calm. Seclusion, restraint only if necessary after previous interventions.

Identify Serious Medical Problems
History, vital signs, physical exam. Review all medications (prescribed, over-the-counter, borrowed). Drug and alcohol screen, CBC, chemistries, LFTs, TFTs, brain imaging for first or atypical presentations, abnormal neuro exam.

Assessment and Tentative Diagnosis
Further treatment dictated by diagnostic category.

Continued Care

1. Continuation of antipsychotics (oral or long-acting intramuscular).
2. Assess for development of side effects, e.g., tardive dyskinesia (5% incidence per year with older antipsychotics); anticholinergic effects, sexual dysfunction, weight gain, sedation, extrapyramidal symptoms: lipid and glucose abnormalities with atypicals.
3. Addition of lithium (Li^{++}), anticonvulsants may benefit some.
4. Psychosocial treatments, including patient and family education, social skills training, residential and day treatment, vocational rehabilitation, supportive psychotherapy.

B. Affective Psychoses: Mania and Psychotic Depression

► H&P Keys

History—Personal and family history of affective disorder; clinical features of mood disorders have been present preceding psychosis; illness course generally episodic; alcohol and drug abuse common.

Physical and Mental Status Exam—Mania: hyperactivity, rapid and pressured speech, flight of ideas, elated or irritable affect with lability, decreased need for sleep, distractibility, impulsivity, poor judgment. Forty percent have psychotic symptoms, e.g., grandiose or paranoid delusions. Depression: psychomotor retardation or agitation, slowed and impoverished speech, signs of weight loss, poor self-care, guilty ruminations, somatic delusions, derogatory hallucinations, suicidal preoccupation. Either mania or depression may present with catatonia.

► Diagnosis

No pathognomonic signs or studies; rule out general medical etiologies (thyroid and adrenal dysfunction, medications [e.g., sympathomimetics, L-dopa, steroids, antidepressants], Parkinson's disease, head injury, multiple sclerosis [MS], dementing illnesses, cerebrovascular accidents [CVAs], pancreatic and other malignancies, epilepsy, lupus, CNS tumors, viral illnesses); psychiatric disorders including personality disorders, substance intoxication or withdrawal (e.g., stimulants, anabolic steroids, alcohol).

► Disease Severity

Mania—Severe hyperactivity can lead to exhaustion, dehydration, cardiac death; impaired judgment, irritability, grandiosity, assaultiveness may result in danger to self/others; assess symptom progression, support system.

Depression—Increased suicide risk (15% overall) with presence of delusions; previous attempt; plan and means (especially firearm); male; concurrent substance abuse; social isolation; recent loss; family history; poor health; unemployment. Assess self-care ability, potential life-threatening medical problem.

Both—Mood-incongruent psychotic features predict poorer prognosis. Mixed and rapid cycling disorders difficult to treat with high suicide risk.

► Concept and Application
See section II.

► **differential diagnosis**

PSYCHOTIC MANIA OR DEPRESSION VERSUS SCHIZOPHRENIA

Psychotic Mania or Depression	Schizophrenia
Premorbid adjustment good	Premorbid adjustment poor in ≥ 50%
Family history of affective disorder	Family history affective disorder less likely
Personality and functioning usually preserved between episodes	Chronic, often deteriorating course
Prior mood episodes	No prior mood episodes
Mood disturbance always present and begins before onset of psychosis	Psychosis usually precedes any mood symptoms
Psychotic features usually reflect underlying mood disturbance (e.g., somatic delusions in depression, grandiose delusions in mania)	Psychotic features often bizarre, persecutory, nihilistic (e.g., mind or body control)

► Treatment Steps

Acute

1. Hospitalization for protection of self/others, treatment (may need involuntary commitment).
2. Rule out general medical, substance-induced etiologies.
3. For mania: may require restraint, IV/IM benzodiazepines; may use loading doses of lithium or valproate; use IM antipsychotic if necessary for control of agitation. Electroconvulsive therapy (ECT) for toxic mania, rapid control, pregnancy. Lamotrigine, carbamazepine, atypical antipsychotics also used for mania.
4. For psychotic depression: ECT most effective and rapid; antidepressant (AD) with antipsychotic also effective; poor response to AD alone.

Continued Care—See section II.

C. Delusional Disorder

► H&P Keys

Fixed, nonbizarre, systematized delusion; common types are erotomanic (one is loved by a famous other), grandiose, jealous, persecutory (most common), somatic. Age of onset and psychosocial functioning variable. No hallucinations.

► Diagnosis

Rule out general medical disorders (early dementias, CNS tumor, endocrine and metabolic disorders, stimulant abuse, basal ganglia trauma).

► Disease Severity

Course is variable; worsens with stress.

► Concept and Application

Increased in immigrants, deafness, severe stress, visuospatial deficits.

► Treatment Steps

Acute

1. Hospitalize for suicidal or homicidal risk; extreme impairment, danger associated with delusions.
2. General medical workup.

3. Supportive and psychoeducational therapies with attention to building trust.

Continued Care
1. Low-dose antipsychotic may decrease delusions.
2. Antidepressants for depression.

D. Other Psychoses

1. Schizoaffective Disorder

▶ **H&P Keys**

Concurrent symptoms of schizophrenia and depression or mania, with at least 2 weeks of psychotic symptoms alone.

▶ **Disease Severity**

Poorer prognosis with depressive subtype, family history of schizophrenia, insidious onset, poor premorbid history, predominance of psychotic symptoms.

▶ **Concept and Application**

Mood syndrome defines subtype (manic versus depressive); depressive subtype thought to be related to schizophrenia; "bipolar" subtype to bipolar disorder.

▶ **Treatment Steps**
1. Hospitalization as in other psychoses.
2. Rule out general medical etiology.

Bipolar Type—Li^{++} and/or other mood stabilizer, e.g., valproic acid (VPA), carbamazepine (CBZ) with antipsychotic if necessary; ECT if necessary. Li^{++}, VPA, CBZ maintenance; atypical neuroleptics also used.

Depressive Type—Antipsychotic with or without AD; ECT, Li^{++}, mood stabilizers also used.

2. Schizophreniform Disorder

▶ **H&P Keys**

History, signs, symptoms, and differential as in schizophrenia but duration < **6 months.**

▶ **Disease Severity**

Better prognosis with acute onset, confusion and disorientation, full affect, good premorbid functioning.

▶ **Treatment Steps**
1. Hospitalize as needed.
2. Antipsychotics for at least 6 months.

3. Brief Psychotic Disorder

▶ **H&P Keys**

Acute-onset psychosis with emotional turmoil and confusion often following obvious stressor, duration < 1 month, full return to premorbid functioning. Young adult. Predisposed by personality disorder, posttraumatic stress disorder (PTSD). Rule out schizophreniform and mood disorders, general medical etiology, factitious disorder, malingering, substance induced.

▶ **Disease Severity**

Prognostic factors as in schizophreniform disorder. Suicide risk.

► Treatment Steps
1. Hospitalization as needed.
2. Antipsychotic or antianxiety agent.
3. Psychotherapy when stabilized.

4. Shared Psychotic Disorder

► H&P Keys
Patient's delusion (usually persecutory) develops in context of submissive, dependent, isolated relationship with person with established delusion. Suicide or homicide pacts.

► Treatment Steps
1. Hospitalize as necessary.
2. Separate the people involved.
3. Antipsychotic medication as indicated.

5. Psychotic Disorder Not Otherwise Specified

► H&P Keys
Psychotic symptoms that do not meet criteria for other disorders or when enough information is unavailable. Includes postpartum psychoses, culture-bound syndromes. Former occurs 2–3 weeks postpartum, usually primipara, carries risk of infanticide or suicide.

► Treatment Steps
1. Ensure safety.
2. Symptomatic treatment.

E. Psychoses Originating in Childhood

1. Autistic Disorder

► H&P Keys
A pervasive developmental disorder (PDD) with severe impairments in reciprocal social interaction; verbal and nonverbal communication; restricted, rigid, self-stimulating, stereotyped behaviors; no prominent hallucinations or delusions. Onset by age 3, boys > girls; associated mental retardation (70%); seizure disorder (25%). Genetic predisposition. May be associated with neurologic or genetic medical disorders. Other PDDs: Asperger's (intact language and cognition), Rett's (severe mental retardation [MR]), childhood disintegrative disorder (degenerative course).

► Diagnosis
Neurologic evaluation. No pathognomonic tests. Screening for hearing and vision, EEG, computed tomography (CT) or magnetic resonance imaging (MRI), heavy metals, serum ceruloplasmin, phenylketonuria (PKU), karyotype. Developmental assessment.

► Disease Severity
Better prognosis with higher intelligence quotient (IQ), language, and social skills.

► Treatment Steps
1. Structured classroom training, behavioral modification, parent training, family support.
3. Antipsychotics may decrease hyperactivity, stereotypies, irritability. Selective serotonin reuptake inhibitors (SSRIs) may help with social interaction, compulsive behaviors.

2. Psychotic Mood Disorders

Bipolar disorder and major depression diagnosed with same criteria used for adults; children may show irritability, somatic complaints, failure to gain weight, behavioral disturbance. Good premorbid functioning, normal IQ, prominent manic symptoms, family history of mood disorder predict bipolar diagnosis in children and adolescents, as does acute onset, psychomotor retardation, hypersomnia, psychosis, and bipolar family history in first-episode depression. Li^{++} or anticonvulsants with careful monitoring, supportive psychotherapy, family education.

II. MOOD DISORDERS

A. Major (Unipolar) Depression

► H&P Keys

Two weeks of sustained depressed mood or loss of interest and pleasure (anhedonia), and at least four of the following: weight and appetite change, insomnia or hypersomnia, fatigue, psychomotor agitation or retardation, low self-esteem or guilt, trouble concentrating, recurrent thoughts of death or suicide. Associated with social withdrawal, loss of libido, constipation, diurnal mood variation, impoverished speech, somatic preoccupation (cardiac, gastrointestinal [GI], genitourinary [GU], back pain, headache), indecisiveness, obsessive rumination, tearfulness, anxiety. "Masked depression" presents with vague physical complaints. Elderly may present with cognitive complaints (pseudodementia). Personal and family history. Females > males; > 50% recurrence rate; pattern may be seasonal. Chronic medical or psychiatric illness, substance abuse predisposes.

► Diagnosis

Clinical diagnosis. Rule out substance, medication, medical etiologies; dysthymia (chronic, less severe); personality disorder (lifelong pattern of mood instability; may be comorbid); dementia (less likely history of affective disorder; deficits stable; patient may try to hide deficits, rather than complain about them; insidious onset); bipolar depression (history of mania); bereavement (self-limiting; lacks morbid preoccupation with worthlessness, suicidal ideation, psychomotor retardation, marked functional impairment). Diagnosis difficult in medically ill due to overlapping symptoms.

► Disease Severity

Same as for affective psychoses; untreated episodes last > 6 months; 60% recover, 30% partially recover, 5–10% develop chronic course. Worse prognosis with late-life onset, concurrent personality, anxiety, substance abuse, chronic medical problems, dysthymic disorder, psychosocial stress. Aggressive treatment reduces suicide risk (15%) and improves comorbid medical disorders. Each recurrence increases risk of further recurrence.

► Concept and Application

Dysregulation of neurotransmitters and neuroendocrine system, especially in HPA axis; decreased serotonergic activity associated with suicide. Late-onset may have subcortical cerebrovascular disease. ADs increase available monoamines at nerve terminals, alter receptor sensitivity and density. Genetic component. Twenty-five percent identify precipitant, often loss. Higher incidence and earlier age of

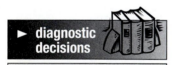

► diagnostic decisions

MAJOR DEPRESSION

Sustained, distinct depressed mood for 2 weeks plus at least four of the following
(SIG E CAPS):

Sleep (increased or decreased)

Interest (loss of interest or pleasure)

Guilt (worthlessness)

Energy (decreased)

Concentration (decreased)

Appetite (increased or decreased)

Psychomotor change (retardation or agitation)

Suicidality (active or passive)

onset in younger age groups (cohort effect) supports psychosocial contribution. Psychiatric or medical illness, substance abuse, and early parental loss predispose.

► Treatment Steps

Acute—See section I.B. for psychotic depression (20%).
1. Hospitalization if suicide risk or incapacity warrants.
2. Rule out general medical, medication, substance induced etiology.
3. Moderate to severe symptoms indication for somatic therapy. ADs successful in 65–75% after 4–6 weeks treatment; good response predicted by vegetative signs, previous response, severe symptoms, acute onset.
4. Serotonin reuptake inhibitors (SRIs) have less toxicity and suicide risk than older classes of ADs, tricyclic antidepressants (TCAs) or monoamine oxidase inhibitors (MAOIs). Other ADs include bupropion, venlafaxine, mirtazapine. AD, Li^{++}, or triiodothyronine (T_3) augmentation for nonresponders. Antipsychotic plus AD for psychotic depression. ECT for psychotic depression drug nonresponders (70–80% respond), previous good response, rapid response, pregnancy, cardiac disease.
5. Psychotherapy alone may be effective for mild major depression; psychotherapy plus ADs more effective than either treatment alone.
6. Seasonal pattern may respond to phototherapy.
7. Diagnose and treat comorbid psychopathology.

Continued Care
1. First episode, continuation of ADs for 6–12 months; recurrent depression indication for long-term maintenance; observe for suicidal thoughts, weight gain, jitteriness, insomnia, sexual dysfunction, dry mouth. Li^{++} prophylaxis also effective.
2. Psychotherapy.

B. Dysthymia

Chronic depression of at least 2 years' duration with at least two of the following: appetite disturbance, sleep disturbance, fatigue, low self-esteem, difficulty concentrating, hopelessness; no history of major depression or manic episode within first 2 years. May be secondary to other psychiatric or general medical illness, chronic stress. Insidious onset childhood through early adulthood; women > men; family history of depression. Rule out major depression, personality disorder (may coexist), chronic illnesses, such as uncontrolled diabetes, hypothyroidism, chronic fatigue syndrome. Ten percent per year develop "double depression" (major depression superimposed on dysthymia), worsens prognosis of both. Treat with ADs, psychotherapy, possibly exercise.

C. Bipolar Disorders

► H&P Keys

See section I.B. above. One or more manic episodes (distinct period of elated or irritable mood with at least three of the following: grandiosity, decreased need for sleep, talkativeness, racing thoughts, distractibility, hyperactivity or increased goal-directed activity, rapid and pressured speech, increased energy, impulsivity [e.g., excessive spending, gambling, promiscuity], causing marked impairment or

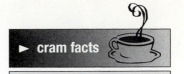

► cram facts

SUICIDE RISK ASSESSMENT

Demographic Factors
- Elderly
- Male
- White
- Adolescent
- Homosexual

Social Factors
- Unemployed
- Isolated
- Access to method (e.g., firearm)

Clinical Factors
- Medical problems
- Prior attempts
- Use of drugs and alcohol
- Psychiatric disorders (mood, schizophrenia, substance, delirium, personality)
- Psychiatric symptoms (command hallucinations, delusions, intoxication)

hospitalization) usually accompanied by one or more major depressive episodes. May be psychotic. Bipolar depressions may have hypersomnia, severe lethargy. Manic episode may be precipitated by psychosocial stressor, sleep deprivation. Subtypes include:

Type I—History of full-blown mania with or without major depression.

Type II—History of hypomania (less severe manic symptoms and impairment) and major depression.

Rapid Cycling—Four or more mood episodes per year (10%).

Mixed—Full symptoms of both mania and depression intermixed or rapidly alternating. Often psychotic. High suicide risk.

► Diagnosis

Same as for affective psychoses. Rapid cycling may be associated with thyroid abnormalities, CNS insult. If onset after age 40, likely general medical etiology.

► Disease Severity

Suicide risk 10–15%. Worse prognosis with substance abuse, early onset, mixed features, rapid cycling, psychosis. Women have more rapid cycling, more depressive episodes, and risk for postpartum episodes. Adolescents at high risk of relapse. Course worsens over time.

► Concept and Application

Strong genetic component. Heterogeneous dysregulations of biogenic amine systems. One theory implicates kindling (sensitization due to repeated subthreshhold stimulation of neuron generating action potential) in limbic system.

► Treatment Steps

Acute Mania—See section I.B.
1. Hospitalize if necessary.
2. Rule out medical, substance-induced causes, e.g., hyper- or hypothyroidism, CNS disorders (head injury, seizures, MS), substance intoxication or withdrawal, medications (e.g., steroids, ADs, stimulants, sympathomimetics).
3. Mood stabilizers: Li^{++} serum levels 1.0–1.2. Family history of affective disorder or Li^{++} responsiveness, euphoric mania predict good response; for rapid cycling or dysphoric mania, VPA, CBZ, lamotrigine, atypicals may be added or substituted. Bipolar depression may respond to Li^{++} or anticonvulsants alone or may need additional AD or ECT. ADs may precipitate mania, increase cycling.

Continued Care
1. Over 80% recurrence without prophylaxis, warranted after second episode (or first in adolescents), high genetic loading, or sudden onset with suicidal or highly disruptive symptoms. Li^{++} levels 0.8–1.0; observe for nausea, diarrhea, vomiting, weight gain, polyuria, polydipsia, tremor, cognitive dysfunction; dysarthria, ataxia, seizures, coma from toxocity; avoid dietary Na^{++} fluctuations; monitor thyroid, renal function. Anticonvulsants for Li^{++} nonresponders, substance abusers, rapid cycling, and mixed forms. Obtain CBC, LFTs, pregnancy test, follow serum levels. ADs may be indicated for bipolar depression unresponsive to mood stabilizers alone.

2. Psychotherapy may increase adaptation, compliance, long-term stability.
3. Family support, education.
4. Stress reduction, maintenance of routine.

D. Cyclothymia

Chronic fluctuating mood disturbance of at least 2 years' duration with symptoms of hypomania and depression insufficient to be diagnosed as major depression or bipolar disorder. Onset adolescence, early adulthood. Family history of affective disorder. Rule out personality disorder, substance abuse. May respond to lithium or anticonvulsants, psychotherapy.

III. ANXIETY DISORDERS

A. Panic Disorder

▶ H&P Keys

History—Recurrent, initially unexpected, sudden episodes of intense fear or discomfort accompanied by autonomic hyperarousal, depersonalization, fears of dying or going crazy; often associated with agoraphobia, fear of situations in which escape is difficult or help unavailable, such as outside the home alone, in a crowd, traveling, on a bridge; may be housebound. Attacks cause anticipatory anxiety, concern about implications, and/or change in behavior (e.g., phobic avoidance). Increased history of separation anxiety disorder, family history of panic disorder, other anxiety disorders. Onset mid-20s, women > men, often associated with stressful event. Nonpsychiatric physicians, emergency departments usually consulted first.

Physical and Mental Status Exam—Trembling, systolic hypertension, sweating, hyperventilation, flushing, tachycardia, palpitations, dilated pupils, piloerection, cold hands; complaints of chest pain, dyspnea, difficulty swallowing, dizziness, nausea, choking, paresthesias; fear of dying, losing control, going crazy, impending doom. Mitral valve prolapse present in 20–50% of cases.

▶ Diagnosis

Rule out general medical etiology (suspect if onset after 35 or if physical > cognitive symptoms): cardiac insufficiency, arrhythmias, hypoxia, hyperthyroidism, hyperparathyroidism, hypoglycemia, asthma, chronic obstructive pulmonary disease (COPD), seizure disorders, pheochromocytoma, vestibular disease, caffeinism, hypoglycemia, carcinoid syndrome, autoimmune disorders, Parkinson's disease, postconcussion syndrome, MS, sedative or alcohol withdrawal, stimulants. Situationally bound (cued) panic attacks occur with phobias, obsessive–compulsive disorder, PTSD.

▶ Disease Severity

Chronic, intermittent course, with disability caused by phobic avoidance, substance use, depression (> 50%), associated with lack of prompt diagnosis, treatment. Excess risk of irritable bowel syndrome, peptic ulcer disease, hypertension, mitral valve prolapse, cardiovascular (CV) mortality, suicide attempts.

▶ Concept and Application

Genetic contribution. Biologic models include disturbances in locus ceruleus (norepinephrine [NE]), serotonergic (5-HT) and γ-aminobutyric acid (GABA) neurotransmission. Benzodiazepines facilitate GABA transmission, and ADs downregulate CNS β-adrenergic receptors.

▶ **Treatment Steps**

Acute
1. Emergency management of panic attack via reassurance, benzodiazepine.
2. Rule out myocardial infarction (MI), pulmonary embolism (PE), substance withdrawal, CNS insult, hypoglycemia, electrolyte abnormalities.
3. Prompt psychiatric referral; avoidance of interminable medical workups.

Continued Care
1. Antidepressants first line; start with low doses and increase slowly; high-potency benzodiazepines also effective but may be difficult to discontinue. Buspirone ineffective. Taper should be attempted in 6–12 months; 70% eventually relapse.
2. Cognitive–behavioral therapy (CBT) effective for agoraphobia and relapse prevention.
3. Support, education.
4. Eliminate caffeine.
5. Diagnose and treat comorbid substance and psychiatric disorders.

B. Generalized Anxiety Disorder

▶ **H&P Keys**

More than 6 months of unrealistic, persistent anxiety and worry unrelated to another psychiatric disorder. Associated with ≥ 3 of the following: restlessness, fatigability, difficulty concentrating, irritability, muscle tension, sleep disturbance. Other somatic complaints common. Often present in primary care.

▶ **Diagnosis**

Differential is same as for panic disorder.

▶ **Disease Severity**

Ninety percent psychiatric comorbidity; 25% develop panic disorder. Depression common.

▶ **Treatment Steps**
1. CBT effective for milder cases.
2. Medications for more severe, chronic disorder; many require prolonged or intermittent treatment. ADs effective, especially with comorbid depression. Buspirone as effective as benzodiazepines without causing sedation, psychomotor impairment, risk of tolerance, abuse potential, rebound; delayed onset of action, headache, nausea, dizziness. Benzodiazepines give immediate relief; abuse rare without substance abuse history.

C. Obsessive–Compulsive Disorder (OCD)

▶ **H&P Keys**

Recurrent intrusive thoughts, impulses, images (obsessions) and perseverative ritualistic behaviors (compulsions), that produce anxiety if resisted. In most cases, experienced as senseless product of own mind (as versus delusion). Typical obsessions involve contamination, sin, aggression, loss of control, order, doubt; common compulsions are washing, checking, counting. Onset childhood through early adulthood; 25% have obsessions only. Comorbid depression (> 50%), other anxiety disorders, Tourette's syndrome (5–7%), alcoholism, anorexia nervosa. Skin problems due to excessive washing.

► Diagnosis
Clinical diagnosis; obsessive–compulsive symptoms in depression, schizophrenia, accompanied by other symptoms of those disorders and respond to specific treatments. "Compulsive" behaviors such as eating, shopping, gambling give pleasure, whereas true compulsions reduce anxiety. Obsessive–compulsive personality lacks true obsessions/compulsions and related anxiety.

► Disease Severity
Chronic intermittent course; worse prognosis with coexisting schizotypal personality, early onset, severe depression, noncompliance with treatment.

► Concept and Application
Biologic illness with genetic contribution. Positron emission tomographic (PET) scans show hypermetabolism in prefrontal cortex and caudate nuclei. Psychobiologic probes suggest abnormality in serotonin system; treated with SSRIs. Autoimmunity to *Streptococcus* linked to some childhood cases (pediatric autoimmune neuropsychiatric disorder associated with group A streptococcal infection [PANDAS]).

► Treatment Steps
1. Rule out temporal lobe epilepsy, postencephalitic states, Tourette's syndrome, MS, basal ganglia lesions, postconcussion syndrome, Sydenham's chorea.
2. Serotonergic ADs (SSRIs, clomipramine); may need higher doses and 4–12 weeks for effect. Observe for nausea, agitation, insomnia (SSRIs); weight gain, sedation, anticholinergic effects (clomipramine); sexual dysfunction (both). Rapid relapse with discontinuation in 90%.
3. Behavioral therapy based on exposure, response prevention; good long-term response in ritualizers. Combined treatment most effective.
4. Support, education.
5. Diagnose and treat comorbid disorders.

D. Posttraumatic Stress Disorder (PTSD)

► H&P Keys
Exposure to markedly stressful event causing terror and helplessness, e.g., combat, rape, sexual abuse, torture, natural disaster. Symptoms from three categories: reexperiencing (e.g., intrusive recollections, nightmares, play in children); emotional numbing (e.g., avoidance, amnesia, restricted affect); autonomic arousal (e.g., insomnia, irritability). Onset may be delayed, with initial presentation of shock, confusion, detachment. Comorbid depression, anxiety, dissociation, substance abuse, personality problems, poor impulse control, suicide attempts.

► Diagnosis
Toxicology, head injury workup as indicated. Chronic PTSD may present with a variety of somatic and psychiatric symptoms; obtain

trauma history routinely. PTSD symptoms following divorce, bereavement, etc., diagnosed as adjustment disorder.

▶ **Disease Severity**

Worse prognosis in children and the elderly; with preexisting psychopathology or brain injury, more severe, repetitive stressor; stressor of human design; insidious onset; poor social support; physical injury.

▶ **Concept and Application**

Traumatic memories may be processed differently from nontraumatic ones, making them more difficult to access and integrate in psychotherapy.

▶ **Treatment Steps**

Acute
1. Rapid evaluation and treatment.
2. Hospitalize for suicide, violence risk.
3. Rape victims require careful documentation of findings, evaluation for sexually transmitted diseases (STDs) and pregnancy, plan for immediate safety, legal advice.
3. CBT, exposure therapy, patient education, group therapy all of value.
4. Cautious use of mild sedation, e.g., with benzodiazepine, as indicated initially.

Continued Care
1. Individual, CBT and supportive therapy, peer group therapy, family education for chronic symptoms.
2. SSRIs are first-line treatment.
3. Treatment of comorbid disorders.

E. Acute Stress Disorder

▶ **H&P Keys**

Symptoms of dissociation (e.g., numbing, detachment, derealization, depersonalization) experienced during/following extreme trauma, followed by reexperiencing, avoidance, and arousal symptoms as in PTSD. Diagnosis predicts development of PTSD. Psychotherapy aims at reducing dissociation and acknowledging trauma. If symptoms still present after 4 weeks, diagnose PTSD.

▶ **Treatment Steps**
1. Psychotherapy.
2. Mild sedation as indicated.

F. Phobias

1. Social Phobia

▶ **H&P Keys**

Fear of scrutiny of others; may be specific (e.g., eating in public, public speaking) or more generalized. Situations avoided or endured with anxiety. Onset in adolescence, chronic course, may develop depression, substance abuse.

▶ **Treatment Steps**
1. CBT.
2. Breathing retraining.
3. ADs (SSRIs, monoamine oxidase inhibitors [MAOIs]) for generalized symptoms; high-potency benzodiazepines also used.
4. β-Blockers used for performance anxiety.

2. Specific Phobia

▶ **H&P Keys**

Irrational, excessive fear and avoidance of object or situation (other than of panic or social situation), e.g., snakes, heights, blood.

▶ **Treatment Steps**

Behavioral and cognitive therapies (systematic desensitization).

IV. ADJUSTMENT DISORDERS

▶ **H&P Keys**

Pathologic, excessive emotional and behavioral responses to recognizable psychosocial stressor resulting in impaired functioning. Stressors within range of normal experience (e.g., school problems, marital discord, job loss, illness). Onset within 3 months, persists no longer than 6 months after termination of stressor. Classified by major symptom: depression, anxiety, mixed emotional features, conduct disturbance, mixed disturbance of conduct and emotions. Adolescents frequently have behavioral symptoms; adults have mood, anxiety symptoms.

▶ **Diagnosis**

PTSD preceded by stressors outside range of normal experience. If one instance in a typical pattern of overreaction, diagnose personality disorder. Rule out substance intoxication, abuse.

▶ **Disease Severity**

Greater vulnerability with history of childhood parental loss, serious medical illness, but 20% of adults and 40% of adolescents have mental disorder at 5-year follow-up. Increased risk of suicide, medical noncompliance.

▶ **Concept and Application**

Vulnerability to stress may be a function of underlying constitution, developmental experiences, temperament, personality structure, severity of stressor.

▶ **Treatment Steps**

1. Evaluate risk of suicide, medical noncompliance, substance abuse.
2. Psychotherapy to help patient clarify concerns, resources, options, develop plan of action.
3. Stress reduction may include social support, exercise, relaxation, cognitive reframing techniques, attention to health habits, peer group support.
4. Antianxiety/antidepressant medication as indicated for short-term symptom relief.

V. PERSONALITY DISORDERS (AXIS II)

▶ **H&P Keys**

Persistent, inflexible, maladaptive patterns of thinking, feeling, and behaving causing dysfunction, subjective distress; frequent interpersonal problems, fragility under stress, depression; traits often egosyntonic. Onset late adolescence. Ten disorders (three clusters) in the *Diagnostic and Statistical Manual of Mental Disorders* (DSM):

Odd, Eccentric

1. **Paranoid:** suspicious, hypervigilant; ascribes malicious intent, hidden meanings to others; hypersensitivity to criticism; nonpsychotic.
2. **Schizoid:** isolated, indifferent to social relationships, restricted affective expression.
3. **Schizotypal:** minor thought disorder (e.g., ideas of reference, magical thinking), peculiar behavior, constricted affect, social anxiety.

Dramatic, Emotional

1. **Antisocial (ASP):** pattern of exploitative, socially irresponsible, destructive, impulsive behavior with no remorse; comorbid substance abuse; conduct disorder in childhood.
2. **Borderline:** problems with intense, unstable relationships; affect regulation; impulse control; identity. Suicide gestures common.
3. **Histrionic:** self-absorbed; seductive, with shallow, labile affect; excess need for praise, reassurance.
4. **Narcissistic:** grandiose, exploitative, entitled, rageful if humiliated, lacks empathy.

Anxious, Fearful, Inhibited

1. **Avoidant:** fearful of rejection, timid, inhibited but desirous of relationships (as versus schizoid); comorbid anxiety disorders.
2. **Dependent:** submissive, passive, clingy; lets others make important decisions; easily hurt; preoccupied with abandonment; predisposed by chronic illness.
3. **Obsessive–compulsive:** preoccupied with rules; rigid, perfectionistic, ambivalent, stingy, controlling, restricted affect; persistent, task-oriented.

▶ Diagnosis

Onset late teens to early twenties. Acute personality changes in adulthood due to Axis I or general medical disorders (e.g., substance intoxication, abuse; CNS disease, e.g., MS; mood disorders; psychosis; psychic trauma); diagnose coexistent Axis I mood, anxiety, psychotic, substance use, eating, somatization disorders. Personality disorders must have long-term, persistent pattern; may need to defer diagnosis in presence of Axis I pathology.

▶ Disease Severity

Hospitalize for protection of self and others (suicide risk significant in borderlines, antisocials, schizotypals, particularly in presence of substance use); psychotic decompensation (borderline, schizotypal, schizoid, paranoid); severe Axis I pathology.

▶ Concept and Application

Personality disorders result from interaction of constitution, temperament, developmental experiences, environment; genetic contribution in antisocial, schizotypal, paranoid; childhood sexual or physical abuse in many borderlines, avoidants, antisocials; nonspecific neurologic abnormalities; decreased CNS serotonin functioning associated with impulsivity, aggression; schizotypals genetically and biologically related to schizophrenia.

▶ Treatment Steps

1. Evaluate suicide and violence risk; hospitalize if necessary.
2. Diagnose and treat comorbid Axis I disorders.

3. Psychotherapy: CBT, interpersonal/psychodynamic, family, group modalities all used depending on specific disorder and patient.
4. Medication for predominant symptoms. Schizotypals may respond to antipsychotics; SSRIs, mood stabilizers, antipsychotics used for borderline personality disorder. Antianxiety, antidepressant medications for anxious, fearful, inhibited disorders.

VI. SOMATOFORM DISORDERS

A. Somatization Disorder

▶ H&P Keys

Recurrent, multiple, unfeigned somatic complaints not fully explained by physical disorder, for which medical attention has been sought. Young women, often with menstrual difficulties. Frequent, vague, dramatic complaints involve chronic pain; GI symptoms, e.g., irritable bowel, vomiting; cardiopulmonary symptoms, e.g., unexplained dyspnea, dizziness; pseudoneurologic symptoms, e.g., paralysis, blindness; reproductive tract, sexual problems. High medical utilizers, multiple doctors; extensive, costly evaluations; may have polysurgeries, e.g., early hysterectomy. Childhood sexual abuse predisposes; at risk for concurrent spousal abuse. Common comorbid disorders: alcohol, analgesic, sedative abuse; depression (80–90%); anxiety (25–45%); personality disorders.

▶ Diagnosis

Rule out disorders that present with vague, multiple, confusing complaints, e.g., MS, porphyria, lupus, hyperparathyroidism; physical symptoms of panic disorder occur only during attacks; conversion disorder involves only pseudoneurologic symptoms; in factitious disorder, person consciously controls production of symptoms.

▶ Disease Severity

Chronic course; suicide associated with substance abuse.

▶ Concept and Application

Both genetic and environmental factors contribute; familial association with substance abuse and antisocial personality in males. Psychologically interpreted as expression of psychological pain, elicits care, secondary gain.

▶ Treatment Steps
1. Regularly scheduled visits with primary care physician; team approach with mental health specialist.
2. Tests, consultations only with evidence of illness.
3. Treat depression, anxiety with ADs.
4. Avoid opiates, benzodiazepines.

B. Pain Disorder

▶ H&P Keys

Persistent preoccupation with pain without adequate physical findings or pathophysiologic mechanism to account for intensity or disabling psychosocial sequelae. Onset usually age 30–50, women > men; high utilizers of medical care, surgery; complaints may be vague, diffuse; frequent analgesic, substance abuse; comorbid depression, anxiety, insomnia; inactivity, invalidism, isolation. Resistant to psychological interpretation.

► **Diagnosis**

Dramatic presentation of pain (due to cultural or personality traits) lacks related impairment; lacks plethora of symptoms of somatization disorder; psychogenic disorders with known pathophysiologic mechanisms, e.g., tension headache, diagnosed as psychological factors affecting physical condition; in malingering, symptoms intentionally produced in pursuit of obvious goal. Rule out reflex sympathetic dystrophy (RSD).

► **Disease Severity**

Prescription drug addiction may require detoxification. Evaluate psychosocial impairment. Suicide associated with severe depression.

► **Concept and Application**

Subjective pain experience has cognitive, affective, behavioral components, which may be modified through cognitive–behavioral interventions; serotonergic, adrenergic, endorphin systems involved in pain may be modulated with ADs, analgesics.

► **Treatment Steps**

1. As with somatization disorder.
2. CBT and supportive therapies (behavioral evaluation, relaxation, contingency management).
3. Nonsteroidal anti-inflammatory agents, TCAs for pain.
4. Family therapy, education.
5. Vocational rehab.

C. Conversion Disorder

► **H&P Keys**

Involuntary psychogenic loss or alteration of functioning suggesting a physical disorder, not limited to pain or sexual disturbance. Temporal relationship between psychologically painful stressor and onset of symptoms. Classic cases involve pseudoneurologic symptoms, e.g., blindness, paralysis, mutism, pseudoseizures, difficulty swallowing because of lump in throat (globus hystericus). Antecedent physical disorder (e.g., seizure disorder), exposure to persons with physical disorders, preexisting gross brain pathology predispose. Women, rural, lower socioeconomic strata. Comorbid somatization, depressive, panic, substance, personality, dissociative disorders.

► **Diagnosis**

Diagnosis of exclusion, requiring careful neurologic exam and testing, psychiatric consultation. May have inconsistency of symptoms with known neuroanatomy and physiology, e.g., glove distribution of anesthesia. Thirty percent subsequently develop neurologic or other illness that explains symptom, e.g., MS, lupus, especially with onset after age 35.

► **Disease Severity**

Improvement or complete resolution associated with abrupt onset, clear precipitant, absence of general medical or psychiatric illness; recurrence predicts chronicity.

► **Treatment Steps**

1. Rule out neurologic, medical disorders (e.g., lupus, MS, HIV encephalopathy).
2. Reassurance, suggestion, attention to any stressful precipitant.
3. Diagnose and treat underlying psychopathology.
4. Hypnosis or amobarbital interview may be helpful.

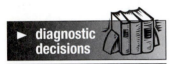

► **diagnostic decisions**

SOMATOFORM AND RELATED DISORDERS

Somatoform Disorders
Symptoms are not intentionally produced. Symptoms not fully explained by medical condition.
Symptoms linked to psychological factors:
  a. Somatization disorder: multiple somanic complaints
  b. Conversion disorder: neurologic symptoms
  c. Pain disorder
  d. Hypochondriasis: fear of specific disease
  e. Body dysmorphic disorder: preoccupation with defect in appearance

Factitious Disorder
Intentional production of symptoms for unconscious psychological reasons (the sick role).

Malingering
Intentional production of symptoms for recognizable gain.

Psychological Factors Affecting a Medical Condition
Known medical condition develops/is exacerbated by psychological factors.

D. Hypochondriasis

▶ H&P Keys

Preoccupation with fear of having serious disease despite medical reassurance to the contrary, not of delusional intensity, duration at least 6 months. Selective attention to and misinterpretation of somatic signs and symptoms. Onset age 20–40. History of doctor shopping, resistance to psychiatric referral. Comorbid depression, anxiety, dependence, hostility. Associated with past experience of illness in self or family member.

▶ Diagnosis

Rule out subtle medical illness; psychotic disorder with somatic (fixed) delusions; in somatization disorder, patients preoccupied with symptoms rather than specific illness; symptoms must not be due to panic attacks or part of OCD.

▶ Disease Severity

Usually chronic, with functional impairment.

▶ Treatment Steps

As for somatization disorder; avoid repeated costly medical workups.

E. Body Dysmorphic Disorder

Excessive preoccupation with imagined or slight defect in appearance, causing marked distress or impairment (not including anorexia nervosa). May be of delusional intensity. Onset adolescence, chronic course. May seek repeated cosmetic surgery. Comorbid depression, delusional disorder, social phobia, OCD. Evaluate social impairment, suicide potential. Psychotherapy, SSRI.

F. Related Disorders

1. Psychological Factors Affecting Physical Condition (Psychosomatic Disorders)

A psychological factor is believed to have contributed significantly to the development or exacerbation of physical symptom or illness, evidenced by temporal relationship with psychologically meaningful stressor; commonly, headaches, peptic ulcer disease, asthma, skin diseases, vomiting, obesity, low-back pain, ulcerative colitis, arrhythmias. Physical condition on Axis III. Stress management, psychotherapy may increase adjustment, reduce medical costs.

2. Factitious Disorders

Intentional (but often compulsive) production of or feigning of physical or psychological symptoms, presumably for psychological reasons unknown to the patient, e.g., unsatisfied dependency needs met in achieving "sick role." Includes reporting or intentionally producing false symptoms, e.g., injection of contaminated substance, surreptitious use of medications, thermometer manipulation, self-induced bruises. Early adult onset; chronic, severe impairment; comorbid severe personality disorders, substance abuse; may have medical occupation, history of illness. Psychiatric consultation, confrontation.

3. Malingering

Intentional production of physical or psychological symptoms for obvious recognizable external incentive, e.g., to avoid military service, financial reward, evading prison, obtaining drugs. Discrepancy with objective findings, vague, uncooperative. Comorbid antisocial personality, substance abuse.

VII. ATTENTION DEFICIT/HYPERACTIVITY DISORDER (ADHD)

► H&P Keys

At least 6 months of age-inappropriate degree of inattentiveness, hyperactivity, and impulsivity; manifested by difficulty following instructions, organizing and completing tasks; easy distractibility; restlessness and fidgetiness; interrupting and talking out of turn; inability to sustain play activity; accident-proneness. Onset before age 7, boys > girls. Associated with academic underachievement, low self-esteem, mood lability, low frustration tolerance, temper outbursts, academic skills disorders, soft neurologic signs, clumsiness. Comorbid conduct disorder, oppositional defiant disorder, anxiety, depression, otitis media. Family history.

► Diagnosis

Clinical diagnosis. Careful neurologic exam, educational testing, teachers' and parents' report using Connors scale; EEG, TFTs, lead level, hearing assessment as indicated. Diagnose specific learning disabilities (LDs). Rule out fragile X, fetal alcohol syndrome, Tourette's disorder, bipolar disorder, chaotic environment.

► Disease Severity

Poorer outcomes associated with more severe symptoms, coexisting conduct disorder, low IQ, mental disorder in parents; many continue symptoms into adulthood; 25% develop antisocial personality disorder; increased rates of substance abuse, arrests, suicide attempts, accidents, comorbid psychiatric disorders, parental abuse. Treatment reduces risks.

► Concept and Application

Genetic contribution. Decreased prefrontal cerebral blood flow possibly mediated by altered dopamine (DA) and NE. Medications increase availability of CNS NE and DA.

► Treatment Steps

1. Medical and psychiatric assessment.
2. Behavioral and environmental management by family, school.
3. Psychostimulant medication, e.g., methylphenidate (10–60 mg/day) or dextroamphetamine (5–40 mg/day). May inhibit growth. Observe also for headache, irritability, insomnia, abdominal pain, dysphoria, tics. Atomoxetine, TCAs, bupropion, clonidine also used.
4. Individual, family therapy as indicated.

VIII. CONDUCT DISORDER

► H&P Keys

Age-inappropriate, persistent violation of societal norms and rights of others, manifested by aggression to people and animals, property destruction, deceitfulness, theft, serious rule violations. May lack empathy, remorse; poor frustration tolerance, irritability, recklessness, low academic achievement. Onset childhood or adolescence. Male-to-female ratio 5:1. Comorbid ADHD, LD, depression, substance abuse.

► Diagnosis

Rule out response to immediate social context, e.g., runaway episodes due to abuse, "adaptive delinquency." Obtain history from multiple sources.

► **Disease Severity**

Early onset, attentional problems, low intelligence, fire setting, family deviance, and large size predict worse prognosis. Forty percent develop ASP as adults; high mortality rates.

► Concept and Application

Genetic, neurodevelopmental, and environmental risk factors, including parental rejection/neglect; harsh and inconsistent discipline and abuse; parental ASP, substance abuse, other psychiatric disorder; poverty; evidence of genetic transmission; neurologic abnormalities, including attention deficits, seizures, perinatal insults, head injuries. Biological markers suggest autonomic underarousal, possibly associated with decreased anxiety or stimulus seeking.

► Treatment Steps

1. Evaluate suicide and violence potential.
2. Containment may involve hospitalization, parents, schools, legal system, residential placement, peers.
3. Aggression may respond to SSRI, mood stabilizers, propranolol, antipsychotics.
4. Individual, group, family therapies, behavioral management, parent training.
5. Evaluate and treat comorbid disorders.

IX. EATING DISORDERS

A. Anorexia Nervosa

► H&P Keys

Refusal to maintain minimal normal body weight (< 85%), intense fear of gaining weight, normal appetite, distorted body image, 3 months' amenorrhea. Associated features: obligate exercise, peculiar food behaviors, bulimic symptoms, emaciation, hypothermia, hypotension, lanugo hair, bradycardia, edema, hair loss, hyposexuality, compulsive behaviors. Onset adolescence, 95% women, mid- to upper socioeconomic strata, premorbid history of perfectionism, inflexibility, need for control, anxiety, possibly sexual abuse. Precipitated by stress, dieting. Comorbid depression, personality, OCD.

► Diagnosis

Rule out weight loss due to depression, AIDS, cancer, GI disorders, substance abuse. In depression, appetite is diminished whereas anorexics have normal appetite; in schizophrenia, bizarre eating patterns related to psychosis; in bulimia, weight does not fall below 85%; underweight persons without anorexia recognize their low weight. May have leukopenia, anemia, electrolyte abnormalities, dehydration, decreased TFTs, prepubertal hormone levels, sinus bradycardia.

► Disease Severity

Thirty percent have chronic course, 5–18% mortality. Poorer outcome associated with longer duration of illness, older age at onset, prior psychiatric hospitalizations, poor premorbid adjustment, comorbid personality disorder. May cause CV problems, impaired renal function, anemia, osteoporosis.

▶ **Concept and Application**

Genetic component; psychologically interpreted as resistance to social or sexual demands of adolescence; cultural preoccupation with extreme slimness rare in nonindustrialized societies. Biologic theories focus on hypothalamic disturbance, supported by amenorrhea preceding weight loss; reduced CNS, serotonin, and NE activity.

▶ **Treatment Steps**

Acute

1. Hospitalize for starvation, dehydration, electrolyte imbalance, hypotension, hypothermia, suicide risk.
2. Monitor and treat metabolic imbalances.
3. Strict enforcement of treatment contract for weight goal with daily weights, nutritional supplements, intake–output, super-

▶ **diagnostic decisions**

SIGNS AND SYMPTOMS OF SUBSTANCE INTOXICATION AND WITHDRAWAL

Substance Category	Intoxication	Withdrawal
CNS depressants: alcohol, sedatives, hypnotics, anxiolytics	Disinhibition, slurred speech, drowsiness, ataxia, confusion, blackouts **Overdose:** respiratory depression, coma, death; barbiturates have low therapeutic index	Autonomic hyperactivity, anxiety, malaise, headache, nausea, vomiting, fever, mydriasis, seizures, delusions, hallucinations, delirium, death; can be life threatening
CNS stimulants: amphetamine, cocaine, other sympathomimetics	Euphoria, alertness, increased energy, loquaciousness, anorexia, insomnia, mydriasis, autonomic hyperactivity **Overdose:** agitation, aggression, fever, chills, arrhythmias, seizures, sudden cardiac death, cerebrovascular accident; paranoid psychosis, hallucinosis, delirium	Fatigue, insomnia or hypersomnia, anxiety, dysphoria, vivid dreams, agitation, drug craving; not life threatening (unless suicidal)
Opioids	Euphoria, analgesia, drowsiness, hypoactivity, miosis, anorexia, constipation, pruritus, nausea, vomiting, ataxia **Overdose:** hypotension, bradycardia, CNS and respiratory depression, pulmonary edema, seizures, coma	Flulike syndrome: myalgias, rhinorrhea, nausea, vomiting, diarrhea, tearing, mydriasis, restlessness, yawning, sweating, piloerection, insomnia, anxiety, tachycardia, hypertension, craving

vised feeding (nasogastric tube as needed), reinforcement, nutrition education.
4. Treat comorbid depression (avoid bupropion because of seizure risk).

Continued Care
1. Residential, partial hospital treatment may prevent relapse.
2. CBT, individual, family therapies with goal of weight maintenance, normalization of eating behaviors.

B. Bulimia Nervosa

► H&P Keys
Recurrent binge eating (2 episodes/wk × 3 months) with lack of control over eating; self-induced vomiting (70–95%), use of laxatives or diuretics, strict dieting, vigorous exercise to prevent weight gain; overconcern with body weight, which is usually normal. Onset late adolescence, early adulthood, often during strict dieting; 95% women; mid- to upper socioeconomic strata. Complications: dental erosion and caries, parotid enlargement, calloused fingers, electrolyte abnormalities (50%), dehydration, weakness, lethargy, GI problems, cardiac arrhythmias; rarely, esophageal tears, gastric rupture, pancreatitis, sudden death. Comorbid anorexia, depression, personality disorders, stealing, substance abuse common.

► Diagnosis
Rule out seizure disorder, CNS tumor, Klüver–Bucy and Kleine–Levin syndromes; obtain ECG, electrolytes, amylase, LFTs.

► Disease Severity
Chronic intermittent disorder with range of impairment.

► Concept and Application
Genetic component; decreased CNS serotonin, NE activity; family history of mood disorders, obesity, substance abuse.

► Treatment Steps
1. Hospitalization for severe electrolyte abnormalities, suicide risk.
2. SSRIs reduce binging. Avoid bupropion.
3. CBT; individual, group, and family therapies.
4. Nutritional counseling, monitor weight.

X. SUBSTANCE-RELATED DISORDERS

A. Overview

Definitions

Abuse—Recurrent maladaptive pattern of use during 12-month period despite physical hazard or legal, social, or occupational problems.

Dependence—Psychological (craving) or physical (withdrawal syndrome, tolerance); loss of control over use; preoccupation with obtaining and using substance; continued use despite adverse social, occupational, or health consequences. Frequent denial, minimization.

Intoxication—Maladaptive behavior associated with recent ingestion.

Withdrawal—Substance-specific syndrome following decreased use or cessation of regular use.

Tolerance—Increasing amount of drug needed to produce intoxication.

▶ H&P Keys

Decrement in work or school performance; absenteeism; fights; family problems; injuries or accidents; acute personality change; driving under the influence (DUI), theft, prostitution; related medical and mental disorders; psychiatric comorbidity, particularly mood, anxiety, personality, schizophrenic, attention deficit disorders; chronic pain; may be self-medicating or symptoms may be caused by substance; defer diagnosis until patient clean ≥ 6 weeks. Needle tracks with IV use. All ages, races, social classes.

▶ Diagnosis

History (from patient and other sources) and physical signs. Drug testing usually done on urine; blood used for alcohol; saliva, sweat, breath, hair also used. Negative test does not rule out diagnosis. Preliminary assays (immunologic) sensitive but less specific than confirmatory tests (chromatography or spectrometry).

▶ Disease Severity

Worse prognosis with long-term use; psychiatric comorbidity; unsupportive milieu; lack of employment, job skills; younger age of onset. May be suicidal, assaultive. Dangerous withdrawal syndromes with alcohol, sedatives; dangerous overdoses with alcohol, narcotics, stimulants, phencyclidine. High blood level without signs of intoxication indicates tolerance. Intravenous drug use may lead to HIV, subacute bacterial endocarditis (SBE), hepatitis, thrombophlebitis, pneumonia, cellulitis; snorting cocaine, heroin may lead to nasal perforation, rhinitis, bleeding; inhaling or smoking marijuana, crack, inhalants may lead to bronchitis, asthma. Relapses common.

▶ Concept and Application

Genetic component to alcohol dependence and possibly others; all abused substances acutely enhance brain reward mechanisms; use reinforced by relief of withdrawal symptoms; environmental learning important.

▶ Treatment Steps

Acute

1. Intoxication: observation and medical treatment for overdose, multiple substance ingestion; protection from injury.
2. Withdrawal: symptomatic treatment; may need to detoxify (especially sedatives, alcohol, opioids) under medical supervision.
3. Diagnosis and treatment of concurrent nonpsychiatric medical problems.

Continued Care

1. Confront denial.
2. Initiate and maintain abstinence (or substitution pharmacotherapy, e.g., methadone), through inpatient, residential, partial and outpatient rehabilitation programs.
3. Individual, CBT, and group therapies; family therapy; self-help groups, e.g., Alcoholics Anonymous (AA).

4. Pharmacologic treatments, e.g., methadone maintenance, disulfiram (Antabuse), naloxone, acamprosate, as indicated.
5. Diagnose and treat comorbid psychiatric problems.

B. Alcohol Dependence

▶ H&P Keys

Early: injuries, accidents, gastritis, diarrhea, headaches, insomnia, absenteeism, blackouts, irritability. Later: nutritional deficiencies, hepatitis, cirrhosis, GI bleeding, pancreatitis, heart disease, hypertension, palmar erythema, acne rosacea, gynecomastia, testicular atrophy, peripheral neuropathy, GI cancers, cardiomyopathy, fetal alcohol syndrome (craniofacial abnormalities, mental retardation, behavior problems, congenital malformations), depression, anxiety, insomnia, neuropsychiatric disorders (below). Onset teens to 30s, men > women, family history. Associated abuse of other substances. Rule out underlying bipolar, anxiety, attention deficit, antisocial disorders. Twenty to 40% of homeless have diagnosis.

▶ Diagnosis

Clinical diagnosis; screen with CAGE (attempts to Cut down, Annoyance with criticism of drinking, Guilt, morning Eye-opener; two positives suggest problem drinking, and three positives give 95% certain diagnosis). Blood level of > 150 mg/dL without intoxication evidence of tolerance. May have increased γ-glutamyl transferase (GGT), mean corpuscular volume (MCV), asparatate transaminase (AST), alanine transaminase (ALT), uric acid, alkaline phosphatase, vertebral or rib fractures, abnormal liver, hepatic disease stigmata, hypertension, peripheral neuropathy on exam.

▶ Disease Severity

One-fourth to one-third have early onset; male, antisocial, family history; poor prognosis; responds best to structured milieu treatments. Two-thirds to three-fourths have later, gradual onset; equal sex distribution; better prognosis. Women have later onset but more virulent course, family and personal history of mood disorder; complications include motor vehicle accidents (MVAs), job loss, assaults, suicide, falls (rule out subdural hematoma), fires, poisonings, drownings.

▶ Concept and Application

Multiple causes: genetic factors, cultural patterns, learning. High heritability in males; nondrinking sons of alcoholics have altered evoked potentials, possibly greater tolerance.

▶ Treatment Steps

Acute
1. Treat withdrawal, detoxification as below.
2. Diagnose and treat acute comorbid medical and psychiatric problems.

Continued Care
1. Confront denial.
2. Inpatient or outpatient rehabilitation programs include group, individual, family, 12-step AA, educational components.
3. Disulfiram, naltrexone, acamprosate, SSRIs used to promote abstinence in some.
4. Anxiety, depression lasting more than 2–4 weeks past detoxification may require specific treatment.

C. Other Alcohol Syndromes

1. Intoxication

Disinhibition, mood lability, irritability, impaired judgment; incoordination, slurred speech, ataxia, nystagmus, flushing; may progress to blackouts, coma, death. Complicated by head injuries, MVAs, delirium, aggressive acts, suicide. Approximate blood alcohol levels for nontolerant person:

- 100–150 mg/dL: incoordination, irritability (legal intoxication)
- 150–250 mg/dL: slurred speech, ataxia (> 250 mg/dL: unconsciousness)
- Blood alcohol level > 150 mg/dL without intoxication evidence of dependence.

Treat supportively; evaluate for subdural, infection, other substances.

2. Alcohol Withdrawal Syndromes

Alcohol Withdrawal—Tremulousness, nausea, vomiting, autonomic hyperactivity, malaise, headache, insomnia, irritability, agitation, transient perceptual disturbance, grand mal seizures (< 3%). Up to 5–7 days postcessation.

Alcohol Withdrawal Delirium (Delirium Tremens)—Recent (2–3 days) cessation/reduction of heavy use in medically compromised patients with 5- to 15-year history of dependence; result of unmasking of downregulation of inhibitory GABA receptors. Delirium, autonomic hyperactivity, vivid auditory, visual and tactile hallucinations, paranoid delusions, agitation, tremor, fever, seizures occurring before delirium ("rum fits"). Treat underlying pneumonia, GI bleed, hepatic failure, subdural hematoma, electrolyte imbalance, dehydration. CBC, chemistries, vitamin B_{12}, folate, LFTs, urinalysis (UA), tox screen, chest x-ray (CXR), ECG; possible blood cultures, lumbar puncture (LP), CT of head, EEG; frequent vital signs, observation. Thiamine 100 mg (give *before* IV glucose), folate 1.0 mg, multivitamin, benzodiazepine, e.g., chlordiazepoxide (or oxazepam with hepatic dysfunction) adjusted to control symptoms and tapered 20–25% daily; phenytoin may be used with history of withdrawal seizures. Decrease stimulation; seclusion, restraint as necessary.

Alcohol Hallucinosis—Vivid, persistent auditory or visual hallucinations without delirium within 48 hours of cessation or reduction; rarely become chronic. Benzodiazepines, IV fluids, nutrition. Antipsychotics if chronic.

3. Alcoholic Encephalopathy (Wernicke's Encephalopathy)

Abrupt onset of nystagmus, ophthalmoplegia, ataxia, confusion due to thiamine deficiency associated with alcoholism; early treatment with thiamine may prevent Korsakoff's syndrome. Give thiamine before giving IV glucose. Diagnose concurrent infection, hepatic failure.

4. Alcohol-Induced Persisting Amnestic Disorder (Korsakoff's Syndrome)

Severe, persistent retrograde and anterograde amnesia, confabulation, apathy, polyneuritis due to thiamine deficiency, following Wernicke's encephalopathy.

5. Alcohol-Induced Persisting Dementia

Dementia following prolonged, heavy ingestion; distinguished from alcohol amnestic disorder by presence of cognitive deficits other than memory; exclude other causes of dementia.

D. Drug Dependence

1. Stimulants (Amphetamines, Cocaine, "Diet Pills," Others)

Highly addictive; ingested, injected, snorted, purified to free-base form and smoked (crack). *Intoxication* produces euphoria, alertness, increased energy, anxiety or panic, talkativeness, psychomotor agitation, impaired judgment, sexual arousal, anorexia, insomnia, pupillary dilatation, hypertension, tachycardia; may progress to hyperpyrexia; nausea and vomiting; visual or tactile hallucinations ("cocaine bugs"); paranoia; seizures, CVA, myocardial infarction (MI), sudden cardiac death. Treat symptomatically, e.g., severe agitation with benzodiazepine, tachyarrhythmia with antiarrhythmic; acidify urine. Assess for suicidality. *Delirium* lasting 1–6 hours with olfactory or tactile hallucinations, may lead to seizures, death. Chronic use and *dependence* associated with tolerance to euphoric effects; severe social, financial, health losses including STD risk through IV use, prostitution, poor judgment; weight loss; depression, irritability, sexual dysfunction, memory impairment, paranoia, persecutory delusions (*delusional disorder*). *Withdrawal* (crash) may be self-treated with sedatives, e.g., alcohol, marijuana; associated with insomnia or hypersomnia, hunger, fatigue, dysphoria, agitation, anxiety, suicidal ideations, craving. Not physically dangerous; assess suicide risk, treat supportively, refer for drug treatment. Treat depression persisting > 2–4 weeks after withdrawal.

2. Opioid Dependence (Heroin, Methadone, Meperidine, Codeine, Pentazocine, Others)

More common in urban settings, males, blacks, health care professionals, chronic pain patients. Opium smoked; heroin snorted, injected IV or SC ("skin popping"); speedball is heroin plus stimulant; pharmaceutic opioids ingested. *Dependence* associated with tolerance, compulsive use, weight loss, hyposexuality, amenorrhea, medical problems (e.g., HIV, SBE, cellulitis), crime, suicide, accidents. *Intoxication* produces euphoria, analgesia, hypoactivity, anorexia, drowsiness, constipation, nausea, vomiting, slurred speech, hypotension, bradycardia, pupillary constriction; CNS and respiratory depression, pulmonary edema, seizures, coma, death in overdose. Treat with IV naloxone, 0.8 mg, double dose q15min × 2 if no response; continue IV administration up to 3 days, support vital functions; diagnose polysubstance overdose. Assess for suicidality. *Withdrawal* severely uncomfortable but not a medical emergency; flulike syndrome of rhinorrhea, myalgias, nausea, vomiting, diarrhea, lacrimation, dilated pupils, restlessness, yawning, sweating, insomnia, piloerection, anxiety, craving, tachycardia, hypertension; methadone 15–25 mg q12h until symptoms suppressed, with gradual taper according to symptoms over 10–14 days; or buprenorphine withdrawal; symptomatic treatment with clonidine, antiemetics, analgesics also used. Methadone maintenance or abstinence; naltrexone used after detoxification to assist abstinence in highly motivated patient; pentazocine detoxified with pentazocine. Comorbid psychiatric disorder (ASP, depression, PTSD) in 80%.

3. **Sedative–Hypnotic Dependence (Benzodiazepines, Barbiturates, Methaqualone, Others)**

Young, polydrug abusers (frequently combined with alcohol, opioids, stimulants) or middle-aged women with iatrogenic dependence. *Dependence* produces tolerance to euphoriant and sedative effects, fatigue, psychomotor impairment, amnesia, depression, headaches, GI disturbances; *intoxication* causes slurred speech, drowsiness, incoordination, ataxia, impaired attention and memory, disinhibition. Flumetrazepam ("roofies") associated with date rape. Barbiturates have low therapeutic index, frequently used in suicide; *overdose* causes respiratory depression, coma; gastric lavage, charcoal, monitor closely, maintain airway and blood pressure. Benzodiazepines have high therapeutic index but may be lethal in combination with other CNS sedatives. Flumazenil (benzo antagonist) does not reverse respiratory inhibition. Mild *withdrawal* syndrome of anxiety, insomnia, headache, anorexia, dizziness common. Severe withdrawal syndrome is a medical emergency: nausea, vomiting, malaise, autonomic hyperactivity, anxiety, photophobia, tremor, hyperreflexia, hyperthermia, insomnia, delirium, seizures, death; short-acting drugs cause most severe syndrome. Pentobarbital challenge test determines substitute phenobarbital or long-acting benzodiazepine dose for gradual withdrawal. Pentobarbital 200 mg PO, then 100 mg q2h (max 500 mg) until intoxication observed; substitute phenobarbital, 30 mg/each 100 mg pentobarbital; taper ≈ 10%/day, adjust for signs of intoxication, withdrawal.

4. **Cannabinoids (THC, Marijuana, Hashish, Bhang, Ganja)**

Intoxication may produce euphoria or dysphoria, heightened sensation, time distortion, increased humorousness, impaired judgment, dry mouth, increased appetite, pupillary dilatation, conjunctival injection, suspiciousness, anxiety, tachycardia, depersonalization, incoordination; rarely hallucinations, mild persecutory delusions. Very high doses may cause prolonged psychosis, mild delirium, panic. Chronic use: apathetic, amotivational syndrome, memory impairment, depression, anxiety, respiratory and reproductive problems. No characteristic withdrawal syndrome. Urine toxicology positive up to 4 weeks after cessation of heavy use.

5. **Hallucinogens (LSD, Mescaline, DMT, Psilocybin, MDMA, Others)**

Eaten, sucked from paper, smoked; intoxication produces hallucinosis, sympathomimetic effects (pupillary dilatation, tachycardia, diaphoresis), perceptual changes, emotional intensity and lability. May cause depression, paranoia, panic reactions with belief that perceptions are real ("bad trips"); treat with reassurance, safe environment; benzodiazepines, antipsychotics for severe symptoms. Prolonged psychosis may develop in vulnerable patients; posthallucinogen perception disorder ("flashbacks") distressing persistent reexperiencing of hallucinations with intact reality testing. Low-dose benzodiazepine acutely, antipsychotic if persistent.

6. **Phencyclidine (PCP, Angel Dust)**

Hallucinogen, smoked with marijuana, eaten, injected, snorted; euphoriant, commonly causes unpredictable, paranoid, agitated, assaultive behavior; accompanied by dysarthria, diaphoresis, vertical and horizontal nystagmus, hypertension, tachycardia, analgesia, injury. May develop muscle rigidity, ataxia, hyperacusis, hyperreflexia, myoclonic jerks, catatonia, seizures, respiratory depression, coma, renal failure, chest pain, palpitations. Pupils normal sized. Elevated creatinine phosphokinase (CPK), myoglobinuria, ALT, blood urea nitrogen (BUN), creatinine. Chronic use may cause psychosis, mood disorder, delirium, long-term neuropsychological damage. Ensure safety in nonstimulating environment; restrain as needed; acidify urine; treat severe hypertension. Use benzodiazepines, antipsychotic symptomatically.

7. **Inhalants (Volatile Glues, Solvents, Gasoline, Cleaners, Nitrates, Others)**

Male adolescents; causes light-headedness, euphoria, disinhibition, dizziness, intensification of orgasm, belligerence, impaired judgment, perceptual disturbances, delusions, ataxia, confusion, disorientation, slurred speech, hyporeflexia, nystagmus, poor judgment, accidents; can progress to delirium, coma; chronic use causes weight loss, fatigue, respiratory problems, facial rash, halitosis, dementia, liver and kidney damage, bone marrow suppression, peripheral neuropathies, immunosuppression. Treat supportively. Substance abuse education, medical and psychiatric evaluation.

8. **Anabolic Steroid Abuse**

Adolescents, athletes; ingested or IM injection; chronic use associated with depression, mania, psychosis, acne, hepatic damage, infection from needle sharing, CVAs, testicular atrophy, and feminization in males, masculinization in females.

9. **Caffeine Dependence (Coffee, Tea, Cola, Chocolate, Over-the-Counter Stimulants, Cold Preps)**

Restlessness, insomnia, diuresis, anxiety, excitement, GI disturbance, flushing with intake > 250 mg/d (two cups brewed coffee); cardiac arrhythmia, muscle twitching, agitation, inexhaustibility with intake > 1 g. Withdrawal symptoms: headache, fatigue lasting 4–5 days.

10. **Nicotine Dependence (Tobacco Smoking, Chewing)**

Strongly conditioned, rapid dependence; assess number of cigarettes smoked/day, use of morning cigarette; dependence causes pulmonary, cardiac, peripheral vascular, neoplastic diseases. Withdrawal associated with craving, irritability, headache, anxiety, difficulty concentrating, restlessness, bradycardia, increased appetite, weight gain, GI distress, increased cough, insomnia, impaired performance. Obtain commitment to stop (motivational enhancement). Counseling, self-help literature, smoking cessation groups, behavioral interventions, nicotine gum or patch for moderate to severe addiction; bupropion also effective, may be used in combination with nicotine replacement. Highly comorbid with other psychiatric, substance use disorders; depression may develop upon withdrawal.

XI. SEXUAL DYSFUNCTIONS

▶ H&P Keys

Disorders of all phases of sexual response cycle causing distress, interpersonal difficulty: *hypoactive sexual desire disorder* (deficient or absent sexual fantasies or desire); *sexual aversion disorder* (revulsion to and avoidance of sexual contact); *female sexual arousal disorder* (inability to attain or maintain adequate sexual excitement and lubrication); *male erectile disorder* (inability to attain or maintain adequate erection); *female and male orgasmic disorders* (persistent or recurrent delay or absence of orgasm following sexual excitement); *premature ejaculation* (persistent ejaculation with minimal stimulation before or shortly after penetration); *dyspareunia* (persistent genital pain with intercourse); and *vaginismus* (involuntary spasm of vaginal musculature during intercourse). May be lifelong or acquired, generalized or situational, due to psychological and/or general medical or substance-induced factors.

▶ Diagnosis
Rule out dysfunction due to another psychiatric disturbance (e.g., depression, PTSD), substance dependence, diabetes, vascular disease, neurologic disease, including MS and trauma, endocrine disorders, hepatic or other systemic disease, surgical procedures; medications, commonly antihypertensives, anticholinergics, antihistamines, ADs, antipsychotics, steroids. Spontaneous erections, morning erections, erections with masturbation rule out organic etiology of impotence. Complete gynecologic or urologic exam, measurement of nocturnal penile tumescence, pudendal nerve latency, penile blood pressure, serum glucose, LFTs, TFTs, prolactin, luteinizing hormone (LH), FSH as indicated.

▶ Disease Severity
Primary and chronic disorders more difficult to treat. May have history of sexual victimization.

▶ Concept and Application
Illnesses, substance abuse, or medications that interfere with normal endocrine, neural, and vascular systems may produce sexual dysfunction. Psychological etiologies include ignorance and misinformation; unconscious guilt, anger and anxiety; conditioned responses; performance anxiety or fear of rejection; lack of communication between partners; physical and psychological stresses.

▶ Treatment Steps
1. Rule out medical or substance-related etiology.
2. Cognitive therapy, specific behavioral therapies, marital therapy, education (e.g., clitoral stimulation for orgasm in women). Behavioral therapies (e.g., sensate focus for erectile dysfunction, squeeze technique for premature ejaculation, directed masturbation for anorgasmia) desensitize patient and decrease performance anxiety.
3. Somatic treatments include alprostadil injections, sildenafil and others for impotence (contraindicated with use of nitrates, heart disease), hormone replacement therapy (HRT), SSRIs for premature ejaculation.

XII. DELIRIUM

▶ H&P Keys
Syndrome of global cognitive impairment with reduced attention; disorganized thought with rambling or incoherent speech; reduced and fluctuating level of consciousness (clear, drowsy, stupor, coma);

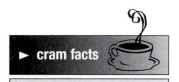

▶ cram facts

SAFE SEX GUIDELINES

Safe Sex Practices
- Masturbation
- Dry kissing
- Hugging, massage
- Use of unshared vibrators, sex toys

Low-Risk Sex Practices
- Wet kissing without mouth sores
- Mutual masturbation
- Intercourse (vaginal or anal) with condom
- Oral sex with use of barrier
- Skin contact with semen, urine with no skin sores or breaks

Unsafe Sex Practices
- Intercourse (vaginal or anal) without condom
- Oral sex without barrier
- Blood contact
- Sharing sex instruments
- Semen, urine, feces in mouth, vagina

► **diagnostic decisions**

DELIRIUM VERSUS DEMENTIA

Delirium
Rapid onset
Fluctuating, clouded consciousness
Often reversible
Perceptual disturbances, sleep–wake cycle
   abnormalities, incoherent speech common

Dementia
Insidious onset
Clear sensorium until late in course
Most irreversible and progressive
These symptoms uncommon until late in
   course

---

sensory (commonly visual) misperceptions, such as illusions, hallucinations; disorientation; disturbed sleep–wake cycle; psychomotor and memory disturbances; rapid onset, fluctuating course, brief duration ending in recovery, dementia, death. May have emotional disturbance (agitated or withdrawn); fearfulness; abnormal movements, e.g., asterixis; autonomic hyperactivity. Increased susceptibility in children, elderly, prior brain damage (e.g., dementia, AIDS). Prevalence 10–15% medical/surgical patients, 30% intensive care unit (ICU) patients.

► Diagnosis

History, physical, lab studies to diagnose underlying problem. Common etiologies include systemic infection; metabolic disorders (hypoxia, hypoglycemia, thyroid disease, electrolyte imbalances, hepatic or renal disease, thiamine deficiency); postoperative states; seizures and postictal states; head injury; substance intoxication, withdrawal syndromes; anticholinergic, sedative, or other medications; toxins; autoimmune disorders; hypertensive encephalopathy; brain neoplasms; focal lesions (right parietal, inferomedial occipital). Psychotic psychiatric disorders lack random fluctuation; problems with attention, orientation, memory; have prior history. Clear sensorium in dementia (may have comorbid dementia). EEG shows background alpha wave slowing or low-voltage fast theta waves.

► Disease Severity

Delirium is a medical emergency, requiring rapid assessment and treatment.

► Concept and Application

Final common pathway for acute brain insult. Dysfunction of brain stem reticular activating system.

► Treatment Steps

1. Diagnose and treat underlying disorder (history, physical, chemistries, CBC, LFTs, UA, erythrocyte sedimentation rate [ESR], toxicologies, HIV, blood cultures, ECG, EEG, CT or MRI of head, LP as indicated.
2. Monitor vital signs, cognitive status (e.g., Mini-Mental State Exam).
3. Treat alcohol, sedative withdrawals as above; anticholinergic delirium treated with physostigmine.
4. Discontinue all unnecessary medications; avoid anticholinergics and sedative–hypnotics.
5. Hydration, nutrition.

6. Reassurance; optimize sensory environment, e.g., night light, soft music, relative or sitter in room, restraint, protection from injury.
7. Low-dose, high-potency antipsychotic for agitation.

XIII. ABUSE SYNDROMES

A. Child Physical and Sexual Abuse

▶ H&P Keys

Risk factors include parental history of child abuse, current substance abuse, depression, impulsivity; premature, hyperactive, emotionally disturbed, physically ill, or otherwise difficult child; stepchild; current toilet training; impairment, unavailability, abuse of mother; familial isolation, stress, poverty, conflict; child's running away. History inconsistent with physical findings or developmental level; inconsistent stories; multiple injuries of different ages; delay in seeking care. Suspect when see linear or geometric marks; old scars; spiral, humerus, or rib fractures; geometric or symmetric lower body burns; ruptured viscera; facial and head trauma; retinal hemorrhages. Genital or anal trauma or lesions; stomach or rectal pain; urinary tract infections with sexual abuse. Signs of disturbed attachment (e.g., lack of physical contact or concern by parent, lack of separation anxiety by child, hypercritical attitude toward child). Delayed development, disturbed play, inappropriate sexual behavior.

▶ Diagnosis

Rule out unintentional trauma, bleeding diathesis, dermatologic conditions, vitamin deficiencies, osteogenesis imperfecta, self-inflicted injuries; thorough physical exam; skeletal series, serologies, bleeding screening, CBC, creatine kinase (CK) as indicated.

▶ Disease Severity

Deaths usually occur only after numerous episodes; psychiatric sequelae (PTSD, depression, substance abuse, personality disorders, dissociative identity disorder, sexual dysfunction, somatic complaints, repetition of abuse, suicidal or self-destructive behavior) worse with early-age onset, chronicity, severe abuse, use of force, multiple perpetrators, abuse by parental figure, lack of support.

▶ Concept and Application

Child may dissociate during abuse episode and later develop dissociative symptoms. Guilt, shame, rage, low self-esteem, self-destructive behavior, developmental delays, anxiety, withdrawal, antisocial behavior common.

▶ Treatment Steps

Acute
1. Interview child alone; expert may be necessary to elicit abuse history; interview parents separately.
2. Document findings, including pictures.
3. All states mandate reporting of suspected abuse (physical, emotional, sexual, severe neglect).
4. Ensure safety of child.

Continued Care
1. Treatment of child for physical, emotional sequelae; individual, group psychotherapy.

2. Treatment for abusers ranges from support (emotional support, social services, education, Parent's Anonymous groups, hotlines) through mandated therapy, removal of parent abuser or child, legal prosecution.

B. Adult Domestic Violence

▶ H&P Keys

Risk factors include pregnancy, younger age, social isolation, child abuse in home; histories of child abuse, substance abuse, criminality in abuser; abused women not shown to have specific predisposing personality traits. History may be incompatible with injury. Trauma repetitive in most; no diagnostic injury pattern; head, face, neck, breast, abdomen frequent injury sites. PTSD symptoms, low self-esteem, somatic complaints, depression, anxiety, substance abuse, suicide attempts.

▶ Diagnosis

Battering present in 20% of women seeking medical care; 22–35% of women presenting to emergency departments; 23% of prenatal patients; 25% of women who attempt suicide; 45–58% of mothers of abused children. Routine inquiry in privacy makes diagnosis.

▶ Disease Severity

Increased risk of severe abuse when abused partner decides to leave; respect victim's judgment regarding her safety. Inquire about presence of firearms. High risk of marital rape.

▶ Concept and Application

Barriers to leaving abusive relationship include shock and denial, self-blame, feelings of helplessness, presence of children, financial dependency, lack of job skills, fear of retaliation.

▶ Treatment Steps

1. Interview victim alone.
2. Treat and document injuries.
3. Evaluate suicide/homicide potential.
4. Ensure confidentiality and safety of victim, children—risk of severe abuse increases when abused partner decides to leave.
5. Assess resources, continued risk (threats, extent of prior injury, presence of weapons, stalking, substance abuse).
6. Referrals for social, legal, medical, psychiatric resources.

C. Elder Abuse

Abuser generally relative/caretaker; victim may fear disclosure due to dependency; family system with frustration, financial or health stress, substance abuse, history of violence; previous injuries, physical deterioration: bruising, head injury, burns, decubiti, contractures, dehydration, lacerations, diarrhea, impaction, malnutrition, urine burns, signs of neglect, sexual assault, PTSD symptoms. Interview privately; social service for assessment of living situation; mandatory reporting in most states.

XIV. BEREAVEMENT

A. Uncomplicated Bereavement

Normal reaction to death of loved one or other significant loss; acute grief characterized by intense emotional distress, somatic symptoms, dissociation, preoccupation with deceased, anger, loss of

▶ **diagnostic decisions**

DEPRESSION VERSUS BEREAVEMENT

Depression	Bereavement
Mood pervasive, unremitting	Mood fluctuates
Pervasive low self-esteem, worthlessness	Self-reproach regarding deceased
May be suicidal	Usually not suicidal
May have sustained psychotic symptoms	May transiently hear voice or see image of deceased
Does not improve without treatment; average episode 6–9 months	Symptoms improve with time; severe symptoms usually gone by 2–6 months
Social withdrawal	Often welcomes social support

habitual patterns of conduct. Mourning can include full depressive syndrome with depressed mood, sleep disturbance, anorexia, guilt, crying, difficulty concentrating, loss of interest, fatigue, anxiety; duration varies, symptoms generally remit spontaneously, anniversary reactions common. Higher risk of general medical and psychiatric illness and mortality. Signs of pathologic grief include marked psychomotor retardation, morbid preoccupation with worthlessness and hopelessness, prolonged functional impairment, persistent suicidal preoccupation; prolonged denial; absence of grief. Encourage expression of feelings, reminiscences; refer to community supports; medication generally contraindicated, but autonomous depressive disorder should be treated.

B. Sudden Infant Death Syndrome (SIDS)

Sudden, unexpected, unexplained death of infant < 1 year old. African Americans and Native Americans have 2–3 times risk. Risk factors include sleeping prone, exposure to cigarette smoke, lack of prenatal care, prematurity. Associated with abnormalities in the arcuate nucleus.

Intense, severe grief reactions frequent in parents, including guilt, anger, hostility, somatic symptoms; delayed mourning; overactivity; social isolation; psychosis; agitated depression. Associated with decline in physical health, marital difficulties, behavioral disturbance in siblings, migration. Contact with dead infant; autopsy may help; education may reduce guilt and blame; parent support groups; involvement of siblings; extended social support; counseling regarding future pregnancy recommended.

BIBLIOGRAPHY

American Psychiatric Association. *Diagnostic and Statistical Manual of Mental Disorders.* 4th ed. Text Revision. Washington, DC: American Psychiatric Association, 2000.

Fauman MA. *Study Guide to DSM-IV-TR.* Washington, DC: American Psychiatric Press, 2002.

Kaplan HI, Sadock BJ. *Synopsis of Psychiatry,* 9th ed. Baltimore: Williams & Wilkins, 2002.

Manley MRS. *Psychiatric Clerkship Guide.* St. Louis: Mosby, 2003.

Taylor MA. *The Fundamentals of Clinical Neuropsychiatry.* New York: Oxford University Press, 1999.

Pulmonary Medicine

16

I. INFECTIOUS DISORDERS

A. Croup

▶ **H&P Keys**

Children under 6 years old following upper respiratory illness. Barking cough, inspiratory stridor, dyspnea, hoarseness, usually worse at night.

▶ **Diagnosis**

X-ray or magnetic resonance imaging (MRI) of upper airway (glottic and subglottic swelling). Diagnosis usually clinical.

▶ **Disease Severity**

Respiratory rate, pulse oximetry, accessory muscle use, stridor.

▶ **Concept and Application**

Glottic and subglottic edema leading to upper airway obstruction. Multiple viral etiologies, including respiratory syncytial virus (RSV), influenza A and B, adenovirus, and rhinovirus.

▶ **Treatment Steps**
1. Humidification of inspired air.
2. Correction of hypoxemia.
3. Aerosol racemic epinephrine, systemic corticosteroids.
4. Intubation if severe (rarely needed).

B. Acute Epiglottitis

▶ **H&P Keys**

Children < 7 years of age most common. High fever, stridor, dyspnea, hoarseness, dry cough, drooling, dysphagia, systemic toxicity, cherry-red epiglottis.

▶ **Diagnosis**

Lateral neck x-ray (enlarged epiglottis), blood culture, throat culture (but see below).

▶ **Disease Severity**

X-ray findings, pulse oximetry, clinical distress, accessory muscle use.

▶ **Concept and Application**

Edema of epiglottis obstructing upper airway. Etiologic agent usually *Haemophilus influenzae* type b.

▶ **Treatment Steps**
1. Antibiotics active against *H. influenzae* (cefuroxime, ampicillin plus clavulanic acid).
2. Endotracheal intubation or tracheostomy in severe cases.

Note: Airway examination and throat culture may provoke laryngospasm and cardiopulmonary arrest!

C. Acute Bronchitis

▶ **H&P Keys**

Severe, prolonged productive cough, fever, dyspnea.

▶ **Diagnosis**

History and physical, sputum culture, chest x-ray (CXR) to rule out bronchopneumonia.

► Disease Severity

Respiratory rate, temperature.

► Concept and Application

Infection and inflammation of large airways. Usually viral (influenza, adenovirus). May be bacterial (*Mycoplasma pneumoniae, Bordetella pertussis, H. influenzae, Streptococcus pneumoniae*).

► Treatment Steps

1. Hydration, cough suppressants.
2. If bacterial: broad-spectrum oral antibiotic (e.g., macrolide, tetracycline derivative, broad-spectrum quinolone).

D. Acute Bronchiolitis

► H&P Keys

Children < 2 years old following upper respiratory infection; tachypnea, inspiratory and expiratory wheezing, intercostal and suprasternal retractions, nasal flaring, hyperresonant chest, inspiratory rales.

► Diagnosis

CXR: hyperinflated lungs, peribronchial thickening; may have concurrent bronchopneumonia. Normal white blood cell (WBC) count. Inspiratory "click."

► Disease Severity

Respiratory rate, intercostal retractions, pulse oximetry.

► Concept and Application

Acute inflammation of small airways causing hyperinflation, obstruction, and atelectasis. Majority associated with RSV.

► Treatment Steps

Oxygen, hydration, aerosol ribavirin for RSV.

E. Pertussis

► H&P Keys

Usually occurs in infants < 2 years old.

Catarrhal Stage—Lasts 1–2 weeks. Presents similarly to viral illness: low-grade fever, injected conjunctiva.

Paroxysmal Stage—Lasts 2–4 weeks. Severe, paroxysmal, short coughs with inspiratory "whoop." Thick, tenacious secretions, usually afebrile.

► Diagnosis

Nasopharyngeal culture (requires special medium), elevated white blood cell (WBC) count (mostly lymphocytes); increased polymorphonuclear neutrophils (PMNs) suggest bacterial superinfection.

► Disease Severity

WBC count. Presence of bacterial superinfection.

► Concept and Application

Infection of tracheobronchial tree with *Bordetella pertussis*. In severe cases, mucopurulent exudate obstructs small airways.

► Treatment Steps

1. Macrolide antibiotic in catarrhal stage (does not help in paroxysmal stage).
2. Supportive care.
3. Antibiotics for treatment of superinfection if present.

F. Bacterial Bronchopneumonia

1. Pneumococcal Pneumonia

▶ **H&P Keys**

Acute onset of rigors, fever, cough productive of "rusty" sputum, tachypnea, respiratory distress, pleuritic chest pain, bronchial breath sounds. Dullness to percussion may indicate accompanying effusion or empyema.

▶ **Diagnosis**

CXR (lobar infiltrate), sputum Gram stain, sputum culture, blood culture, WBC.

▶ **Disease Severity**

Pulse oximetry, arterial blood gases (ABG), tachypnea, CXR. Multi-lobed involvement, low WBC count, positive blood culture, and older age associated with worse prognosis.

▶ **Concept and Application**

Infection caused by *Streptococcus pneumoniae*. Most common cause of community-acquired pneumonia. Elderly, infants, asplenic, and immunocompromised patients at highest risk.

▶ **Treatment Steps**

1. Begin antibiotic immediately (penicillin G, erythromycin, broad-spectrum quinolone). Use vancomycin or quinolone if penicillin resistance is present or suspected.
2. Chest tube drainage if empyema present. Pneumococcal vaccine for high-risk individuals after acute episode resolves.

2. Staphylococcal Pneumonia

▶ **H&P Keys**

Fever, dyspnea, cough with purulent sputum.

▶ **Diagnosis**

CXR (multifocal infiltrates, abscess, pneumatocele, effusions), other tests as above for pneumonia.

▶ **Disease Severity**

Pulse oximetry, ABG, tachypnea, CXR. Metastatic infection (central nervous system [CNS], bone, endocarditis, sepsis).

▶ **Concept and Application**

Pulmonary infection caused by *Staphylococcus aureus*. Seen after influenza infection, chronic obstructive pulmonary disease (COPD), hematogenous spread from staphylococcal endocarditis (especially in intravenous drug abusers with right heart endocarditis), nosocomial infection.

▶ **Treatment Steps**

1. *Begin antibiotic immediately* (β-lactamase–resistant penicillin; if resistant: vancomycin or linezolid).
2. Oxygen if hypoxic.

3. *Haemophilus influenzae* Pneumonia

▶ **H&P Keys**

Young children, chronic lung disease, alcoholics. Fever, cough, dyspnea, purulent sputum. Subacute presentation over several weeks possible.

► **Diagnosis**

CXR (multilobar patchy infiltrates), as above for pneumonias.

► **Disease Severity**

Pulse oximetry, ABG, respiratory rate, CXR. Empyema is rare.

► **Concept and Application**

Pulmonary infection caused by *H. influenzae*. More common in COPD and smokers.

► **Treatment Steps**

Begin antibiotic immediately (broad-spectrum quinolone if > 18 years of age, cefuroxime, ampicillin/clavulanic acid, others).

4. Gram-Negative Bacillary Pneumonias

► **H&P Keys**

Usually nosocomial, fever, chills, dyspnea, cough productive of purulent and sometimes bloody sputum.

► **Diagnosis**

CXR (lobar or multilobar, cavitary infiltrates), as above for pneumonia.

► **Disease Severity**

Pulse oximetry, ABG, respiratory rate, CXR (multilobed involvement and cavitation). High mortality.

► **Concept and Application**

Aspiration of gram-negative bacilli from colonized oropharynx. *Klebsiella pneumoniae, Acinetobacter* and *Pseudomonas* species, Enterobacteriacae genera; common in immunocompromised and hospitalized patients. *Klebsiella* common in alcoholics.

► **Treatment Steps**

1. Third-generation cephalosporin, semisynthetic penicillin (ticarcillin, piperacillin), or carbopenem plus either an aminoglycoside or a broad-spectrum quinolone.
2. Check antibiotic sensitivities and adjust for resistance.

G. Atypical Pneumonias

1. Legionnaire's Disease

► **H&P Keys**

Lethargy, headache, fever, rigors, anorexia, myalgias, nonproductive cough, GI symptoms. Rales and rhonchi, abdominal tenderness, relative bradycardia.

► **Diagnosis**

CXR (lobar, nodular, or patchy subsegmental), low sodium and phosphate, elevated WBC. Sputum culture (requires special media), serologic titers, urinary antigen.

► **Disease Severity**

Symptoms, respiratory rate, pulse oximetry, ABG, CXR.

► **Concept and Application**

Infection with *Legionella* species; transmitted through contaminated water system (not person to person). More common in immunocompromised, chronic disease, dialysis, alcoholics.

▶ Treatment Steps
1. Begin antibiotic immediately (macrolide, tetracycline, or quinolone).
2. Add rifampin in severe cases.

2. *Mycoplasma pneumoniae* Infection

▶ H&P Keys
Fever, chills, persistent nonproductive cough, headache, sore throat. Common in young adults.

▶ Diagnosis
Gram stain (many WBCs without predominant organism), CXR (interstitial or diffuse alveolar infiltrates), cold agglutinins, serum complement fixation titers.

▶ Disease Severity
Usually does not require hospitalization.

▶ Concept and Application
Extrapulmonary manifestations common, including bullous myringitis, pharyngitis, meningitis.

▶ Treatment Steps
Macrolide antibiotic, quinolone, or tetracycline.

3. *Pneumocystis jiroveci* (formerly *carinii*) Pneumonia

▶ H&P Keys
Opportunistic infection most commonly related to HIV or other immunodeficiency states. Subacute onset fever, dyspnea, nonproductive cough, tachypnea, tachycardia, diffuse rales.

▶ Diagnosis
Induced sputum cytology, bronchoscopic lavage or biopsy, elevated lactic dehydrogenase (LDH), HIV test, CD4 count, CXR (diffuse interstitial or alveolar infiltrates, may be atypical or even clear).

▶ Disease Severity
Pulse oximetry, ABG, respiratory rate, and clinical appearance.

▶ Concept and Application
Molecular genetic data suggest organism is fungal.

▶ Treatment Steps
1. Trimethoprim and sulfamethoxazole (TMP-SMZ) or pentamidine.
2. Oxygen and systemic corticosteroids if hypoxic.
3. Prevent in susceptible patients with TMP-SMZ, dapsone, or aerosolized pentamidine. Aerosol less effective; risk of upper lobe disease.

4. Influenza Pneumonia

▶ H&P Keys
Abrupt onset fever, chills, headache, myalgias, and malaise. Nonproductive or productive cough, tachypnea and dyspnea follow.

▶ Diagnosis
Sputum Gram stain (many WBCs without organisms); CXR (bilateral diffuse midlung and lower-lung infiltrates), viral cultures of nose and throat, acute and convalescent serum titers.

► **Disease Severity**

Respiratory rate, clinical appearance.

► **Concept and Application**

Viral pneumonia caused by influenza A.

► **Treatment Steps**

1. Zanamivir, oseltamivir, or rimantadine if administered within 48 hours of onset; otherwise, symptomatic treatment.
2. Prophylactic influenza vaccine for high- and moderate-risk groups.
3. Consider postexposure prophylaxis of high-risk patients with zanamivir, oseltamivir, rimantadine, or amantadine.

H. Pulmonary Tuberculosis

► **H&P Keys**

Fever, malaise, weight loss, dyspnea, night sweats; productive cough with hemoptysis, rales in area of involvement; amphoric breath sounds may indicate cavity.

► **Diagnosis**

CXR (upper-lobe cavitary disease if reactivation, lower-lobe infiltrates in primary infection, upper-lobe scarring may indicate latent infection). Sputum culture, acid-fast smear; bronchoscopy if unable to get diagnosis on sputum studies. Purified protein derivative (PPD) (tuberculin) skin test.

► **Disease Severity**

CXR. Extrapulmonary involvement (lymphatic, pleural, peritoneal, genitourinary, miliary, bone and joint, meningeal) may be more problematic.

► **Concept and Application**

Inhalation of *Mycobacterium tuberculosis* leads to primary lower-lobe infection. Localized inflammatory response usually halts infection. Reactivation disease occurs in upper lobes of lung or other areas of high oxygen content.

► **Treatment Steps**

Prophylaxis—Isoniazid for 6–12 months in appropriate patients with inactive infection (Table 16–1).

Treatment
1. Isoniazid and rifampin for 6 months, with pyrazinamide plus either ethambutol or streptomycin for first 2 months. In locales with frequent drug resistance, therapy may be started with five or six drugs. Drug-resistant strains require longer treatment with additional antibiotics.
2. Directly observed therapy highly recommended.

I. Fungal Pneumonias

1. Histoplasmosis

► **H&P Keys**

Mostly asymptomatic, can have abrupt onset of flulike illness, with fever, chills, substernal chest pain, nonproductive cough with myalgias, arthralgias, and headache.

► **Diagnosis**

CXR: acute disease often normal, hilar adenopathy with lower-lobe alveolar infiltrates, leading to chronic calcification). Progressive

16-1

INTERPRETATION OF A POSITIVE PPD

1. A reaction of > 5 mm is classified as positive in the following groups of patients:
   - HIV positive
   - Recent close contact
   - Fibrotic changes on CXR c/w old TB
   - Organ transplant recipient or immune suppressed (equivalent of ≥ 15 mg/day prednisone ≥ 1 mo)
2. A reaction of > 10 mm is classified as positive in persons who have other risk factors for tuberculosis or are in high-prevalence situations. These include:
   - Injection drug users
   - Diabetes mellitus
   - High-risk job or environmental exposure
   - Hematologic, head, neck malignancies
   - Chronic renal failure
   - Weight > 10% below ideal body weight
   - Silicosis
   - Gastrectomy
   - Recent immigrant (≤ 5 yrs) from high-prevalence country
   - Resident/employee of high-risk setting
   - Child/adolescent
   - Prison inmate
   - Medical caregiver
   - TB lab personnel
3. Reactions > 15 mm are classified as positive in all other persons.

Sources: American Thoracic Society (ATS)/Centers for Disease Control and Prevention (CDC). Diagnostic standards and classifications of tuberculosis in adults and children. *Am J Respir Crit Care Med* 161:1376–1395, 2000; and ATS/CDC. Targeted tuberculin testing and treatment of latent tuberculosis infection. *Am J Respir Crit Care Med* 161 (4 Pt 2):S221–47, 2000.

form mimics tuberculosis. Diagnosis with sputum culture. Progressive disseminated histoplasmosis: blood and bone marrow culture. Serologic testing (acute and convalescent titers; poor sensitivity).

▶ Disease Severity
Progressive and progressive disseminated more severe. Latter associated with T-cell dysfunction (acquired immune deficiency syndrome [AIDS]).

▶ Concept and Application
Infection with *Histoplasma capsulatum*. Inhalation of spores from soil (bat and bird droppings) evolve into pathogenic yeast form. Endemic areas: Ohio and Mississippi River valleys and neighboring states.

▶ Treatment Steps

Acute—None needed.

Progressive Cavitary Disease
1. Itraconazole.
2. Alternative: ketoconazole.

Progressive Disseminated Disease—Amphotericin B.

Chronic Suppression (for Patients with AIDS)—Itraconazole.

2. Blastomycosis

▶ H&P Keys
Abrupt fever, chills, cough with mucopurulent sputum, arthralgias, and myalgias. Signs of consolidation, erythema nodosum.

▶ Diagnosis
KOH preparation of expectorated sputum; culture, complement fixation. CXR (round densities, may cavitate).

▶ Disease Severity
CXR, evidence of extrapulmonary involvement.

▶ **Concept and Application**

Infection with *Blastomyces dermatitidis*. Yeast form pathogenic. Manifestations vary: asymptomatic to severe, life-threatening, disseminated illness. Midwest and south central United States, midwestern Canada.

▶ **Treatment Steps**

Progressive Pulmonary, Nonsevere
1. Itraconazole.
2. Alternative: ketoconazole.

Disseminated or Severe Disease—Amphotericin B.

3. Coccidioidomycosis

▶ **H&P Keys**

Cough, fever, pleuritic chest pain, headache (may be indicative of meningitis); erythematous rash, "valley fever": erythema nodosum, erythema multiforme, arthralgias.

▶ **Diagnosis**

CXR (patchy pneumonitis, hilar adenopathy, "coin lesions," cavitary lesions), KOH preparation of sputum, lung biopsy, complement fixation, skin test.

▶ **Disease Severity**

Disseminated disease (meningitis, skin lesions, bone, etc.). Dissemination more common in AIDS, steroids, malignant disease, African-Americans, Native Americans, Mexicans.

▶ **Concept and Application**

Infection with *Coccidioides immitis*. Spherules are pathogenic form. Mostly mild, self-limited, but can be life threatening and disseminated. Southwestern United States and California valley regions, northern Mexico.

▶ **Treatment Steps**

Nonmeningeal Disease
1. Fluconazole or amphotericin B.
2. Alternative: ketoconazole, itraconazole.

Disseminated Disease or Meningitis
1. Fluconazole, miconazole, or amphotericin B.
2. Intrathecal amphotericin if fluconazole fails.

4. Cryptococcosis

▶ **H&P Keys**

Pneumonia—Usually asymptomatic, but may have fever, malaise, chest pain, cough.

Meningitis—Subacute fever, confusion, headache. May be fulminant. Cranial nerve palsies.

▶ **Diagnosis**

Cerebrospinal fluid (CSF) examination (India ink stain, latex particle agglutination), lung biopsy, CXR (variable, large and small round lesions).

▶ **Disease Severity**

Disseminated disease (CNS), presence of meningitis, CXR.

► Concept and Application

Cryptococcus neoformans, found in bird droppings and soil. Increased risk in immunocompromised states.

► Treatment Steps

None needed in noncompromised host with isolated pulmonary disease.

> *Immunocompromised Host or Disseminated Disease*
> 1. Amphotericin B plus flucytosine.
> 2. Alternatives: fluconazole, itraconazole.

5. Invasive Aspergillosis

► H&P Keys

Immunosuppressed patient on multiple antibiotics, high fever, pleuritic chest pain, pleural friction rub.

► Diagnosis

Cultures of sputum and nasal swab (suggestive, not diagnostic), lung biopsy.

► Disease Severity

CXR (lobar, peripheral wedge-shaped infiltrates, often cavitary), pulse oximetry, ABG.

► Concept and Application

Opportunistic infection with *Aspergillus fumigatus* causing pneumonia, pulmonary infarction.

► Treatment Steps

1. Amphotericin B; alternatives: voriconazole or caspofungin.
2. Add flucytosine if metastatic infection.
3. Consider surgical resection if focal but severe disease.

6. Phycomycosis

► H&P Keys

Occurs in diabetic ketoacidosis, with glucocorticosteroids, cytotoxic agents, burn victims. Rhinocerebral disease, acute pneumonia with pleuritic chest pain and hemoptysis.

► Diagnosis

CXR (multiple wedge-shaped infiltrates), tissue biopsy.

► Disease Severity

Life-threatening disease.

► Concept and Application

Infection with *Mucor* (most common), also *Rhizopus* or *Absidia.*

► Treatment Steps

1. Amphotericin B and aggressive resectional surgery.
2. Prognosis extremely poor.

II. OBSTRUCTIVE PULMONARY DISEASES

A. Pulmonary Function Tests (PFTs)

See Table 16–2.

> *Obstruction*—Low forced expiratory volume in one second (FEV_1), low or normal forced vital capacity (FVC), reduced FEV_1:FVC ratio (< 70%), normal to increased total lung capacity (TLC).

16-2

CHARACTERISTIC CHANGES IN LUNG VOLUMES AND FLOW RATES IN PATIENTS WITH RESTRICTIVE, OBSTRUCTIVE, AND COMBINED VENTILATORY DISORDERS

Test	Restrictive	Obstructive	Combined
Forced vital capacity (FVC)	Decreased	Decreased or normal	Decreased
Total lung capacity (TLC)	Decreased	Increased or normal	Decreased
FEV_1	Decreased	Decreased	Decreased
FEV_1/FVC ratio	Increased or normal	Decreased	Decreased

Restriction—Defined by reduced TLC. Pure restriction will also have low FEV_1, FVC with normal or elevated FEV_1:FVC ratio.

Combined Obstruction and Restriction—Reduced FEV_1, FVC, TLC, and reduced FEV_1:FVC ratio.

B. Asthma

▶ H&P Keys

Acute onset of dyspnea, wheezing, cough that remit spontaneously or with treatment.

▶ Diagnosis

PFT (obstructive), response to bronchodilators, response to bronchoconstricting provocational agents.

▶ Disease Severity

PFT, use of accessory muscles, ABG, paradoxical pulse, respiratory rate, pulse oximetry, symptoms.

▶ Concept and Application

Bronchospasm, inflammation, hyperreactivity to inhaled antigens and irritants, mucus plugging. Obstruction may improve to normal with treatment.

▶ Treatment Steps

Acute

1. Bronchodilators:
   - Inhaled β-agonist, inhaled ipratropium bromide.
   - If fails, consider subcutaneous epinephrine, and/or intravenous aminophylline.
2. Anti-inflammatory agents: systemic corticosteroids; use if severe.

Chronic

1. Bronchodilators: β-Agonists (inhaled, subcutaneous, oral) as "rescue," theophylline.
2. Anti-inflammatory agents:
   - Inhaled corticosteroids, cromolyn sodium, nedocromil sodium, or oral leukotriene blocker (montelukast, zafirlukast). Omalizumab (anti–immunoglobulin E [IgE] antibody) if sensitivity to perennial aeroallergens and high IgE level.
   - Choose one as "controller"; may add a second for poor control. Combining inhaled steroid with long-acting inhaled β-agonist improves control.
3. Avoidance of causative agents.

C. Chronic Obstructive Pulmonary Diseases

Term is usually applied to patients with chronic bronchitis or emphysema who have obstruction on PFTs. The obstruction may be partially reversible.

1. Chronic Bronchitis

▶ H&P Keys

Defined as presence of chronic productive cough for *3 months in 2 successive years* without other discernible cause. Dyspnea, recurrent productive cough, "blue bloater"; cyanosis with edema, wheezes.

▶ Diagnosis

PFTs (obstructive), history, CXR (usually clear or hyperinflated). Sputum cultures for acute exacerbations.

▶ Disease Severity

PFTs, pulse oximetry, ABG.

▶ Concept and Application

In pure form, pathologic conditions in bronchi and airways, not alveoli. Tobacco smoke a causative agent. Bacterial infections may exacerbate (pneumococcus, *Haemophilus,* others).

Simple Chronic Bronchitis—Symptoms fit criteria for chronic bronchitis but no obstruction on PFTs (therefore not truly a form of COPD).

Obstructive Chronic Bronchitis—Symptoms fit criteria for chronic bronchitis, reduced FEV_1 percent with no or partial bronchodilator response (this is a form of COPD). Obstruction caused by hypertrophic glands in airway, mucous hypersecretion.

▶ Treatment Steps

1. Smoking cessation.
2. Ipratropium bromide.
3. Add inhaled β-agonist bronchodilator if needed.
4. Influenza and pneumococcal vaccination.
5. Antibiotics for acute bacterial exacerbation.
6. Oxygen if saturaton ≤ 88% or Po_2 ≤ 55 (or ≤ 60 with cor pulmonale).
7. Corticosteroids if severe.

2. Emphysema

▶ H&P Keys

Dyspnea, wheezing, cough. "Pink puffer": thin, not cyanotic, tachypneic. Diminished breath sounds, hyperinflated chest, hyperresonant to percussion.

▶ Diagnosis

Obstructive PFTs (TLC may be increased), CXR, history, and physical. Serum protein electrophoresis or α_1-protease inhibitor level if deficiency suspected.

▶ Disease Severity

PFTs, ABG, exercise tolerance.

▶ Concept and Application

Defined pathologically: enlarged respiratory air spaces beyond terminal bronchioles, with destruction of alveoli. Smoking a major risk factor; α_1-protease inhibitor deficiency a rare cause.

► Treatment Steps

Same as for chronic bronchitis, above. α_1-protease inhibitor if deficiency proven.

3. Cystic Fibrosis (CF)

► H&P Keys

Persistent cough, recurrent pneumonia and bronchitis, recurrent abdominal pain, meconium ileus, failure to thrive, steatorrhea, infertility, diabetes, family history. Usually diagnosed in childhood.

► Diagnosis

Sweat chloride test (> 60 mEq/L before age 20; < 80 in adults) diagnostic. Genetic testing available for more common genotypes of CF. Mucoid *Pseudomonas* lung infection, unexplained azoospermia, and obstruction on PFTs suggests diagnosis. CXR (hyperinflation, enlarged pulmonary arteries, bronchiectasis, cystic areas).

► Disease Severity

PFTs, pulse oximetry, ABG, CXR.

► Concept and Application

Autosomal recessive disorder; CF gene locus located on long arm of chromosome 7; genetic defect in chloride permeability in exocrine glands due to cystic fibrosis transmembrane regulator protein (CFTR); affects all exocrine secretions; frequent *Pseudomonas* and *Staphylococcus* infections.

► Treatment Steps

1. Chest physiotherapy.
2. Inhaled β-agonist and mucolytic agents (DNase, acetylcysteine).
3. Antibiotics prn; aerosol tobramycin for chronic *Pseudomonas*.
4. Influenza vaccine.
5. Pancreatic enzymes.
6. Lung transplant in selected cases.

4. Bronchiectasis

► H&P Keys

Chronic cough, copious purulent sputum, recurrent fever, weakness, weight loss, hemoptysis, clubbing, cyanosis, edema.

► Diagnosis

History, CXR, high-resolution computed tomographic (CT) scan, bronchography (rarely used), sputum culture.

► Disease Severity

PFTs (obstructive), stigmata of cor pulmonale.

► Concept and Application

Abnormal dilatation of bronchi from inflammation and destruction of bronchial wall. Often associated with infection, bronchial obstruction, immotile-cilia syndrome, CF, allergic bronchopulmonary aspergillosis, immunoglobulin deficiency.

► Treatment Steps

1. Chest physiotherapy.
2. Antibiotics for infection.
3. Steroids for allergic bronchopulmonary aspergillosis if present.
4. Surgery or bronchial artery embolization for severe hemoptysis.

III. RESTRICTIVE PULMONARY DISEASES

A. Idiopathic

1. Sarcoidosis

▶ H&P Keys

May be asymptomatic. Dyspnea, cough, wheezing, hemoptysis, skin lesions (erythema nodosum, nodules, plaques), eye pain, arthralgias, cardiac arrhythmias, cranial nerve palsies. More common in African-Americans, Scandinavians.

▶ Diagnosis

CXR (bilateral hilar adenopathy, interstitial lung disease), tissue biopsy (noncaseating granuloma). Elevated serum calcium or angiotensin-converting enzyme suggestive. Exposure history to rule out occupational granulamatous disease or intravenous injection of foreign matter (i.e., talc).

▶ Disease Severity

PFTs (restriction, low diffusion), CXR, gallium scan (reflects disease activity); presence of CNS and cardiac involvement.

▶ Concept and Application

Granulomatous disorder of unknown etiology.

▶ Treatment Steps

1. May be self-limited.
2. Corticosteroids for significant pulmonary, CNS, or cardiac disease.
3. Hydroxychloroquine or topical steroids for skin involvement.
4. Alternative agent: methotrexate.

2. Idiopathic Pulmonary Fibrosis

a. Usual Interstitial Pneumonitis (UIP)

▶ H&P Keys

Insidious onset of dyspnea (may progress over many years), nonproductive cough, clubbing, fine crackles.

▶ Diagnosis

CXR (diffuse interstitial infiltrates), lung biopsy, PFTs (restriction, low diffusion).

▶ Disease Severity

PFTs, high-resolution chest CT scan, ABG.

▶ Concept and Application

Pulmonary fibrosis of unknown etiology leading to hypoxia and cor pulmonale.

▶ Treatment Steps

1. Corticosteroids.
2. Treat cor pulmonale with diuretics, oxygen.
3. Lung transplant.

b. Desquamative Interstitial Pneumonitis (DIP)—Predominant alveolar component, more responsive to drugs, mostly in smokers.

▶ **Diagnosis**

CXR (diffuse interstitial infiltrates), lung biopsy, PFTs (restriction, low diffusion).

▶ **Disease Severity**

PFTs, high-resolution chest CT scan, ABG.

▶ **Treatment Steps**

1. Stop smoking.
2. Corticosteroids.
3. Treat cor pulmonale with diuretics, oxygen.

B. Pneumoconiosis

1. Silicosis

▶ **H&P Keys**

Sandblasters, miners, stoneworkers. Asymptomatic, or progressive dyspnea, cough.

▶ **Diagnosis**

Exposure history, CXR (upper lobe nodules, "eggshell calcification" of hilar nodes), PFTs (restriction).

▶ **Disease Severity**

CXR and PFTs. Progressive massive fibrosis: coalescence of small nodules into larger conglomerate lesions.

▶ **Concept and Application**

Inhalation of quartz particles causes reactive fibrosis. Increased risk for tuberculosis.

▶ **Treatment Steps**

1. Avoidance of further exposure.
2. No medical treatment known to be effective.
3. Lung transplantation in severe cases.

2. Asbestosis

▶ **H&P Keys**

History of asbestos exposure (mining, shipbuilding, insulation workers, construction). Asymptomatic, or progressive dyspnea, persistent cough, basilar inspiratory crackles, clubbing.

▶ **Diagnosis**

Clinical diagnosis: interstitial disease with exposure history. CXR (lower-lobe linear infiltrates, pleural plaques and thickening); high-resolution chest CT scan, PFTs (restriction), ferruginous bodies (hemosiderin-coated asbestos fibers) in sputum, alveolar lavage fluid, or lung tissue suggestive but not diagnostic.

▶ **Disease Severity**

CXR, PFTs.

▶ **Concept and Application**

Inhalation of asbestos fibers releases damaging enzymes and inflammatory mediators. Increased risk of lung cancer, especially in smokers.

▶ **Treatment Steps**

1. Avoidance of further exposure.
2. Stop smoking.

Other Asbestos-Related Diseases
- Mesothelioma: malignant tumor of the mesothelial cells of the pleura. Usually associated with severe chest wall pain.
- Pleural plaques: benign, asymptomatic fibrous plaques detected on CXR. Most common finding in asbestos exposure.
- Pleural thickening: asymptomatic, detected on CXR.
- Acute benign pleural effusions.

3. Coal Workers' Pneumoconiosis

► H&P Keys
Coal miners, carbon manufacturers.

Simple Coal Workers' Pneumoconiosis—Asymptomatic radiographic finding.

Complicated Coal Workers' Pneumoconiosis (Progressive Massive Fibrosis—PMF)—Dyspnea, signs of cor pulmonale.

Chronic Obstructive Lung Disease—Dyspnea, wheezing, productive cough.

► Diagnosis
Occupational exposure, CXR (small round opacities, usually upper lobes), PFTs. X-ray findings are not necessary for the diagnosis.

► Disease Severity
PFTs (usually normal in simple disease; restrictive in PMF, obstructive in COPD), CXR. Simple has small round opacities; PMF has enlarging, irregular nodular infiltrates, which may cavitate.

► Concept and Application
Pulmonary nodules resulting from exposure to coal dust. PMF probably caused by an immunologic response. Effects of coal dust inhalation and concomitant smoking are additive on COPD severity. Increased risk for tuberculosis. COPD from coal dust exposure may be present even absent radiographic findings.

► Treatment Steps
1. Avoidance.
2. Surveillance for COPD, PMF, tuberculosis.
3. Stop smoking.
4. Treatment of COPD if present.

4. Hypersensitivity Pneumonitis

► H&P Keys
Acute—Fever, chills, dyspnea, malaise 4–6 hours after exposure to antigen, lasting 18–24 hours.

Subacute—Insidious onset of cough, progressive dyspnea, fatigue, and weight loss, diffuse crackles.

Chronic—Insidious onset of progressive dyspnea over years.

► Diagnosis
Exposure history key to diagnosis. Common antigens include thermophilic *Actinomyces* (farmer's lung: moldy hay; bagassosis: moldy sugar cane); avian secretory proteins (pigeon breeder's disease). Serum precipitins can help identify agent but are not diagnostic of disease. High-resolution CT pattern suggestive.

► Disease Severity

CXR (interstitial and alveolar infiltrates); PFTs (restriction, decreased diffusion).

► Concept and Application

Immune complex–mediated and cell-mediated hypersensitivity responses to inhaled antigen.

► Treatment Steps

1. Removal and avoidance of offending antigen.
2. Corticosteroids for severe attacks or if symptoms persist.

IV. PLEURAL DISEASES

A. Pleural Effusion

► H&P Keys

Asymptomatic or signs and symptoms of underlying cause. Dyspnea, pleuritic chest pain. Decreased breath sounds, dullness to percussion.

► Diagnosis

CXR with lateral decubitus views. Pleural fluid chemistries (LDH, protein, glucose) (Table 16–3), cell count, cultures.

► Disease Severity

CXR.

► Concept and Application

Transudate—Increased hydrostatic pressure or decreased systemic oncotic pressure.

• Diagnosis: pleural protein:serum protein < 0.5, pleural LDH:serum LDH < 0.6, pleural LDH less than two thirds of the upper limit of normal for serum LDH.
• Examples: congestive heart failure, nephrotic syndrome.

Exudate—Intrapulmonary or abdominal inflammation adjacent to pleura.

• Diagnosis: Pleural:serum protein > 0.5, pleural:serum LDH > 0.6, pleural LDH greater than two thirds upper limit of normal for serum LDH.
• Examples: Parapneumonic effusion, empyema, malignant disease, collagen vascular diseases.

16-3

CHARACTERISTIC CHEMISTRIES OF PLEURAL EFFUSIONS

	Exudate	Transudate
Protein	> 3 g/dL	< 3 g/dL
Pleural/serum protein	> 0.5	< 0.5
LDH	> 200	< 200
Pleural/serum LDH	> 0.6	< 0.6

► Treatment Steps
1. Treatment of underlying disease.
2. Drainage of fluid with thoracentesis or chest tube if symptomatic or infected.
3. Pleurodesis for recurrent effusions.

B. Pleurisy (Pleuritis)

► H&P Keys
Pleuritic chest pain (sharp pain on inspiration), usually rapid onset, dyspnea, low-grade fever.

► Diagnosis
CXR, history and physical.

► Disease Severity
Usually self-limited.

► Concept and Application
Inflammation of pleura.

> *Pleurodynia*—Epidemic infection with coxsackie B or echovirus.

> *Pleuritis*—Pleural inflammation, which may be due to infection, pulmonary infarction, collagen vascular disease, etc.

► Treatment Steps
1. Nonsteroidal anti-inflammatory agents.
2. If fails—corticosteroids if indicated.

C. Pneumothorax

► H&P Keys
Chest pain, dyspnea, enlarged hemithorax, hyperresonance to percussion, absent or reduced breath sounds and fremitus on involved side, tracheal shift away from involved side.

► Diagnosis
CXR (air in pleural space).

► Disease Severity
CXR, pulse oximetry and ABG, pulse rate, respiratory rate, blood pressure.

► Concept and Application
Communication between lung or atmosphere and pleural space.

> *Spontaneous Pneumothorax*—Rupture of subpleural blebs or bullae; also seen with COPD and interstitial lung diseases.

> *Traumatic Pneumothorax*—Direct or indirect chest trauma.

> *Tension Pneumothorax*—Intrapleural pressure exceeds atmo-spheric pressure, decreases venous return, which drops cardiac output and blood pressure.

► Treatment Steps
1. Observation if stable.
2. Chest tube if large, symptomatic, or if tension pneumothorax is present or suspected.

V. DISEASES OF PULMONARY CIRCULATION

A. Cardiogenic Pulmonary Edema (Congestive Heart Failure)

▶ **H&P Keys**

Dyspnea, diaphoresis, wheezing, tachycardia, cyanosis, diffuse crackles or rales, edema, cough with frothy sputum, fine and coarse crackles, S3, displaced point of maximal impulse (PMI), peripheral edema.

▶ **Diagnosis**

History and physical, CXR (diffuse alveolar infiltrates, enlarged heart, Kerley B lines), echocardiogram or nuclear multiple-gated arteriography (MUGA) scan, electrocardiogram (ECG) (ischemic changes), pulmonary artery catheterization (elevated pulmonary artery and pulmonary artery occlusion pressures).

▶ **Disease Severity**

ABG, clinical appearance, vital signs, pulmonary artery occlusion pressure.

▶ **Concept and Application**

Increased hydrostatic pressure from left ventricular failure (ischemia, myocardial infarction [MI]) or fluid overload.

▶ **Treatment Steps**

1. Oxygen.
2. Diuresis.
3. Venodilators (nitroglycerin, morphine), afterload reduction agents (intravenous nitroglycerin, sodium nitroprusside; angiotensin-converting enzyme [ACE] inhibitors).
4. Dobutamine.
5. Treatment of ischemia if present.

B. Adult Respiratory Distress Syndrome

▶ **H&P Keys**

Acute onset of severe dyspnea, tachypnea, cough productive of frothy sputum, diffuse rales and rhonchi, cyanosis.

▶ **Diagnosis**

CXR (bilateral alveolar infiltrates), ABG (hypoxemia $Pa_{O_2} < 50$ mm Hg with $F_{IO_2} > 0.6$), pulmonary artery catheterization (pulmonary artery occlusion pressure > 18) in setting of known risk factor.

▶ **Disease Severity**

CXR and ABG.

▶ **Concept and Application**

Pulmonary edema from increased permeability across the alveolar and capillary walls. Risk factors: sepsis, diffuse pulmonary infection, trauma, aspiration, drowning, toxic inhalations, hypertransfusion, others.

▶ **Treatment Steps**

1. Treatment of underlying cause (e.g., antibiotics for sepsis).
2. Supportive measures: mechanical ventilation, oxygen, and positive end-expiratory pressure (PEEP).
3. Use of low tidal volumes on ventilator (5–8 mL/kg) improves outcome.

C. Newborn Respiratory Distress Syndrome (Hyaline Membrane Disease)

► H&P Keys

Neonate, usually premature, with dyspnea, tachypnea, poor air movement; chest wall retractions occur shortly after birth.

► Diagnosis

CXR (diffuse granular or ground-glass infiltrate), pulse oximetry, ABG.

► Disease Severity

Clinical appearance of respiratory distress, ABG.

► Concept and Application

Decreased pulmonary surfactant leading to reduced lung compliance and atelectasis.

► Treatment Steps

1. Prevention of premature labor and use of prenatal steroid therapy.
2. Oxygen.
3. Continuous distending airway pressure (CDAP or CDP).
4. Mechanical ventilation.
5. Surfactant replacement therapy.

D. Pulmonary Embolism

► H&P Keys

Acute onset of dyspnea and pleuritic chest pain. Cough, hemoptysis, tachypnea, tachycardia; look for pleural rub, edema, or tenderness in lower extremity (Fig. 16–1).

► Diagnosis

ABG (acute respiratory alkalosis, usually decreased Po_2), CXR (clear, or wedge-shaped infiltrate, effusion), ECG (sinus tach, or S1, Q3, T3 inversion pattern), ventilation perfusion lung scan (perfusion defect with normal ventilation), noninvasive (e.g., duplex ultrasound) or venogram studies for deep vein thrombosis (DVT) in lower extremities, pulmonary angiogram, contrast helical "spiral" CT, quantitative D-dimer levels (if < 500 ng/mL, PE unlikely).

► Disease Severity

ABG, vital signs.

► Concept and Application

Venous thrombus, usually from lower extremity, embolizes to pulmonary artery. Pregnancy, use of birth control pills, smoking, malignant disease, obesity, immobilization (hip fracture) at highest risk for DVT.

► Treatment Steps

1. Anticoagulation (heparin, then warfarin for 3–6 months).
2. Thrombolytic agents for massive embolism with shock.
3. Embolectomy in unresponsive cases.
4. Vena caval interruption if anticoagulation is contraindicated (vena caval clip, Greenfield filter, others).
5. Prophylaxis of high-risk patients with subcutaneous low-dose heparin, warfarin, or compression boots.

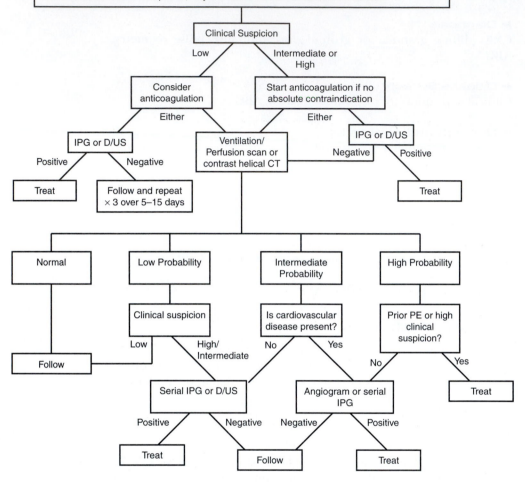

Figure 16–1. Management of Acute Pulmonary Thromboembolism. (Adapted, with permission, from Schulman ES. Management of acute pulmonary thromboembolism. In: Sherman MS, Schulman ES, eds. *The Pocket Doctor 2001.* Educational Communications, Mt. Kisko, NY, 2001 and www.pocketdoctor.com.)

E. Pulmonary Vasculitis

▶ H&P Keys

Dyspnea; symptoms of underlying disease process.

▶ Diagnosis

CXR, ABG, urinalysis, creatinine, serologic studies for systemic vasculitic processes (ANA, ANCA, hepatitis B and C, rheumatoid factor, cryoglobulins, complement). Tissue biopsy usually required.

▶ Disease Severity

ABG, exercise tolerance, serologic studies of underlying disease.

▶ Concept and Application

Inflammation of pulmonary blood vessels.

> *Leukocytoclastic Vasculitis*—Neutrophilic inflammation caused by drugs, neoplasms, infection.

Granulomatous Vasculitis—Lymphocytic infiltration, e.g., Wegener's granulomatosis (renal involvement), allergic granulomatosis (asthma, eosinophilia; "Churg–Strauss syndrome").

Collagen Vascular Diseases

▶ Treatment Steps

Leukocytoclastic Vasculitis
1. Usually self-limited.
2. Steroids if hypoxemia present.

Wegener's Granulomatosis—Cyclophosphamide with or without corticosteroids.

Allergic Granulomatosis, Collagen Vascular Diseases
1. Corticosteroids; azathioprine or cyclophosphamide in severe cases.
2. Progressive systemic sclerosis usually does not respond.

F. Goodpasture's Syndrome

▶ H&P Keys

Hemoptysis, hematuria, fever, dyspnea.

▶ Diagnosis

Antiglomerular basement membrane antibodies, renal biopsy (linear immunofluorescence pattern).

▶ Disease Severity

Amount of hemoptysis, CXR, blood urea nitrogen (BUN), creatinine, ABG.

▶ Concept and Application

Circulating glomerular basement membrane antibodies damage glomerular and alveolar basement membranes.

▶ Treatment Steps

Corticosteroids plus cyclophosphamide or azothioprine; plasmapheresis.

G. Cor Pulmonale

Defined as right ventricular failure secondary to pulmonary disease.

▶ H&P Keys

Breathlessness, hepatic discomfort, symptoms of underlying disease. Right ventricular heave, loud split S2, peripheral edema, ascites.

▶ Diagnosis

CXR (large pulmonary artery, right ventricular hypertrophy [RVH]); ECG (RVH, pulmonale), echocardiogram (RVH, elevated pulmonary artery pressures), PFTs (reflect underlying disease).

▶ Disease Severity

ABG, cardiac catheterization (direct measurement of pulmonary artery pressures), symptoms, and exercise tolerance.

▶ Concept and Application

Hypoxic vasoconstriction leads to pulmonary hypertension and hypertrophy of right ventricle. Occurs in severe primary pulmonary diseases, including COPD, interstitial lung diseases, and sleep apnea.

► Treatment Steps
1. Oxygen, diuretics.
2. Treatment of underlying disease.
3. Endothelin receptor antagonist (Bosentan) in selected cases (i.e., primary pulmonary hypertension or scleroderma pulmonary vasculopathy).

VI. PULMONARY NEOPLASTIC DISEASES

A. Bronchogenic Carcinoma

► H&P Keys

Smoking, asbestosis produce highest risk. Asymptomatic or cough, hemoptysis, dyspnea, chest pain, fever, weight loss, hoarseness, focal wheezing or decreased breath sounds, adenopathy.

► Diagnosis

CXR (coin lesion or mass, adenopathy), CT scan, bronchoscopic or percutaneous needle biopsy or cytologic aspiration.

► Disease Severity

Severity depends on stage, cell type, and patient's general condition.

► Concept and Application

Adenocarcinoma—Usually peripheral; glandlike structure on path.

Squamous Cell—Usually central, often cavitates, best prognosis.

Oat Cell (Small Cell)—Usually central, high metastatic potential.

Alveolar Cell—Subtype of adeno, originates in terminal bronchioles or alveoli, peripheral. Mimics pneumonia on CXR.

Large Cell—Poorly differentiated, tends to be peripheral, rapid-growing with high metastatic potential.

► Treatment Steps

Non–Small Cell
1. Staging, surgery if resectable.
2. Radiation for palliation.

Small Cell
1. Chemotherapy.
2. Rarely resectable (usually metastatic when discovered).

All
1. May metastasize to other lung, mediastinum, brain, adrenal glands, other organs.
2. Watch for superior vena cava syndrome, hypercalcemia.

B. Carcinoid Tumors

► H&P Keys

Asymptomatic or wheezing, cough, hemoptysis, obstruction. Carcinoid syndrome (episodic flushing, bronchospasm, and diarrhea) is rare.

► Diagnosis

CXR (clear, mass, or obstructive pneumonia). Lung biopsy, urine 5-hydroxyindoleacetic acid.

► Disease Severity

Metastatic workup.

► Concept and Application

Tumors are slow growing with low metastatic potential. Classified as "neurosecretory," but cellular origin is now unclear.

► Treatment Steps

1. Surgical resection.
2. Chemotherapy or radiation for recurrent or metastatic disease.

C. Metastatic Malignant Tumors

► H&P Keys

Often asymptomatic, or cough, hemoptysis, wheezing, dyspnea, pain, symptoms of obstructive pneumonia. Signs and symptoms of primary malignant disease.

► Diagnosis

CXR (single or multiple masses or nodules, pleural effusion, hilar or mediastinal adenopathy), biopsy of pulmonary lesion or primary lesion.

► Disease Severity

Metastatic workup.

► Concept and Application

Metastatic tumor cells enter via hematogenous or lymphatic route. Colon, breast, lymphoma, testicular, kidney, thyroid, melanoma, others.

► Treatment Steps

1. Surgical excision for single metastases if possible.
2. Otherwise, systemic therapy determined by primary tumor cell type and site.

VII. ILL-DEFINED SYMPTOM COMPLEX

A. Cough

► H&P Keys

Smoking history, sputum characteristics (color, viscosity), postnasal drip, throat clearing, reflux symptoms, wheezing, occupational history, medication.

► Diagnosis

History and physical, PFTs, bronchoprovocation challenge tests, CXR, sputum culture, trial of medication. Common causes of cough:

Postnasal Drip—History of rhinitis, frequent throat clearing.

Asthma—Wheezing may not be present. Diagnose by history, bronchoprovocation challenge.

COPD

Gastroesophageal Reflux—Worse at night and recumbent.

Others—Recurrent aspiration, lung carcinoma, congestive heart failure (CHF), medications (β-blockers, ACE inhibitors), bronchiectasis, others.

► **Disease Severity**

Cough intensity and number.

► **Concept and Application**

Nonspecific symptom caused by (1) direct stimulation of cough receptors (foreign body, tumor); (2) increased sensitivity of cough receptors (asthma); (3) inadequate glottic closure (aspiration, reflux); or (4) altered mucus quantity or quality (chronic bronchitis, bronchiectasis).

► **Treatment Steps**

1. Treatment of underlying disorder if identified.
2. Therapeutic trials of bronchodilators, antacids, antihistamines, proton pump inhibitors, or decongestants may be diagnostic.
3. Guaifenesin, dextromethorphan, or codeine may alleviate symptoms.

B. Dyspnea

► **H&P Keys**

Shortness of breath, chest tightness, air hunger, signs and symptoms of underlying disease.

► **Diagnosis**

History and physical examination, PFTs, exercise testing, ECG, CXR. Differential diagnosis of dyspnea includes pulmonary diseases, CHF, neuromuscular disease, anemia, hyperventilation disorders (e.g., metabolic acidosis, psychogenic).

► **Disease Severity**

Exercise tolerance, symptom scores. Usually dyspnea correlates with degree of pulmonary dysfunction.

► **Concept and Application**

Sensation of increased respiratory effort.

► **Treatment Steps**

1. Specific treatment of underlying disease.
2. General supportive measures include oxygen, nutritional and psychological support.
3. Pulmonary rehabilitation.

C. Chest Pain

► **H&P Keys**

Quality of pain, location, and relationship to breathing keys to diagnosis. Signs and symptoms of underlying disease.

► **Diagnosis**

Breathing-Associated Pain—Pleuritis, lung infection, pulmonary embolism, pneumothorax, musculoskeletal pain, pericarditis.

Pain Not Associated with Breathing—Pulmonary hypertension, airway or mediastinal inflammation, cardiac ischemia, dissecting aortic aneurysm, esophagitis, costochondritis.

► **Disease Severity**

Symptoms, exercise test, CXR, PFTs, ECG.

► **Concept and Application**

Sensation of pain resulting from tissue injury or inflammation.

► Treatment Steps

1. Diagnostic workup to identify source of pain.
2. Specific therapy of underlying disease.
3. Analgesics, therapeutic trial of antacids, nitrates, nonsteroidal anti-inflammatory drugs when diagnostic workup is unrevealing.

D. Hemoptysis

► H&P Keys

Cough productive of bloody or blood-tinged sputum.

► Diagnosis

Differential diagnosis (common causes).

- *Tracheobronchial disorders:* Acute or chronic bronchitis, bronchogenic carcinoma, bronchiectasis, cystic fibrosis, trauma.
- *Cardiovascular disorders:* Pulmonary infarction, mitral stenosis, CHF, atrioventricular malformation, aneurysm, others.
- *Hematologic disorders:* Anticoagulation, thrombocytopenia, hemophilia, disseminated intravascular coagulation.
- *Parenchymal lung disorders:* Bacterial pneumonia, tuberculosis, paragonimiasis, contusion.
- *Vasculitic disorders:* Systemic lupus erythematosus, Goodpasture's syndrome.

► Disease Severity

Massive hemoptysis: > 600 mL blood/24 hr.

► Concept and Application

Damage to pulmonary parenchyma, tracheobronchial tree, or pulmonary vasculature; defects in coagulation, increased hydrostatic pressure.

► Treatment Steps

1. Diagnostic workup (CXR, complete blood count [CBC], platelet count, prothrombin time [PT], partial thromboplastin time [PTT], sputum culture, cytology, acid-fast bacilli [AFB] smear, cytology).
2. Quantitate hemoptysis.
3. Bronchoscopy to localize source.
4. Treatment of coagulation abnormalities and CHF if present.
5. Cough suppressant (codeine).
6. Antibiotic if infection present.
7. Surgical excision of bleeding segment or angiographic embolization if persists.

E. Wheezing and Stridor

► H&P Keys

Audible, continuous, musical adventitial sound. Location and timing to respiratory cycle help in diagnosis.

► Diagnosis

PFT, flow volume loop, bronchoprovocation challenge, CXR, soft-tissue neck films, bronchoscopy.

Stridor—Inspiratory "wheeze" heard best over trachea and upper airway (e.g., epiglottitis, croup, tracheal stenosis, angioedema, laryngeal ("psychogenic") asthma.

Focal Inspiratory and Expiratory Wheeze—Bronchogenic tumor, foreign body.

Diffuse Expiratory Wheeze—Asthma, COPD, CHF.

► Disease Severity
Clinical symptoms, PFT.

► Concept and Application
Sound caused by vibrations of airway narrowed by bronchospasm, inflammation, mass, or edema.

► Treatment Steps
Treatment of underlying disease, bronchodilators, oxygen if hypoxic.

F. Solitary Pulmonary Nodule (Coin Lesion)

► H&P Keys
Asymptomatic, or cough and hemoptysis. Smoking history, occupational exposures, previous malignant disease.

► Diagnosis
CXR (single round lesion 1–6 cm), old CXR, CT scan, bronchoscopic or transthoracic needle biopsy or aspirate, open biopsy.

► Disease Severity
Lung biopsy.

► Concept and Application
Round mass may be benign or malignant tumor, tuberculoma, granuloma, artifact, cyst, resolving pneumonia, others.

► Treatment Steps
1. Locate old films: if lesion unchanged more than 2 years, probably benign. If unavailable or new lesion, CT scan and biopsy mass. Unless a firm benign diagnosis can be made, surgical excision usually required. Laminated or solid calcification suggests benign granuloma. A negative positron emission tomography (PET) scan also suggests a benign lesion.
2. Consider periodic CXRs over 2 years if nonsmoker, age < 45, with nonspiculated lesion < 2.2 cm.

G. Sleep Apnea Syndrome

► H&P Keys
Daytime sleepiness, restlessness, unrefreshed sleep, morning headaches, neuropsychiatric changes, signs and symptoms of cor pulmonale. Hypothyroidism, use of sedatives, ethanol should be ruled out.

► Diagnosis
Physical examination (obesity, narrowed pharyngeal opening); polysomnography.

► Disease Severity
Polysomnography, degree of nocturnal oxygen desaturation.

► Concept and Application

Central Sleep Apnea—Defective central drive causing transient apneic periods.

Obstructive Sleep Apnea—Occlusion of oropharyngeal upper airway during sleep.

▶ Treatment Steps

Central Sleep Apnea—Oxygen, respiratory stimulants (acetazolamide), noninvasive mechanical ventilation (bilevel positive airway pressure [BiPAP]).

Obstructive Sleep Apnea—Nasal continuous positive airway pressure (CPAP), tracheostomy, weight reduction, avoidance of sedatives and alcohol.

BIBLIOGRAPHY

American Thoracic Society/Centers for Disease Control and Prevention. Diagnostic standards and classifications of tuberculosis in adults and children. *Am J Respir Crit Care Med* 161:1376–1395, 2000.

Fishman AP, ed. *Pulmonary Diseases and Disorders,* 3rd ed. New York: McGraw-Hill, 2002.

Light RW. *Pleural Diseases,* 4th ed. Philadelphia: Williams & Wilkin, 2001.

Murray JF, Nadel JA, eds. *Textbook of Respiratory Medicine,* 3rd ed. Philadelphia: W.B. Saunders, 2000.

NHLBI/WHO workshop report: Global Strategy for Asthma Management and Prevention, 2002 update. NIH Pub No. 02-3659.

Diseases of the Renal and Urologic Systems

17

I. INFECTIOUS DISEASES AND INFLAMMATORY CONDITIONS

A. Urinary Tract Infection (UTI)

► H&P Keys

Dysuria, urgency, frequency, nocturia, suprapubic pain, back or flank pain, tenesmus, voiding of small volumes of urine, urethral discomfort.

► Diagnosis

Urinalysis (UA): pyuria, white blood count/high-power field, bacteriuria, hematuria. Urine culture, dip-slide method. Cystoscopy, voiding cystourethroscopy, intravenous (IV) urography in chronic cases.

► Disease Severity

Gross hematuria, pain, ascending infection, fever and chills, initial or persistent or recurrent infection, pregnancy status, renal function.

► Concept and Application

Male–female difference because of anatomy; bacterial–mucosal adherence principal reason for recurrent infection. Urinary stasis, *Escherichia coli* is principal pathogen. Fecal flora are primary source during indwelling or short-term catheterization. Asymptomatic bacteriuria in pregnant females (3–15%).

► Treatment Steps

1. Uncomplicated: trimethoprim–sulfamethoxazole (TMP-SMZ) for 5–7 days; also nitrofurantoin monohydrate macrocrystals, 100 mg bid for 7–10 days. Three-day regimens effective. Persistent/recurrent infection: chronic or prophylactic use of antibiotics.
2. Timed voiding, urodynamics, and imaging for complicated cases.
3. Rule out nonbacterial causes such as tuberculosis, chlamydia, and yeast.

B. Painful Bladder and Urethral Syndromes

► H&P Keys

Urinary urgency and frequency or dysuria, absence of documented chronic UTI, negative neurologic findings, absence of carcinoma.

► Diagnosis

Cystoscopy: hydrodistention, urodynamics, bladder biopsy. Diagnosis of exclusion.

► Disease Severity

Degree of *urinary* frequency, level of pain, and bladder capacity and deterioration of quality of life.

► Concept and Application

Etiology undefined; grouping of syndromes rather than specific disease. Theories of mast-cell activity and glycosaminoglycan layer defects. Epithelial permeability.

► Treatment Steps

1. Cystoscopy, hydrodistention.
2. Pentosan polysulfate 100 mg tid.
3. Anticholinergics.
4. Therapies for chronic pain.

C. Prostatitis

▶ H&P Keys

Slow or sudden onset, perineal discomfort, voiding dysfunction, prostate tenderness on digital rectal exam, UTI.

▶ Diagnosis

Urine culture and sensitivity, extraprostatic secretion culture, UA (pyuria).

▶ Disease Severity

Fever or rigors, urinary retention, constant or intermittent discomfort, degree of voiding dysfunction.

▶ Concept and Application

Distinguish true bacterial prostatitis (acute and chronic) from nonbacterial (inflammatory states, chlamydia) and prostatodynia. Acute bacterial prostatitis responds dramatically to antibiotics. Fifty percent empiric response to antibiotics in other conditions. Prostatodynia associated with pelvic floor or sphincter spasm.

▶ Treatment Steps

1. Acute bacterial infection requires culture-appropriate antibiotics.
2. Chronic bacterial or nonbacterial infection requires ciprofloxacin or levofloxacin or tetracyclines for 4–6-week course.
3. Warm soaks and nonsteroidal anti-inflammatory drugs (NSAIDs).
4. Chronic pain evaluation for prostatodynia.

D. Epididymitis

▶ H&P Keys

Pain, tenderness, discomfort distinct from testis parenchyma. Normal testis, palpable epididymal discomfort. Slow or sudden onset. No trauma, sexual activity, voiding symptoms, genitourinary (GU) instrumentation.

▶ Diagnosis

Pyuria; culture and sensitivity are usually negative. Scrotal ultrasound or Doppler good flow state, inflammation of epididymis.

▶ Disease Severity

Fever or rigors, testis and epididymis are indistinguishable, scrotal induration, incapacitation.

▶ Concept and Application

Rule out torsion or tumor in young men (Prehn's sign is unreliable). Bacterial infection in older men with voiding dysfunction; chlamydia in younger men. Irritative urine reflux in acute or chronic states. Most respond to antibiotics in 3–6 weeks.

▶ Treatment Steps

1. Intermediate course of antibiotics (ciprofloxacin or tetracyclines).
2. NSAIDs.
3. Warm soaks, elevation.

E. Urethritis

▶ H&P Keys

Purulent or mucoid discharge. Dysuria and frequency during urination. History of sexual activity.

► Diagnosis

Gonococci (GC) culture in Thayer–Martin media, gram-negative diplococci, or specific chlamydia culture.

► Disease Severity

Ranges from painless discharge to severe voiding symptoms, epididymal and testicular involvement, systemic illness.

► Concept and Application

Generally gonococcal and nongonococcal (*Chlamydia trachomatis, Ureaplasma urealyticum, Trichomonas*) complications of urethral stricture or Reiter's syndrome.

► Treatment Steps

1. Gonococcal infection: ceftriaxone, 250 mg intramuscularly (IM); levofloxacin, 500 mg, one dose.
2. Nongonococcal infection: tetracycline, 500 mg qid; doxycycline, 100 mg bid for 7–10 days; or levofloxacin, 250–500 mg qd for 7–10 days.
3. Metronidazole for *Trichomonas;* acyclovir for herpes.

F. Orchitis

► H&P Keys

Rapid or slow onset, fever and malaise, absence of trauma. Scrotal contents can be normal, inflamed, or distorted (torsion). Sexual or voiding dysfunction. Child or adolescent versus adult.

► Diagnosis

Pyuria, scrotal ultrasound, urine culture.

► Disease Severity

Scrotal induration, fistula, abscess on ultrasound, rule out torsion–hyperemic blood flow and systemic infection.

► Concept and Application

Rule out torsion in young men; bacterial infection in older men and sexually transmitted disease (STD) in younger men. Mumps orchitis in children and adolescents. Chronic orchalgia can be present without infection.

► Treatment Steps

1. Four to six weeks of ciprofloxacin, levofloxacin, doxycycline.
2. NSAIDs, warm soaks, and elevation.

G. Gonorrhea

► H&P Keys

Sexual exposure; thick, creamy urethral discharge; urethritis. May involve epididymis.

► Diagnosis

Gram-negative diplococci. GC culture in Thayer–Martin media.

► Disease Severity

Severity of pain and discharge; associated epididymitis or orchitis.

► Concept and Application

β-Lactamase plasmid–penicillin resistance. Pili contribute to virulence. Different infection rate per exposure (male 20%, female 90%). Coexisting chlamydial infection.

► Treatment Steps

Ceftriaxone, 125 mg IM; ciprofloxacin, 500 mg PO, single dose, plus azithromycin, 1 g PO single dose, and doxycycline, 100 mg bid for 7 days.

H. Syphilis

► H&P Keys

Sexual activity. Painless genital ulcer, lack of vesicles. Negative travel history.

► Diagnosis

Rapid plasma reagin (RPR) and fluorescent treponemal antibody-absorption test (FTA-ABS) for syphilis, patient's history.

► Disease Severity

Primary, secondary, or tertiary disease; systemic symptoms, neurosyphilis; cardiovascular changes.

► Concept and Application

Treponema pallidum or spirochete family of bacteria. Three stages of disease with different systemic findings.

► Treatment Steps
1. Benzathine, 2.4 million units IM, one dose.
2. Erythromycin base, 2 g/day for 2 weeks.
3. Late latent: benzathine, 2.4 million units IM weekly for 3 weeks.

I. Chlamydia

► H&P Keys

Sexual activity, younger age group, clear or mucoid discharge.

► Diagnosis

No routine culture; tissue culture 8–10 days, fluorescent antibody stains, history.

► Disease Severity

Pain, spread to testis or prostate.

► Concept and Application

Obligate intracellular parasite. Cannot produce adenosine triphosphate. Antibiotics effective. Neonatal infection is serious—conjunctivitis or pneumonitis. Think of mycoplasma and ureaplasma in differential diagnosis.

► Treatment Steps

Doxycycline; tetracycline; quinolones; azithromycin, 1 g PO, single dose.

J. Herpes

► H&P Keys

Genital ulcer, painful vesicles, multiple lesions.

► Diagnosis

Tzanck test with Wright or Giemsa stain and cell culture.

► Disease Severity

Pain, coalesced vesicles, persistence or recurrence of infection.

▶ Concept and Application

Double-strand DNA virus. Subclinical infections, systemic complications—aseptic meningitis, fever, urinary retention in women, and, in rare cases, hepatitis or pneumonia.

▶ Treatment Steps

1. Oral acyclovir, 200 mg 5 times/day for 10 days. Topical application for pain relief.
2. Suppressive treatment, acyclovir, 400 mg PO bid.

K. Human Immunodeficiency Virus (HIV/AIDS)

▶ H&P Keys

Night sweats, fever, adenopathy, weight loss, opportunistic infections.

▶ Diagnosis

HIV antibody test. Western blotting.

▶ Disease Severity

HIV positivity versus systemic disease.

▶ Concept and Application

RNA virus, AZT therapy. Lymphocyte counts.

▶ Treatment Steps

1. Per current therapy.
2. Evaluation of GU symptoms as per uninfected patients. Minimize invasive procedures in immunocompromised patients.

II. BENIGN CONDITIONS OF THE GENITOURINARY TRACT

A. Cryptorchidism

▶ H&P Keys

Immature birth, absence of testis on scrotal exam. If hypospadias is present, consider sex ambiguity.

▶ Diagnosis

Physical exam. In adults, consider computed tomographic (CT) scan.

▶ Disease Severity

Retractile testis; inguinal canal versus intra-abdominal, unilateral, or bilateral.

▶ Concept and Application

Maldescent of testes hormonally controlled. Gubernaculum provides path of descent with or without mechanical assistance. Rule out retractile, ectopic, or absent testis (blind-ending vas deferens at exploration).

▶ Treatment Steps

1. Surgical correction at 6–12 months of age.
2. Hormonal manipulation.

B. Testicular Torsion

▶ H&P Keys

Common scrotal swelling in children. Acute severe onset. Possible nausea and vomiting, abdominal pain.

▶ Diagnosis

Negative UA, distorted or rotated gonad, Doppler ultrasound, nuclear flow scan.

▶ Disease Severity

Degree of pain and scrotal swelling. Duration (less than or more than 5 hours). Absence of contralateral testis.

▶ Concept and Application

Twisting of spermatic cord with mechanical ischemia. Congenital tunica vaginalis attachment is irregular; thus favors twisting (bell-clapper deformity). Contralateral side at risk.

▶ Treatment Steps

Surgical correction in 5 hours. Bilateral orchiopexy with permanent suture.

C. Intersex

▶ H&P Keys

Salt loss, salt retention. Phallic enlargement. Precocious pubic hair, early masculinization, early epiphyseal closure (congenital adrenal hyperplasia [CAH]). Sparse axillary and pubic hair (testicular feminization). Penile scrotal hypospadias and bilateral cryptorchidism. Groin mass (gonad).

▶ Diagnosis

Buccal smear, karyotype. Metabolic studies for CAH. Genitography, ultrasound gonadal histology.

▶ Disease Severity

Degree of underdevelopment or ambiguity of genitalia. Neonatal versus pubertal diagnosis. Reproductive and gender role dysfunction.

▶ Concept and Application

Four major groups:

1. Female pseudohermaphrodites, normal ovaries, 46,XX, virilization (CAH).
2. Male pseudohermaphrodites, normal testis, 46,XY, failure to masculinize (testicular feminization), androgen insensitivity (receptor block, other 5α-reductase deficiency.
3. True hemaphrodites, testicular and ovarian tissue. Appearance and karyotype variable.
4. Dysgenetic gonads, replaced by fibrous stroma, mosaicism with XY,XX (Turner's syndrome) and XO lines.

▶ Treatment Steps

1. Variable. Treatment depends on specific syndrome and time of recognition.
2. Possible gender reassignment, usually male to female.
3. Support in assigned role (testicular feminization).

D. Infertility

▶ H&P Keys

Failure to conceive after 1 year of unprotected intercourse. Asymmetric or undescended testicles. Testicular mass. Varicocele. Secondary sexual characteristics. Drug and chemical exposure. Stress.

▶ Diagnosis

Semen analysis (> 20 million/cc, 1.5–5 cc volume). UA, semen fructose (obstruction/dysfunction of seminal vesicles). Luteinizing hormone (LH), follicle-stimulating hormone (FSH), and testosterone level. Sperm function tests.

▶ Disease Severity

Mild disorders of semen parameters (motility or morphology) to azoospermia (total absence of sperm).

▶ Concept and Application

Need to distinguish treatable (blockage, varicocele) from untreatable (gonadal failure, FSH three times normal) conditions.

▶ Treatment Steps

1. Varicocele repair.
2. Repair of anatomic blockage.
3. Clomiphene citrate administration (idiopathic infertility).
4. Assisted reproductive techniques.
5. Adoption.

E. Hydrocele and Varicocele

▶ H&P Keys

Hydrocele—Painless scrotal mass; fluid accumulation in tunical layer of testis; symmetrical swelling, occasionally bilateral; transillumination.

Varicocele—Spermatic venous varices; "bag of worms" palpation; commonly occurs on left side; occasionally, painful or heavy sensation.

▶ Diagnosis

Physical exam, UA, scrotal ultrasound. Check tumor marker in young men if diagnosis is questionable.

▶ Disease Severity

Hydrocele—Cosmetic deformity.

Varicocele—Deformity, pain, testicular atrophy, infertility problems.

▶ Concept and Application

Hydroceles—Benign; membranes actively secrete serumlike fluid. Reaccumulation with simple drainage.

Varicoceles—Gonadal venous valve insufficiency; occasionally subclinical on right side. Unclear mechanisms for effect on fertility in some men. Most men with varicoceles do not have fertility problems. Sperm parameters improve after procedure in two-thirds of infertile men.

► Treatment Steps

Hydrocele
1. Drainage with sclerotherapy or surgical correction (5–15% recurrence).
2. Observation.

Varicocele
1. Venous ligation or embolization.
2. Observation.

F. Benign Urethral Stricture

► H&P Keys

Prior history of STD or urinary instrumentation, decreased force of stream, meatal stenosis.

► Diagnosis

Physical exam, UA, retrograde urethrogram, cystoscopy.

► Disease Severity

Blood urea nitrogen (BUN) and creatinine, degree of voiding dysfunction, dysuria.

► Concept and Application

Usually occurs at meatus, fossa navicularis (glans–shaft border), or bulbar urethra; bulbar is site for most STD infections. Ischemia from instrumentation or catheterization while on cardiopulmonary bypass.

► Treatment Steps
1. Dilatation.
2. Optical internal urethrotomy.
3. Plastic staged repair. Biopsy irregular stricture to rule out neoplasia.

G. Peyronie's Disease

► H&P Keys

Painless, firm, nonindurated area on penile shaft.

► Diagnosis

Physical exam. Color-flow Doppler ultrasound.

► Disease Severity

Firm area, degree of pain with erection, deformity of erection, impotence.

► Concept and Application

Idiopathic fibrosis of tunic of corpora cavernosa. Asymmetric thickening leads to erectile thickening and pain. Natural history is unclear. Ten percent are associated with Dupuytren's contracture.

► Treatment Steps
1. Observation.
2. Oral antioxidants.
3. Surgical excision and graft repair.

H. Erectile Impotence

► H&P Keys

Neurological disease, diabetes, peripheral vascular disease, medications, radical pelvic surgery, Peyronie's plaque, psychological factors.

► Diagnosis

History and physical exam, color-flow Doppler ultrasound, nocturnal penile tumescence studies, hormone profile (testosterone), LH, FSH, prolactin.

► Disease Severity

Occasional or permanent inability to attain erection sufficient for vaginal penetration.

► Concept and Application

Vascular, muscular, or neurologic etiology is the site of primary dysfunction; psychogenic issues much less common.

► Treatment Steps

1. Sildenafil, 25 to 100 mg PO.
2. Intracavernosal injection (prostaglandin E_1 or papaverine–regitine).
3. Vacuum suction device.
4. Penile prosthesis.

I. Hypospadias

► H&P Keys

Ectopic position of urethral meatus on ventral shaft of penis. Lack of ventral foreskin. Check for undescended testicles.

► Diagnosis

Physical examination.

► Disease Severity

Glandular position to more proximal location on shaft (penile or scrotal). Associated anomalies.

► Concept and Application

Occurs at the rate of 1 in 300 live male births. Failure of mesothelial folds to close in the midline. Epispadias (dorsal urethral opening) is extremely rare. Associated with midline closure defects.

► Treatment Steps

Surgical correction.

J. Vesicoureteral Reflux

► H&P Keys

Associated family history. Occurs in 50% of infant UTIs and 30% of childhood UTIs; recurrent UTIs in infancy and childhood.

► Diagnosis

Ultrasound, IV urography, renal nuclear scan.

► Disease Severity

Grades 1–5, international classification.

► Concept and Application

Ectopic ureteral bud leading to lateral placement of ureter in bladder. Decreased flap-valve mechanism. May improve with maturity. High-pressure voiding states also can overwhelm normal anatomy. Goal is to preserve upper tracts. Avoid renal scarring and hypertension.

► Treatment Steps

1. Prophylactic antibiotics: TMP-SMZ, nitrofurantoin. Initial medical management of grades 1–3; grade 4, medical or surgical; grade 5, surgery. Cohen reimplant.

2. Breakthrough infection, noncompliance, reflux persistent at puberty are indications for surgery.

K. Urolithiasis

▶ **H&P Keys**
Prior history of stone, geography, metabolic disorders, flank or groin tenderness.

▶ **Diagnosis**
Urinalysis, IV urogram, ultrasound.

▶ **Disease Severity**
Stone burden on imaging studies; degree of urinary obstruction or renal impairment; pain, nausea, vomiting.

▶ **Concept and Application**
Most stones are "idiopathic" calcium oxalate. Struvite stones are associated with infections *(Proteus)* and uric acid; cysteine is less common.

▶ **Treatment Steps**
1. Small calculi: hydration, pain control, spontaneous passage.
2. Upper tract: extracorporal shockwave lithotripsy.
3. Lower tract: ureteroscopic extraction or lithotripsy.

L. Neurogenic Bladder

▶ **H&P Keys**
Neurologic exam, palpable bladder, rectal exam. Rule out stricture disease.

▶ **Diagnosis**
Urodynamics: pressure-flow, cystometrogram, electromyography, uroflowmetry, cystoscopy.

▶ **Disease Severity**
Voiding dysfunction versus complete retention, total incontinence, chronic UTIs, deterioration of renal function.

▶ **Concept and Application**
Several classification schemes: (1) failure to empty versus failure to store is most functional scheme, (a) emptying failure resulting from decompensated detrusor mechanical obstruction or overactive sphincters (smooth and striated), (b) failure to store because of overactive detrusor or incompetent sphincters; and (2) motor versus sensory. Classification of uninhibited versus autonomous is used least often.

▶ **Treatment Steps**
1. Failure to empty (detrusor): clean intermittent catheterization; bethanechol is ineffective.
2. Failure to empty (mechanical): cystoscopy to rule out stricture or enlarged prostate.
3. Failure to empty (sphincter dyssynergia): α-blockage, bladder neck incision, sphincterotomy. Failure to store (detrusor): anticholinergics, surgical bladder augmentation. Failure to store (sphincter incompetence): bladder sling surgery, collagen injections, artificial sphincter placement.

Note: Diabetes can induce a sensory neurogenic bladder. Initial good motor function can be maintained with *timed* voiding.

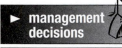

▶ **management decisions**

GENITOURINARY TRACT

Urolithiasis
Size and location of stone. Observe with spontaneous passage, extracorporeal shock wave lithotripsy (ESWL), ureteroscopy for lower ureter. Chronic/recurrent stones—medical management.

Prostate Cancer
Patient age, disease stage and performance status: Local disease: younger patients (< 70) surgery > radiation, older patients radiation > surgery. Androgen ablation in advanced disease.

Vesicoureteral Reflux
Initial antibiotic therapy (grades 1–3), surgery (ureteral reimplant) higher grade or failed medical therapy.

Enuresis
Reassurance with spontaneous resolution, behavioral modification, intranasal DDAVP.

Chronic overdistention creates dilated myopathy with motor decompensation as well. Treatment involves intermittent catheterization.

M. Stress-Related Urinary Incontinence

► H&P Keys

Childbirth, pelvic surgery (total abdominal hysterectomy), loss of urine with cough or movement.

► Diagnosis

Incontinence cystogram, urodynamics, cystoscopy.

► Disease Severity

Occasional leakage to gravity incontinence.

► Concept and Application

Forms of failure to store: type 1, hypermobility of urethra and mild leakage; type 2, descensus of bladder and cystocele; type 3, nonfunctional bladder neck.

► Treatment Steps

1. Initial management is conservative: pelvic floor strengthening exercises, possible biofeedback training, use of α-agonists to tighten bladder neck (phenylpropanolamine, 50 mg daily).
2. Then consider bladder neck suspension. Type 3 is treated with collagen injections or bladder sling surgery.

N. Enuresis

► H&P Keys

Lack of neurologic history, structural disorder that precludes normal toilet training, polyuria.

► Diagnosis

UA and culture and sensitivity. Radiography if infection is present, wetting is diurnal and present beyond age 12 years.

► Disease Severity

Frequency and persistence into adolescence.

► Concept and Application

Persistence of immature reflex pattern of bladder emptying.

► Treatment Steps

1. Reassure patient about spontaneous resolution. Restrict fluids in evening.
2. 1-deamino-8-D-arginine vasopressin, 10–40 µg intranasally.

O. Ureteropelvic Junction Obstruction

► H&P Keys

Flank pain or abdominal pain or mass.

► Diagnosis

Renal ultrasound, cystoscopy as indicated, retrograde pyelogram.

► Disease Severity

Renal function, preserved renal parenchyma. Can occur with or without dilation of collecting system.

► Concept and Application

A dynamic segment of ureter, patent but functionally obstructive. Can occur at ureteral vesical junction (megaureter). Severe prostatism, neurogenic bladder, or ureteral reflux can cause general hydronephrosis.

▶ Treatment Steps
1. Surgical correction, open or endoscopic, of ureteropelvic junction.
2. Megaureter: observation or surgery. Treat prostatism or reflux according to recommendations.

P. Urologic Trauma

▶ H&P Keys
Cardiovascular stability, hematuria, pelvic stability, prostate location on rectal exam. Penile and scrotal ecchymosis, blood at urethral meatus, blunt or penetrating trauma.

▶ Diagnosis
Urinalysis, CT scan, IV urogram, retrograde urethrogram, cystogram. Ultrasound for oliguria.

▶ Disease Severity
Mild contusions treated with observation. Renal fracture involving collecting system, ureteral disruption, intra- versus extraperitoneal bladder extravasation. Penile or testicular fracture.

▶ Concept and Application
Much renal trauma can be managed conservatively; ureteral injuries usually iatrogenic (ureteroscopy or gynecologic); urethral disruption and pelvic hematoma mitigate against immediate repair. Diagnosis of genital injury is aided by ultrasound.

▶ Treatment Steps
Renal (stable):

1. Observation and bed rest, serial imaging; renal (unstable). Diversion of urine with stent; ureteral (major). Catheter drainage; bladder (extraperitoneal). Drainage and later repair in most cases. Debridement and repair.
2. Surgery or angiography. Ureteral (minor). Early or immediate repair (major, delayed diagnosis). Open repair. Urethra (suprapubic): Penile–testicular.
3. Urine diversion with later repair. Bladder (intraperitoneal).

III. NEOPLASIAS OF THE GENITOURINARY TRACT

A. Benign Prostatic Hyperplasia (BPH)

▶ H&P Keys
Hesitancy, decreased force of stream, postvoid dribbling, nocturia, urgency, frequency. Enlarged prostate. Rule out palpable bladder.

▶ Diagnosis
Uroflowmetry, postvoid residual urine, UA, pressure-flow urodynamics if indicated, cystoscopy if indicated, serum prostate-specific antigen (PSA).

▶ Disease Severity
American Urological Association symptom score of 0–35. UTIs, renal deterioration, urinary retention.

► **on rounds**

UROLOGIC DISORDERS

Prostate Cancer
- Diagnosis by digital rectal exam and PSA followed by needle biopsy, bone scan.
- Staging: Jewett–Whitmore A–D.
    A = Local, nonpalpable
    B = Palpable, confined
    C = Extracapsular
    D = Lymph node or distant mets
- Treatment if local includes radical prostatectomy or radiation.
- Treatment if extracapsular is radiation.
- Treatment for advanced disease includes androgen ablation (orchiectomy, LH-releasing hormone agonists).

Wilms' Tumor
- Pediatric tumor (peak age 3), flank mass, hematuria.

Bladder Cancer
- Risk factors include exposure to tobacco, cyclophosphamide, and aniline dyes.

Hydrocele
- Painless scrotal mass, transillumination, fluid in tunical layer of testes, a cosmetic problem.

Varicocele
- Spermatic venous varicies, "bag of worms" feel, pain, infertility.

Testicular Torsion
- Scrotal swelling in children, acute severe onset, nausea, abdominal pain.

► Concept and Application

Testosterone and aging are principal factors in enlargement. Static component is enlarged gland; dynamic component is smooth muscle tone in prostate, prostate capsule, and bladder neck.

► Treatment Steps

1. Expectant management.
2. Decrease tone with α-blocker (several) hs.
3. Medical bulk reduction with finasteride.
4. Surgical bulk reduction with transurethral resection of prostate (TURP).

B. Prostate Cancer

► H&P Keys

Digital rectal exam and serum PSA. Ultrasound is not part of routine exam. Hematuria and obstruction symptoms are less specific.

► Diagnosis

Needle biopsy of prostate. Staging: Bone scan. Endorectal coil magnetic resonance imaging (eMRI) investigational. CT scan and MRI of body are not useful.

► Disease Severity

Tumor grade and stage (Jewett–Whitmore, A-D, TNM [tumor, node, metastasis] system). (A/T1) local, PSA, or incidental biopsy, nonpalpable disease; (B/T2) palpable organ, confined disease; (C/T3) extracapsular disease; (D/T4, N+, M+) lymph node or distant metastasis.

► **Concept and Application**

There are 31,900 cancer-related deaths per year. Etiology is unknown. Adenocarcinoma. Disparity in racial incidence: high in African-American men, low in native Asians. PSA plus digital rectal exam detects more cancer than either test alone. True value of screening awaits long-term follow-up, indirect data supports it. Androgen-sensitive and androgen-resistant tumor.

► **Treatment Steps**

Prostate cancer is a progressive disease. Slow rate of progression suggests that active observation is an option in patients with local disease and expected life span of < 10 years. *Local disease:* radical prostatectomy or radiation therapy. *Extracapsular disease:* radiation therapy. *Advanced disease:* androgen ablation (orchiectomy, LH-releasing hormone agonists with or without antiandrogen). Brachytherapy and cryosurgery for local disease is investigational. Palliative therapy for hormone-refractory disease.

C. Bladder Carcinoma

► **H&P Keys**

Gross or microscopic hematuria. Irritative voiding symptoms. Occasionally, pelvic pain. Exposure to tobacco, cyclophosphamide, analine dyes.

► **Diagnosis**

IV urogram, cystoscopy, barbitage cytology. Transurethral resection biopsy of bladder lesion.

► **Disease Severity**

Key determinant is presence or absence of muscle invasion by the tumor. Degree of hematuria does not correlate with tumor stage. TNM staging system. Patients with gross nodal and distant disease do poorly.

► **Concept and Application**

Cancer-related deaths per year: 10,000. Two-thirds of tumors are superficial and treated by resection; two-thirds of these will recur, and 10–20% progress to muscle-invasive disease. Associated carcinoma in situ is a bad prognostic feature regarding recurrence and progression. Tumor grade is strong indicator of recurrence.

► **Treatment Steps**

Superficial

1. Resect initial tumor and observe, on standard schedule (see below), multiple tumors or recurrence. Treat with intravesical bacillus Calmette–Guérin (BCG).
2. Mitomycin decreases papillary recurrence, decreases recurrence and progression in carcinoma in situ.

Cysto Schedule—Every 3 months for 1 year, every 6 months for 1 year, yearly thereafter. Recurrence resets schedule.

Muscle Invasive

1. Radical cystectomy and urinary tract reconstruction (ileal conduit or continent neobladder).
2. Radiation therapy, and chemotherapy used in combination.
3. Transurethral resection.

Advanced Disease

1. Methotrexate, vinblastine, Adriamycin, and cisplatin (MVAC), with 40–50% response and 15% sustained complete remission.
2. Paclitaxel or combinations.

D. Renal Cell Carcinoma

► H&P Keys

Classically called "internists' tumor" because it was found after workup for general weight loss, fatigue, and so on. Now, it is usually discovered as incidental mass on an imaging study. Classic hematuria, flank pain, and mass are present in only 11% of patients.

► Diagnosis

Mass on IV urogram, ultrasound, CT, or MRI. Angiography rarely performed now. CT criteria: mass with slight increase in Hounsfield units after contrast. Paraneoplastic effect of hypercalcemia and elevated liver function tests (LFTs) (Stauffer's syndrome) does not indicate metastases. Anemia is more common than erythrocytosis.

► Disease Severity

Robeson or TNM tumor stage. Weight loss, fatigue, and large-mass organ-confined disease easily treated with surgery. Metastatic disease responds poorly to therapy.

► Concept and Application

Annual mortality rate is 12,000. Arises from proximal tubule. Exposure to tobacco increases the relative risk twofold. Surgical disease; not responsive to irradiation, chemotherapy.

► Treatment Steps

1. Radical nephrectomy is treatment of choice if no evidence of metastatic disease.
2. Interleukin-2 or 5-fluorouracil (FUDR), or research protocol.
3. Progesterones are used for palliation and have few side effects. Some positive results with biological response modifiers.

E. Wilms' Tumor

► H&P Keys

Pediatric tumor. Noticed as flank mass on exam. Hematuria.

► Diagnosis

History and physical exam, CT scan or ultrasound, IV urogram.

► Disease Severity

Clinical staging, performance status.

► Concept and Application

Arises from metanephric blastema tissue. Occurs in young children (peak age 3 years); rarely presents in adolescents and adults.

► Treatment Steps

1. Radical nephrectomy for localized or regional disease and chemotherapy (actinomycin and vincristine).
2. Radiation therapy for advanced disease.

F. Testicular Carcinoma

▶ H&P Keys

Painless testicular mass, testis rupture after mild trauma. Advanced disease includes gynecomastia, shortness of breath, adenopathy, abdominal mass.

▶ Diagnosis

Scrotal ultrasound, tumor markers (β-human chorionic gonadotropin [β-hCG] and α-fetoprotein [AFP]). Diagnosis by radical orchiectomy (inguinal incision).

▶ Disease Severity

Marker level, retroperitoneal CT scan, organ confined versus subdiaphragmatic lymph nodes versus pulmonary/visceral disease.

▶ Concept and Application

Annual mortality rate, 350. Major distinction: seminoma versus non-seminomatous lesion (e.g., embryonal, teratoma, choriocarcinoma). Nonseminoma: any elevated AFP and more than twice the normal β-hCG. Tumors sensitive to platinum-based chemotherapy.

▶ Treatment Steps

Radical orchiectomy. Staging. Seminoma (local): 2,500 cGy of radiation; seminoma (node positive): chemotherapy. Nonseminoma (local): retroperitoneal lymph node dissection (RPLND); nonseminoma (advanced, six positive nodes or > 2.5 cm): chemotherapy followed by salvage RPLND. Bleomycin, etoposide, and cisplatin (BEP).

Seminoma
1. Radical orchiectomy and radiation.
2. Chemotherapy.

Nonseminoma
1. Radical orchiectomy.
2. RPLND for localized.
3. Chemotherapy and RPLND; advanced: BEP, usually 3 cycles.

G. Penile, Urethral, and Scrotal Carcinoma

▶ H&P Keys

If patient is not circumcised, check under foreskin and look for bloody urethral stricture and scrotal mass. Check for inguinal adenopathy.

▶ Diagnosis

Physical exam and biopsy.

▶ Disease Severity

Degree of penile shaft destruction, adenopathy, weight loss.

▶ Concept and Application

Rare cancer in developed world; usually squamous in origin. Adenopathy may be secondary to infection.

▶ Treatment Steps
1. Local excision.
2. Inguinal lymph node disection.
3. Bleomycin-based chemotherapy.

IV. RENAL DISORDERS

A. Pyelonephritis

▶ **H&P Keys**

History of UTIs, voiding dysfunction, flank pain, fever, malaise. Differentiate acute from chronic pyelonephritis.

▶ **Diagnosis**

Urine culture, urinalysis (pyuria, white blood cell casts), renal ultrasound to rule out obstruction by stone or other cause.

▶ **Disease Severity**

Discomfort to frank sepsis. Acute infection versus chronic deterioration (renal scarring, insufficiency, proteinuria, hypertension).

▶ **Concept and Application**

Ascending UTI can cause significant initial damage in pediatric population (usually associated with reflux). Infection and obstruction enhance renal damage. Can be associated with stone disease. Usually standard pathogens.

▶ **Treatment Steps**
1. Rule out obstruction and calculus.
2. Treat with culture-appropriate antibiotics.
3. Monitor renal function in chronic patients.

B. Acute Renal Failure

▶ **H&P Keys**

Increased creatinine and BUN, edema, hypertension, toxicity exposure, rhabdomyolysis, hemolysis.

▶ **Diagnosis**

Urine diagnostic indexes, renal failure index, electrolyte measurements, possible renal biopsy.

▶ **Disease Severity**

Acute progression versus rapid progression; oliguric versus non-oliguric. Rate of improvement and associated pathology.

▶ **Concept and Application**

Prerenal, 55%; intrinsic, 40%; and postrenal causes, 5%. Conversion of oliguric to nonoliguric state improves management and may improve outcome. Prerenal conditions include congestive heart failure (CHF), hypovolemia, plasma protein deficiency. Hepatorenal syndrome probably reflects renal response to prerenal circulatory environment. Intrinsic disease caused by restricted blood flow to glomeruli, decreased basement membrane permeability, tubular plugging, disrupted tubules. Intrinsic disease; also acute glomerular nephritis and allergic interstitial nephritis. Acute anuria suggests urologic origin. Also consider solitary kidney. Acute tubular necrosis. Mortality can range between 25% and 70%.

▶ **Treatment Steps**

Assess clinical and laboratory parameters.

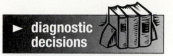

▶ **diagnostic decisions**

RENAL DISORDERS

Polycystic Kidney Disease
Positive family history in 75%, clinical (bilateral flank masses, elevated BP, uremia).

Alport's Syndrome
Hematuria, proteinuria, hearing loss, ocular disorders.

Acute Scrotum
Patient age: torsion in younger patients, hyperacute onset; orchitis in older patients, gradual onset. Orchitis in younger patients due to chlamydia, *E. coli* in older population. Rule out trauma or chronic mass; varicocele, hydrocele.

Flank Pain
Acute obstruction—stone, papillary necrosis, fungus ball. Rule out pyelonephritis or renal abscess; consider vascular occlusion, renal vein thrombosis, or arterial emboli.

Voiding Dysfunction
Failure to empty/failure to store, irritative versus obstructive symptoms. Look for associated neurologic disease or history of infection.

Prerenal
1. Restore adequate circulating plasma volume.
2. Correct nonrenal pathology.

Renal
1. Convert to nonoliguric state, remove toxins, dialyze as needed.
2. Urologic evaluation (ultrasound, cystoscopy, retrograde stent placement) as needed.

C. Chronic Renal Failure

▶ H&P Keys
Diabetes, hypertension, pericarditis, glomerulopathy, obstructive uropathy, edema, anemia, pruritus, osteodystrophy (osteitis fibrosa).

▶ Diagnosis
Shrunken kidneys on imaging; uremia; creatinine clearance; edema; hyperkalemia; normochromic, normocytic anemia.

▶ Disease Severity
Creatinine clearance, edema, electrolyte derangement, neurologic complications of uremia.

▶ Concept and Application
Multiple causes, majority of cases involve hypertension, diabetes mellitus, and glomerulonephritis. Early reduction of glomerular filtration rate (GFR) (30–50%) compensated. Azotemia between 20% and 35% GFR, and overt renal failure below 20% of normal.

▶ Treatment Steps
1. Initial dietary restriction of protein.
2. Control hypertension.
3. Correct electrolyte imbalances.
4. Dialysis and transplantation.

D. Tubulointerstitial Disease

▶ H&P Keys
Toxin exposure (analgesics, heavy metal), immune disorders, neoplasia, vascular disease, family history of renal disorders.

▶ Diagnosis
Electrolyte irregularities, eosinophilia, impaired creatine clearance, renal biopsy.

▶ Disease Severity
Acute or chronic, tubular defects versus marked GFR deterioration.

▶ Concept and Application
Pathology is morphologically in tubules and interstitium, not glomerulus. *Acute disease:* inflammation, tubule necrosis, edema. *Chronic forms:* fibrosis is common. Condition has many causes. Look for dysfunction in tubular transport. Proteinuria usually not severe. Eventual GFR dysfunction.

▶ Treatment Steps
1. Remove offending agent.
2. Compensate tubular defect.
3. Treat primary disease.

E. Renal Transplant Rejection

► **H&P Keys**

Oliguria, azotemia, graft tenderness, fever, proteinuria.

► **Diagnosis**

Ultrasound to rule out obstruction, urine output, proteinuria, renal scan, renal biopsy.

► **Disease Severity**

Mild azotemia, frank renal failure, rapidity of onset and progression.

► **Concept and Application**

Immunologic reaction, cellular and humoral. Hyperacute, acute accelerated, acute, and chronic rejection.

► **Treatment Steps**

Hyperacute and Acute Accelerated—Rare, nephrectomy.

Acute
1. Immunosuppression.
2. Methylprednisolone.
3. Cyclosporine.

Chronic
1. Rule out obstruction, no treatment.
2. Kidney-sparing diet.

F. Nephrotic Syndrome

► **H&P Keys**

Edema.

► **Diagnosis**

Urinalysis, proteinuria, 24-hour collection, hypoalbuminemia, renal biopsy.

► **Disease Severity**

Rapid versus chronic course. Degree of proteinuria/renal insufficiency.

► **Concept and Application**

Albuminuria, hypoalbuminemia, hyperlipidemia, and edema. Minimal change disease, mesangial proliferative immunoglobulin A (IgA) glomerulonephritis (Berger's disease), focal and segmental glomerulosclerosis, membranous Berger's disease.

► **Treatment Steps**

Treatment with combination of steroids, cytotoxic drugs, cyclosporine.

G. Glomerulonephritis

► **H&P Keys**

Infectious disease, primary renal disease, multisystem disease. Abrupt azotemia, oliguria, edema, hypertension.

► **Diagnosis**

Serum electrolytes, proteinuria, urinalysis for hematuria, red cell casts.

► Disease Severity

Degree of edema, renal insufficiency, acute versus rapidly progressing disease.

► Concept and Application

Glomerular damage, capillary wall damage (anionic charge/pore size), vascular changes resulting from vessel damage and surrounding inflammation.

► Treatment Steps

Acute Supportive Disease
1. Diuresis.
2. Bed rest.
3. Antihypertension drugs as needed.

Rapidly Progressing Disease
1. Glucocorticoid
2. Pulse treatment.
3. Cytotoxic agents.
4. Plasma exchange.

H. Diabetic Nephropathy

► H&P Keys

History of diabetes, diabetic stigmata, edema, hypertension.

► Diagnosis

BUN and creatinine, creatinine clearance, oliguria.

► Disease Severity

Degree and duration of diabetes, level of renal impairment.

► Concept and Application

Microangiopathy of renal system and glomeruli (Kimmelstiel–Wilson lesions), nodular deposits in glomeruli.

► Treatment Steps
1. *Early:* compensate for electrolyte-fluid derangement.
2. *Later:* dialysis or transplantation.

I. Renal Osteodystrophy

► H&P Keys

Renal insufficiency, growth retardation, rickets. Bone pain or proximal muscle weakness in adults.

► Diagnosis

Calcium and phosphorus levels. Parathyroid activity. Plain film findings.

► Disease Severity

Renal dwarfism versus growth retardation or maturation, degree of orthopedic disability in adults. Extent of calcium imbalance, pathologic calcification.

► Concept and Application

Impaired vitamin D metabolism, parathyroid hormone overproduction. Dialysis accelerates bone pathology secondary to aluminum deposition. Osteitis fibrosa cystica, renal rickets, osteosclerosis.

► Management

Early treatment to reduce morbidity.

1. Reduce dietary phosphate with calcium carbonate as phosphate binder.
2. Balanced dialysate. Keep PO_4 at 4.5 mg/dL and Ca at 10 mg/dL.

J. Papillary Necrosis

► H&P Keys

Hematuria and flank pain, patient may be asymptomatic, disease often associated with severe infection and other conditions.

► Diagnosis

Urinalysis, culture, filling defect on urogram; ring shadow may be present.

► Disease Severity

Asymptomatic or flank pain infection, obstructive uropathy with papillary sloughing.

► Concept and Application

Infection or microangiopathy of renal pyramids. Associated with diabetes, alcoholism, sickle cell anemia.

► Treatment Steps
1. Asymptomatic finding: treat primary disease.
2. Mechanical removal of obstruction.

K. Renovascular Hypertension

► H&P Keys

Hypertension, rapid onset, poorly controlled, epigastric bruit.

► Diagnosis

Renal vein renin sampling (ratio > 1.5); angiography (classic, digital, MRI); occasionally, IV urogram (not a screening test).

► Disease Severity

Pharmacologic control, severity of stenosis on imaging.

► Concept and Application

Usually secondary to atherosclerotic vascular disease; several forms of fibromuscular hyperplasia.

► Treatment Steps
1. Medical.
2. Angioplasty.
3. Surgical repair.

L. Preeclampsia

► H&P Keys

Pregnancy related, edema, proteinuria, and hypertension after 24th week of pregnancy.

► Diagnosis

Blood pressure 140/90, proteinuria, 30 mm Hg systolic or 15 mm Hg diastolic relative to earlier pregnancy readings.

► Disease Severity

Progression to eclampsia; need for intervention beyond bed rest.

► Concept and Application

Etiology unknown. Glomerular capillary endotheliosis is major pathologic alteration.

► Treatment Steps

1. Bed rest.
2. Antihypertensives (hydralazine), delivery.
3. Magnesium sulfate, 4–6 g, then 1–2 g/hr.

M. Eclampsia

► H&P Keys

Preeclampsia and seizures.

► Diagnosis

Preeclampsia and seizure evaluation.

► Disease Severity

Proteinuria, level of hypertension and degree of seizure activity.

► Concept and Application

Etiology unknown.

► Treatment Steps

Control blood pressure and seizures.

N. Polycystic Kidney Disease

► H&P Keys

Flank mass, renal insufficiency, family history.

► Diagnosis

Azotemia, uremia, CT scan, proteinuria.

► Disease Severity

Age of onset, infection, hypertension, rate of renal deterioration, abdominal distension.

► Concept and Application

Ten percent of end-stage renal failure. Cortical and medullary cysts. Hepatic cysts, cerebral aneurysms. Presents in third and fourth decades. Hypertension in 75%. Autosomal dominant disease (usually adult, wide range and penetrance). Two genes identified. Autosomal recessive, infancy or childhood (renal failure or portal fibrosis), medullary ductal ectasia.

► Treatment Steps

1. Hypertension control.
2. Dialysis or transplantation.

O. Nephrosclerosis

► H&P Keys

Mild, moderate, or malignant hypertension; neurologic signs; papilledema.

► Diagnosis

UA, proteinuria, renal imaging (size).

► Disease Severity

Mild sclerosis with mild to moderate physiologic changes (slight azotemia, exaggerated natriuresis with fluid challenge versus malignant hypertension, neurologic symptoms.

► Concept and Application

Mild to moderate secondary changes of essential hypertension, vascular atherosclerotic changes (afferent arterioles). Severe disease with fibrinoid necrosis and hyperplastic arteriolitis.

► Treatment Steps

Control hypertension (acute and chronic).

P. Lupus Nephritis

► H&P Keys

Associated history of systemic lupus erythematosus (SLE) and physical exam, edema.

► Diagnosis

Urinalysis, azotemia, low C_3 and C_4 concentrations. Positive double-stranded DNA antibody, proteinuria, nephrotic syndrome, renal biopsy.

► Disease Severity

Asymptomatic, clinical SLE, mild to severe renal status.

► Concept and Application

Renal involvement in 35–90% of SLE patients, deposition of circulating immunocomplexes, autoantibody activity.

► Treatment Steps

1. Steroids.
2. Cyclophosphamide.
3. Azathioprine.

V. ELECTROLYTE AND ACID–BASE DISORDERS

A. Hyponatremia

► H&P Keys

Nausea, confusion, lethargy, coma, seizures, decreased deep tendon reflexes.

► Diagnosis

Serum sodium < 130 mg/dL.

► Disease Severity

Abnormal laboratory value to severe clinical derangement.

► Concept and Application

Free-water retention, exogenous free water, TURP or water intoxication, syndrome of inappropriate secretion of antidiuretic hormone (SIADH), renal and cardiac decompensation.

► Treatment Steps

Restrict free water, replace salt.

B. Hypernatremia

► H&P Keys

Dehydration, hyperpnea, oliguria, thirst, hypotension.

► Diagnosis

Serum sodium > 145 mg/dL.

▶ **Disease Severity**

Laboratory finding to severe clinical derangement.

▶ **Concept and Application**

Impaired thirst mechanism, excessive water loss, solute and free-water loss (diabetic ketoacidosis).

▶ **Treatment Steps**

Slow replacement of free water to avoid cerebral edema.

C. Hypokalemia

▶ **H&P Keys**

Dysrhythmia, rhabdomyolysis, muscle weakness or cramps.

▶ **Diagnosis**

Serum potassium < 3.5 mg/dL. Changes in electrocardiogram (ECG): wide decrease in T wave, U wave, atrioventricular block.

▶ **Disease Severity**

Laboratory finding to severe clinical derangement.

▶ **Concept and Application**

Inappropriate gastrointestinal (GI) or GU loss, cellular sequestration, decreased intake. Because of body stores, small decrease in serum value can indicate significant total-body depletion.

▶ **Treatment Steps**

1. Oral replacement for chronic loss (diuretic use).
2. IV replacement is not advised except in monitored situation (keep below 20 mEq/hr).

D. Hyperkalemia

▶ **H&P Keys**

Renal insufficiency, diarrhea, weakness.

▶ **Diagnosis**

Laboratory findings, ECG: widened QRS waves and peaked T waves.

▶ **Disease Severity**

Laboratory value or severe clinical derangement.

▶ **Concept and Application**

Reduced renal excretion of potassium; adrenal insufficiency, excessive intake; hyperchloremic acidosis.

▶ **Treatment Steps**

1. Limit exogenous potassium.
2. Correct underlying acidosis.
3. Exchange resin, insulin/D_{50} glucose.
4. Dialysis.

E. Volume Depletion

▶ **H&P Keys**

Decreased skin turgor, orthostasis, thirst, coma, sunken eyes.

▶ **Diagnosis**

Serum electrolytes, increased sodium, BUN, osmolality increased.

▶ **Disease Severity**

Laboratory derangement to severe clinical compromise.

▶ Concept and Application

Third spacing, insufficient replacement of free water, excessive loss of free water.

▶ Treatment Steps

1. Slow replacement of free water.
2. Replace sodium as needed.

F. Volume Excess

▶ H&P Keys

Renal insufficiency, CHF, pathologic free-water consumption (water intoxication), syndrome of inappropriate antidiuretic hormone secretion (SIADH), nausea, seizures, weakness, coma.

▶ Diagnosis

Serum electrolytes, clinical scenario.

▶ Disease Severity

Mild electrolyte disturbance to severe clinical derangement.

▶ Concept and Application

Excessive exogenous free water or poor elimination of free water.

▶ Treatment Steps

Restrict fluids.

G. Metabolic Alkalosis

▶ H&P Keys

GI loss, renal loss, H^+ translocation (hypokalemia), $NaHCO_3$ administration.

▶ Diagnosis

Elevation of arterial pH, increase in plasma HCO_3, compensatory hypoventilation (increased P_{CO_2}).

▶ Disease Severity

Compensated disturbance or severe metabolic derangement.

▶ Concept and Application

Generally a loss of H^+, retention of bicarbonate, or contraction alkalosis.

▶ Treatment Steps

1. Correct primary cause.
2. Compensate electrolyte abnormality.

H. Respiratory Alkalosis

▶ H&P Keys

Hypoxemia, CHF, pulmonary disease, severe anemia, gram-negative sepsis, hepatic failure.

▶ Diagnosis

Elevated arterial pH, hypocapnea, plasma HCO_3 decreased.

▶ Disease Severity

Mild compensated disorder or severe metabolic derangement.

▶ Concept and Application

Hyperventilation caused by hypoxemia or central stimulation of respiration. Primary respiratory disease and mechanical ventilation also a cause.

▶ **management decisions**

ELECTROLYTE AND ACID–BASE DISORDERS

- - - - - - - - - - - - - -

Metabolic Acidosis
Correct primary pathology (anion gap or nonanion gap causes), assess renal function and GI function, evaluate for lactic acidosis or ketoacidosis.

Hypercalcemia
Discern appropriate etiology—neoplasia, hyperparathyroidism, sarcoidosis; evaluate ECG; saline hydration and furosemide diuresis; calcitonin or bisphosphonates.

▶ Treatment Steps
1. Correct underlying medical defect.
2. Rebreathing (increase P_{CO_2}).

I. Metabolic Acidosis

▶ H&P Keys
Low arterial pH, reduced plasma HCO_3 concentration, compensatory hyperventilation.

▶ Diagnosis
Electrolytes, blood gas, associated metabolic disorders.

▶ Disease Severity
Mild electrolyte disturbance to severe metabolic derangement.

▶ Concept and Application
Generally characterized as anion gap (ingestions, ketoacidosis, lactic acidosis, renal failure, rhabdomyolysis), and hyperchloremic (normal anion gap) renal dysfunction, GI loss of HCO_3, renal loss of HCO_3, ingestion.

▶ Treatment Steps
1. Correct primary etiology.
2. Replace HCO_3 with accompanying additional cation load (Na^+).

J. Respiratory Acidosis

▶ H&P Keys
Medications, acute cardiac arrest, obesity, upper-airway obstruction, chest wall pathology, adult respiratory distress syndrome, and chronic obstructive pulmonary disease.

▶ Diagnosis
Blood gas and electrolytes. Elevated serum HCO_3, reduced arterial pH. Elevated P_{CO_2}.

▶ Disease Severity
Mild disorder to severe decompensation.

▶ Concept and Application
Inability to excrete respiratory CO_2, multiple mechanical and structural disorders.

▶ Treatment Steps
Correct primary ventilatory defect.

K. Hypomagnesemia

▶ H&P Keys
Alcoholism, malnutrition, diuretics, diabetic ketoacidosis, lethargy, delirium, irritability of central nervous system.

▶ Diagnosis
Low serum magnesium (< 1.1 mEq/dL); ECG, prolonged QT waves; hypokalemia; hypocalcemia.

▶ Disease Severity
Electrolyte abnormality to severe neurologic decompensation.

▶ Concept and Application
Metabolism similar to calcium; generally difficult to deplete body stores.

► **Treatment Steps**

IV or IM exogenous replacement.

L. Hypercalcemia

► **H&P Keys**

Carcinoma, hyperparathyroidism or hyperthyrosis, sarcoidosis, milk alkali syndrome.

► **Diagnosis**

Serum free calcium > 2.9 mEq. ECG: short QT and long PR waves.

► **Disease Severity**

Abnormal electrolytes to tetany and cardiac arrest.

► **Concept and Application**

Inappropriate calcium storage mobilization, hormonal etiology, neoplasia. Excretion linked to sodium and state of hydration.

► **Treatment Steps**

1. Saline infusion, furosemide.
2. Diuresis.
3. Calcitonin, mithramycin.
4. Sodium etidronate.

M. Hypocalcemia

► **H&P Keys**

Renal failure, hypoparathyroidism, vitamin D deficiency, malabsorption, Chvostek's sign, Trousseau's sign, perioral paresthesias, muscle cramps.

► **Diagnosis**

Serum calcium (free Ca < 2.2 mEq).

► **Disease Severity**

Electrolyte finding to tetany, neurologic, cardiovascular complications.

► **Concept and Application**

Secondary to parathyroid surgery, poor absorption, inability to access bone stores.

► **Treatment Steps**

1. Correct underlying defect.
2. Administer exogenous calcium and vitamin D.

BIBLIOGRAPHY

Gillenwater J, Grayhack J, Howards S, Duckett JW. *Adult and Pediatric Urology*, 4th ed. St. Louis: Mosby, 2002.

Walsh PC, Retik AB, Vaughn ED, Wein AJ (eds.). *Campbell's Urology*, 8th ed. Philadelphia: W.B. Saunders, 2002.

Surgical Principles

I. DISORDERS OF THE SKIN AND SUBCUTANEOUS TISSUE

A. Cellulitis

► **H&P Keys**

Erythematous and edematous skin; red or tender streaks; indistinct advancing edge; history of venous or lymphatic insufficiency.

► **Diagnosis**

Physical examination, culture blister aspirate.

► **Disease Severity**

Malaise, high fever, lymphangitis, bullae, necrosis, sepsis.

► **Concept and Application**

Injury to skin, bacterial invasion of skin and subcutaneous tissue (*Streptococcus, Staphylococcus,* anaerobes); lymphatic spread.

► **Treatment Steps**

1. Warm packs, rest, limb elevation.
2. Antibiotics.
3. Remove the infective source (e.g., intravenous [IV] line, infected bullae).

B. Lipoma

► **H&P Keys**

Soft subcutaneous lobulated mass.

► **Diagnosis**

Physical examination; excisional biopsy.

► **Disease Severity**

Hard mass, rapid growth.

► **Concept and Application**

Benign tumor of mature fat cells (malignant counterpart: liposarcoma).

► **Treatment Steps**

Surgical excision (cosmesis, local symptoms, persistent growth).

C. Hemangioma

► **H&P Keys**

Red or bluish, raised lesion; present soon after birth; regress spontaneously.

► **Diagnosis**

Physical examination.

► **Disease Severity**

Degree of disfigurement, ulceration, high-output cardiac failure (arteriovenous shunting), intravascular coagulation.

► **Concept and Application**

True neoplasm or malformation of normal vascular structures, mostly capillaries. The most common head and neck tumor in children.

▶ Treatment Steps
1. Observation.
2. Partial or complete surgical excision (do not biopsy secondary to hemorrhage risk).
3. Embolization (useful for inaccessible lesions or in cases in which resection would cause significant deformity).
4. Injection sclerotherapy.
5. Corticosteroids, interferon-2α.
6. Radiation.

D. Neurofibroma

▶ H&P Keys
Mass, pain, sensory deficit, muscular weakness. Multiple in von Recklinghausen's disease (neurofibromatosis, café au lait spots).

▶ Diagnosis
Physical examination, nerve conduction studies, magnetic resonance imaging (MRI).

▶ Disease Severity
Peripheral nerve dysfunction, malignant transformation, involvement of craniospinal axis.

▶ Concept and Application
Proliferation of perineurial/endoneurial fibroblasts and Schwann cells.

▶ Treatment Steps
Observation or surgical excision (for malignant transformation, functional impairment, cosmesis).

E. Basal Cell Carcinoma

▶ H&P Keys
Lesion on face or other sun-exposed areas; bleeding; pearly nodule; central ulceration; rolled or raised edge. Most common skin cancer.

▶ Diagnosis
Physical examination, biopsy.

▶ Disease Severity
Size and site of lesion, involvement of adjacent tissue, recurrent disease.

▶ Concept and Application
Ultraviolet B light exposure, fair-skinned persons. Slow growth and local invasion.

▶ Treatment Steps
1. Surgical excision: 3–4-mm margin (preferred).
2. Mohs' micrographic surgery (facial lesion).
3. Radiation, topical chemotherapy.

F. Squamous Cell Carcinoma

▶ H&P Keys
Erythematous plaque or nodule, ulceration with raised edges. Second most common form of skin cancer. Precursor lesion: actinic keratosis.

► Diagnosis

Physical examination; biopsy.

► Disease Severity

Burn-scar carcinoma (Marjolin's ulcer); fixed to surrounding structures, immune status, regional lymphadenopathy.

► Concept and Application

Invasive neoplasm devised from keratinocytes, ultraviolet exposure, impaired immunity, chronic irritation or granulomas. Lower lip, ears, and genitalia have higher metastatic potential. In situ squamous cell carcinoma is called Bowen's disease.

► Treatment Steps

1. Surgical excision, regional lymph node excision (if clinically palpable.
2. Radiotherapy.

G. Melanoma

► H&P Keys

Increase in size or change in color of mole or any pigmented nevus, bleeding, itching, pain, family history. Risk factors: sun exposure, dysplastic nevus syndrome, xeroderma pigmentosum, > 50 moles, history of nonmelanoma skin cancer.

► Diagnosis

Physical examination, excisional biopsy.

► Disease Severity

Lymphatic and hematogenous metastatic spread; most common sites: liver and lung.

► Concept and Application

Malignant tumor of melanocytes. Majority arise de novo; up to 50% in existing nevi; 90% occur in skin (other sites: eye, anus, viscera).

► Treatment Steps

1. Wide surgical excision, elective lymph node dissection for intermediate-thickness lesions (sentinel node biopsy in selected cases).
2. Chemotherapy, immunotherapy.
3. Regional hyperthermic limb perfusion for recurrent or unresectable extremity lesions.

► cram facts

MELANOMA: POOR PROGNOSTIC FACTORS

- Head, neck, or trunk lesion
- Thick tumor (Breslow classification)
- Multiple, congenital, or dysplastic nevi
- Ulceration
- Lymphadenopathy
- Vertical growth
- Subungual lesions

► cram facts

BRESLOW THICKNESS PROGNOSIS AND MARGIN OF EXCISION

- < 0.76 mm—1-cm margin of excision—< 10% 10-year mortality.
- 0.76 mm—4-mm to 2-cm margins of excision—intermediate prognosis.
- > 4 mm—2-cm margins of excision—worst prognosis, > 50% 10-year mortality.

H. Sarcoma

► **H&P Keys**

Painless discrete mass in limb, abdominal/flank mass. Patient often gives an antecedent history of trauma.

► **Diagnosis**

MRI, computed tomography (CT) scan, needle or incisional biopsy.

► **Disease Severity**

Histologic grade; tumor size, depth, and site; metastatis.

► **Concept and Application**

Invasive neoplasm derived from mesodermal connective tissue. Radiation exposure, oncogenic viruses, human immunodeficiency virus (HIV), neurofibromatosis. Hematogenous metastasis: lung is most common site.

► **Treatment Steps**

1. En bloc resection.
2. Radiotherapy, chemotherapy.
3. Hyperthermic limb perfusion.

I. Decubitus Ulcer

► **H&P Keys**

Blanching erythema, shallow or extensive dermal defects, fever, cellulitis. Immobilized patient.

► **Diagnosis**

Physical examination, x-ray of ulcer to assess osteomyelitis and subcutaneous extension (air).

► **Disease Severity**

Depth and size of defect, underlying osteomyelitis.

► **Concept and Application**

Microcirculatory ischemia from prolonged pressure due to immobilization. Malnutrition and incontinence contribute. Muscle necrosis always more extensive than skin (more sensitive to ischemia).

► **Treatment Steps**

1. Prevention: offloading and mobilization (e.g., turn patient frequently, use air or foam mattress), improve nutrition.
2. Definitive: drainage of infected spaces, debridement, musculocutaneous flaps or skin grafts.

J. Venous Ulceration

► **H&P Keys**

Ulceration proximal to medial malleolus; history of deep vein thrombosis (DVT); saphenofemoral or perforator incompetence, incompetence; brawny, hyperpigmented skin in distal, medial leg; lipodermatosclersosis; dependent edema; cellulitis (stasis dermatitis).

► **Diagnosis**

Clinical examination, Doppler ultrasound, plethysmography to assess for venous reflux.

► **Disease Severity**

Cellulitis, subfascial perforator incompetence, obesity, cardiac failure.

► Concept and Application

Venous hypertension from reflux and/or obstruction causes peri-capillary fibrin deposition, protein accumulation, leukocyte rapping, inflammatory mediator release, and ulceration.

► Treatment Steps

Subdural—Elevation, gradient-compression hosiery, compressive dressing (Unna's boot), antibiotics for cellulitis.

Surgical (For Recurrent or Nonhealing Ulcers)—Ligation of incompetent perforators; possible skin graft.

K. Arterial Ulcer

► H&P Keys

Smoking, claudication, pain at rest, increased low-density lipoprotein (LDL), diabetes. Punched-out appearance of ulcer, absent pulses, painful ulcer. Ulcer location at toes or pressure point.

► Diagnosis

Ankle–brachial index (ABI < 0.5), digital pressures (< 35 mm Hg), arteriography (for intervention plans only).

► Disease Severity

Pain at rest, gangrene, diabetes, previous bypass.

► Concept and Application

Skin ischemia and impaired healing from limited perfusion due to atherosclerotic arterial occlusive disease.

► Treatment Steps

Angiography, debridement, and closure or skin graft after revascularization (bypass or angioplasty).

II. BREAST DISORDERS

A. Benign Breast Mass

► H&P Keys

Breast lump; mastalgia; bloody nipple discharge (ductal papilloma or cancer). Any discrete mass in a postmenopausal woman, or that persists through the follicular phase of the menstrual cycle in a premenopausal woman, requires evaluation for cancer.

► Diagnosis

Regular self-examination; bilateral mammograms further define lesion features and assess contralateral breast. Fine-needle aspiration cytology; ultrasound; core or excisional biopsy.

► Disease Severity

A mass that is discrete, hard, fixed, irregular, or associated with lymphadenopathy or skin changes is suggestive of breast cancer. Fever and fluctuation indicate abscess.

► Concept and Application

Proliferative breast lesions with atypia (ductal and lobular hyperplasia) have increased risk for breast cancer.

► Treatment Steps
1. Fluid-filled, cystic lesions are aspirated and followed clinically.
2. Discrete nodules require close follow up or excisional biopsy.
4. For nonimproving mastitis, consider "inflammatory cancer."

B. Breast Cancer

► H&P Keys

History of previous breast cancer; family history (first- and second-degree relatives); early menarche; late menopause; nulliparity. Palpable breast mass, hard, irregular; dimpling of the skin; nipple retraction; brawny, edematous, indurated skin (inflammatory carcinoma); lymphadenopathy.

► Diagnosis

Annual screening mammography recommended for women over age 50. Fine-needle cytology, stereotactic core biopsy, excisional biopsy, tumor markers.

► Disease Severity

Inflammatory carcinoma, skin ulceration, chest wall invasion, metastasis to regional lymph nodes, distant metastasis (most common: bone, lung, liver).

► Concept and Application

Malignant transformation of breast epithelial cells is strongly influenced by hormones—breast cancer is more than 150 times more common in women than men. Mutations in tumor-suppressor genes such as p53, BRCA-1, and BRCA-2 have been implicated in 10% of breast cancers.

► Treatment Steps
1. Stages I and II: either modified radical mastectomy (MRM) or lumpectomy with axillary dissection and postoperative radiotherapy.
2. Stage III: MRM or radical mastectomy.
3. Stage IV: palliative procedures.
4. Adjuvant chemotherapy for node-positive or high-risk patients: premenopausal: chemotherapy with or without tamoxifen; postmenopausal: tamoxifen.
5. Sentinel node biopsy allows more precise surgical intervention with decreased morbidity. Only patients with positive sentinel node require axillary dissection. Contraindicated in patients with clinically positive nodes.

► **diagnostic decisions**

BREAST MASS

Cystic
If aspirate is bloody, cytology is suspicious, or cyst does not resolve, excisional biopsy is indicated.

Solid
If clinical breast examination, mammogram, and fine-needle aspiration *all* are negative, can be followed clinically ("triple diagnosis"). Otherwise, excisional biopsy—the "gold standard" for diagnosis of breast cancer—is mandatory.

► **cram facts**

BREAST CANCER STAGES

Stage	General Description
Stage I	Tumor < 2 cm; no nodes
Stage II	Tumor 2–5 cm and moveable regional lymph node metastasis
Stage III	Fixed axillary lymph node metastasis or locally advanced tumor
Stage IV	Distant metastasis

Note: Clinical trials show no survival difference for breast conservation therapy versus mastectomy. Radiation following lumpectomy decreases local recurrence but does not change survival.

III. DISEASES OF THE ENDOCRINE SYSTEM

A. Thyroid Neoplasm

► H&P Keys

Neck mass, dysphagia, dysphonia, respiratory difficulty, hoarseness, vocal cord paralysis, female patient, childhood neck irradiation, lymphadenopathy, goiter. Medullary cancer in multiple endocrine neoplasia type II (MEN II) syndrome.

► Diagnosis

Serum thyroid-stimulating hormone (TSH) level, fine-needle aspiration cytology, high-resolution ultrasound, radioisotope scan, calcitonin if suspect medullary thyroid cancer. Four types of primary thyroid cancer: papillary (85%), follicular (10%), medullary (4%), and anaplastic (1%).

► Disease Severity

Symptoms of local invasion, metastatic disease, older age, size of tumor, histology, lymphadenopathy, cellular differentiation. Anaplastic carcinoma—poor prognosis. Papillary and follicular cancer—good prognosis.

► Concept and Application

1. Genetic predisposition, neck radiation, preexisting goiter.
2. Etiology of goiter: environmental (iodine deficiency), immunologic, genetic, neoplastic, and drug induced (lithium, amiodarone).
3. Differential diagnosis of thyroid nodule: multinodular goiter (50%), adenoma (33%), carcinoma (10%), cyst, inflammatory thyroid disease, and developmental abnormalities.

► Treatment Steps

1. Lobectomy, total thyroidectomy, cervical lymph node dissection.
2. Thyroxine (to suppress TSH), radioiodine.

B. Hyperparathyroidism

► H&P Keys

Lethargy, confusion, depression, peptic ulcer, muscle weakness, recurrent nephrolithiasis, renal insufficiency.

► Diagnosis

Hypercalcemia with elevated or normal level of parathyroid hormone (PTH), hypophosphatemia, ultrasonography, sestamibi scan.

► Disease Severity

Renal failure, hypertension, recurrent disease.

► Concept and Application

Excess PTH production, from parathyroid adenoma, hyperplasia (all four glands), and rarely parathyroid carcinoma.

► Treatment Steps

Medical
1. IV fluids.
2. Furosemide.

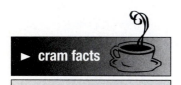

INDICATION FOR SURGERY IN A THYROID NODULE

- Malignant lesions
- Indeterminate on biopsy
- Hypofunctioning lesions
- Local symptoms
- Neck disfigurement

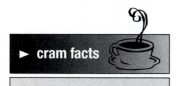

ETIOLOGY OF HYPERPARATHYROIDISM

Primary: Adenoma 80%
Secondary:
- Renal failure
- Carcinoma with bone metastases
- Multiple myeloma
- Osteogenesis imperfecta
- Paget disease
Tertiary: Renal transplant patients

3. Stop thiazide or vitamin D.
4. Severe cases: bisphosphonates, estrogen/progesterone.

Surgical
1. Adenoma resection.
2. Three and one-half gland excision or total parathyroidectomy with autotransplantation for hyperplasia; consider MEN evaluation.

C. Cushing's Disease/Cushing's Syndrome

▶ **H&P Keys**

Cushing's syndrome is caused by an excess of adrenocortical hormones from any source. Cushing's disease refers to pituitary hypersecretion of adrenocortical hormone (ACTH). Signs: "mooning" of face, central obesity, wide purple striae, spontaneous ecchymosis, hirsutism, buffalo hump, impotence or amenorrhea, hypertension, diabetes.

▶ **Diagnosis**

Twenty-four-hour urine cortisol and low-dose dexamethasone suppression test confirm Cushing's syndrome; plasma ACTH levels; high-dose dexamethasone suppression test distinguishes between pituitary (suppresses) and ectopic sources (does not suppress) of ACTH; isotope-scanning, CT scan of abdomen, angiography, venous sampling, MRI, NP.59 (iodocholesterol scanning).

▶ **Disease Severity**

Hypertension, stroke, diabetes mellitus, muscle wasting, osteoporosis (pathologic fractures).

▶ **Concept and Application**

1. Excess cortisol production: pituitary adenoma producing ACTH, adrenal adenoma or carcinoma, ACTH-secreting tumors.
2. Ectopic ACTH secretion results from bronchial carcinoid, thymic carcinoid, or pulmonary neoplasm.
3. High ACTH indicates pituitary or ectopic ACTH tumor.
4. Low ACTH indicates hypersecretion from adrenal source.

▶ **Treatment Steps**

Medical
1. Mitotane for metastatic adrenal cancer (blocks β_2 hydroxylation, reversible adenolytic).
2. Lifelong mineralo- and glucocorticoid replacement after bilateral adrenalectomy.
3. Temporary steroid replacement after unilateral adrenalectomy (because of contralateral atrophy).

Surgical
1. Pituitary ablation (transsphenoidal), adrenalectomy (laparoscopic if < 6 cm).
2. Postoperative corticosteroid therapy.

D. Pheochromocytoma

▶ **H&P Keys**

Classic triad—hypertension, palpitation, diaphoresis.

▶ **Diagnosis**

Twenty-four-hour urine catecholamines, metanephrine, vanillylmandelic acid (VMA), serum catecholamine, CT scan of abdomen, metaiodobenzylguanidine (MIBG) isotope scanning (for extra-abdominal or malignant pheochromocytoma).

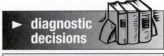

▶ **diagnostic decisions**

CUSHING'S SYNDROME

Adrenal Hyperplasia
High plasma ACTH, secondary to pituitary hypersecretion, pituitary tumor (image with MRI), or ectopic tumor.

Adrenal Adenoma
Low plasma ACTH. Abdominal CT scan or MRI to localize.

Adrenal Carcinoma
Low ACTH. Palpable abdominal mass. Markedly elevated urinary 17-ketosteroids and plasma dehydroepiandrosterone (DHEA).

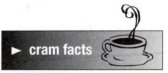

▶ **cram facts**

ETIOLOGY OF CUSHING'S SYNDROME

1. Autonomous adrenal tumor (20%)
2. Pituitary adenoma (60%)
3. Ectopic ACTH production (10%)
4. Iatrogenic Cushing's
5. Adrenocortical cancer (rare)

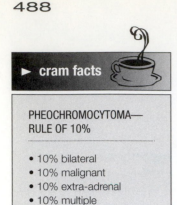

PHEOCHROMOCYTOMA—
RULE OF 10%

- 10% bilateral
- 10% malignant
- 10% extra-adrenal
- 10% multiple
- 10% children

► Disease Severity

Myocardial infarction, arrhythmias, renal failure, pregnancy, stroke.

► Concept and Application

There are four adrenergic receptors: α_1, α_2, β_1, and β_2. Tumors of adrenal medulla and chromaffin tissue, associated MEN II; excess catecholamine production (1/1,000 of hypertensives have pheochromocytoma). Extra-adrenal pheochromocytoma does not produce epinephrine (most common site: organ of Zuckerkandl).

► Treatment Steps

Preoperative

1. α-Adrenergic blockade first (phenoxybenzamine).
2. Then β-adrenergic blockade.
3. Volume replacement.
4. Blood pressure control (nitroprusside, calcium channel blockers).

Note: If the β-blocker is administered first, a hypertensive crisis may result because of unopposed α-adrenergic vasoconstriction.

Surgical—Adrenalectomy with hemodynamic monitoring, volume and blood pressure control.

IV. DISORDERS OF THE KIDNEY AND URINARY TRACT

A. Testicular Tumors

► H&P Keys

Asymptomatic painless swelling (85%), history of cryptorchidism (15%), associated hydrocele (5%).

► Diagnosis

Physical examination, ultrasound, orchiectomy.

► Disease Severity

Staging: CT scan (chest, abdomen), tumor markers (β-human chorionic gonadotropin [β-hCG], and α-fetoprotein [α-FP]).

► Concept and Application

Ninety-five percent are germ cell tumors (seminomas most common).

► Treatment Steps

1. Orchiectomy by inguinal approach.
2. For seminoma: radiation to retroperitoneum.
3. For nonseminoma germ-cell tumor: retroperitoneal lymphadenectomy, adjuvant chemotherapy.

B. Carcinoma of the Bladder

► H&P Keys

Hematuria, pyuria, frequency; tobacco, β-naphthylamine and para-aminodiphenyl exposure.

Risk factors for bladder squamous cell carcinoma: chronic indwelling catheter or infection, bladder stone/strictures, infection with *Schistosoma hematobium*.

Risk factors for bladder transitional cell carcinoma: exposure to aromatic amines, benzidine, naphthylamine, dyes, rubber, textiles, and plastics; cigarette smoking; dietary nitrosamines.

► Diagnosis

Urinary cytology, cystoscopy with biopsy, CT scan and MRI to detect local invasion and distant metastases.

► Concept and Application

Staging: cell type (transitional, squamous, adenomatous), grade, depth of invasion.

► Treatment Steps

Carcinoma In Situ
1. Intravesical therapy (bacillus Calmette–Guérin [BCG], doxorubicin, mitomycin C).
2. Intravesical fulguration.

Superficial
1. Intravesical chemotherapy, local immunotherapy (BCG).
2. Transurethral endoscopic resection.
3. Recurrence common, may require cystectomy.

Invasive—Radical cystectomy, chemotherapy.

C. Prostate Cancer

► H&P Keys

Often asymptomatic; average age 73 years. Dysuria, urinary frequency or retention, hematuria. Risk factors: age, race (African-Americans twofold increase), family history.

► Diagnosis

Digital rectal examination, prostate-specific antigen (PSA). Confirmation by needle biopsy, transrectal ultrasound.

► Concept and Application

Adenocarcinoma (95%). At diagnosis, 40% of tumors have metastasized. Common site for metastasis: obturator lymph nodes, lumbar spine.

► Treatment Steps

Stages A and B (Confined to Prostate)—Radical prostatectomy or interstitial/external radiation. Postop impotence 50%, incontinence 10–30%.

Stage C (Disease Outside Capsule)—Radiation.

Metastatic Carcinoma—Castration: orchiectomy or luteinizing hormone–releasing hormone (LHRH) agonist (goserelin).

D. Renal Cell Carcinoma

► H&P Keys

Flank mass, pain, gross hematuria (10% of patients with classic triad), hypertension, fever, anemia, erythrocytosis, paraneoplastic syndromes.

► Diagnosis

CT scan, MRI, renal ultrasound, cystoscopy (for hematuria).

► Concept and Application

Adenocarcinoma from proximal convoluted tubule is most common type.

► Treatment Steps

1. Stages I and II (local tumor, minimal nodes): radical nephrectomy (partial nephrectomy for tumor < 4 cm).
2. Stage III (advanced tumor, nodal spread): radical nephrectomy, possible adjuvant immunotherapy.
3. Stage IV (metastatic): radical nephrectomy; surgical excision of isolated lung or brain metastasis

E. Renal Calculi

► H&P Keys

Excruciating pain (upper back to testicle or vulva) secondary to dilation of urinary tract, hematuria, nausea, vomiting, urinary frequency or urgency.

► Diagnosis

Urinalysis (UA): hematuria, crystals; ultrasound: hydronephrosis or acoustic shadow, noncontrast CT scan.

► Disease Severity

Recurrent calculi, hyperparathyroidism, decreased renal function, hydronephrosis.

► Concept and Application

Three theories of ureteric stone formation: nucleation, stone matrix, decreased urinary crystallization inhibitors. Infection-related calculi: struvite stones associated with urea-splitting bacteria (e.g., *Proteus*).

► Treatment Steps

Medical (50% Pass Spontaneously)
1. Analgesics.
2. Diuretics, cholestyramine (oxalate-binding resin).
3. Fluids, low-purine diet, alkali, and allopurinol for uric acid stones.

Surgical (Indicated for Infection, Complete Obstruction, Intractable Pain, Progressive Renal Damage)
1. Shock wave lithotripsy.
2. Transurethral extraction if < 4 mm.
3. Nephrostomy.

F. Benign Prostatic Hypertrophy (BPH)

► H&P Keys

Increased urinary frequency, nocturia, decreased force and difficulty initiating stream (retention).

► Diagnosis

Digital rectal examination, UA, PSA.

► Disease Severity

Indication for biopsy of BPH prostate: PSA > 4.

► Concept and Application

Obstruction of outflow in the aging male, stromal and epithelial hyperplasia.

► Treatment Steps

Medical

1. α-Blockade—decreases smooth muscle tone; 5α-reductase blockade (Proscar).
2. Hormonal manipulations; antiandrogen, LHRH agonist.

Surgical—Transurethral resection of the prostate (TURP) or open prostatectomy.

Note: Postoperative TURP syndrome is due to opening of venous sinuses and excess absorption, and is characterized by seizure, sodium loss, cerebral edema, and hypervolemia.

V. TRAUMA

A. Multiple Injuries

► H&P Keys

Blunt Trauma—Mechanisms: compression, crushing, deceleration); alcohol and drug use; prehospital care; localized pain or neurologic deficit; bruises; deformities.

Penetrating Trauma—Type of agent and energy (missile caliber and velocity, proximity to vital structures.

► Diagnosis

Primary Survey (Includes Initiating Appropriate Treatment)—ABCs: **A**irway, with control of cervical spine; **B**reathing and ventilation; **C**irculation with control of obvious bleeding and insertion of IV lines; **D**isability (alert, responds to verbal stimuli, responds to painful stimuli, or unresponsive; see Glasgow Coma Scale); **E**xposure and control of environmental factors.

Secondary Survey—AMPLE: **A**llergies, **M**edications, **P**ast illness and surgery, **L**ast meal, **E**vents related to the trauma. Complete physical examination, diagnostic tests (complete cervical spine x-ray series or CT scan, CT chest/abdomen, ultrasound, blood test results).

► Disease Severity

Presence of immediately life-threatening conditions, old age, preexisting diseases, intoxication (alcohol, drugs), multiple systems affected, hypothermia, severe neurologic deficit.

► Concept and Application

Death and sequelae may result from initial injury (e.g., aortic transection, severe brain damage) or complications (e.g., brain edema, sepsis, renal failure).

► Treatment Steps

1. ABCs (airway, breathing, circulation), oxygen, fluid replacement, warming; tetanus toxoid, antibiotics.
2. Treatment of life-threatening conditions and management according to specific injuries.

B. Cranial Injury

► H&P Keys

Loss of consciousness, amnesia, headache, lethargy, seizures, weakness, scalp laceration or hematoma, hemotympanum, rhinorrhea, otorrhea, periorbital or mastoid ecchymosis.

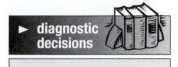

► **diagnostic decisions**

GLASGOW COMA SCALE

Eye opening	(4) Spontaneous
	(3) To voice
	(2) To pain
	(1) None
Verbal response	(5) Oriented
	(4) Confused
	(3) Inappropriate words
	(2) Incomprehensible sounds
	(1) None
Motor response	(6) Obeys commands
	(5) Localizes pain
	(4) Withdrawal, to pain
	(3) Flexion, to pain
	(2) Extension, to pain
	(1) None

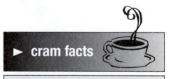

► **cram facts**

CLUES FOR THORACIC AORTIC INJURY

- Severe deceleration mechanism
- Hypotension
- Left hemothorax; apical pleural hematoma
- Fractures: ribs, sternum, clavicle, scapula
- Widened mediastinum
- Obliteration of aortic knob contour
- Deviated nasogastric tube

► management decisions

LIFE-THREATENING CONDITIONS REQUIRING IMMEDIATE TREATMENT

Airway Obstruction
Signs: respiratory distress; cyanosis. Treatment: avoid tongue drop (most common cause), remove blood, foreign body. If face, oropharynx, or larynx severely damaged, emergency surgical airway is required (cricothyroidotomy or tracheostomy).

Tension Pneumothorax
Signs: respiratory distress, cyanosis, hypotension, tracheal deviation to the contralateral side, unilateral absence of breath sounds, neck vein distention. Insert large-bore needle into anterior chest (2nd intercostal), followed by tube thoracostomy.

Open Pneumothorax
"Sucking chest wound," occurs when a chest wall defect is greater in diameter than two-thirds of the trachea. Requires closure of the defect and tube thoracostomy.

Flail Chest
Unstable chest wall from sternum or rib fractures. Intubation and ventilation. Treat associated hemo- or pneumothorax.

Exsanguinating Hemorrhage
Stop obvious bleeding by applying direct pressure. Establish large-bore IV lines. Massive hemothorax—shock, loss of breath sounds, shifting of mediastinum—require chest tube drainage and urgent thoracotomy.

Cardiac Tamponade
Penetrating parasternal or upper abdominal trauma. Cyanosis, hypotension, distended neck veins, and muffled heart sounds. Needle pericardiocentesis for temporary relief; sternotomy or thoracotomy for definitive treatment.

► cram facts

CRITERIA FOR BRAIN DEATH

Preconditions
- Coma with known cause
- Documentation of irreversible structural brain injury

Exclusions (Preclude Diagnosis of Coma)
- Hypotension
- Hypothermia
- Hypoxemia
- Metabolic derangements

Tests
- Absence of brain stem function
- Pupillary corneal, oculovestibular, gag, cough reflexes absent
- Apnea (strict definition)

► Diagnosis

Neurologic examination, CT scan of the head, cervical spine x-rays.

> *Subdural Hemorrhage*—Venous in origin, occurs in elderly, and shows a smooth semilunar white density on the head CT scan.

> *Epidural Hemorrhage*—Arterial in origin, marked by a concave focal white density on the head CT scan; may have lucid interval.

► Disease Severity

Age, low Glasgow Coma Scale score, focal neurologic deficits, hypoxia, associated injuries, hypertension, bradycardia, loss of gag or cough reflex.

► Concept and Application

Sudden movement of brain relative to skull (deceleration injury), cerebral laceration, diffuse axonal injury, intracranial hemorrhage, brain edema, raised intracranial pressure (ICP).

► Treatment Steps

1. Secure airway; correct hypoxia; restore blood pressure (ABCs).
2. Monitor ICP (maintain adequate cerebral perfusion pressure).
3. Appropriate surgical intervention, suture scalp laceration; perform craniotomy for bleeding/decompression.

C. Abdominal Injury

► H&P Keys

Abdominal pain, distention, tenderness, guarding; mechanism of injury.

► Diagnosis

Serial physical examinations; UA, upright chest x-ray (CXR), abdominal ultrasound (focused abdominal sonogram for trauma [FAST] exam), CT scan.

► Disease Severity

Indicators of surgical injury: persistent hypotension, no response to therapy, peritonitis, evisceration, blood on nasogastric aspirate or rectal examination, positive ultrasound.

► Treatment Steps

Exploratory laparotomy; inspect all intra-abdominal organs.

Spleen

1. Can manage nonoperatively if blood pressure and hematocrit stable (Fig. 18–1).
2. Embolization of splenic artery.
3. Splenorrhaphy, splenectomy.

Liver

1. Pringle maneuver, direct ligation of bleeding vessels, hepatic lobectomy, insertion of atriocaval shunt for control of hepatic vein or caval injury, drainage, packing.
2. Nonoperative management with red cell replacement and serial CT scans in hemodynamically stable patients.

Biliary Tract—Cholecystectomy, T-tube in common bile duct, choledochojejunostomy.

Pancreas

1. Drainage, debridement of devitalized pancreas, ligation of main duct if visualized, internal drainage, pancreaticoduodenectomy.
2. Also can manage expectantly with serial CT scans in stable patient without evidence of ductal injury.

Gastrointestinal (GI) Tract—Primary repair, drainage. Colon resection and colostomy with gross contamination.

Kidney

1. Observation, serial imaging.
2. Partial or total nephrectomy.

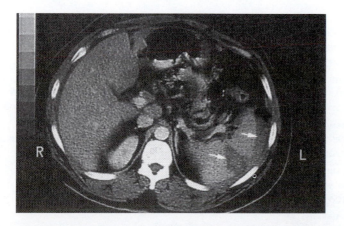

Figure 18–1. Computed tomography (CT) scan showing ruptured spleen following abdominal trauma in patient with human immunodeficiency virus (HIV) infection and splenomegaly. Note intra- and perisplenic hematoma *(arrows)*.

VI. POSTOPERATIVE INFECTIONS

A. Wound Infections

▶ **H&P Keys**

Fever, wound pain, malaise, anorexia, tachycardia, local redness, tenderness, crepitance, swelling, discharge (bloody, serous, or purulent), postoperative days 3–7 most commonly.

▶ **Diagnosis**

Physical examination, wound exploration, culture.

▶ **Disease Severity**

Abscess, fascial dehiscence, evisceration, poor nutrition.

▶ **Concept and Application**

Contamination of wound at surgery, postoperative formation of hematoma or seroma, foreign body, wound-tissue ischemia, enterocutaneous fistula.

▶ **Treatment Steps**
1. Evacuate pus, debridement.
2. Antibiotics.
3. Local wound care.
4. Optimize nutrition/hemodynamics.

▶ **management decisions**

POSTOPERATIVE INFECTIONS

Wound
Erythema, edema, pain/tenderness, drainage, fever. Open and pack the wound. Antibiotics if extensive cellulitis present or patient immunocompromised. Check for foreign body or fistula.

Respiratory Tract
Productive cough, yellow or green sputum; fever, tachycardia, tachypnea; leukocytosis; CXR infiltrate. Treat with intensive respiratory physiotherapy and IV antibiotics.

IV Lines
Superficial phlebitis (erythema, and tenderness over IV line insertion area): Remove line; treat with warm compresses and analgesic anti-inflammatory drugs. *Central venous catheter infection* (positive blood cultures): remove line and give antibiotics if infection persists or patient immunocompromised.

Intra-abdominal
Peritonitis requires exploratory laparotomy or laparoscopy. Abscess may be drained percutaneously. Both require IV antibiotics that cover enteric gram-negatives and anaerobes.

Genitourinary
History of catheterization or instrumentation of urinary tract. Remove catheters if possible. Maintain diuresis. Oral or IV antibiotics depending on severity of infection.

Gastrointestinal
Fever, leukocytosis, and diarrhea. Stool culture and *Clostridium difficile* toxin assay. Treat with metronidazole or vancomycin.

Prosthetic device
Fever, leukocytosis, and bacteremia. CT scan, MRI, radionuclide scan, blood cultures. Give IV antibiotics. Definitive treatment is removal of prosthesis.

B. Urinary Tract Infection (UTI)

► **H&P Keys**

Dysuria, frequency, suprapubic or flank pain and tenderness, fever.

► **Diagnosis**

UA, urine Gram stain and culture, blood cultures.

► **Disease Severity**

High fever, mentation changes.

► **Concept and Application**

Contamination of urinary tract, urine stasis, urinary tract instrumentation.

► **Treatment Steps**

Adequate hydration, remove catheter (if possible), antibiotics.

C. Atelectasis and Pneumonia

► **H&P Keys**

Early postoperative period, pain, shallow breathing. Fever, dyspnea, cough, tachypnea, cyanosis, decreased breath sounds. Purulent sputum suggests pneumonia.

► **Diagnosis**

Physical examination, arterial blood gases (ABGs), sputum culture, CXR.

► **Disease Severity**

Cyanosis, tracheal deviation, dyspnea at rest, hypoxia.

► **Concept and Application**

Obstruction of tracheobronchial airway, abnormality of surfactants, loss of lung volume (atelectasis), secondary bacterial infection (pneumonia). Pain-induced decreased lung volumes.

► **Treatment Steps**

1. Deep breathing or coughing exercises, ambulation, intermittent positive-pressure breathing, bronchoscopy, nasotracheal suctioning.
2. Pain control is mandatory.

VII. DISEASES OF THE CIRCULATORY SYSTEM

A. Carotid Artery Disease

► **H&P Keys**

Definitions
- **Transient ischemic attack (TIA):** brief paresis or numbness of an arm or leg contralateral to the affected carotid territory (< 24 hours in duration).
- **Amaurosis fugax (AF):** transient episode of monocular or partial blindness.
- **Stroke:** permanent neurologic deficit.

Symptoms—TIAs, amaurosis fugax, or resolving or permanent neurologic deficit. Vertebrobasilar artery symptoms consist of vertigo, drop attacks, or dizziness due to cerebellar or brain stem ischemia.

Signs—Carotid bruits, presence of Hollenhorst plaques (both are nonspecific). Significant disease can exist without signs or symptoms.

► Diagnosis
• Duplex ultrasound: 95% accurate and 90% sensitive.
• Arteriography: used selectively (Fig. 18–2).
• Magnetic resonance angiography (MRA): anatomic study; also images intracranial segments.

► Disease Severity
Crescendo TIAs and stroke in evolution mandate urgent anticoagulation and intervention.

► Concept and Application
Ulceration of atherosclerotic plaque causes microemboli (usually platelets), resulting in ischemia and infarct of cerebral parenchyma. Risk of microbmeoli correlates with degree of stenosis.

► Treatment Steps
1. Medical therapy is indicated for patients with stenosis < 60%: aspirin, clopidogrel.

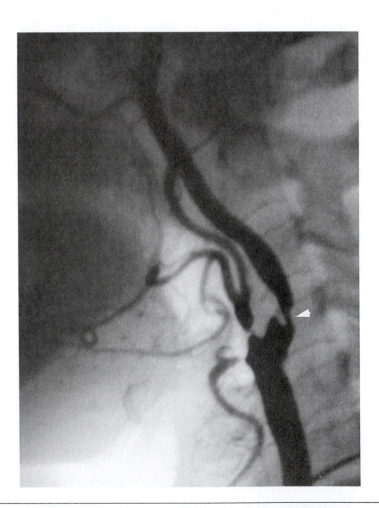

Figure 18–2. Carotid angiogram showing a high-grade stenosis of the origin of the internal (arrow) as well as the external carotid artery. This study is currently reserved for recurrent carotid artery stenosis (atherosclerotic or radiation therapy related), high carotid bifurcation, stenotic "string sign" lesion of the internal carotid artery, or if the patient is being considered for carotid angioplasty and stenting.

2. Carotid endarterectomy reduces the risk of stroke in:
   • Symptomatic patients with > 60% stenosis.
   • Asymptomatic patients with > 80% stenosis.
3. Carotid stenting may be useful in selected cases:
   • High-surgical-risk patients.
   • Hostile neck (previous radiation, high bifurcation).

Indications for Operation—Symptoms (TIA, amaurosis, nonhemorrhagic stroke, asymptomatic high-grade stenosis.

Contraindication to Operation—Fixed dense stroke, total occlusion of carotid.

B. Renovascular Disease

► H&P Keys

Renal artery stenosis can cause hypertension and/or renal insufficiency. Clinical clues: accelerated hypertension, uncontrolled blood pressure on multiple meds, early-onset hypertension, deterioration of renal function (especially after starting angiotensin-converting enzyme [ACE] inhibitor), abdominal/flank bruit.

► Diagnosis

Renal Artery Duplex—No contrast, elevated arterial velocity indicates renal artery stenosis.

Renal Vein Renins—Ratio of renin from involved compared to uninvolved kidney is > 1.5.

Renal Arteriography—Contrast study used for operative planning or endovascular intervention.

► Disease Severity

Conditions associated with favorable response to therapy: unilateral disease, renal length > 8 cm, fibromuscular dysplasia (FMD), acute onset versus chronic hypertension or azotemia.

► Concept and Application

Renin–angiotensin system (RAS) releases renin that increases angiotensin I and II causing vasoconstriction, sodium retention, and hypertension. Renal insufficiency is caused by hypoperfusion, microembolization, parenchymal changes.

► Treatment Steps

Medical—Control hypertension with antihypertensive drugs, ACE inhibitors (must monitor renal function), diuretics, β-blockers.

Surgical
1. Percutaneous balloon angioplasty is most successful in FMD. Stenting has reasonable success rates for renovascular hypertension. Long-term outcome and restenosis remain controversial.
2. Bypass: aortorenal (first choice), hepatorenal, splenorenal, iliorenal.

C. Peripheral Arterial Occlusive Disease

► H&P Keys

Definitions
• **Claudication:** deep ache or cramping (most commonly in the calf) secondary to muscle ischemia during exercise.
• **Rest pain:** burning pain usually in the forefoot; indicates severe disease.

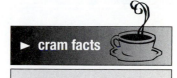

► cram facts

CAUSES OF RENAL ARTERY STENOSIS

• Atherosclerosis (90%): age > 55 years; cardiovascular risk factors.
• Fibromuscular dysplasia (FMD): 20- to 40-year-old women

- **Tissue loss:** necrosis or failure to heal an open wound secondary to inadequate blood flow.
- **Distal aortic occlusion (Leriche's syndrome):** claudication of the hip, thigh, and buttock muscles; leg atrophy, impotence, and diminished or absent femoral pulses.

Risk Factors—Smoking, hypertension, diabetes, hyperlipidemia.

▶ Diagnosis

Physical Examination—Diminished or absent pulses distal to the arterial stenosis, pallor on elevation, rubor with dependency.

Noninvasive Vascular Tests—ABI, segmental pressures with pulse volume recordings or Doppler waveforms, arterial duplex.

Imaging Studies—Arteriography reserved for preoperative patients to define the site of arterial obstruction and delineate arterial anatomy. MRA provides arterial anatomy without contrast, but may overestimate stenosis.

▶ Disease Severity

Heart disease, previous bypasses, small-vessel disease (limits revascularization attempts).

▶ Concept and Application

Atherosclerotic narrowing (stenosis) causes decreased blood flow during exercise (mild disease, claudication) or at rest (severe disease, rest pain).

▶ Treatment Steps

Medical
1. Reduction of risk factors (smoking cessation is most important), exercise program.
2. Antiplatelet and vasodilatory agents (cilostazol).

Surgical
1. Indication: incapacitating claudication or limb salvage.
2. Aortoiliac or aortofemoral reconstruction: 80% patency after 5 years. Iliac angioplasty (stenting) also has good results. Extra-anatomic bypass (femorofemoral, iliofemoral, or axillobifemoral) for high-risk patients.
3. Femoropopliteal and infrapopliteal reconstruction ideally with ispsilateral greater saphenous vein. Reconstructions to the tibial, peroneal, or pedal arteries are generally performed for limb salvage.

D. Aneurysms of the Thoracic Aorta

▶ H&P Keys

Majority are asymptomatic. Chest pain and pressure, hoarseness, superior vena cava syndrome, and cough and dyspnea from tracheobronchial obstruction. Hemoptysis may indicate erosion into the trachea and mainstem bronchus.

▶ Diagnosis

CT scan and MRI; echocardiography and anteriography; transesophageal echo is a sensitive diagnostic method.

▶ Disease Severity

Ascending Aortic—Mortality of surgical repair < 10%.

Aortic Arch—Mortality rate 10–15%; neurologic complications 10%.

Descending Aortic—Mortality rate 10%; paraplegia, 5–20%.

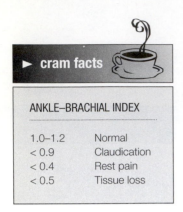

▶ cram facts

ANKLE–BRACHIAL INDEX

1.0–1.2	Normal
< 0.9	Claudication
< 0.4	Rest pain
< 0.5	Tissue loss

▶ Concept and Application

Etiology: atherosclerosis, cystic medial degeneration, dissection, trauma, and poststenotic dilatation. Syphilitic aortitis is rare. Incidence of aneurysm increases with age. Rupture is the most common cause of death.

▶ Treatment Steps

1. Aneurysms > 6 cm should be repaired in patients with reasonable surgical risk.
2. Vascular reconstruction with interposition bypass graft.

   Ascending Aortic—Reconstruction with prosthetic graft, and repair of aortic valve, if necessary.

   Aortic Arch—Reconstruction during deep hypothermic circulatory arrest.

   Descending Aortic—Reconstruction during partial cardiopulmonary to lower complications of paralysis and organ failure.

E. Aortic Dissection

▶ H&P Keys

Severe, sudden-onset pain radiating to the back. May exhibit neurologic deficit, dyspnea, pulmonary edema, nausea, and vomiting. More common in men; typical age 45–70. Hypertensive history in 80–90%. Shock, pulmonary edema, and a murmur of aortic insufficiency may be noted.

Differential diagnosis: myocardial infarction, cerebrovascular accident, pulmonary embolism, aortic thrombosis, and acute abdominal disorders.

▶ Diagnosis

CXR may show a dilated aorta, widened mediastinum, pulmonary edema, or mass effect with or without pleural effusion (rupture). CT (Fig. 18–3A), MRI, and transesophageal echocardiogram. Aortogram usually shows splitting of contrast column (Fig. 18–3B).

▶ Disease Severity

Dissections classified as ascending (usually involve the entire aorta or descending aorta distal to the left subclavian artery).

▶ Concept and Application

Degeneration of medial layer can be caused by hypertension, atherosclerosis, coarctation, endocrine factors, Marfan's syndrome, trauma. Hemodynamic forces, shear stress, and weakened arterial wall lead to development of an intimal tear. A hematoma forms within the torn aorta and dissects distally and proximally within the media.

▶ Treatment Steps

Ascending Dissections—Repair surgically using median sternotomy and cardiopulmonary bypass.

Descending Dissections
1. Control blood pressure with nitroprusside.
2. Begin β-blockers and oral antihypertensives after stabilization.
3. One-third of patients require surgery for enlarging aneurysm over time.
4. Immediate surgery indicated for expanding aneurysm; rupture; neurologic deficit; or visceral, renal, or lower extremity ischemia.

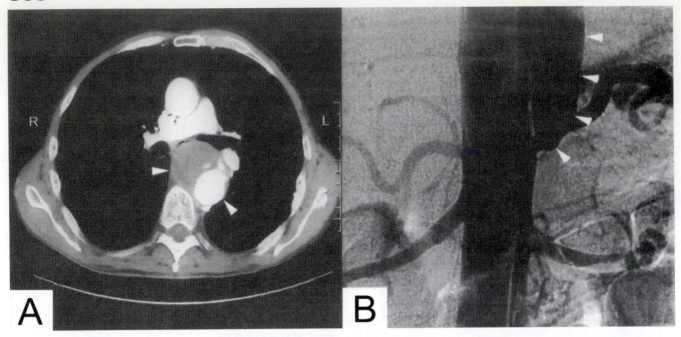

Figure 18–3. Dissecting thoracoabdominal aneurysm in a 70-year-old man with history of hypertension. (A) Contrasted computed tomography (CT) scan of descending thoracic aorta showing dilatation (arrowheads), double lumen, and mural thrombus. (B) Aortogram demonstrating true and false lumina, separated by a septum. The dissection column (arrowheads) extends to the suprarenal portion of the aorta. (Courtesy of Dr. Oswaldo Yano, Mount Sinai School of Medicine, New York, NY.)

F. Abdominal Aortic Aneurysmal Disease

▶ H&P Keys

Most patients are asymptomatic. Symptoms of rupture: acute abdominal pain radiating to the back and hypotension. Exam discloses pulsatile supraumbilical mass.

▶ Diagnosis

Ultrasound to assess size of aneurysm (most rapid diagnosis). CT scan to assess size of aneurysm as well as extent (Fig. 18–4). Aortography used selectively to define suprarenal involvement, suspected renovascular disease, visceral arterial involvement or stenosis, possible distal occlusive disease.

▶ Disease Severity

Risk of rupture increases with increasing diameter. Majority of aneurysms enlarge slowly over time (2–4 mm/yr). Risk of rupture 5–7%/yr for aneurysms 5–7 cm; 20%/yr for aneurysms > 7 cm.

▶ Concept and Application

Aneurysmal dilatation secondary to combination of factors: genetic (collagen abnormalities); proteolytic (matrix metalloproteinases); atherosclerotic (disordered remodeling).

▶ Treatment Steps

1. Recommend repair of all aneurysms ≥ 5 cm in diameter in reasonable-risk patients.
2. Aortic replacement with prosthetic grafts.
3. Endovascular repair for high-risk patients.

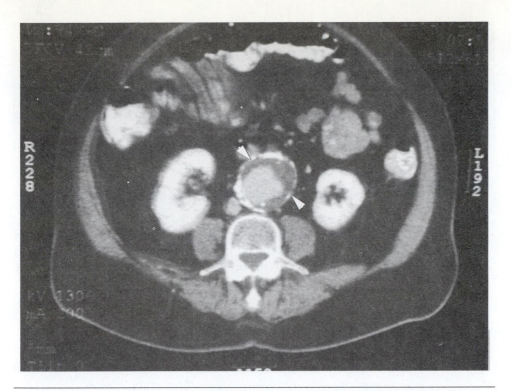

Figure 18–4. Abdominal CT scan with IV contrast showing an abdominal aortic aneurysm *(arrows).* Note the white inner lumen surrounded with a darker mural thrombus and an outer white ring of calcification around the aneurysm.

G. Thoracic Outlet Syndrome (TOS)

▶ H&P Keys

History of clavicle or rib trauma, exercise or occupational injury, poor posture. Symptoms dependent on compression of brachial plexus, subclavian/axillary artery or vein.

▶ Diagnosis

Adson maneuver: positive if radial pulse is lost when patient turns head to affected side and inhales deeply. Costoclavicular compression maneuver; elevated-arm stress test. Diagnostic studies include plain x-rays to assess cervical ribs or other bony abnormalities; venogram to demonstrate compression or obstruction of the subclavian/axillary vein; arteriograms to show partial or complete arterial occlusion with positioning. Electromyography may detect compression of peripheral nerves (conduction delay).

▶ Disease Severity

Three basic types of TOS: neurogenic (95%), venous (2%), and arterial (1%).

▶ Concept and Application

Compression areas include interscalene triangle, scalenus anticus space (between first rib and clavicle), costocoracoid fascia, and pectoralis minor tendon. Compression may be associated with cervical ribs or long process of C7.

▶ Treatment Steps

1. Physical therapy if no evidence of vascular occlusion, distal embolization, or poststenotic aneurysm.
2. Surgical treatment can include resection of the first rib, anterior and/or scalenectomy; removal of a cervical rib if present.

TOS Type	Signs and Symptoms
Neurogenic	Weakness, paresthesia, pain, numbness (ulnar distribution)
Arterial	Weak or absent pulses, delayed capillary refill, gangrene
Venous	Distended veins on chest, arm, hand; arm edema; cyanosis

H. Infrainguinal Aneurysmal Disease

► H&P Keys

Femoral and popliteal aneurysms are often asymptomatic. They may appear as a groin or popliteal mass. Bilateral in 50–75%; coexistent abdominal aortic aneurysm present in 60% of popliteal aneurysms.

► Diagnosis

Ultrasound delineates size of the aneurysm. Angiography to define distal runoff is indicated in all operative candidates.

► Disease Severity

Risk of amputation increases when repair of aneurysm is performed emergently because of thrombosis or distal embolization.

► Concept and Application

Infrainguinal aneurysms are at risk for thrombosis, embolization, and rupture (rarely). Pseudoaneurysms (does not include all layers of the arterial wall) are more common than true aneurysms and are usually iatrogenic (prior femoral catherization); also caused by trauma (blunt or penetrating); infection, especially associated with IV drug abuse.

► Treatment Steps

Femoral Artery Aneurysm—Excision and replacement with autologous conduit (preferable) or prosthetic.

Popliteal Artery Aneurysm—Proximal and distal ligation of native popliteal artery, with bypass using saphenous vein.

I. Arterial Embolism/Thrombosis

► H&P Keys

Acute occlusion: six Ps—pulselessness, pallor, paresthesia, pain, paralysis, and poikilothermia. Irreversible limb loss may occur within 6–8 hours.

► Diagnosis

ABI; angiography; echocardiography because cardiac system is most common source of emboli.

► Disease Severity

Embolism usually secondary to cardiac source (atrial fibrillation, myocardial infarction, congestive heart failure).

► Concept and Application

Embolic occlusion is more common than thrombotic. Thrombosis generally occurs in area of atherosclerotic disease. Compromise of oxygenation leads to anaerobic metabolism, acidosis, membrane destabilization, and cellular edema and death.

► Treatment Steps
1. Heparinization.
2. Embolectomy.
3. Thrombolytic agents (tissue plasminogen activator [tPA]) are used when thrombus has progressed into small vessels.
4. Fasciotomy for reperfusion after prolonged ischemia
5. Maintenance of urine output recommended to prevent renal injury from reperfusion of ischemic limb.

J. Deep Vein Thrombosis (DVT)

► H&P Keys

Patient can be asymptomatic or exhibit the classic findings of calf swelling and tenderness, elevated temperature. Phlegmasia cerulea dolens is massive swelling, pain, and cyanosis that occurs with complete iliofemoral venous occlusion (may progress to venous gangrene).

► Diagnosis

Clinical findings are often inaccurate. Duplex scan has become the standard test for diagnosis (sensitivity and specificity for above-the-knee thrombi: 90–100%).

► Concept and Application

Thrombosis is related to three factors—endothelial abnormalities, blood stasis, and hypercoagulability (Virchow's triad).

► Treatment Steps
1. Prevent with exercise, elastic or pneumatic stockings, and early ambulation after surgery. Important role for DVT prophylaxis with anticoagulant medications in patients at high risk (orthopedic procedures, etc.).
2. Bed rest with leg elevation to reduce the edema after DVT.
3. Drug therapy to prevent propagation of the thrombus and pulmonary embolus includes IV unfractionated heparin or low-molecular-weight heparin. Warfarin therapy is then initiated, and continued for 3–6 months.
4. Vena cava filter placement is indicated when anticoagulation is contraindicated or patient has pulmonary embolism or recurrent DVT on adequate anticoagulation.
5. Thrombolytic therapy is used in selected cases of iliofemoral DVT to decrease the late sequelae of venous thrombosis (valvular incompetence, chronic venous insufficiency).

K. Varicose Veins

► H&P Keys

Affect 10–20% of the population. Patients may be asymptomatic or complain of aching, swelling, heaviness, cramps, itching; occasionally hemorrhage. Physical findings: dry, scaling skin; edema and brawny induration; dilated, tortuous, subcutaneous veins of the thigh and leg.

► Diagnosis

Valvular competence of the deep, superficial, and perforating veins must be determined and can be performed most accurately with a duplex ultrasound examination.

► Concept and Application

Caused by incompetent valves and abnormalities in the structure of the vein wall.

► cram facts

DVT RISK FACTORS

- Previous DVT
- Traumatic injury
- Immobilization
- Postoperative (especially orthopedic and neurosurgery)
- Cancer
- Hypercoagulable disorders

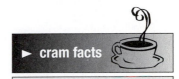

► cram facts

PULMONARY EMBOLISM

Signs and Symptoms
- Dyspnea
- Tachypnea
- Pleuritic chest pain
- Hemoptysis
- Bulging neck veins

Specific Diagnostic Tests
- Ventilation–perfusion lung scan
- Spiral CT scan
- Pulmonary arteriography

▶ Treatment Steps
1. Nonoperative management consists of improving venous return and reducing venous pressure by elevation and graduated elastic stockings.
2. Surgical therapy is indicated for severe symptoms, large varicosities, superficial phlebitis, hemorrhage, ulceration, and cosmesis. It consists of saphenous vein ablation (stripping, radiofrequency, or laser) and removing branch varicosities.
3. Sclerotherapy is used for small and "spider" varicosities.

L. Superficial Thrombophlebitis

▶ H&P Keys
History of IV catheters or drug abuse. Cancer may cause recurrent or migratory superficial thrombophlebitis (Trousseau's sign). Signs include erythema, pain, induration, heat, tenderness along the course of a superficial vein.

▶ Diagnosis
History and physical examination.

▶ Disease Severity
Disease usually has a short and uncomplicated time course.

▶ Concept and Application
Introduction of bacteria with either IV catheters or IV drug abuse. Local infection and inflammatory response result in thrombosis.

▶ Treatment Steps
1. Conservative measures: nonsteroidal anti-inflammatory agents, local heat, and elastic compression bandages.
2. If inflammation of saphenous vein involves the saphenofemoral junction, pulmonary embolism may result, and ligation of the greater saphenous vein or anticoagulation is indicated.
3. In cases of suppuration, surgical excision of involved vein is indicated.

VIII. DISEASES OF THE GASTROINTESTINAL (GI) TRACT

A. Zenker's Diverticulum

▶ H&P Keys
Dysphagia, regurgitation of undigested food, coughing, mass on the left side of the neck.

▶ Diagnosis
Barium swallow showing cricopharyngeal bar and hypopharyngeal diverticula.

▶ Disease Severity
Pulmonary complications, poor nutrition, weight loss, size of pouch. Most common esophageal diverticulum.

▶ Concept and Application
Abnormal cricopharyngeus muscle (more scar, smaller opening dimensions) exerts increased hypopharyngeal bolus pressure during swallowing.

► Treatment Steps
Diverticulectomy, cricopharyngeal myotomy.

B. Midesophageal Traction Diverticulum

► H&P Keys
Often associated with mediastinal granulomatous disease. Most commonly asymptomatic and incidentally discovered.

► Diagnosis
Barium esophagogram.

► Concept and Application
Mediastinal adenopathy from tuberculosis (TB) or histoplasmosis adheres to the esophagus, "dragging" its wall and creating a diverticulum.

► Treatment Steps
Indicated for severe symptoms; suspend diverticula, add myotomy if motor abnormality also present.

C. Achalasia

► H&P Keys
Dysphagia, regurgitation of undigested food, weight loss, dyspnea, cough.

► Diagnosis
Barium esophagogram showing dilated esophagus with tapered distal end ("bird's beak"), esophagoscopy, esophagomanometry.

► Disease Severity
Aspiration, pneumonia, old age, recurrent dysphagia. Increased risk for squamous cell carcinoma.

► Concept and Application
Dilatation, absent esophageal peristalsis, incomplete relaxation of lower esophageal sphincter, hypertensive lower esophage-al sphincter, decreased ganglion cells in Auerbach's plexus.

► Treatment Steps

Medical—Calcium channel blockers, esophageal balloon dilatation.

Surgical—Distal esophagomyotomy (Hellar myotomy) and antireflux procedure (laparoscopic or open).

D. Esophageal Varices

► H&P Keys
Hematemesis, melena, signs of liver failure (ascites, encephalopathy, clonus, jaundice, hepatomegaly, palmar erythema, cachexia). History of alcohol abuse.

► Diagnosis
Esophagogastroduodenoscopy.

► Disease Severity
Recurrent bleeding. Child's classification.

► Concept and Application
Significant elevation of portal pressures. Shunting of blood through left gastric vein (coronary vein) into submucosal plexus. Majority of

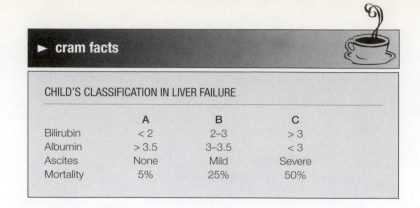

► cram facts

CHILD'S CLASSIFICATION IN LIVER FAILURE

	A	B	C
Bilirubin	< 2	2–3	> 3
Albumin	> 3.5	3–3.5	< 3
Ascites	None	Mild	Severe
Mortality	5%	25%	50%

patients have cirrhosis or had extrahepatic portal obstruction in childhood.

► Treatment Steps
1. Fluid resuscitation, vasopressin, β-blockers, endoscopic banding sclerotherapy, balloon tamponade.
2. Transjugular intrahepatic portosystemic shunt (TIPS).
3. Surgery: portosystemic shunt if TIPS and endoscopy fail or are unavailable.

E. Cancer of the Stomach

► H&P Keys
Anorexia, epigastric pain (unrelieved by food), weight loss, dysphagia (esophagogastric junction), vomiting, hematemesis.

► Diagnosis
Gastroscopy with multiple biopsies, barium meal, CT scan of abdomen.

► Disease Severity
Advanced stage, tumor histology, depth of invasion, cachexia, ascites, degree of local extension, associated adenopathy.

► Concept and Application
Adenocarcinoma most common (95%). Premalignant conditions are atrophic gastritis, intestinal metaplasia, dysplastic gastric polyp, and pernicious anemia.

► Treatment Steps
Radical gastric resection and chemotherapy.

F. Gastric Volvulus

► H&P Keys
Abdominal pain; retching with inability to vomit; inability to pass nasogastric tube.

► Diagnosis
Upper GI series, endoscopy.

► Disease Severity
Perforation or gangrene of stomach, shock.

► Concept and Application
Presence of diaphragmatic defect (paraesophageal hernia in adults). Rotation around the longitudinal axis (organoaxial) or vertical axis (mesenteroaxial).

► Treatment Steps

Acute—Surgery to uncoil stomach, repair diaphragmatic defect, anterior gastropexy or gastrostomy tube.

Chronic—Anterior gastropexy and antireflux procedure (open or laparoscopic).

G. Appendicitis

► H&P Keys

Periumbilical pain shifting to right lower quadrant, anorexia, tender right lower quadrant, tender on rectal examination.

► Diagnosis

History and physical, leukocytosis, ultrasound (especially in children). Fecalith (uncommon), CT scan with oral or rectal contrast.

► Disease Severity

Perforation and abscess. Marked leukocytosis, high fever, peritonitis, elderly, pregnancy, delayed diagnosis.

► Concept and Application

Obstruction of appendix lumen and bacterial invasion.

► Treatment Steps

1. Fluid resuscitation, antibiotics.
2. Appendectomy (open or laparoscopic).

H. Ulcerative Colitis

► H&P Keys

Diarrhea, rectal bleeding, weight loss, abdominal cramps/tenderness.

► Diagnosis

Colonoscopy, barium enema; rectum always involved; continuous, uninterrupted inflammation.

► Disease Severity

Dehydration, malnutrition, cecal perforation, massive lower GI bleeding, total colonic involvement. Increased risk of colon carcinoma.

► Concept and Application

Etiology unclear; immunologic injury to colon mucosa, defect of suppressor T cells in intestinal wall.

► Treatment Steps

Acute

1. Bed rest, sulfasalazine, steroids, nothing by mouth.
2. Total parenteral nutrition.
3. Subtotal colectomy and ileostomy (if fails medical management, persistent GI bleeding, or toxic megacolon).

Chronic—Sulfasalazine, steroids, immunosuppressive agents, proctocolectomy with ileoanal pull-through and J-pouch.

I. Crohn's Disease

► H&P Keys

Abdominal pain, diarrhea, weight loss, perianal fistula and abscess.

► Diagnosis

Small-bowel series, endoscopy, cobblestone mucosa, skip lesions, fistula.

► cram facts

COMPARISON OF CROHN'S DISEASE AND ULCERATIVE COLITIS

	Crohn's Disease	Ulcerative Colitis
Pathology	Transmural inflammation; granulomas	Mucosal inflammation
Anatomic extent	Segmental; skip lesions	Contiguous; rectum always involved
Gross bleeding	Absent in 25–30%	Universal
Complications	Fistula, abscess, perforation, stricture	Toxic megacolon, hemorrhage
Role of surgery	Palliative; treat complications, preserve bowel	Curative; remove colon and rectum

► Disease Severity

Severe anal disease, extraintestinal manifestations, malnutrition, abdominal mass, intra-abdominal abscesses, amount of small bowel and colon involved.

► Concept and Application

Possible immunologic mechanism that leads to inflammatory reaction and transmural damage.

► Treatment Steps

Medical

1. Bowel rest.
2. Low-residue, high-protein diet.
3. Sulfasalazine, metronidazole, aminosalicylates orally or rectally.
4. 6-Mercaptopurine and cyclosporin in refractory cases.

Surgical

1. Small-bowel resection, segmental colectomy, stricturoplasty.
2. Surgery is indicated only for complications (obstruction, perforation, GI bleeding, failure of medical therapy, malignancy).
3. Unlike ulcerative colitis, surgery is not definitive treatment.

J. Acute Mesenteric Ischemia

► H&P Keys

Abdominal pain (out of proportion to physical findings), rectal bleeding, atrial fibrillation.

► Diagnosis

Leukocytosis, elevated lactic acid, angiography (definitive).

► Disease Severity

Peritonitis (bowel infarction).

► Concept and Application

Four mechanisms—embolic, thrombosis, vasoconstriction, venous thrombosis (see Cram Facts).

► Treatment Steps

1. IV fluids, antibiotics, thromboembolectomy, bowel resection, anticoagulation, intra-arterial papaverine.

> **cram facts**

ACUTE MESENTERIC ISCHEMIA

Mechanism	Treatment
Embolic occlusion (Fig. 18–5)	Embolectomy; control dysrhythmia
Thrombosis of preexisting stenosis	Thrombectomy; endarterectomy or bypass
Severe splanchnic vasoconstriction due to low flow state	Intra-arterial papaverine; improve hemodynamics
Mesenteric vein thrombosis	Anticoagulation

2. Treatment of cardiac etiologic findings with arrhythmia control.
3. Long-term anticoagulation.

K. Small-Bowel Obstruction

► H&P Keys
Colicky abdominal pain, vomiting, failure to pass flatus or feces; abdominal distention, dehydration, previous surgery.

► Diagnosis
Plain abdominal x-rays (distended small bowel with air–fluid levels) (Fig. 18–6), barium small-bowel follow-through, CT scan.

► Disease Severity
Poor urine output, leukocytosis, unremitting pain, high fever, peritonitis.

► Concept and Application
Narrowing or occlusion of bowel lumen, proximal bowel distention with gas and fluid. Distention leads to increased intestinal wall pressure, ischemia, and gangrene. Adhesions, hernia, and tumor are the most common causes.

► Treatment Steps
1. Fluid and electrolyte resuscitation, nasogastric decompression.
2. Laparotomy, with correction of cause with or without bowel resection.

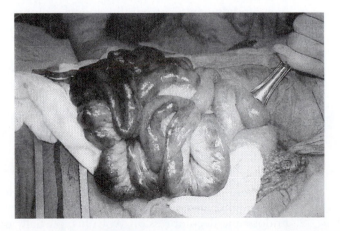

Figure 18–5. Acute mesenteric ischemia in a 74-year-old man with history of atrial fibrillation and heart failure, who developed acute abdominal pain and shock. Exploratory laparotomy disclosed extensive areas of intestinal necrosis and embolic occlusion of the superior mesenteric artery.

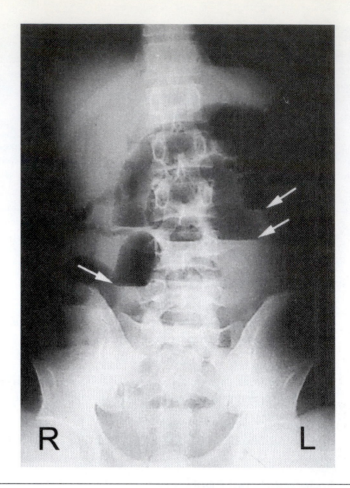

Figure 18–6. Upright abdominal x-ray showing small-bowel obstruction secondary to Crohn's disease. Note distended loops of small-bowel and multiple air–fluid levels *(arrows)*.

L. Large-Bowel Obstruction

► H&P Keys

Crampy abdominal pain, nausea, obstipation; abdominal distention; abdominal tenderness.

► Diagnosis

Plain x-ray of abdomen, Gastrografin enema, colonoscopy. Evaluate for volvulus.

► Disease Severity

Low urine output, leukocytosis, obstructing tumor, peritonitis.

► Concept and Application

Five percent of large-bowel obstruction is caused by volvulus, a twisting of bowel on mesenteric axis.

► Treatment Steps

Medical

1. Fluid and electrolyte resuscitation, nasogastric decompression, monitor urine output.
2. Endoscopic decompression (volvulus, partially obstructing lesion).

Surgical

1. Decompression (colostomy or cecostomy).

2. Colectomy with colostomy or primary anastomosis.
3. Sigmoid colectomy for sigmoid volvulus; right hemicolectomy for cecocolic volvulus.

M. Diverticulitis

▶ **H&P Keys**

Abdominal pain, left lower quadrant tenderness, constipation, low-grade fever.

▶ **Diagnosis**

History and physical, CT scan of abdomen and pelvis, water-soluble contrast enema (rarely).

▶ **Disease Severity**

Perforation, abscess formation, fecal peritonitis, septic shock.

▶ **Concept and Application**

Raised intracolonic pressure leading to pulsion diverticulum; entrapped fecalith causes obstruction of the diverticulum with resulting inflammation and potential perforation.

▶ **Treatment Steps**

Medical (Indicated for Uncomplicated Initial Episode)
1. Systemic antibiotics.
2. Fluid resuscitation.
3. Bowel rest.

Medical (Indicated for Complicated or Recurrent Diverticulitis)
1. Drainage of abscess (may be percutaneous).
2. Colectomy (Hartman's procedure).
3. Colectomy with primary anastomosis (can be done laparoscopically).

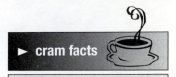

▶ **cram facts**

UNCOMPLICATED
DIVERTICULITIS

Medical Management
• Bowel rest
• IV fluid resuscitation
• Antibiotics (ciprofloxacin and metronidazole)
• High-fiber diet after resolution of symptoms

Indications for Surgery
• Second episode of uncomplicated diverticulitis
• Mass or abscess
• Fistula
• Perforation
• Obstruction
• Bleeding

N. Benign Neoplasm of the Small Bowel

▶ **H&P Keys**

Asymptomatic, occult GI bleeding, bowel obstruction.

▶ **Diagnosis**

Small-bowel follow-through, CT scan of the abdomen and pelvis.

▶ **Disease Severity**

Massive GI bleeding, intussusception, obstruction.

▶ **Concept and Application**

Most common tumor type is GI stromal tumor (GIST); made up of spindle and epithelioid cells. Other benign tumors: adenoma, lipoma, hamartoma, hemangioma.

▶ **Treatment Steps**

Enucleation, wedge excision, depending on size and symptomatology.

O. Benign Neoplasm of the Colon

▶ **H&P Keys**

Rectal bleeding, altered bowel habits, mucous discharge from rectum, rectal mass, heme-positive stools, anemia.

▶ **Diagnosis**

Colonoscopy, barium enema (Fig. 18–7).

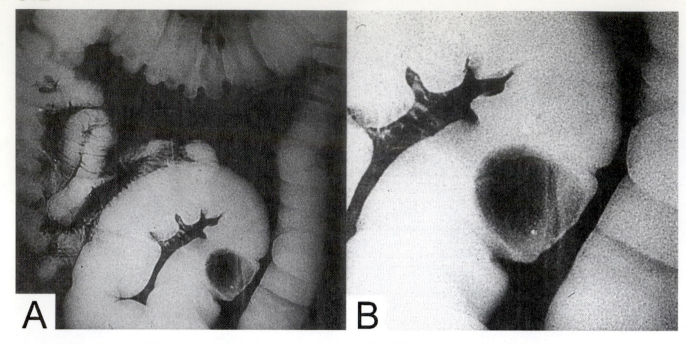

Figure 18–7. Benign tumor of sigmoid colon (submucosal lipoma) in a 35-year-old man. Note regular and smooth appearance of the lesion and normal distensibility of the colonic wall.

▶ **Disease Severity**

Family history of polyposis or colon cancer, size of polyp, degree of dysplasia, multiple adenomas.

▶ **Concept and Application**

Neoplasia of intestinal epithelium (tubular, villous), abnormal mixture of normal tissue (hamartomas), other benign growths (e.g., lipoma).

▶ **Treatment Steps**

Polypectomy, bowel resection, panproctocolectomy and J-pouch (for familial polyposis).

P. Colon Cancer

▶ **H&P Keys**

Familial polyposis, inflammatory bowel disease, adenomatous polyps. Anemia, changes in bowel habits, weight loss. Palpable abdominal mass (right colon, sigmoid) or rectal mass.

▶ **Diagnosis**

Proximal Colon—Anemia, bulky tumor.

Distal Colon—Luminal narrowing and obstruction. Carcinoembryonic antigen (CEA) is useful to detect recurrence after resection.

▶ **Disease Severity**

Depth of tumor according to a modified Dukes' classification—A, muscularis propria; B, serosa; C, regional lymph nodes; D, liver metastasis; or TNM classification.

▶ **Concept and Application**

Adenoma–cancer sequence: colorectal cancer evolves from benign polyp to invasive carcinoma. Larger polyps have higher risk of can-

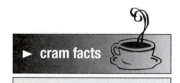

▶ **cram facts**

TNM CLASSIFICATION FOR COLORECTAL CANCER

T1	Involves the submucosa
T2	Muscularis mucosa
T3	Through the wall
T4	Involves the adjacent organs
N1	1–3 nodes
N2	> 4 nodes
N3	Para-aortic, vascular involvement
M1	Distant metastasis

cer; villous adenomas are more prone to malignant transformation than tubular adenomas.

► Treatment Steps

1. Surgical resection usually indicated—segment of colon along with regional lymph nodes.
2. Resection of liver metastases can contribute to cure.
3. Radiotherapy useful for rectal tumors.
4. Chemotherapy indicated for Dukes' C stage or distant metastasis (5-fluorouracil/leukovorin).

Q. Rectal Tumor

► H&P Keys

Rectal bleeding, mucous discharge, change of bowel habits, tenesmus, rectal mass.

► Diagnosis

Colonoscopy, rigid proctoscopy, endorectal ultrasound (to determine depth of invasion), MRI with endorectal coil, CT scan.

► Disease Severity

Anemia, abnormal liver function tests (LFTs), sphincter destruction, lymph node involvement, fixed tumor.

► Concept and Application

Malignant change in adenoma, genetic predisposition, mutation of genes by carcinogenic agents.

► Treatment Steps

1. Local excision for superficial lesions.
2. Low anterior resection or abdominoperineal resection.
3. Radiation, chemotherapy (often preoperatively for tumor downstaging).

R. Hemorrhoids

► H&P Keys

Rectal bleeding, mucous discharge, prolapse spontaneously or with defecation.

► Diagnosis

Rectal examination, proctosigmoidoscopy.

► Disease Severity

Degree of hemorrhoidal prolapse, thrombosis.

► Concept and Application

Prolapse of normal mucosal cushion, increased anal canal pressure. Portal hypertension causes increased pressure in the inferior mesenteric vein.

► Treatment Steps

1. Evaluate for coexistent rectal or sigmoid pathology (e.g., cancer), sigmoidoscopy.
2. High-fiber diet, warm sitz baths.
3. Rubber band ligation.
4. Hemorrhoidectomy.

S. Perirectal Abscess

► **H&P Keys**

Deep buttock or rectal pain, fever, perianal mass.

► **Diagnosis**

Rectal–perianal examination, CT scan sometimes indicated.

► **Disease Severity**

Coexisting Crohn's disease, extension into adjacent anatomic space, complex fistula.

► **Concept and Application**

Infection in anal gland starts as intersphincteric abscess; can spread to become supralevator, perianal, or ischioanal abscess.

► **Treatment Steps**

1. Examination under anesthesia.
2. Incision and drainage.
3. Warm sitz baths and local wound care.

T. Anorectal Fistula

► **H&P Keys**

Chronic purulent discharge from perianal opening, history of perianal abscess.

► **Diagnosis**

Rectal examination, anoproctoscopy, rectal ultrasound, fistulography.

► **Disease Severity**

Coexisting Crohn's, complex or high fistulas, TB, incontinence, HIV.

► **Concept and Application**

Injury or infected anal crypts. Epithelialization of fistulous tract.

► **Treatment Steps**

1. Examination under anesthesia.
2. Lay open the fistula and use seton.

U. Pilonidal Cyst

► **H&P Keys**

Purulent drainage from sacrococcygeal sinus; pain, tender mass, induration.

► **Diagnosis**

Physical examination.

► **Disease Severity**

Multiple tracts, multiple recurrences.

► **Concept and Application**

Macerated skin, suction effect of buttock when walking, loose hair embedded in skin.

► **Treatment Steps**

1. Incision and drainage of abscess; wide local excision of sinus tract, down to sacral fascia.
2. Healing by primary closure (if not infected), secondary intention, local flaps.

IX. CONGENITAL ABNORMALITIES

A. Duodenal Atresia

▶ H&P Keys

Congenital, diagnosed shortly after birth; bile-stained vomiting, post-feeding vomiting, distended upper abdomen, antepartum polyhydramnios, stigmata of Down's syndrome (30%).

▶ Diagnosis

Plain x-ray ("double-bubble" sign), upper GI series and follow-through, barium enema, evaluate cardiac system with echocardiography.

▶ Disease Severity

Prematurity, associated anomalies (e.g., congenital heart disease), low birth weight, trisomy 21.

▶ Concept and Application

Hypoplasia or atresia of duodenum at level of ampulla. Evaluate for annular pancreas.

▶ Treatment Steps

1. Elevate head of bed, nasogastric decompression.
2. Correct fluid and electrolyte imbalance.
3. Duodenoduodenostomy, decompression gastrostomy; correct associated malrotation.

B. Biliary Atresia

▶ H&P Keys

Jaundice, dark urine, pale-colored stools, hepatomegaly, splenomegaly, usually in 2- to 4-week-old infants.

▶ Diagnosis

Technetium-iminodiacetic acid (Tc-IDA) hepatobiliary scan, conjugated hyperbilirubinemia, abdominal ultrasound; needle biopsy of liver, exploratory laparotomy. Must differentiate from α-antitrypsin deficiency.

▶ Disease Severity

Jaundice, fever, cirrhosis, sepsis, esophageal varices, liver failure, delayed diagnosis, age (< 12 weeks).

▶ Concept and Application

Absence of patent bile ducts, periportal fibrosis, cirrhosis.

▶ Treatment Steps

1. IV fluids, vitamin K.
2. Roux-en-Y hepaticojejunostomy, liver transplantation.

C. Malrotation

▶ H&P Keys

Biliary vomiting, hematemesis, heme-positive nasogastric aspirate, failure to thrive, mild abdominal distention.

▶ Diagnosis

Plain x-ray of abdomen, upper GI series, barium enema.

▶ Disease Severity

Peritonitis, tachycardia, hypotension.

► Concept and Application

Abnormality of usual embryonic intestinal rotation and fixation.

► Treatment Steps

1. Fluid and electrolyte correction, nasogastric decompression, antibiotics.
2. Surgical derotation of bowel, division of Ladd's bands, widen base of mesentery, fixation of cecum, appendectomy.

D. Hirschsprung's Disease

► H&P Keys

Failure to pass meconium, chronic constipation, bile-stained vomiting, reluctance to feed, diarrhea, irritability, abdominal distention, palpable stool in lower abdomen, male infant.

► Diagnosis

Plain abdominal x-ray, barium enema, rectal biopsy, and rectal manometry.

► Disease Severity

Enterocolitis, malnutrition, length of bowel involved.

► Concept and Application

Interrupted development of myenteric nervous system (lack of ganglion cells in distal intestine) causes a functional obstruction; rectum always involved.

► Treatment Steps

1. Rectal tube and colonic washing.
2. Colostomy, endorectal pull-through.

E. Imperforate Anus

► H&P Keys

Anal dimple but no orifice; ectopic anal opening or fistula; meconium in vagina, urethra, or urine.

► Diagnosis

Physical examination, test urine for meconium, ultrasound of kidneys and heart, sacrum x-ray.

► Disease Severity

Associated anomalies (70%)—VACTERL (vertebral, anorectal, cardiac, tracheal, esophageal, renal, limb), acidosis, neurologic deficit, agenesis of sacral vertebrae, incontinence.

► Concept and Application

Abnormal growth and fusion of embryonic anal hillocks, faulty division of the cloaca by urorectal septum.

► Treatment Steps

1. Posterior sagittal anoplasty, sigmoid colostomy, division of fistula.
2. Repeated anal dilation.

F. Diaphragmatic Hernia

► H&P Keys

Gasping respiration, cyanosis, absent breath sound on left, bowel sounds on affected hemithorax, scaphoid abdomen.

► Diagnosis

CXR, antenatal ultrasound, upper GI series.

► Disease Severity

Associated anomalies, cyanosis, prolonged mechanical ventilation.

► Concept and Application

Incomplete diaphragm, persistence of pleuroperitoneal hiatus, impaired pulmonary development.

► Treatment Steps

1. Nasogastric tube decompression, mechanical ventilation, extracorporeal membrane oxygenation (ECMO).
2. Surgery to reduce herniated bowel and repair diaphragmatic defect.

X. DISEASES OF THE GALLBLADDER AND LIVER

A. Acute Cholecystitis

► H&P Keys

Right upper quadrant pain, tenderness, guarding, subscapular radiation, nausea and vomiting, anorexia, fever, history of fatty food intolerance.

► Diagnosis

Ultrasound, plain x-ray of abdomen (radiopaque stones), hepatobiliary iminodiacetic acid (HIDA) scan, LFTs.

► Disease Severity

Unremitting fever, leukocytosis, elevated amylase, palpable gallbladder suggesting empyema or pericholecystic abscess, chills, common duct stones, diabetes.

► Concept and Application

Obstruction of cystic duct with stone, secondary bacterial invasion.

► Treatment Steps

1. IV fluids, antibiotics, and cholecystectomy.
2. Cholecystostomy if patient is too ill for cholecystectomy (Fig. 18–8).

B. Choledochal Cyst

► H&P Keys

Abdominal pain, episodic jaundice, mass in right upper quadrant, fever.

► Diagnosis

Ultrasound and CT scan of abdomen, endoscopic retrograde cholangiopancreatography (ERCP), percutaneous transhepatic cholangiography (PTC).

► Disease Severity

Fever, recurrent pancreatitis.

► Concept and Application

Persistence of embryonic hepaticopancreatic duct, regurgitation of pancreatic juice in bile duct, cystic changes in bile duct, fibrosis, inflammation. If untreated, risk of carcinoma is increased.

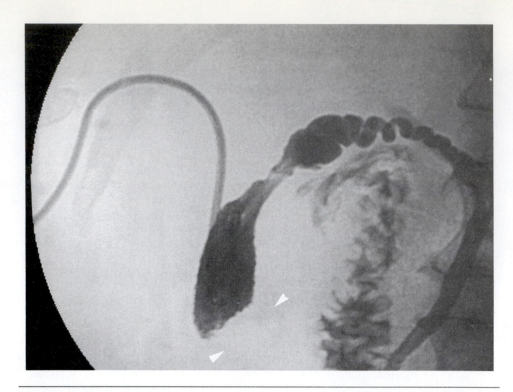

Figure 18–8. A cholecystostomy tube cholangiogram showing a somewhat decompressed gallbladder filled with gallstones. Arrows point to the portion of the gallbladder containing stones. This patient had calculus cholecystitis in the setting of severe hemodynamic instability and was too sick for an open cholecystectomy.

► Treatment Steps
1. Excision of choledochal cyst.
2. Cholecystectomy and biliary reconstruction with a Roux-en-Y limb.

C. Choledocholithiasis

► H&P Keys
Biliary colic, pruritus, chills, fever, jaundice, dark urine, pale stools, right upper quadrant tenderness.

► Diagnosis
LFTs, ultrasound, ERCP, PTC, amylase, lipase.

► Disease Severity
Cholangitis: fever, right upper quadrant pain, jaundice (Charcot's triad).

► Concept and Application
Secondary stones originate in gallbladder (more common); primary stones arise in intrahepatic duct or common bile duct.

► Treatment Steps
1. IV fluids, IV antibiotics.
2. ERCP and sphincterotomy, cholecystectomy and common bile duct exploration with possible transduodenal sphincteroplasty, or choledochoduodenostomy.

D. Carcinoma of the Gallbladder

► H&P Keys
Right upper quadrant pain and mass, jaundice, weight loss.

▶ Diagnosis

Ultrasound, CT scan of abdomen and pelvis.

▶ Disease Severity

Weight loss, malnutrition, depth of tumor invasion, nonresectability. Calcification of gallbladder wall (porcelain gallbladder) has higher incidence of cancer.

▶ Concept and Application

Adenocarcioma most common, lymphatic spread, most involve liver at diagnosis.

▶ Treatment Steps

Cholecystectomy, radical regional lymphadenectomy and wedge excision of gallbladder bed (usually palliative).

E. Hepatic Adenoma

▶ H&P Keys

Right upper quadrant pain, palpable liver mass, use of oral contraceptives, female gender.

▶ Diagnosis

Ultrasound, CT scan of the abdomen, technetium colloid sulfur scan, MRI.

▶ Disease Severity

Abdominal distention, guarding, large adenoma, spontaneous rupture, hemoperitoneum.

▶ Concept and Application

Encapsulated homogeneous mass of hepatocyte, no bile ducts or central vein present.

▶ Treatment Steps

1. < 6 cm: observation, discontinue oral contraceptive.
2. > 6 cm: surgical resection.

F. Focal Nodular Hyperplasia

▶ H&P Keys

Most often asymptomatic, much less tendency to hemorrhage than adenomas.

▶ Diagnosis

Ultrasound, CT scan, biopsy.

▶ Disease Severity

Extension, compression of adjacent structures, symptoms.

▶ Concept and Application

Histologically normal-appearing hepatocytes, bile ducts, Kupffer cells.

▶ Treatment Steps

Conservative, observation with imaging follow-up.

G. Primary Hepatobiliary Cancer

▶ H&P Keys

Fatigue, weight loss, abdominal discomfort, jaundice. Palpable liver mass, signs of cirrhosis and portal hypertension.

► Diagnosis

Elevated α-fetoprotein (AFP), alkaline phosphatase, direct bilirubin. Ultrasound, CT scan, or MRI. Percutaneous or laparoscopic needle biopsy.

► Disease Severity

Hepatocellular carcinoma (HCC) can undergo spontaneous rupture. Invasion of diaphragm and adjacent organs. Metastases to lymph nodes, lung, bone, adrenals, and brain.

► Concept and Application

HCC is the most common fatal cancer worldwide; risk factors include hepatitis, cirrhosis, aflatoxin exposure. Cholangiocarcinoma involves the biliary tree and is often unresectable. Hepatoblastoma is a distinctive tumor of infants and children.

► Treatment Steps

1. Liver resection, radiotherapy, chemotherapy.
2. Liver transplantation may be indicated in select patients.

H. Liver Metastasis

► H&P Keys

History of cancer, especially GI (portal drainage). Anorexia, fatigue, weight loss, abdominal and shoulder pain. Jaundice, hepatomegaly, ascites.

► Diagnosis

High alkaline phosphatase. Ultrasound, CT scan (Fig. 18–9), needle biopsy.

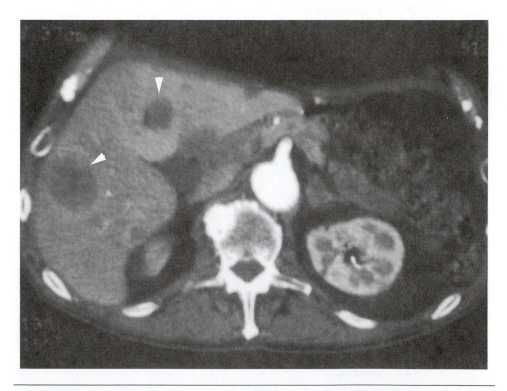

Figure 18–9. Abdominal CT scan of a cachectic patient showing bilobar liver metastatic lesions *(arrows)*. This patient will be managed nonsurgically.

► Disease Severity
Multiplicity, involvement of both liver lobes. Prognosis depends on the primary tumor type.

► Concept and Application
Large size of liver and portal and systemic blood supply contribute to metastatic seeding.

► Treatment Steps
1. Palliative chemotherapy and radiation.
2. Resection is only curative method, most often indicated for select patients with colorectal or endocrine tumors.

XI. DISEASES OF THE PANCREAS

A. Acute Pancreatitis

► H&P Keys
Epigastric and back pain, nausea and vomiting, retching, hypotension, fever, left pleural effusion, abdominal tenderness, abdominal mass, jaundice, abdominal distention, Cullen's sign (periumbilical ecchymosis). Alcohol abuse.

► Diagnosis
Amylase, lipase, ultrasound, CT scan.

► Disease Severity
Predicted mortality increases with number of Ranson's criteria.

► Concept and Application
Enzymatic digestion of gland, duct obstruction (gallstones and protein), chemical injury to the gland. Most common causes: alcohol ingestion, gallstones.

► cram facts

RANSON'S CRITERIA (PREDICTING THE SEVERITY OF ACUTE PANCREATITIS)		
On Admission:		
W	WBC	> 16,000/mm^3
A	Age	> 55 yr
G	Glucose	> 200 mg/dL
A	AST	> 250 IU/dL
L	LDH	> 350 IU/L
At 48 hrs:		
B	Base deficit	> 4 mEq/L
E	Estimated fluid gain	> 6 L
C	Calcium	< 8 mg/dL
H	Hct fall	> 10%
U	Urea rise	> 5 mg/dL
P	PaO$_2$	< 60 mm Hg

Mortality rate in acute pancreatitis closely related to the number of positive Ranson signs (1% if up to 2 signs, 15% if 3–4, 40% if 5–6, and 100% if 7–8 signs present).
NOTE: Amylase is not part of the Ranson's criteria.

▶ Treatment Steps

1. Fluid replacement, GI rest, calcium and magnesium replacement.
2. ERCP; analgesia; cholecystectomy; biliary drainage; debridement of necrotic, infected pancreatic tissue.

B. Pancreatic Carcinoma

▶ H&P Keys

Vague abdominal pain, back pain, weight loss, pruritus, painless jaundice, hepatomegaly, migratory thrombophlebitis.

▶ Diagnosis

Ultrasound, CT scan (Fig. 18–10), ERCP, endoscopy, magnetic resonance cholangiopancreatography (MRCP), biopsy of pancreatic mass.

▶ Concept and Application

Malignant change in ductal epithelium, increased risk with severe smoking.

▶ Treatment Steps

Curative—Pancreaticoduodenectomy, total or distal pancreatectomy, external-beam radiation, multidrug chemotherapy.

Palliative—Bilioenteric bypass, biliary stent, celiac plexus nerve block.

C. Gastrinoma

▶ H&P Keys

Severe peptic ulcer symptoms, diarrhea, previous ulcer operation.

▶ Diagnosis

Basal acid output/maximal acid output ratio, serum gastrin level, secretin provocative test, intraoperative endoscopic ultrasound, gastri-

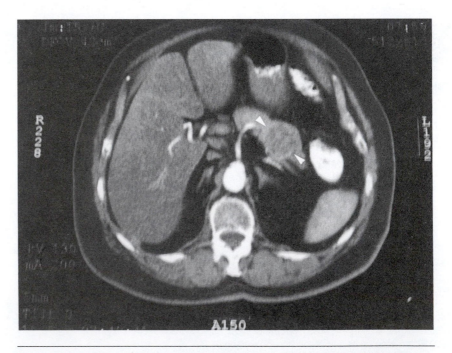

Figure 18–10. Abdominal CT scan showing an oval-shaped, distal pancreatic mass *(arrows)*. This patient will be managed with a distal pancreatectomy and possible adjuvant therapy depending on the stage of the tumor.

noma triangle (cystic duct, junction of second and third portions of the duodenum and junction of the head and neck of the pancreas).

► **Disease Severity**
Refractory peptic ulcer disease, hemorrhage, perforated ulcer, extremely high gastrin levels, multiple tumors, associated MEN type I. Malignant potential in 50–70%.

► **Concept and Application**
Hypersecretion of gastric acid caused by excessive production of gastrin by tumor.

► **Treatment Steps**
1. Omeprazole, H_2-receptor antagonist, streptozocin and 5-fluorouracil (for malignancy), gastrectomy.
2. Resection of the tumor.

XII. HERNIA

A. Inguinal Hernia

► **H&P Keys**
Aching in groin, bulge or lump in groin. Symptoms may be precipitated by exercise or straining.

► **Diagnosis**
Physical examination.

► **Disease Severity**
Hernia complications: incarceration (sac contents not reducible); strangulation (loss of blood supply to sac contents leading to infarction/necrosis).

► **Concept and Application**
Persistent peritoneal diverticulum, increased intra-abdominal pressure (more severe in chronic obstructive pulmonary disease [COPD], chronic constipation, prostatism), weakness of transversalis fascia, patent process vaginalis.

► **Treatment Steps**
Standard or laparoscopic herniorrhaphy.

B. Femoral Hernia

► **H&P Keys**
Groin discomfort; mass below inguinal ligament, medial to femoral vessels. Rule out lymphadenopathy.

► **Diagnosis**
Physical examination, ultrasound.

► **Disease Severity**
Intestinal obstruction, irreducible hernia, compression and/or thrombosis of femoral vein.

► **Concept and Application**
Protrusion of intra-abdominal contents through femoral canal.

► **Treatment Steps**
1. Excision of sac, closure of femoral canal.
2. For intestinal obstruction, exploratory laparotomy, and possible bowel resection.

C. Umbilical Hernia

► **H&P Keys**

Bulge in umbilicus; fascial defect felt.

► **Diagnosis**

Physical examination.

► **Disease Severity**

Associated diseases such as cirrhosis and intra-abdominal tumor; pregnancy.

► **Concept and Application**

Gradual yielding of the umbilical scar tissue.

► **Treatment Steps**

1. < 6 years: observation.
2. > 6 years: repair fascial defect.

D. Incisional Hernia

► **H&P Keys**

Pain; swelling adjacent to scar.

► **Diagnosis**

History and physical examination.

► **Disease Severity**

Large multiple defects, bowel obstruction, steroids, malnutrition, history of COPD.

► **Concept and Application**

Disruption of fascial suture resulting from surgical technique, wound infection, suture material, poor nutrition.

► **Treatment Steps**

Tension-free repair, usually with mesh.

E. Hernia with Obstruction

► **H&P Keys**

Pain at site of hernia, abdominal pain, vomiting, obstipation, fever, abdominal distention, oliguria.

► **Diagnosis**

Physical examination, leukocytosis, plain x-ray, high-resolution ultrasound scan.

► **Disease Severity**

Fever, low urine output, tachycardia, hypotension, abdominal guarding, advanced age.

► **Concept and Application**

Intra-abdominal contents present within hernial sac; fascial neck compromises blood supply.

► **Treatment Steps**

1. Fluid resuscitation, nasogastric tube decompression, correction of electrolyte imbalance.
2. Surgery to release hernia content, resect bowel, repair hernia.

BIBLIOGRAPHY

Brunicardi CF. *Schwartz's Principles of Surgery,* 8th ed. New York: McGraw-Hill, 2005.

Cameron J. *Current Surgical Therapy,* 8th ed. Philadelphia: Mosby, 2004.

Greenfield LJ. *Surgery: Scientific Principles and Practice,* 3rd ed. Philadelphia: Lippincott-Raven, 2001.

Mattox KL. *Trauma,* 5th ed. New York: McGraw-Hill, 2003.

Townsend CM. *Sabiston Textbook of Surgery: The Biological Basis of Modern Surgical Practice,* 17th ed. Philadelphia: W.B. Saunders, 2004.

Otolaryngology and Respiratory System Diseases

19

I. DISEASES OF THE EAR

A. Infectious Otitis Externa

▶ **H&P Keys**

Pain in the external canal that can be enhanced by tragal pressure or by tugging on the auricle. Erythema of the ear canal and evidence of debris and swelling within the canal on otoscopy, occasional erythema of the pinna, and swelling in the postauricular space. History of mild ear canal trauma, exposure to high humidity, or swimming. Sensations of fullness, tinnitus, and hearing loss; occasional sensations of disequilibrium, itching of external canal.

▶ **Diagnosis**

Direct examination, identification of offending organism by Gram stain and/or culture.

▶ **Disease Severity**

Pain, fever, degree of swelling, closure of ear canal, regional soft-tissue swelling and erythema, and lymphadenopathy.

▶ **Concept and Application**

Contamination of the external canal by contaminated water or trauma of the ear canal by manipulation permits invasion of offending organism; organisms are usually mixed, bacterial, or fungal. Implies failure of the piloapocrine system and the protective effect of cerumen.

▶ **Treatment Steps**

1. Acute: Cleansing of ear canal, inspect eardrum to rule out middle-ear disease, place a wick to carry otic drops to the canal and maintain in place (otic drops usually contain 2% acetic acid to change pH of canal), hydrocortisone to reduce inflammation and swelling, and a specific topical antibiotic usually to cover gram-positive as well as gram-negative organisms. Pain management is important, and antibiotics should be administered if the infection has extended beyond the confines of the canal to produce lymphadenopathy, soft-tissue involvement, and fever.
2. Subsequent prophylaxis requires keeping the ear dry and using prophylactic (acetic acid or alcohol) drops to decontaminate the ear after bathing or swimming in the future.

B. Malignant Otitis Externa

▶ **H&P Keys**

Auricular pain, discharge, hearing loss, feeling of fullness, granular tissue within the external auditory canal. Usually a history of immunocompromise such as diabetes mellitus, old age, or human immunodeficiency virus (HIV) infection. Presence of lymphadenopathy and evidence of infiltration into surrounding soft tissues; loss of cranial function, including facial nerve (VII) and cranial nerves X, XI, XII.

▶ **Diagnosis**

Should include culturing the external auditory canal for offending organism, computed tomographic (CT) scan to determine extent of bony destruction and infiltration into surrounding soft tissues. Possibly, subsequent magnetic resonance imaging (MRI) to evaluate presence of intracranial disease, and gallium and technetium scans to detect presence of bony involvement of surrounding structures.

► **Disease Severity**

Expanding soft-tissue involvement with intracranial spread and decreased function of cranial nerve.

► **Concept and Application**

Severe infection of periauricular soft tissue and bone in immunocompromised host, with rapidly expanding and infiltrating infection with potential for cranial nerve destruction, central nervous system (CNS) involvement. Most common organism is *Pseudomonas aeruginosa.*

► **Treatment Steps**

1. Intravenous antibiotics, with judicious debridement as necessary.
2. Despite aggressive treatment, still significant percentage of mortality.

C. Acute Otitis Media

► **H&P Keys**

This infection usually occurs in all age groups but is more prevalent in children ages 3 months to 7 years. Occurs more frequently during winter months and is associated with upper respiratory tract and viral infections. Symptoms and signs normally include hyperemia of the tympanic membrane with erythema, exudate within the middle-ear space, and, at times, purulent discharge from the external canal as well as pain and dizziness with decreased appetite in young children. Other signs and symptoms are hearing loss, tinnitus, and, on occasion, imbalance; fever also is a key point.

► **Diagnosis**

Direct inspection via otoscopy, culture of any purulent debris from the external canal, and tympanocentesis in infants under 3 months of age.

► **Disease Severity**

Degree of fever, pain, hearing loss, and duration of otorrhea when present. Postauricular swelling indicates spread of disease process to mastoid air cell system; the presence of adenopathy within the parotid and upper neck indicates extension into soft tissues in surrounding regions. Necrotizing otitis media, β-hemolytic streptococci seen in patients with concomitant disease process or immunocompromise.

► **Concept and Application**

The basic etiology is eustachian tube dysfunction with bacterial spread through the eustachian tube from the nasopharynx into the middle-ear space. Most common organisms include *Streptococcus pneumoniae* and *Haemophilus influenzae;* also *Branhamella catarrhalis, Streptococcus pyogenes* and *Staphylococcus aureus,* but less commonly; in infants gram-negative organisms such as *Escherichia coli* must be identified during tympanocentesis (most common in infants < 6 weeks old).

► **Treatment Steps**

1. Systemic antibiotics, usually amoxicillin (30–40 mg/kg/day for uncomplicated infections and for children under age 12; other antibiotics used are amoxicillin–clavulanate, erythromycin, sulfa for children allergic to penicillin, and trimethoprim–sulfamethoxazole and cephalosporins as necessary.

2. Myringotomy may be indicated to determine bacteriology as well as tympanocentesis (as mentioned).

3. When purulent discharge and tympanic membrane perforation exist, topical antibiotic drops in addition to systemic antibiotics are useful.

4. Acute otitis media may benefit from prophylactic antibiotics as well as possible myringotomy and tube placement.

D. Chronic Otitis Media

▶ H&P Keys

Chronic otitis media is a rare complication of acute otitis media. It is manifested by the presence of a tympanic membrane perforation or development of a cholesteatoma in the middle-ear space, particularly in the area of the pars flaccida. The physical findings are drum perforations with persistent otorrhea, hearing loss, tinnitus, presence of retraction pockets with epithelial debris, and occasional sensations of disequilibrium and vertigo.

▶ Diagnosis

Diagnostic studies include direct otoscopy, with careful cleansing of tympanic membrane area to identify presence or absence of perforation, its position and size. The character of the middle-ear mucous membrane is seen through the perforation and the presence or absence of epithelial debris either within the middle ear or in the pars flaccida area. Tuning fork studies will suggest the reversal of the Rinne, with lateralization to the side of greatest conduction loss; and audiogram, tympanogram, CT scans of temporal bone, both axial and coronal views without contrast, help delineate the degree and severity of disease and location of bone destruction and cholesteatoma if present. Cultures are helpful in determining antibiotic therapy; chronic otitis media is produced most commonly by *P. aeruginosa* and staphylococcal organisms; not uncommonly *Proteus mirabilis* and *E. coli* may be present. Culture sensitivity is needed to determine the offending organism.

▶ Disease Severity

Degree of perforation and otorrhea, vertigo, degree of hearing loss, presence of facial nerve paralysis, or headache indicate the possibility of intracranial extension of middle-ear and mastoid disease.

▶ Concept and Application

Recurrent acute otitis media or a single episode of acute necrotizing otitis media produces obstruction of tympanic membrane and chronic changes in the mucous membrane of the middle ear and mastoid concomitant with eustachian tube obstruction. Organisms involved are *P. aeruginosa* (most commonly) and *S. aureus;* occasionally, *Proteus* species as well as *E. coli* may be isolates. In immunocompromised patients, acid-fast and fungal disease must be considered.

▶ Treatment Steps

1. Antibiotics directed at gram-negative organisms; treatment with antibiotics for 3–6 weeks; concomitant use of otic drops with broad-spectrum antibiotics, acidifying agents (2% acetic acid), and often steroids to reduce inflammation.

2. In patients with perforation, the ear must be kept dry during washing and bathing; swimming is not allowed.

3. If cholesteatoma is present, this is a surgical disease requiring extirpation of the cholesteatoma and sealing of the eardrum by

means of tympanoplasty, with or without reconstruction of the ossicular chain if it is involved.

E. Otitis Media with Effusion (Serous Otitis Media)

▶ H&P Keys

History is associated with multiple bouts of acute otitis media with slow resolution. Condition also should be suspected in children with language delay and decreased response to auditory cues. Signs and symptoms include decreased hearing, retracted eardrum, dullness to the tympanic membrane, and straw-colored fluid with bubbles within the middle-ear space.

▶ Diagnosis

Direct visualization via otoscopy and insufflation during pneumatic otoscopy; also tympanometry and audiometry.

▶ Disease Severity

Degree of hearing loss, as noted on audiometry, and disability in response to auditory cues.

▶ Concept and Application

Eustachian tube blockage, with subsequent negative pressure within the middle-ear space changing the surface tension and producing metaplasia of epithelium of middle ear to a secretory epithelium migrating from the eustachian tube orifice of the middle ear.

▶ Treatment Steps

1. Initial management should be observation for approximately 3 months, during which 90% resolve.
2. Generally, antibiotics are offered initially; some suggest that antihistamine decongestants are not uniquely helpful. In adults with serous otitis media, if unilateral, one must pay careful attention to the nasopharynx to rule out nasopharyngeal lesions—again, particularly in immunocompromised hosts.
3. If the serous otitis media does not resolve and hearing loss persists after a period of careful observation and treatment, myringotomy with aspiration of the middle ear content and subsequent placement of ventilation tubes is the treatment of choice. In adults, attempts at autoinflation with Valsalva's maneuver is often effective in resolving serous otitis media; in children with recurrent nonresolving serous otitis media, adenoidectomy with or without tonsillectomy is often recommended.

F. Cerumen (Earwax) Impaction

▶ H&P Keys

The patient will often complain of a history of feeling of fullness in the ear; decreased hearing, often after washing; pressure in the ear; and occasional pain in the external ear.

▶ Diagnosis

Direct visualization via otoscopy.

▶ Disease Severity

Quality of hearing loss and degree of cerumen impaction. Rule out foreign body within the external canal, particularly in children and retarded patients.

► Concept and Application

Often occurs with physical manipulation of the ear canal, particularly with the use of cotton applicators and digging in the ears. Narrow canal with increased cerumen production and possible foreign body.

► Treatment Steps

Removal of cerumen by mechanical irrigation when an intact tympanic membrane is known, or use of instruments, suction, or both as appropriate to degree of impaction and quality of cerumen.

G. Vertigo

► H&P Keys

Vertigo is a complex complaint; it must be determined whether the vertigo is otologic, central, or medical in origin. Determining whether the disease is peripheral is made easier by the symptom of definite sensation of movement, most often rotatory. When the vertigo is paroxysmal and severe, it is more likely to be peripheral; attacks may last minutes to hours (seldom longer) and may be associated with vegetative signs such as sweating, nausea, and vomiting. Patient never loses consciousness. Conversely, central vertigo is more often mild and described as a sensation of light-headedness or unsteadiness. It is vague, without specific onset or termination, and may be constant; attacks may last weeks or months, often without an obvious nystagmus. Associated symptoms of vertigo may be nystagmus (with peripheral pathology, the nystagmus can often be seen); with irritative lesions, nystagmus is often to the side of involved ear; nystagmus with changing of direction is more often central than peripheral. Causes of vertigo of otologic origin are acute otitis media, serous otitis media, head trauma with involvement of labyrinthine apparatus, and trauma to middle ear by penetrating wound, with dislocation of ossicles and production of vertigo and hearing loss, Cogan's syndrome, vestibular neuronitis, temporal bone fractures, acute barotrauma with perilymph fistulas, and endolymphatic hydrops (Ménière's disease). Ménière's disease is a disease process involving abnormal absorption or production of endolymph, which produces a quadrad or triad of symptoms of tinnitus, vertigo, fluctuant hearing loss, and sensations of fullness or blockage in the ear; the disease process may begin suddenly with tinnitus or any of the other symptoms; vertigo is severe and unrelenting for minutes to hours; nausea and vomiting are often present.

► Diagnosis

History of fluctuant hearing loss, tinnitus, vertigo, neurosensory hearing loss on audiometric evaluation, evidence of canal paresis with vestibular studies involving the affected ear, negative examinations with intracranial MRI with gadolinium for cranial nerve VIII and neurovascular bundles. Electronystagmography (ENG) documenting canal paresis or hypoactivity of affected ear.

► Disease Severity

Severity of vertigo, length of episodes, frequency of attacks, degree of hearing loss.

► Concept and Application

Temporal bone studies indicate presence of hydrops of the endolymphatic space with destruction of neuroepithelium thought to be secondary to abnormality of stria vascularis, endolymphatic sac mechanism, or both.

► Treatment Steps

1. For acute cases, benzodiazepam-like drugs are effective if nausea and vomiting are not a problem.
2. For long-term management of Ménière's disease, diuretics and low-sodium diet are often effective.
3. In patients with continuing sensations of disequilibrium who fail to respond to medical therapy, endolymphatic sac decompression; cranial nerve VIII section; or, in patients who have nonfunctioning ears from auditory standpoint and unilateral disease for > 5 years, labyrinthectomy is procedure of choice; diazepam and antihistamine group such as meclizine hydrochloride, diphenhydramine hydrochloride (Benadryl), or dimenhydrinate (Dramamine).

H. Otalgia

► H&P Keys

Otalgia may represent pain of otologic origin or of distant disease referred to the ears, such as dental infection, pharyngitis, or tonsillitis. Symptoms include ear pain (sharp, constant, dull, or burning). Determination of duration of pain and exacerbating and remitting factors are essential. Physical examination includes inspection of the external ear, otoscopy with examination of external canal and tympanic membrane with middle ear; examination of the temporomandibular joints with direct pressure both externally and on the pterygoid muscles within the oral cavity; and complete examination of the upper aerodigestive tract, nasopharynx, oropharynx, tongue, larynx, and hypopharynx.

► Diagnosis

If cause is not obvious, diagnostic studies such as CT scan and MRI of upper aerodigestive tract and neck are useful. Studies also include direct laryngoscopy, nasopharyngoscopy, audiologic testing, and tympanometry, as well as palpation of tonsillar fossae, tongue base, and neck. Direct laryngoscopy and cervical esophagoscopy also may be indicated.

► Disease Severity

Presence of tumors or lesions in the upper aerodigestive tract referring pain to the ear are of potentially great concern and may be life threatening.

► Concept and Application

Direct stimulation of nerves supplying sensation to the ear via inflammatory process or direct pressure, transmission via the same nerves through the temporomandibular joint and mechanism of referred pain via myositis and muscle spasm from associated joint musculature. Referred pain from tongue base, larynx, or pyriform sinus occurs via the vagus or glossopharyngeal nerve.

► Treatment Steps

1. Management will vary, depending on underlying disease process.
2. It may be as simple as cerumen removal or as complex as cancer extirpation and adjunctive treatments.

I. Hearing Loss

► H&P Keys

Obvious loss of hearing acuity is noted either by patient or by friends and family; may be associated with other otologic signs such as tinnitus or vertigo or with associated exposure to loud noise or head trauma. Hearing loss may be mild, moderate, or severe; patient may have congenital hearing loss as a result of either congenital or acquired disease, a history of head injury or recurrent ear infection, exposure to ototoxic drugs, exposure to loud noise, or infectious processes such as meningitis. Physical examination begins with an interview to determine degree of hearing loss; then otoscopy to rule out disease process in external canal or middle ear and tuning fork studies with Rinne and Weber studies as primary modalities.

► Diagnosis

Audiometry, including air, bone, and speech discrimination studies; brain stem evoked potential studies when indicated; tympanometry. In children with congenital losses or rapidly progressive neural losses, CT scan of temporal bone and serologic studies for autoimmune disease as well as congenital or acquired syphilis.

► Disease Severity

Careful evaluation of the individual's ability to communicate. Degree of hearing loss is evinced on audiometry.

► Concept and Application

Conductive hearing losses are manifested primarily by evidence of congenital findings of abnormal pinna and microtia, atresia, and periauricular tags and stenosis. Concomitant congenital abnormalities such as cleft palate, cardiac disease, and kidney abnormalities should trigger search for otic abnormality. Conductive hearing loss in children is most often of congenital or traumatic origin in infancy. In acquired disease, acute otitis media and serous otitis media affect more than 30% of children at some point. Most common disease in young adults is otosclerosis, with gradual fixation of the stapes foot plate; it is a genetically determined disease process (Mendelian dominant with variable penetrance; Fig. 19–1). Other conductive hearing losses can occur as result of longitudinal fractures of the temporal bone and barotrauma with middle-ear bleeding; effusion also produces conduction hearing losses. Congenital sensorineural hearing losses may be of genetic origin (e.g., Waardenburg's syndrome) or caused by congenital syphilis. Acquired neural losses may be secondary to head or ear trauma, meningitis, an autoimmune disease process, acoustic tumors, or syphilis. In the aging population, pres-

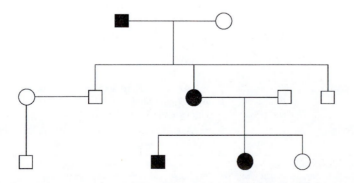

Figure 19–1. Pedigree of a typical family with autosomal dominant hearing loss. Note the multiple affected family members; transmission can be either maternal or paternal. ■, ● Affected male, female; □, ○ unaffected male, female.

bycusis or a gradual high-frequency sensorineural hearing loss is most often seen after age 60.

► Treatment Steps

1. For sensorineural hearing losses of acquired type and of mild to moderate or even severe degree, amplification by means of hearing aid is available.
2. For profound losses not amenable to amplification, cochlear implant surgery is available.
3. For conductive hearing losses secondary to middle-ear disease, aspiration of fluid and myringotomy (as noted), ossicular reconstruction by means of stapes surgery or ossiculoplasty, and tympanoplasty for correction of tympanic membrane perforations.

J. Sudden Hearing Loss

► H&P Keys

History of abrupt hearing loss for minutes to hours. Presence of tinnitus and vertigo and their severity should be determined by clinical history. History should include infection, trauma, vascular problem, otologic problem, neurologic problem, history of neurotoxic drugs, possible diabetes mellitus, autoimmune disorders, etc.

► Diagnosis

Audiometric testing, including air and bone conduction, ENG and calorics, testing of auditory brain responses, CT scan and MRI of the temporal bone, blood sugar, fluorescent treponemal antibody absorption (FTA-ABS) testing and sedimentation rate, and direct examination.

► Disease Severity

Degree of hearing loss as determined by audiogram; presence or absence of vertigo or tinnitus and patient's disability.

► **diagnostic decisions**

SUDDEN HEARING LOSS

Indications	Testing
All patients	Audiologic/tympanometric testing
Acoustic neuroma/skull base lesions	MRI or CT with contrast
Autoimmune inner-ear disease	Lymphocyte transformation testing
	Western blot immunoassay
Syphilis	FTA-ABS
	MHA-TP
Bacterial infections	Appropriate culture and Lyme disease titer
Viral infections	Appropriate titers
	HIV testing
Miscellaneous	ENG, ABR, ECoG, perilymphic fistula test, CBC, blood chemistries, metabolic studies

ABR, auditory brain stem evoked responses; CBC, complete blood count; CT, computed tomography; ECoG, electrocochleography; ENG, electronystagmography; FTA-ABS, fluorescent treponemal antibody absorption; HIV, human immunodeficiency virus; MHA-TP, microhemagglutination assay for *Treponema pallidum*; MRI, magnetic resonance imaging.

► **Concept and Application**

Multiple etiologies with multiple mechanisms of disease: infection, including mumps, herpes zoster, syphilis, meningitis, otitis media encephalitis; vascular lesions, including embolic phenomenon, coagulopathy, cerebrovascular accident; trauma, including temporal bone fracture, barotrauma, or noise-induced trauma; otologic, including Ménière's disease, perilymph fistula, chronic otitis media, and acoustic neuroma; neurologic disease, including multiple sclerosis, Cogan's syndrome; and metabolic disorders, including diabetes mellitus, drug toxicity, and autoimmune disorders.

► **Treatment Steps**

1. After treatment of the underlying etiology when the hearing loss is idiopathic, high-dose steroids (prednisone, 60 mg/day) tapered over 2–3 weeks may be beneficial.
2. Other numerous therapies have been employed depending on suspected etiology (see Management Decisions).

K. Barotrauma

► **H&P Keys**

History of recent scuba diving or air flight with inability to equalize pressure between external environment and middle ear; pain, tinnitus, hearing loss, and vertigo. Physical examination may reveal hemotympanum, eardrum perforation, nystagmus, nausea, vomiting, and hearing loss.

► **Diagnosis**

Direct inspection of ear via otoscopy and pneumatic otoscopy; audiologic and tympanometric testing; vestibular testing, including ENG.

► **Disease Severity**

Degree of vertigo and patient's functioning, including hearing loss and duration of symptoms.

► **Concept and Application**

Acute changes in barometric pressure and failure of the eustachian tube to function properly. A large pressure gradient across the middle ear may result in trauma and the destruction of middle ear, inner ear, or both. Eustachian tube dysfunction may be a result of infectious, anatomic, or neoplastic abnormalities. The difference in barometric pressure may result in rupture of round or oval window seals, causing acute inner-ear abnormalities that lead to hearing loss or vertigo. Disruption of the tympanic membrane or vessels within middle ear may result in tympanic membrane perforation or hemotympanum.

► **Treatment Steps**

1. For uncomplicated barotrauma, appropriate nasal decongestants, systemic decongestants, and watchful waiting for resolution of hemotympanum or tympanic membrane perforation.
2. For inner-ear dysfunction, bed rest for 24 hours may result in resolution if no significant hearing loss or vertigo is present; should these symptoms persist, middle-ear exploration with patching of oval and round windows is treatment of choice.
3. Prevention of barotrauma can be helped with appropriate use of nasal decongestants and systemic decongestants before scuba diving or flying. Patients' tolerance to these medications

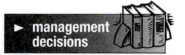

► **management decisions**

TREATMENT MODALITIES UTILIZED FOR SUDDEN SENSORINEURAL HEARING LOSS

Anti-inflammatory and Immunologic Agents
Steroids
Prostaglandin

Antivirals
Acyclovir

Calcium Antagonists
Nifedipine

Diuretics
Hydrochlorothiazide
Furosemide

Vasodilators
Carbogen
Papaverine
Nicotinic acid
Pentoxifylline

Volume Expanders
Hydroxyethyl starch
Dextran

Other Therapies
Vitamins
Acupuncture
Procaine

should be determined prior to use in conjunction with any diving activities.

L. Tinnitus

▶ H&P Keys

History of noise in the ear, which is generated endogenously, not from the environment. Complaints are about continuous humming, hissing, or whistling. Pulsatile tinnitus that is synchronous with heartbeat may accompany hearing loss or vertigo.

▶ Diagnosis

Tinnitus that is bilateral, symmetrical, and of reasonably long standing is most often benign and requires audiometry. Unilateral tinnitus or pulsatile tinnitus requires workup with MRI, magnetic resonance angiography (MRA), auscultation of the chest and neck to determine presence of transmitted or carotid bruits, auscultation within the ear to determine presence or absence of lesions, and CT scan to rule out vascular lesions of the ear.

▶ Disease Severity

Tinnitus may be extremely loud and produce inability to concentrate, sleep, or function. Tinnitus matching audiogram, CT scan, MRI, auscultation of neck, ultrasound, noninvasive studies of great vessels of neck, and transcranial Dopplers. Examination of the ear for vascular lesions involving middle ear.

▶ Concept and Application

Tinnitus may result from cochlear disease secondary to acoustic trauma, ototoxic drugs, viral or vascular disease of the cochlea, otosclerosis, conductive hearing loss such as ossicular discontinuity secondary to trauma, and serous otitis media. Tinnitus also may be of central origin, with brain stem lesions or eighth-nerve lesions secondary to acoustic tumors. Patient should have temporomandibular joint examination as well.

▶ Treatment Steps
As per etiology.

II. DISEASES OF THE MOUTH AND THROAT

A. Herpes Simplex of the Oral Cavity

▶ H&P Keys

History of prodromal fever, headache, irritability, malaise, nausea, vomiting, halitosis, and tender adenopathy. Usually includes children ages 2–5 years.

▶ Diagnosis

Clinical examination with Giemsa stain evaluation of vesicular fluid revealing syncytial giant cells with intranuclear inclusions.

▶ Disease Severity

Degree of symptoms listed above.

▶ Concept and Application

Initial herpesvirus type I. Infection usually occurs in children ages 2–5 years.

▶ Treatment Steps

1. Symptomatic therapy includes saltwater gargles and irrigations, soft diet, antipyretics, and topical anesthetics as needed.
2. Intravenous (IV) hydration for severe debilitation.

B. Oral Thrush (Candidiasis, Moniliasis)

▶ H&P Keys

Tends to occur in patients who are immunocompromised, debilitated, diabetic, or HIV positive; have used antibiotics or steroids for prolonged periods; or are receiving radiotherapy. Also seen in normal infants. Signs and symptoms include oral pain, odynophagia, and dysphagia. Physical examination reveals erythematous and edematous mucosa with soft, white exudate, which is easily scraped, revealing red, slightly ulcerated surface. Fever and adenopathy are unusual.

▶ Diagnosis

Physical examination, Gram stain revealing yeast forms, culture on Saboraud's agar.

▶ Disease Severity

Depends on underlying etiology.

▶ Concept and Application

Candida albicans occurs on 25% of normal mucosa; a normal saprophytic organism becomes pathogenic in circumstances mentioned.

▶ Treatment Steps

1. Includes nystatin oral suspension (200,000 units/cc, 2–3-cc swish and swallow) q4h until inflammation is controlled.
2. Mycelex troches or other antifungal agents also can be used.

C. Masses in the Nasopharynx

▶ H&P Keys

History of nasal obstruction, bleeding, hearing loss, pain, and neck masses.

▶ Diagnosis

Direct examination of nasopharynx by anterior rhinoscopy, flexible intranasal endoscopy, rigid endoscopy, mirror laryngoscopy, lateral x-rays of the nasopharynx, CT scan, and MRI with gadolinium for more careful delineation. Biopsy of lesion when found with tissue diagnosis. Determination of presence or absence of immunocompromising disease process, acquired immune deficiency syndrome (AIDS), diabetes, post chemotherapy for malignancy.

▶ Disease Severity

Hearing loss, nasal obstruction, epistaxis, cranial nerve neuropathies and involvement, cervical lymphadenopathy, distant metastases.

▶ Concept and Application

Numerous lesions may involve nasopharynx, including lymphoepithelioma (poorly differentiated squamous cell carcinoma), chordoma, angiofibroma, lymphoma and other age-related tumors, serous otitis media secondary to eustachian tube blockage and infiltration by tumor. Tumor may invade skull base with third-nerve palsy as well as other cranial nerve involvements; metastasis to regional lymph nodes produces lymphadenopathies.

▶ Treatment Steps

1. Depends on type of lesion noted.
2. Benign processes respond most often to conservative management or surgical extirpation.
3. Malignancies may require extirpation and irradiation, chemotherapy, or both.
4. Lesions of the ear secondary to masses in the nasopharynx may require myringotomy and tube placement to correct serous otitis media.

D. Malignant Neoplasms of the Oropharynx and Hypopharynx

▶ H&P Keys

Usual history of tobacco and ethanol use. More common in men than women; usually occurs between ages of 50 and 80 years. Symptoms may include globus sensation, odynophagia, dysphagia, irritation with foods, referred otalgia, lump in neck, alteration of voice, weight loss. More advanced lesions may include respiratory distress with stridor. Physical examination includes complete examination of upper aerodigestive tract, including indirect mirror examination and flexible fiber-optic nasopharyngolaryngoscopy as well as bimanual palpation of the oral cavity and neck.

▶ Diagnosis

Careful clinical examination of upper aerodigestive tract, including direct laryngoscopy, cervical esophagoscopy, nasopharyngoscopy, and bronchoscopy, with appropriate histologic examination of biopsy material. Additional studies include CT scan and MRI of head and neck region.

▶ Disease Severity

TNM (tumor, node, metastasis) staging and extent of tumor with its location, yielding extreme variation in disease severity.

▶ Concept and Application

Vast majority are squamous cell carcinoma of the involved mucosa and muscle, with varying degrees of tissue involvement based on stage and invasion. Initial spread of primary tumor tends to be in cervical lymph nodes, followed by distant metastasis should disease process continue.

▶ Treatment Steps

Combined treatment using surgery, irradiation, and chemotherapy as dictated by size and extent of tumor.

E. Hoarseness

▶ H&P Keys

Presence of infectious disorder, local use/abuse, history of smoking and ethanol use, history of arthritis, history of trauma and intubation, possible endocrinopathy, benign and malignant neoplasms, functional disorders, reflux symptomatology. Physical examination includes indirect mirror examination and direct laryngoscopy as well as complete physical examination of the upper aerodigestive tract. Symptoms include possible referred otalgia, possible throat/laryngeal pain, dysphagia, dyspnea, cough, etc.

▶ Diagnosis

Thorough examination of the larynx using indirect and direct methods, complete examination of the upper aerodigestive tract; adjunctive radiologic studies include CT scan, MRI scan, barium swallow, thyroid function tests, biopsy as appropriate.

▶ Disease Severity
Due to vast etiologic sources, a large variety of disease severity occurs.

▶ Concept and Application
Disruption of normal mucosal wave of the vocal cords with creation of turbulent air flow resulting in hoarseness, edema, vocal masses and irregularities, as well as limited function or hyperfunctioning of the vocal cords.

▶ Treatment Steps
Directed toward etiology.

F. Strep Throat (Acute Tonsillitis/Pharyngitis)

▶ H&P Keys
Sore throat, fever, malaise, anorexia, and odynophagia; occurs more commonly in children. Physical findings include erythema of the pharynx and tonsils, purulent debris in tonsillar crypts and pharynx, malodorous purulence causing halitosis and bad taste, peritonsillar swelling and limited motion of the uvula and soft palate, dysphagia (with severe infections), and palpable and tender adenopathy with severe infections.

▶ Diagnosis
Direct physical examination with visualization of the tonsils and pharyngeal walls, culture of offending organisms.

▶ Disease Severity
Fever, tonsillar hypertrophy, dehydration, referred otalgia, odynophagia, dysphagia, dehydration, peritonsillar abscess, retropharyngeal abscess, and airway compromise. Response to therapy.

▶ Concept and Application
Bacterial infection involving the tonsils, pharynx, or both. Most common are β-hemolytic strep, *Streptococcus pyogenes, Haemophilus influenzae, Haemophilus parainfluenzae, Corynebacterium diphtheriae,* and *Streptococcus pneumoniae.* Other possibilities include viral diseases such as adenovirus and mononucleosis.

▶ Treatment Steps
1. Appropriate antibiotics, oral or IV hydration, incision and drainage of peritonsillar or retropharyngeal abscesses, if present.
2. IV hydration and antibiotics for recalcitrant infections.
3. Recurrent tonsillitis (six episodes per calendar year) is best treated with tonsillectomy.
4. Pain management, oral rinses, and antipyretics for fever are important.

G. Cancer of the Larynx

▶ H&P Keys
History of heavy tobacco and ethanol use or possible asbestos exposure. Occurs in males between the ages of 50 and 70 years. Symptoms include hoarseness, throat and neck pain, dysphagia, dyspnea, hemoptysis, weight loss, referred otalgia, neck mass. Physical examination may include visualization of tumor on indirect and flexible direct laryngoscopy, palpation of neck for masses, and detectable stridor, wheezing, and hoarseness.

► Diagnosis

Complete examination of the upper aerodigestive tract, including indirect and direct laryngoscopy, bimanual palpation, CT scan of neck and larynx, MRI.

► Disease Severity

Depends on TNM staging and extent of disease process.

► Concept and Application

Squamous cell carcinoma is most frequent malignant neoplasm of the larynx (95%). Tumor initially remains confined to the larynx, then spreads to cervical lymph nodes and ultimately metastasizes to distant areas.

► Treatment Steps

Management includes surgery, radiation therapy, and chemotherapy, depending on extent and stage of disease.

III. DISEASES OF THE RESPIRATORY SYSTEM

A. Acute Sinusitis

► H&P Keys

History of recent upper respiratory tract infection associated with purulent rhinorrhea, headache, pain, and pressure over the affected sinus (cheek—maxillary, forehead—frontal, periorbital—ethmoid, and occipital—sphenoid). Other signs and symptoms include purulent postnasal drip, pressure and headache, nasal obstruction, referred otalgia, and orbital pain.

► Diagnosis

Nasal endoscopy, both standard and endoscopic; culturing of purulent discharge; sinus x-rays or CT scan of sinuses; sinus tap to determine presence of pus for culture and treatment.

► Disease Severity

Fever, chills, sinus pressure and pain; possible periorbital cellulitis, edema, proptosis, blindness, headache; intracranial complication such as meningitis, brain abscess, or cavernous sinus thrombosis.

► Concept and Application

Obstruction of ostea of sinuses in middle meatus (osteomeatal complex) leading to negative pressure, transudate followed by exudate, and acute infection. Presence of anatomic abnormalities such as septal deviation, concha bullosa, turbinate hypertrophy, nasal polyposis, and allergic rhinitis. Bacteriology is similar to that of acute otitis media, including *H. influenzae*, *S. aureus*, group A β-streptococcus, pneumococcus, and more unusual organisms in immunocompromised hosts.

► Treatment Steps

1. Antibiotics such as amoxicillin, ampicillin, or amoxicillin with clavulanic acid to cover suspected organisms; both systemic and topical decongestants to nasal mucosa.
2. Surgical drainage of affected sinuses as indicated by severity of disease and degree of patient's illness.
3. Steroids, antihistamines, or both for patients with a significant allergic component to their sinusitis.

B. Chronic Sinusitis

▶ H&P Keys

Symptoms are persistent rhinorrhea, postnasal discharge, pressure, headache, foul smell or taste. Physical examination reveals presence of changes in nasal mucosa; history of allergy is predisposing factor; erythema and swelling of nasal mucosa and purulence are present.

▶ Diagnosis

Intranasal examination after careful vasoconstriction both by direct examination and by fiber-optic endonasal examination, with particular reference to middle meatus, osteomeatal complex to rule out presence of polypoid changes and presence or absence of occlusion of maxillary sinus and sphenoid ethmoid sinus complex. Plain x-rays are not as valuable as axial and coronal CT scans without contrast of sinuses to determine degree of sinus involvement, which sinuses are in fact involved, and presence of anatomic abnormalities. Cultures for offending organism.

▶ Disease Severity

Persistence of purulent rhinorrhea, pain, pressure, fatigue, halitosis; presence of complications of chronic sinusitis with orbital or intracranial complications.

▶ Concept and Application

Patients who have had poorly treated acute sinusitis and patients with allergic nasal disease with edema and polypoid changes of mucous membrane that block ostea outflow tracts are predisposed to sinusitis. Anatomic abnormalities such as septal deviations and pneumatization of turbinates with blockage of osteomeatal complex.

▶ Treatment Steps

Long-term antibiotics (3–6 weeks) with concomitant use of intranasal steroid sprays, nasal decongestants, and correction of intranasal anatomic abnormalities. In patients who fail conservative medical management, as described above; functional endoscopic sinus surgery (FESS) to remove the offending tissue blocking osteomeatal complex with ethmoidectomy, maxillary sinus antrostomy, sphenoidotomy, and frontal sinus duct reconstruction. Children refractive to conservative therapy should undergo adenoidectomy prior to consideration of endoscopic sinus surgery (see Management Decisions).

C. Fungal Sinusitis

▶ H&P Keys

Immunocompromised patients, patients with chronic sinusitis, or both; presence of unremitting sinusitis following vigorous local therapy; pain and swelling about the ethmoid and eyelid areas.

▶ Diagnosis

Diagnostic studies include biopsy, Gram stain and culture of suspicious material for septate versus nonseptate hyphae, CT scan for evidence of calcifications within the sinuses, and skin testing for *Aspergillus.*

▶ Disease Severity

Evidence of bone-destructive, foul-smelling rhinorrhea, with swelling of soft tissues of cheek, eyelid, lateral face; involvement of infraorbital nerve; systemic manifestations of fatigue and debility.

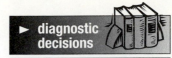

▶ **diagnostic decisions**

TYPICAL LOCATION OF HEADACHES AND PAIN WITH ACUTE SINUSITIS

Sinus	Location of Symptoms
Maxillary	Behind cheeks and face, upper teeth, under eyes.
Ethmoid	Between eyes, nasal bridge and sides.
Frontal	Forehead, eyebrows.
Sphenoid	Occipital region, vertex, retro-orbital.

▶ **management decisions**

INDICATIONS FOR FESS IN CHILDREN WITH CHRONIC SINUSITIS

1. Persistent symptoms despite adenoidectomy; *and*
2. CT evidence of chronic sinus disease, osteomeatal obstruction associated with sinusitis; *and*
3. Discussion of FESS with child's treating primary and specialty physicians; *and*
4. Committed postoperative follow-up for at least 1 year; *and*
5. Realistic parental expectations and understanding of potential complications.

FESS—function endoscopic sinus surgery.

► Concept and Application

Patients with immunocompromised states following chemotherapy for malignant disease or with diabetes or HIV infection have decreased ability to mount immunologic response to these secondary fungal infections; decreased ability also may be secondary to prolonged use of antibiotics with overgrowth of fungi as consequence.

► Treatment Steps

1. Surgical debridement.
2. Use of appropriate antifungal agents such as amphotericin.
3. Correction of underlying immunocompromising mechanism if possible.

D. Chronic Rhinitis

► H&P Keys

Long-term nasal obstruction, postnasal discharge, sneezing, rhinorrhea, and possible purulence. Patients may complain of seasonal symptoms or have symptoms referable to emotional or temperature change. Physical examination reveals erythema of mucous membrane, often with crusting and bleeding and occasional purulence.

► Diagnosis

Gram stain of nasal smears for eosinophils or polymorphonuclear cells; sinus x-rays, CT scan, or both to rule out occult sinusitis. Allergy studies to rule out allergic disease as primary causative factor.

► Disease Severity

Persistence of nasal obstruction, postnasal discharge, pressure and pain, inability to sleep because of nasal obstruction, fatigue, loss of concentration, and loss of time from work.

► Concept and Application

Symptoms may be of allergic, infectious, or vasomotor origin. Determination of presence or absence of purulence by culture sensitivities. Presence of allergy by allergy studies and by history. Nasal obstruction secondary to temperature change mechanism, positioning of head, or emotional factors (fear, anger, passion, sadness); mechanism is endogenous release of vasoactive histaminelike substances that trigger vasodilatation and activation of goblet cells within the nasal and sinus mucous membranes.

► Treatment Steps

Determination of etiology and direction of therapy to allergic, infectious, or vasomotor disease process; also included in therapy would be antihistamine decongestants, steroid nasal sprays, cromolyn sodium as a nasal spray, systemic steroids, and intranasal medicaments such as lubricating drops when indicated.

E. Allergic Rhinitis

► H&P Keys

Nasal obstruction and congestion, nasal pruritus, rhinorrhea, sneezing, and symptoms related to seasons. History of presence or absence of animals, specific plants, flowers, molds, and conditions (e.g., feather pillows) that would support the growth of molds or allergies. Physical examination may reveal swollen, pale blue nasal mucosa and turbinates with nasal obstruction and generally clear rhinorrhea, and swollen (cobblestone-like) lymphoid tissue in the posterior pharyngeal wall.

► Diagnosis
Nasal smears to detect the presence of eosinophils, immunoglobulin E levels, and total eosinophil count. Allergic skin testing, radioallergosorbent testing (RAST), food diary with confirmation of symptoms related to specific food allergens.

► Disease Severity
Degree of function during allergic periods (i.e., potential loss of school or work time).

► Concept and Application
The antigen/antibody reaction causing degranulation of mass cells and basophils releasing histamines, prostaglandins, and other vasoactive elements leading to symptoms of rhinorrhea, nasal congestion, pruritus, etc.

► Treatment Steps
1. If possible, avoiding specific allergen is most useful for mild to moderate symptoms.
2. Treatment with antihistamines, nasal steroids, systemic steroids, sympathomimetic medications as well as sodium cromolyn nasal spray are indicated.
3. Also, immunotherapy with allergy shots for desensitization as well as diet control are useful adjuncts.

F. Epistaxis (Nosebleed)

► H&P Keys
Episode can be intermittent or acute; bleeding may be from anterior nares or may produce postnasal bleeding. Patient may give history of digital trauma to nose or history of nasal obstruction, particularly in boys < 15 years old. Bleeding may respond to anterior nares pressure or may require intranasal packing, posterior nasal packing, or both.

► Diagnosis
Direct examination of nose after careful intranasal vasoconstriction and local anesthesia permits examination of anterior nares, particularly in Kiesselbach's (Little's) area (Fig. 19–2). Postnasal space can be examined by fiberscope under local anesthesia; sinus x-rays or CT scans should be done to rule out intrasinus occult malignancies.

► Disease Severity
Minor intermittent bleeding stops spontaneously with gentle pressure. Severe postnasal bleeding is life threatening and requires postnasal packing, hospitalization, and intensive care observation; necessity for blood transfusion and surgical intervention with ligation of sphenopalatine or maxillary artery.

► Concept and Application
Most common cause is simple drying and crusting of nasal mucosa with neovascularization of Kiesselbach's area. Sphenopalatine artery bleeding is often associated with hypertension; patients may have Rendu–Osler–Weber disease or hereditary telangiectasia. Bleeding in young male children is produced by juvenile angiofibromas and other bleeding diatheses involving platelet or other coagulation

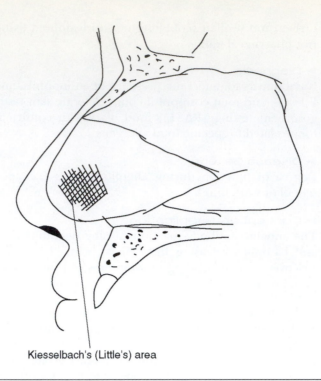

Kiesselbach's (Little's) area

Figure 19–2. Epistaxis.

deficit secondary to either primary platelet involvements or other blood dyscrasias.

▶ Treatment Steps

1. Bleeding from anterior Kiesselbach's area responds well to gentle pressure or, in recurrent involvements, to cauterization using trichloroacetic acid or other oxidizing agents such as silver nitrate in dilute solutions; significant bleeding requires anterior nasal packs.

2. Posterior bleeding requires posterior packing or intranasal balloons.

3. Unresponsive bleeding requires transfusion, ligation of offending vessels, hospitalization, and intensive care management.

4. For Rendu–Osler–Weber disease, bleeding from affected telangiectatic areas is controlled with cauterization or argon laser. Juvenile angiofibromas and neoplastic lesions of the sinuses require extirpation.

G. Disorders of Olfaction and Taste

▶ H&P Keys

Anosmia (loss of sense of smell) and lack of taste and secondary to upper respiratory infection, nasal obstruction, trauma, viral infections, tumors, exposure to irritative fumes such as ammonia or other industrial pollutants.

▶ Diagnosis

Intranasal examination after careful intranasal vasoconstriction to rule out obstructive lesions of nasal cavity and nasal vault. CT scan of sinuses to rule out sinus and intranasal involvement and MRI with gadolinium to rule out involvement of the olfactory bulb and olfactory projections into the hippocampus and temporal lobe. Taste and smell testing and examination of the tongue to rule out atrophy or abnormality of taste buds.

▶ Disease Severity

Inability to function in environment because of inability to detect crucial odors, loss of appetite, malnutrition secondary to loss of appetite, psychic trauma because of loss of sense of taste and smell.

▶ Concept and Application

Olfactory fibers project into the nose from the olfactory bulb through the area of the cribiform plate; lesions of nose that obstruct air flow to these critical fibers produce a relative anosmia. Head injury with a commotio injury in the brain case may result in forces that shear the olfactory fibers from the olfactory nerve. Viral infections most often produce reversible neuritic change in olfactory fibers, preventing their ability to respond to olfactory stimuli. Irritation secondary to industrial solvents and pollutants also may injure the neural epithelium in the same fashion. Loss of taste most often is olfactory in origin; majority of patients do not lose chorda tympani function, which monitors salty, sour, sweet, and bitter taste. Chorda tympani function can be lost following middle-ear or mastoid surgery or trauma to the temporal bone or head.

▶ Treatment Steps

1. Use of topical steroids for inflammatory process, removal of obstructive lesions of nose and nasal vault.
2. Removal from environment containing noxious and polluting substances.
3. Treatment of infectious processes when appropriate.
4. Return of olfactory function may take from 3 weeks to 18 months.

H. Acute Upper Respiratory Infection (Most Common in Winter Months)

▶ H&P Keys

Manifested by coryza, rhinorrhea, nasal obstruction, pharyngitis, cough, conjunctivitis, headache. Physical examination reveals conjunctivitis; nasal obstruction with boggy, pale turbinates; and, initially, clear rhinorrhea. Later, purulence may occur; pharynx is diffusely red without exudate; low-grade fever and, occasionally, small, mild to moderate cervical lymphadenopathy are present.

▶ Diagnosis

Physical examination, determination of febrile state.

▶ Disease Severity

Degree of nasal obstruction, ear discomfort, throat pain, dysphagia, musculoskeletal symptoms.

▶ Concept and Application

Acute upper respiratory infections are viral in origin in both adults and children, most commonly in winter months. More than 120 adenoviruses produce coryza-like symptoms; none confer any specific long-term immunity and none respond to antibiotic therapy.

▶ Treatment Steps

1. In acute phase, nasal and oral decongestants, steam or cool-mist vaporization, antihistamines, antipyretics, and anti-inflammatory

agents such as acetaminophen in young children, and aspirin or nonsteroidal anti-inflammatory agents in adults.

2. Chicken soup and other fluids; bed rest when indicated.

3. Purulent phase lasts 3–5 days and should not require antibiotics. If it lasts longer, one must consider the possibility of sinusitis as a consequence of the acute upper respiratory infection; acute otitis media may occur in conjunction as well.

I. Wegener's Granulomatosis

► H&P Keys

Lesion of upper respiratory tract may involve ear, nose, sinus, soft palate, hard palate, tongue, and larynx—most often close to midline. Patients generally have systemic symptoms, including cough, and often renal symptoms.

► Diagnosis

CT scans of sinuses and ear to determine presence of lesion, biopsy of specific lesions showing Wegener's granulomas, chest x-ray (CXR) to determine presence of vasculitis. Biopsies of pulmonary lesions and renal biopsies also are indicated.

► Disease Severity

Wegener's granulomatosis may progress rapidly and may involve the ear, with both facial and auditory nerve involvement; may involve the sinuses and eyes, with changes in vision; and may involve the upper airway, with airway compromise.

► Concept and Application

Wegener's granulomatosis is a disease of unknown etiology manifested by the involvement of upper respiratory, pulmonary, and renal systems. Biopsies show classic granulomas and vasculitis.

► Treatment Steps

Use of cyclophosphamide and steroids in combination for long-term and supportive systemic therapy.

J. Cystic Fibrosis

► H&P Keys

Chronic recurrent upper and lower respiratory dysfunction with nasal obstruction, nasal purulence, loss of pulmonary function, dyspnea, chronic cough, production of purulent secretions with cough. Examination reveals debilitated child or adolescent; watery nasal polypoid tissue can be seen intranasally, often extending into the nasopharynx.

► Diagnosis

Direct examination shows multiple polypoid changes in young children; CT scans show polypoid and polycystic changes in all sinuses. Sweat colloid study and CXR.

► Disease Severity

The degree of nasal obstruction and purulence and their impact on patient's pulmonary status with increased dyspnea, cough, cyanosis, and recurrent infection.

► Concept and Application

Mucous membrane abnormalities with loss of salivary function, mucous membrane reactivity with polypoid changes within the nose

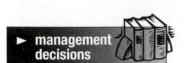

► management decisions

RECOMMENDED MEDICAL TREATMENT FOR WEGENER'S GRANULOMATOSIS

Nonsystemic Localized Disease
Upper airway: nasal steroids, saline irrigations, antibiotics for superimposed bacterial infections
Lower airway: systemic antibiotic therapy, systemic steroid therapy

Systemic Disease
Cyclophosphamide therapy
Steroid therapy
Systemic antibiotic therapy

and sinuses, production of abnormal mucoid elements and increased tenacity and viscosity block sinus outflow tracts and involve pulmonary system.

▶ Treatment Steps
1. Systemic antibiotics.
2. Intranasal removal of polyps with recurrence and sinusitis, and functional endoscopic sinus surgery for recurrent sinusitis with polyp formation.
3. Supportive systemic therapy.

BIBLIOGRAPHY

Cummings C, Fredrickson JM, Horker LA, Krause CA, Schuller DE. *Otolaryngology: Head and Neck Surgery,* 4th ed. St. Louis: Mosby, 2004.

Lee KJ, ed. *Essential Otolaryngology: Head and Neck Surgery,* 8th ed. New York: McGraw-Hill, 2003.

Seiden AM. *Otolaryngology: The Essentials.* New York: Thieme Medical Publishers, 2002.

Wilson W. *Clinical Handbook of Ear, Nose and Throat Disorders.* New York: Parthenon, 2002.

Index